Clinical Pediatric Arrhythmias

Clinical Pediatric Arrhythmias

2nd Edition

Paul C. Gillette, M.D.
Medical Director, Pediatric Cardiology
Cook Children's Medical Center
Fort Worth, Texas

Arthur Garson, Jr., M.D., M.P.H.
Professor of Pediatrics,
Senior Vice President, and Dean for Academic Operations
Baylor College of Medicine
Vice President
Texas Children's Hospital
Houston, Texas

W.B. SAUNDERS COMPANY
A Division of Harcourt Brace & Company
Philadelphia London Toronto Sydney

W.B. SAUNDERS COMPANY
A Division of Harcourt Brace & Company

The Curtis Center
Independence Square West
Philadelphia, Pennsylvania 19106

Library of Congress Cataloging-in-Publication Data

Clinical pediatric arrhythmias / [edited by] Paul C. Gillette, Arthur Garson, Jr.—2nd ed.

p. cm.

Rev. ed. of: Pediatric arrhythmias, electrophysiology, and pacing. 1990.

Includes bibliographical references and index.

ISBN 0-7216-6629-9

1. Arrhythmia in children. I. Gillette, Paul C. II. Garson, Arthur. III. Pediatric arrhythmias, electrophysiology, and pacing. [DNLM: 1. Arrhythmia—in infancy & childhood. 2. Arrhythmia—diagnosis. 3. Arrhythmia—therapy. 4. Cardiac Pacing, Artificial—in infancy & childhood. 5. Electrophysiology—in infancy & childhood. WG 330 C6417 1999]

RJ426.A7P39 1999 618.92′128—dc21

DNLM/DLC 98-40585

CLINICAL PEDIATRIC ARRHYTHMIAS ISBN 0-7216-6629-9

Printed in the United States of America.

Last digit is the print number: 9 8 7 6 5 4 3 2 1

To our wives, Vicki and Suzan, and our children, Noella, Caltresine, Lauren, and Kathleen

CONTRIBUTORS

Robert H. Anderson, M.D., F.R.C.Path.

Joseph Levy Professor of Paediatric Cardiac Morphology, Section of Paediatrics, National Heart and Lung Institute, Royal Brompton Campus, Imperial College School of Medicine; Honorary Consultant, Royal Bromptom Hospital, London, United Kingdom
Morphology of the Cardiac Conduction System

Seshadri Balaji, M.B.B.S., M.R.C.P.(UK)

Assistant Professor (Pediatrics), Division of Pediatric Cardiology, Medical University of South Carolina College of Medicine, Charleston, South Carolina
Chronic Postoperative Arrhythmias

Henry L. Blair, C.-C.P.T.

Clinical Assistant for Electrophysiology, Cook Children's Medical Center, Fort Worth, Texas
Intracardiac Electrophysiology Studies

Beth Bubolz, M.D.

Assistant Professor, Tufts University School of Medicine; Director of Pediatric Electrophysiology, Boston Floating Hospital for Children, Boston, Massachusetts
Noninvasive Diagnostic Techniques

Christopher L. Case, M.D., D.M.D.

Associate Director, Pediatric Cardiology, Cook Children's Medical Center, Fort Worth, Texas
Noninvasive Diagnostic Techniques; Catheter and Surgical Ablation Therapies; Fetal Arrhythmias

John M. Clark, M.D.

Assistant Professor of Clinical Pediatrics, Northeastern Ohio Universities College of Medicine, Rootstown; Director, Pediatric Arrhythmia Center, Division of Pediatric Cardiology, Children's Hospital Medical Center of Akron, Akron, Ohio
Fetal Arrhythmias

Fred A. Crawford, Jr., M.D.

Horace Smithy Professor of Surgery and Chairman, Department of Surgery, Medical University of South Carolina College of Medicine, Charleston, South Carolina
Catheter and Surgical Ablation Therapies

John Deanfield, M.D.

Professor of Cardiology, University College; Consultant Cardiologist, Great Ormond Street Hospital for Sick Children, London, England
Chronic Postoperative Arrhythmias

Arthur Garson, Jr., M.D., M.P.H.

Professor of Pediatrics, Senior Vice President, and Dean for Academic Operations, Baylor College of Medicine; Vice President, Texas Children's Hospital, Houston, Texas
Ventricular Arrhythmias; Arrhythmias and Sudden Death; Palpitations; Chronic Postoperative Arrhythmias

Paul C. Gillette, M.D.

Medical Director, Pediatric Cardiology, Cook Children's Medical Center, Fort Worth, Texas
Intracardiac Electrophysiology Studies; Atrioventricular Block and Bundle Branch Block; Catheter and Surgical Ablation Therapies; Cardiac Pacing; Advanced Electrical Management of Atrial and Ventricular Tachyarrhythmias; Chronic Postoperative Arrhythmias

Jeffrey S. Heinle, M.D.

Associate Medical Director, Cardiovascular Surgery, Cook Children's Medical Center, Fort Worth, Texas
Cardiac Pacing

Siew Yen Ho, Ph.D., F.R.C.Path.

Senior Lecturer, Section of Paediatrics, National Heart and Lung Institute, Royal Brompton Campus, Imperial College School of Medicine, London, United Kingdom
Morphology of the Cardiac Conduction System

Ronald J. Kanter, M.D.

Associate Professor of Pediatrics, Duke University School of Medicine; Director, Pediatric Electrophysiology, Duke University Medical Center, Durham, North Carolina
Acute Treatment of Arrhythmias; Catheter and Surgical Ablation Therapies; Syncope

John D. Kugler, M.D.

Professor of Pediatrics and Chief, Joint Division of Pediatric Cardiology, University of Nebraska College of Medicine and Creighton University School of Medicine; Children's Memorial Hospital, Omaha, Nebraska
Sinus Node Dysfunction

Ameeta B. Martin, M.D.

Assistant Professor of Pediatrics, Joint Division of Pediatric Cardiology, University of Nebraska College of Medicine and Creighton University School of Medicine; Children's Memorial Hospital, Omaha; St. Elizabeth's Regional Medical Center, Lincoln, Nebraska
Sinus Node Dysfunction

Brian K. O'Connor, M.D.

Assistant Professor, New York University School of Medicine; Director, Pediatric Electrophysiology, New York University Medical Center, New York, New York
Arrhythmias in Long QT and WPW Syndromes

John Papagiannis, M.D.

Associate Director, Department of Pediatric Cardiology, Onassis Cardiac Surgery Center, Athens, Greece
Acute Treatment of Arrhythmias

James C. Perry, M.D.

Director of Cardiology, Director of Electrophysiology and Pacing, Children's Hospital and Health Center, San Diego, California
Medical Antiarrhythmic Therapy

Bertrand A. Ross, M.D.

Associate Professor of Pediatrics, Eastern Virginia Medical School of the College of Hampton Roads; Director, Pediatric Cardiology, Children's Hospital of the King's Daughters, Norfolk, Virginia
Atrioventricular Block and Bundle Branch Block

Michael J. Silka, M.D.

Professor of Pediatrics/Cardiology, Oregon Health Sciences University School of Medicine, Portland, Oregon
Ventricular Arrhythmias; Advanced Electrical Management of Atrial and Ventricular Tachyarrhythmias

Mary C. Sokoloski, M.D.

Assistant Professor of Pediatrics, Hahnemann University Hospital; Director of Electrophysiology, St. Christopher's Hospital for Children, Philadelphia, Pennsylvania
Tachyarrhythmias Confined to the Atrium

George F. Van Hare, M.D.

Director, Pediatric Arrhythmia Center, Stanford Health Care; Associate Professor of Pediatrics, Stanford University School of Medicine, Stanford; Associate Clinical Professor of Pediatrics, University of California, San Francisco, San Francisco, California
Supraventricular Tachycardia

Amy Todd Winslow, R.N., M.S.N., P.N.P.

Pediatric Electrophysiology Nurse Practitioner, Cook Children's Medical Center, Fort Worth, Texas
Acute Treatment of Arrhythmias

Vicki Zeigler, R.N., M.S.N.

Arrhythmias Case Manager, Cook Children's Medical Center, Fort Worth, Texas
Cardiac Pacing

PREFACE

Although this book is considered a second edition, most sections have been completely revised and specific chapters deleted to reflect the changes in the field of cardiac arrhythmias in children. *Clinical Pediatric Arrhythmias*, second edition, is intended not only to assist the clinician for evaluating and understanding arrhythmias in children but also as a reference for determining appropriate treatment strategies. The information presented in this edition is more succinct and understandable than in the previous edition, as evidenced in the chapter Morphology of the Cardiac Conduction System by Siew Yen Ho and Robert H. Anderson. It is hoped that this edition will be of great assistance to those who care for children with cardiac arrhythmias.

The diagnostic technique of invasive electrophysiology testing, which was the benchmark of the 1980s, is now directed toward interventional electrophysiology, which is in most cases curative. Noninvasive means of identifying arrhythmias have become more commonplace, with surface electrocardiographic criteria being used with increasing frequency as a means of identifying those patients at risk for sudden death.

The clinical arrhythmias seen in children remain somewhat the same, although many strides have been made in determining etiology. In most sections of this book, we have attempted to address issues ranging from those that are critical to the youngest neonate to those of the young adult with postoperative congenital heart disease. Although we have tried to present different views of controversial points, we know that in some cases we have our own biases. Everything presented here has not been proven as fact, since there are still many gaps in our overall knowledge.

Although tremendous improvements have been made in the diagnosis and management of children with cardiac arrhythmias, we predict even more improvements in the next millenium. Our intent for our readers is to help them to better understand pediatric arrhythmias in order to provide the most appropriate treatment strategies and to ensure a higher quality of life for children, young adults, and their families.

PAUL C. GILLETTE, M.D.
ARTHUR GARSON, JR., M.D.

NOTICE

CONTENTS

SECTION I

Techniques

CHAPTER 1

MORPHOLOGY OF THE CARDIAC CONDUCTION SYSTEM

Siew Yen Ho and Robert H. Anderson

Although it is now just more than 100 years since His[1] and Kent[2] concurrently claimed to have demonstrated the anatomic substrates of muscular conduction across the atrioventricular junction, it is only within the last decade that the direct treatment of arrhythmias by means of intervention rather than pharmacology has become a medical rather than a surgical preserve. Thus, it remains a prerequisite for surgeons to understand the morphology of the cardiac conduction system so as to avoid it, but it is now an equal prerequisite for pediatric cardiologists to have this information if they are to ablate or modify the substrates of abnormal conduction. Those who are interested in this field, presumably represented by the readers of this book, should also be well aware that the intervening period since the discoveries of His and Kent has not been devoid of controversy. Even the initial descriptions[1, 2] were far less than adequate, because as distinguished a morphologist as Sir Arthur Keith[3] had been unable to rediscover the bundle of His until prompted by the epochal investigations of Sunao Tawara.[4] Tawara,[4] subsequently followed in short order by Keith himself,[5] set the ground rules for what we now know to be the disposition of the cardiac conduction system. Subsequent controversies[6–8] largely reflect the fact that not all investigators have appreciated that the morphologist, looking down the microscope, cannot predict the function of a cell during its life from its autopsy appearance. Morphologic criteria are needed for definition of discrete conducting pathways, and such criteria were established by Mönckeberg[9] and Aschoff.[10] In essence, if a tract is to be considered specialized in morphologic terms, it must be insulated from its surrounding nonspecialized myocardial environment and must be recognizable histologically in serial sections. The paradigm for such a conduction system is the His bundle and its branches. Cells and tracts specialized in this morphologic fashion may not always coincide with areas considered to show physiologic specialization. However, this is the problem confronting the morphologist: cells showing a specialized action potential may be identical morphologically to those exhibiting "working" potentials.[11]

This is the background against which we describe our understanding of the normal and abnormal conduction system, and introduce some of the known substrates for pediatric arrhythmias. We start by reviewing the gross disposition of the normal conduction system and set that in the context of normal anatomy before considering the abnormal arrangements.

NORMAL CONDUCTION SYSTEM

In the normal heart, the atrial musculature constitutes a separate myocardial mass relative to the ventricular musculature apart from one muscular connection: the bundle of His. Normal cardiac electrical activity, therefore, depends on activation of the atrial musculature from the sinus node, but then insulation of the atrial mass from the ventricles at all points apart from the penetration of the histologically specialized atrioventricular bundle. This insulation occurs within the atrioventricular junctions, the areas of contiguity (but no electrical continuity) between atrial and ventricular muscle masses around the orifices of the atrioventricular valves. These anatomic junctions and the septum separating them must be distinguished from, but set in context with, the *specialized* atrioventricular junction. This latter term is used to describe the atrioventricular conduction system described by Tawara,[4] which starts in the histologically discrete transitional cells of the atrioventricular node, continues into the compact node, and, having penetrated into the ventricles, continues as the insulated ventricular conduction axis (Fig. 1–1). A major role of this specialized system is to conduct rapidly the impulse to the ventricles, but equally important is the delay induced within the system, predominantly within the atrial components of

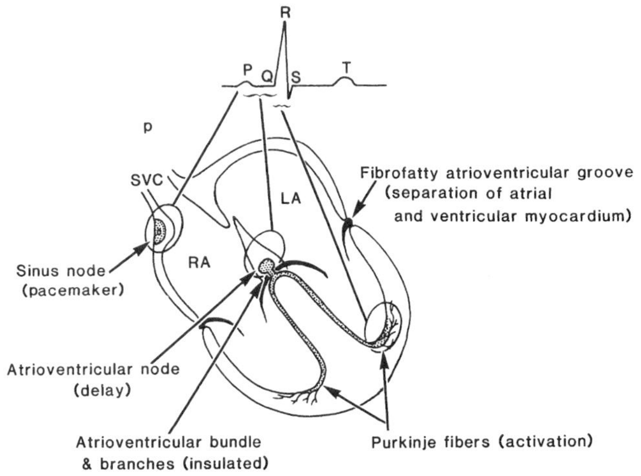

FIGURE 1–1. Components of the cardiac conduction system. (SVC, superior vena cava; RA, right atrium; LA, left atrium.)

the conduction axis. With increasing electrophysiologic knowledge, we now know that the myocardial atrial approaches to the morphologically specialized area are important as the so-called slow and fast pathways. As we see, however, these pathways show no evidence of gross morphologic specialization, as judged within the criteria proposed by Mönckeberg[9] and Aschoff.[10] Preferential conduction in these pathways, as with the remainder of the atrial myocardium, is almost certainly underscored by the orderly arrangement of the myocardial fibers, perhaps influenced by the degree and extent of intercellular communications.

SINUS NODE AND INTERNODAL MYOCARDIUM

In the normal heart, the sinus node is usually located immediately subepicardially in the terminal groove (sulcus terminalis) on the lateral margin of the junction between the superior caval vein and the right atrium. It is spindle-shaped,

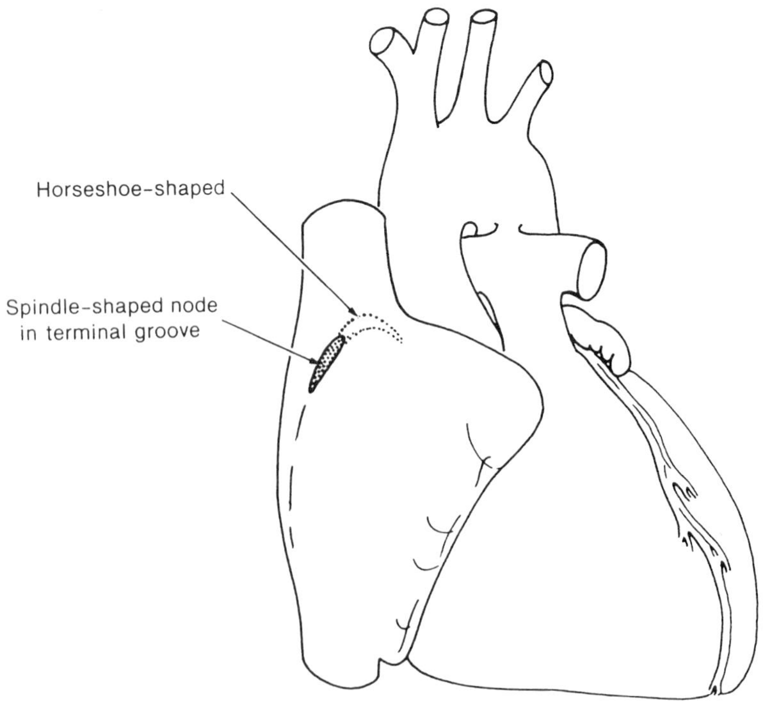

FIGURE 1–2. Usual spindle shape of the sinus node occupying a lateral position in the terminal groove. Occasionally, the node is horseshoe shaped and occupies a more medial position.

with a tapering tail in the majority of hearts (Fig. 1–2). In about one tenth of individuals, it is shaped like a horseshoe and straddles the crest of the right atrial appendage. The nodal cells, smaller than ordinary (working) atrial myocytes, are grouped into clusters, enmeshed in a matrix of fibrous tissue (Fig. 1–3). A prominent artery, or its branches, usually passes through the body of the node. The origin and course of the artery supplying the node are highly variable.[12, 13] The borders of the node are not surrounded by a uniform zone of transitional cells. In places, the nodal cells are adjacent to working myocytes. In others, short tongues of transitional cells interdigitate with ordinary musculature (see Fig. 1–3).

The tail of the sinus node penetrates posteroinferiorly into the musculature of the terminal crest to varying distances. Apart from the occasionally long tail, and the tongues of transitional cells, no histologically specialized pathways are seen in the internodal musculature. In consequence of the location of the orifices of the great veins, along with the oval fossa in the atrial septum, the atrial myocardium between the cardiac nodes is arranged in broad bands of musculature. These bands, composed of ordinary myocytes, have been shown to allow preferential spread of excitation from the sinus node.[14, 15] Considering only the right atrium, its internal aspect shows bands of musculature anterosuperior and posteroinferior to the oval fossa, together with the terminal crest. The latter passes from a position anterosuperior to the junction of the superior caval vein with the right atrium to a posteroinferior position near the orifice of the inferior caval vein, continuing into the posteustachian sinus inferior to the coronary sinus. All along its length, it gives origin to an array of branching pectinate muscles, which occupy the major part of the parietal right atrial wall. Between the pectinate muscles, the atrial wall is thin and crisscrossed by fine muscle bundles. Pectinate muscles can be traced all around the tricuspid vestibule to the cardiac crux at the so-called atrial isthmus. Dissections of the subendocardial fibers show fibers of the pectinate muscles in this area to run perpendicularly to the annular insertion of the tricuspid valve but turning to become circular in the vestibular portion, passing anterosuperiorly to the apex of the triangle of Koch (Fig. 1–4). Variations in this area of the isthmus are seen in some hearts.[16] These areas correspond to the sites targeted for ablation of the slow pathway in patients with atrioventricular nodal re-entrant tachycardia and also in patients with the common form of atrial flutter. The subendocardial fibers show more variation in arrangement in the area anterosuperior to the apex of the triangle of Koch, where fibers from the sinus septum (separating the coronary sinus from the inferior caval vein) meet fibers from the anterior rim of the oval fossa. This is the area purported to be the fast pathway of the atrioventricular nodal re-entrant circuit. The different orientations of the fibers could account for variations in propagation of impulses, but, as expressed earlier, this morphologic variability needs to be correlated with electrophysiologic studies.

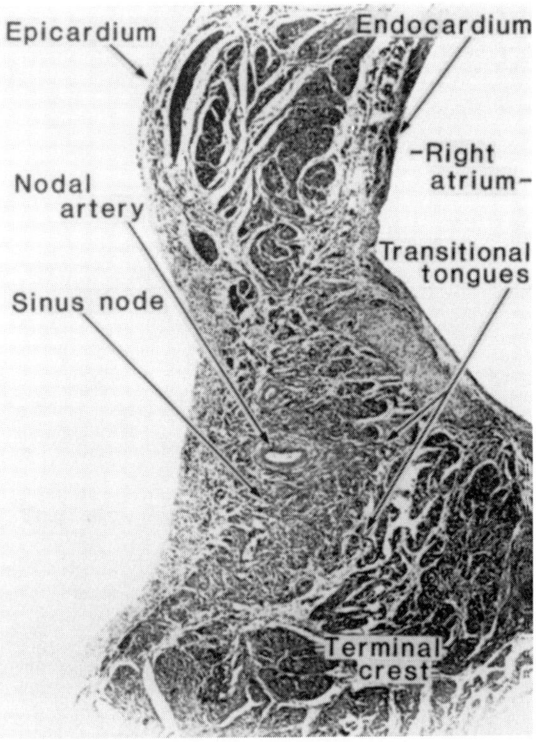

FIGURE 1–3. Cross-section of a neonatal sinus node. Note the subepicardial position.

GROSS ANATOMY OF THE ATRIOVENTRICULAR JUNCTION

As we have already discussed, it was the histologic studies of Tawara[4] in 1906 that set a milestone in the localization of the specialized atrioventricular conduction system. Tawara demonstrated in exquisite detail that the atrioventricular bundle is the only pathway of myocardial continuity between atrial and ventricular muscular masses. Koch[17] subsequently emphasized the gross landmarks to the position of the atrioventricular node. Viewed from the right atrial aspect,

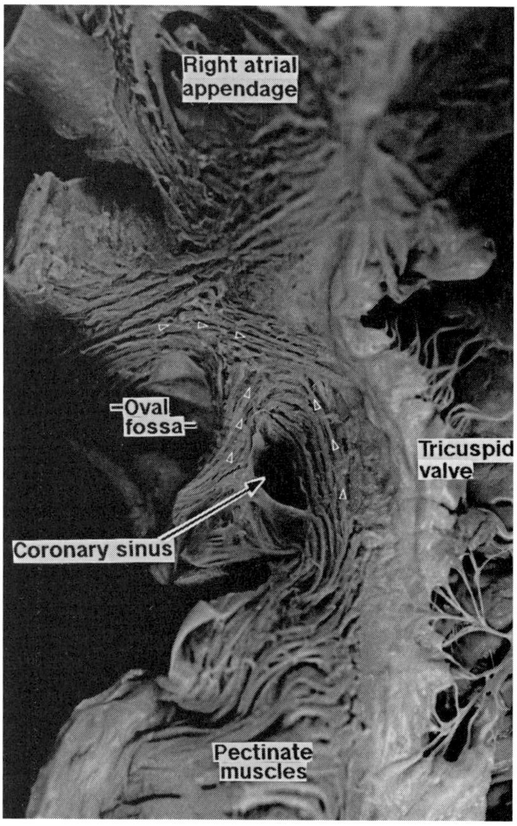

FIGURE 1–4. Prominent muscle bundles with different fiber orientations *(arrowheads)* are seen in the area of the triangle of Koch. (Photograph kindly provided by Damian Sanchez-Quintana, MD.)

Koch's triangle is delimited on one side by the continuation of the commissures guarding the openings of the inferior caval vein and the coronary sinus (the tendon of Todaro) and on the other side by the hinge of the septal leaflet of the tricuspid valve. The mouth of the coronary sinus is usually taken as the base of the triangle, with the atrioventricular node located at the apex. Variation in size of the mouth of the coronary sinus, however, is well recognized.[18] Whether or not it is associated with persistence of the left superior caval vein, a large coronary sinus conceivably reduces the distance between the sinus and the location of the atrioventricular node.[19]

Because of the more apical insertion of the septal leaflet of the tricuspid valve relative to the mitral valve, well seen in sections through the four chambers of the heart, the surface of the triangle of Koch is the right atrial component of the atrioventricular muscular septum (Fig. 1–5). This superficial part is a thin layer of atrial musculature that extends into the vestibule to the tricuspid valve. The tendon of Todaro passes through the sinus septum and continues between the coronary sinus and oval fossa, inserting anterosuperiorly into the atrioventricular component of the membranous septum (part of the central fibrous body). This fibrous area separates the cavity of the right atrium from the extensive recess of the left ventricular outflow tract underneath the aortic valve. The penetrating portion of the conduction axis passes through the angle to reach the muscular crest of the ventricular septum.

Gross examination of this part of the atrioventricular junction, as seen through a right atriotomy, suggests an extensive septal continuum, which has been divided by electrophysiologists into purported "anterior septal," "posterior septal," and "midseptal" components (Fig. 1–6). In reality, only the midseptum part is truly septal

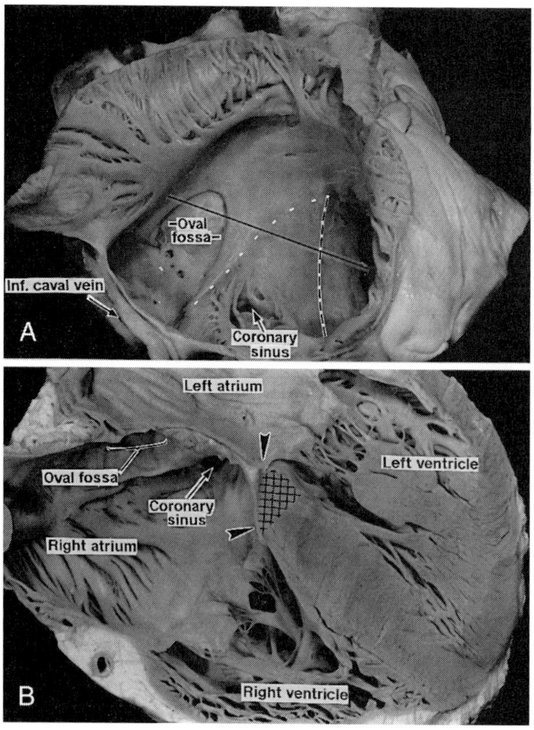

FIGURE 1–5. *A,* The right atrium is viewed through a right atriotomy. The angle between the tendon of Todaro *(white broken line)* and the attachment of the septal leaflet of the tricuspid valve *(black broken line)* marks the apex of the triangle of Koch. The solid line represents the approximate plane of section used to produce the heart specimen shown in *B. B,* View of muscular atrioventricular septum *(hatched area)* between the offset attachments of the mitral and tricuspid valves *(arrowheads)*. In this area, the vestibule of the tricuspid valve is a thin layer overlying the atrioventricular septum.

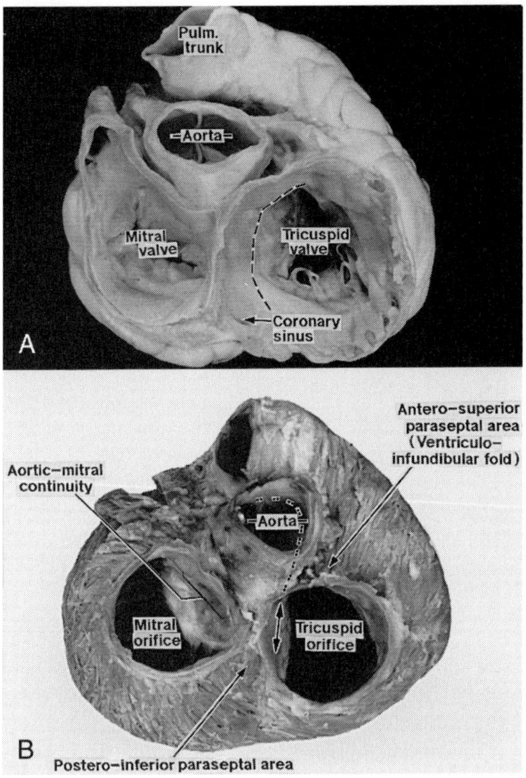

FIGURE 1–6. Two views of the atrioventricular junction from the base of the heart. The septal area in *A* appears very extensive *(broken line)*. *B,* The true septal area *(double arrows)* is revealed after removal of all the atrial walls and epicardial tissues. The broken line indicates the orientation of the ventricular septum.

in that it separates cavities of adjacent cardiac chambers from each other. The remainder of the purported septal area separates the cavity of the right atrium from the outside of the heart. The midseptal area, or the true septum, corresponds to the atrial aspect of the overlapping muscular atrioventricular region. The anterosuperior extent of the midseptum is the central fibrous body, which contains the penetrating bundle (of His), and the membranous septum, which lies beyond. In this area, the conduction bundle usually passes from the nearly subendocardial location of the compact atrioventricular node in the right atrium to run leftward into the central fibrous body. This leftward shift, which can be as much as 0.5 cm in the adult heart, gives the penetrating and common atrioventricular bundle some degree of protection from assaults by ablative lesions placed on the right atrial aspect to disrupt so-called para-Hisian pathways. The branching bundle, although sandwiched between the membranous septum and the muscular ventricular septum, is disposed toward the left in many hearts, resulting in the right bundle branch taking an intramyocardial course. In some hearts, the branching bundle is well off the septal crest.

Because the so-called anterior septum denotes the region anterosuperior and to the right of the membranous septum, and because it separates the cavity of the right atrium from pericardial space, it is in reality no longer septal. The ventricular septum, in fact, curves leftward as it extends anterosuperiorly, passing toward the subpulmonary infundibulum (see Fig. 1–6). On the left side, the aortic valve interposes between atrial musculature and the ventricular septum. Thus, catheters placed to ablate so-called anteroseptal pathways are frequently positioned to the right, lateral to the anteroseptal commissure of the tricuspid valve. This area corresponds with the supraventricular crest of the right ventricle. When the hinge of the septal leaflet is traced anterosuperiorly, it can be followed across the membranous septum, dividing it into atrioventricular and interventricular components, and then it veers away from the septum (Fig. 1–7). In this region, the musculature of the right atrium has a close relationship with the aortic root, with the transverse sinus intervening. This area, described as the aortic mound, is the anteromedial wall of the right atrium. As indicated previously, on the ventricular aspect, this part of the atrioventricular junction corresponds to the parietal and rightward extension of the supraventricular crest of the right ventricle. In this area, the proximal portion of the right coronary artery courses obliquely through the fatty tissues of the atrioventricular groove. Thus, the "anterior septum" is more accurately described as the *anterosuperior paraseptal area.*

Similarly, the term *posterior septum* is a misnomer. From the atrial aspect, much of this area is the floor of the coronary sinus, which is separated from diverging ventricular walls by the fatty tissues of the posterior atrioventricular groove (see Fig. 1–6). It is through this fatty tissue that the artery to the atrioventricular node passes forward from the characteristic obtuse angle bend of the dominant coronary artery at the cardiac crux. Anterosuperiorly, the vestibular portions of the left and right atrial walls turn in to converge on the atrial layer overlying the muscular ventricular septum in the midseptal area. Posteroinferiorly, the vestibular portions diverge, following the diverging ventricular walls, with the left atrial vestibule anterosuperior to the coronary sinus. From an anatomic stance, left-sided accessory pathways are closer to the coronary sinus than the orifice of the tricuspid valve.

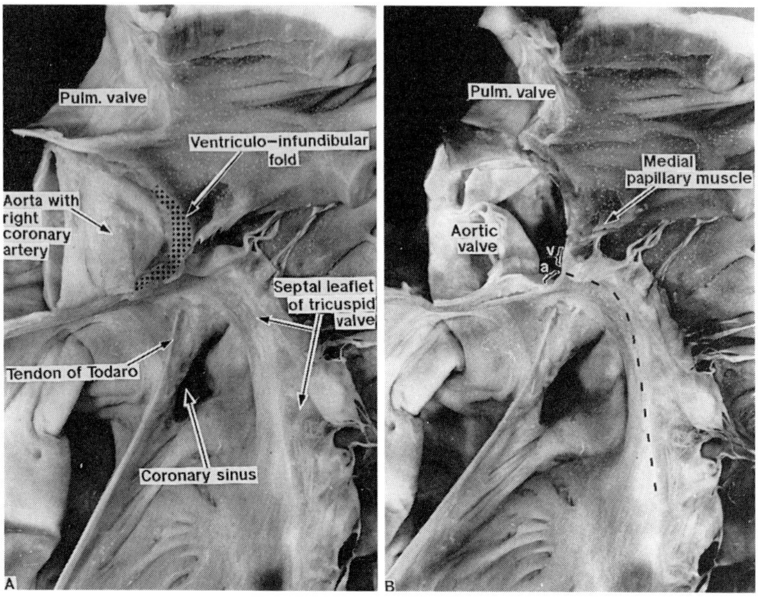

FIGURE 1–7. *A*, The right side of the heart is dissected to show the muscular separation between the tricuspid and pulmonary valves. The ventriculoinfundibular fold is a right heart structure. When incised *(stippled area)*, left-sided heart structures are not entered. *B*, A deeper cut into the septum reveals the aortic valve and the left ventricular outflow tract. This incision also reveals the membranous septum, which is divided by the attachment of the tricuspid valve *(broken line)* into atrioventricular (a) and interventricular (v) components.

The area as a whole is the posteroinferior paraseptal space.

Labeling the anterosuperior and posteroinferior *paraseptal* areas as septal, therefore, obfuscates their true anatomic relationships.[20] The only septal area, as described previously, is the muscular atrioventricular septum and the adjoining membranous septum. The left and right parietal areas comprise the remainder of the atrioventricular junctions (see Fig. 1–6). The left parietal junction is that which embraces the major part of the hinge of the mural leaflet of the mitral valve. On the epicardial aspect, this is also the area through which courses the great cardiac vein leading to the coronary sinus, together with the circumflex artery. The remaining part of the left atrioventricular junction is the area of fibrous continuity between the aortic (anterior) leaflet of the mitral valve and the leaflets of the aortic valve. This area is usually devoid of ventricular musculature. Expansions of fibrous tissue at either end of this area form the left and right fibrous trigones. The right trigone is in continuity with the membranous septum, the two structures together constituting the central fibrous body. At the hinge of the mitral valve, a collagenous structure surrounds much of the valvar orifice, helping to separate atrial from ventricular myocardium.

Around the orifice of the tricuspid valve, however, a firm collagenous ring is rarely found. Instead, atrial and ventricular myocardial masses are separated by small aggregates of fibrous tissue at some points but, most often, by fibrofatty tissues. The right parietal junction is infolded to a greater extent than on the left side, resulting in a deeper wedge of tissue occupying the atrioventricular groove. At the insertion of the atrial myocardium into the junction, it is also common to find nodelike remnants of histologically specialized tissues, especially in the area of the acute margin. These structures are the "nodes" observed and illustrated by Kent.[21, 22] They do not, in the normal heart, form muscular connections with ventricular myocardium.

ATRIOVENTRICULAR CONDUCTION SYSTEM

The classic works of early workers like Tawara[4] and Keith and Flack[5] clearly demonstrated the presence of the specialized muscular system, which conducts impulses from atrial to ventricular myocardium. This specialized conduction system comprises the transitional atrial zone, compact atrioventricular node, penetrating bundle, branching bundle, and ventricular bundle branches (see Fig. 1–1). The atrial portion of this so-called specialized atrioventricular junctional area is composed of the compact atrioventricular node and its zone of transitional cells (Fig. 1–8). In terms of function, nonetheless, we must now recognize also that the nodal approaches of working atrial myocardium are part of the electrophysiologically specialized area, because they constitute the slow and fast pathways. Histologically, the compact node itself is made up of

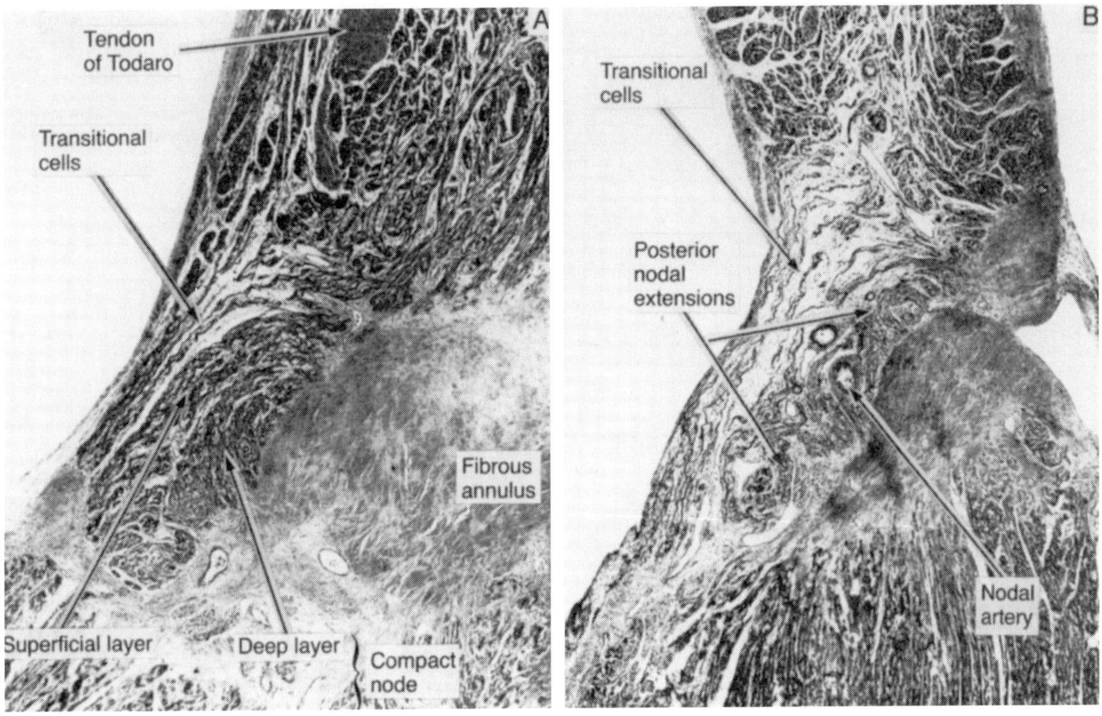

FIGURE 1–8. Histologic sections through the atrioventricular junctional area. *A*, Components of the atrioventricular node. *B*, Posterior extensions of the nodes.

interweaving fascicles of small cells. The compact node is stratified in many hearts into deep and superficial layers[23]; the superficial layers are arranged in more circumferential fashion. The node is club shaped, but in infants and children appears in cross-section as a distinctive half-oval structure. It lies against the central fibrous body, inclining more to the right than the left atrium as an interatrial structure.[24] Although described as the compact node, archipelagos or loops of specialized tissue can extend into the central fibrous body (Fig. 1–9). These extensions are commonly found in hearts from young children. They have been implicated as substrates of instability causing sudden death in infancy,[25] but our own studies failed to provide evidence to substantiate this claim.[26] Posteroinferiorly, the cells of the compact node diverge to receive the nodal artery. The entire compact node is surrounded by a diffuse zone of transitional cells that approach from the posteroinferior and anterosuperior parts of the nodal triangle. Transitional cells are slender, wavy myocytes interposed between ordinary "working" atrial myocytes and the specialized cells of the compact node. This transitional zone has already been recognized in the earliest works[4] and was stressed again by Taussig[27] in 1931, writing on the boundaries of the cardiac nodes. The region is also described as nodal fiber extensions[23] and nodal approaches.[28] Transitional cells, which pass from the area of the floor of the anterior wall of the coronary sinus to the divergent and posterior parts of the compact node, make up the posterior transitional zone. Anterosuperiorly, cells from the left side of the atrial septum are described as the deep transitional cells. Superficial transitional cells, which are the continuations of the right atrial myocytes from the sinus septum and the anterior rim of the oval fossa, pass over the body of the compact node. Other atrial cells, described as overlay cells, also descend from the anterior rim of the oval fossa to pass over the node as the musculature of the atrial vestibule to the insertion of the tricuspid valve (see Fig. 1–8).

The myocardium of the atrial approaches to the node is now of particular interest, because these are the areas important as the substrates for the dual pathways recognized electrophysiologically in humans and other animals. Although most morphologic studies have not attempted to ascribe specialized characteristics to this area, a few do continue to promote the concept of "atrionodal tracts," describing these as insulated pathways that represent the substrates for arrhythmias associated with dual atrioventricular

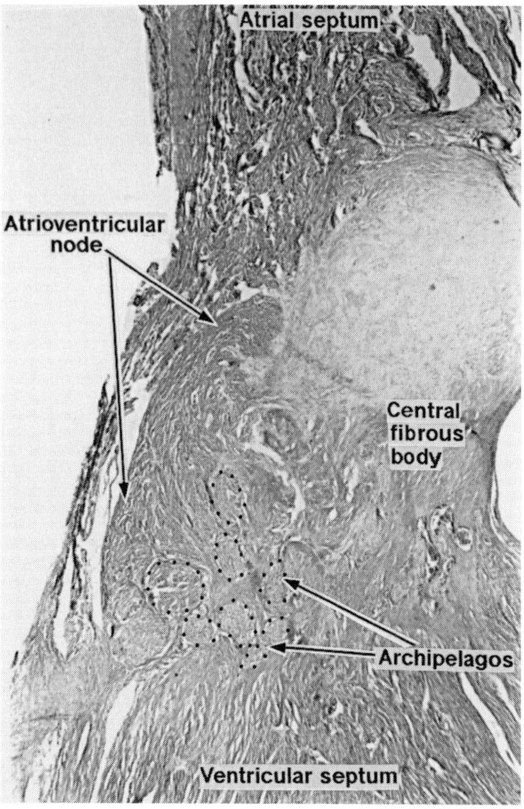

FIGURE 1–9. Histologic section through the atrioventricular node of an infant shows excursions of specialized tissues into the central fibrous body.

nodal inputs.[29] In concurrence with other investigators, our studies in dogs and in humans have shown bands of histologically ordinary myocardium in this area.[30, 31] There are certainly no myocardial tracts that can be judged as specialized by the criteria of Mönckeberg[9] and Aschoff.[10] It is already well recognized that the mode of conduction of impulses within the muscular walls of the atrium reflects the arrangement of well-developed muscle bands, although these bands are not insulated from the rest of the atrial myocardium.[14, 32] On this basis, the orderly arrangement of the myocardial fibers must be important in effecting preferential conduction through the bands. Variations in the orientation of the fibers in the atrial approaches, together with the arrangement and extent of intercellular communications, must play a role in influencing the input of impulses to the node. It is then, perhaps, of significance that, as described previously, variations in gross architecture are particularly evident in the areas corresponding to the so-called slow and fast pathways.

Returning to consider the histologically specialized area, the node progresses anterosuperiorly to become the penetrating bundle, with only a gradual and marginal increase in cellular size. Following the precedent of Tawara,[4] we take the point at which the conduction axis becomes completely surrounded by the tissues of the central fibrous body as the transition from compact node to penetrating atrioventricular bundle (of His) (Fig. 1–10). The "last" atrial fiber[33] to join the axis before penetration can come from the superficial transitional fibers on the right or from the deep fibers from the left side of the septum.

At the distal end of the penetrating bundle, the cells become oriented in a more parallel fashion. In most hearts, the conduction bundle begins to branch as soon as it passes into the ventricular component. In some hearts, nonetheless, there is a short intervening nonbranching segment. The cells making up the branching bundle are similar in size to the ventricular myocytes, but are sheathed by fibrous tissue in their proximal portions. Pale or swollen cells, described as Purkinje's cells are, in our experience, rarely observed in hearts from children. As soon as the bundle branches lose their fibrous sheaths, the distal ramifications become practically indistinguishable from ordinary ventricular myocytes.

The left bundle branch is the first to take off from the branching bundle. Its proximal portion is immediately subendocardial in the left ventricular outflow tract. It originates as a sheet of cells over a considerable length of the branching bundle and then fans out into major fascicles as it descends along the septal surface. As originally described by Tawara,[4] there are three major fascicles, although others have suggested a bifascicular arrangement. More distally, the fascicles are interconnected by a subendocardial network before ramifying into the ventricular myocardium.

Because the branching bundle is usually positioned to the left of the septal crest, the right bundle branch turns intramyocardially to reach the septomarginal trabeculation of the right ventricle (Fig. 1–11). On the right ventricular septal aspect, the right bundle branch emerges at the base of the medial papillary muscle. Unlike the left bundle branch, the right bundle is a thin, cordlike structure. It runs subendocardially from the medial papillary muscle toward the apex of the ventricle, and passes through the moderator band to reach the parietal wall. The right bundle branch is usually the terminal portion of the nodal bundle axis, but, in some neonatal hearts, the axis itself continues along the septum and terminates in an anteriorly situated bundle termed the *dead-end tract*.[34]

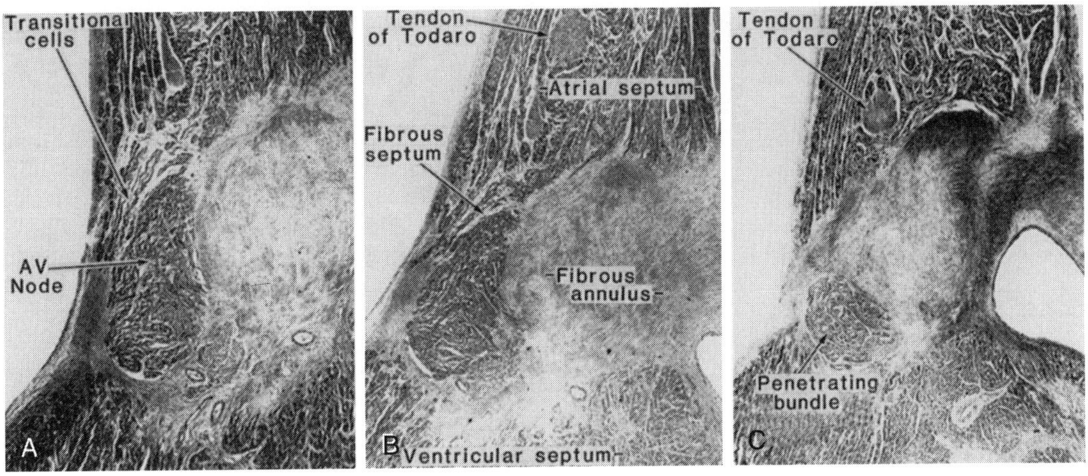

FIGURE 1–10. A series of histologic sections showing the transition from atrioventricular (AV) node to penetrating bundle. *A,* Nodal cells are still in contact with superficial transitional cells. *B,* This contact is lost when a fibrous septum intervenes. The axis then becomes the penetrating bundle, although the histologic appearance is similar to that in *A.* The penetrating bundle is more readily recognized in *C,* where it is surrounded by a prominent fibrous collar.

CONDUCTION SYSTEM IN CONGENITALLY MALFORMED HEARTS

Both the sinus node and the atrioventricular conduction system can be abnormally positioned in malformed hearts,[35] but it is convenient to describe them separately.

SINUS NODE

The majority of malformed hearts have the atrial chambers in their usual position (so-called situs solitus). This arrangement is associated with a regular location of the sinus node. Abnormal positions of the sinus node have been found in hearts with juxtaposition of the atrial appendages and in hearts with an atrial arrangement other than the usual.

Juxtaposition exists when the atrial appendages lie to the same side of the arterial pedicle rather than to either side at the base of the heart. Right juxtaposition, in which the left atrial appendage lies alongside the right atrial appendage to the right side of the pedicle, is uncommon. This distortion of atrial anatomy does not seem to affect the location of the sinus node. In contrast, left juxtaposition is a more common anomaly. The terminal crest is deviated by the distortion.[36] In these cases, the sinus node is also displaced (Fig. 1–12).

Abnormal arrangement of the atrial chambers themselves also affects the locations of the sinus node. When the atria are arranged in mirror image (situs inversus), the right atrium and the sinus node are on the left side of the patient (Fig. 1–13). In hearts with isomeric arrangement of the morphologically right atrial appendages (asplenia), there are bilateral terminal crests and, correspondingly, bilateral sinus nodes. Terminal crests, however, are mostly lacking in hearts with isomeric arrangement of the morphologically left atrial appendages (polysplenia). The majority of these hearts lack a histologically recognizable sinus node. When found, the node is hypoplastic and located posteroinferiorly, far from the orifice of the superior caval vein.[37, 38]

ATRIOVENTRICULAR CONDUCTION SYSTEM

Most types of congenital heart defects are simple holes in the cardiac septa, valvar stenosis, or abnormal ventricular origins of the great arteries. In these, the disposition of the atrioventricular conduction system generally follows the normal pattern when there is normal arrangement of the cardiac chambers and alignment between the atrial and ventricular septa. When there is mirror-image arrangement of the atria with concordant atrioventricular connections, the conduction system is also arranged in mirror-image fashion.

HEART DEFECTS WITH NORMALLY ALIGNED SEPTAL STRUCTURES

The more relevant malformations in this group are hearts with an isolated ventricular septal de-

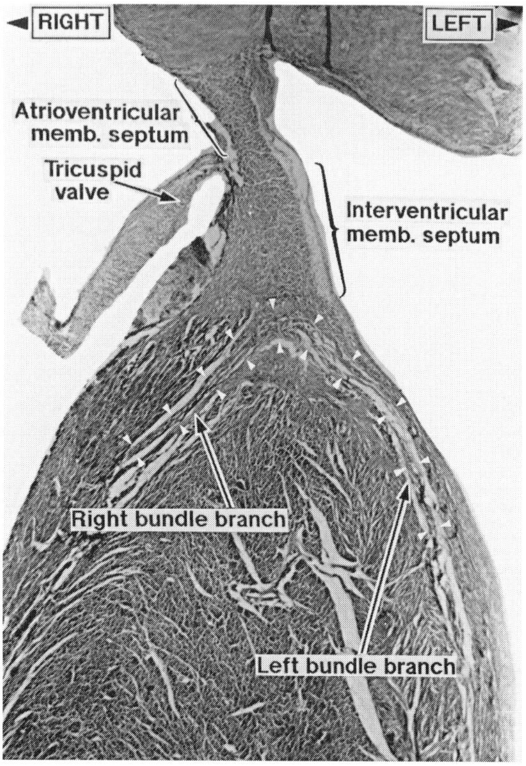

FIGURE 1–11. The branching component of the conduction axis (between *white arrowheads*) is sandwiched between the membranous septum and the muscular ventricular septum. The right bundle branch passes through the septal musculature as it descends from the left side of the septum.

fect, with atrioventricular septal defect, and with tetralogy of Fallot. Except for those hearts with atrioventricular septal defect, the triangle of Koch remains a good landmark for the location of the atrioventricular node.

In terms of distribution of the atrioventricular conduction axis, hearts with tetralogy of Fallot are directly comparable to hearts with isolated ventricular septal defect, because a defect in the ventricular septum is a cardinal feature of tetralogy of Fallot. Most ventricular septal defects, whether in isolation or otherwise, are located in the environ of the membranous septum. These are termed *perimembranous defects*, and they have a fibrous component to their borders (Fig. 1–14). The fibrous part is usually seen as a remnant of the membranous septum (the membranous flap) situated in the region of fibrous continuity between the atrioventricular valves and, usually, an arterial valve. The nonbranching bundle is considerably longer than in normal hearts. The normal leftward shift of the axis, nonetheless, still brings the bundle into the left ventricular outflow tract directly underneath the membranous septal remnant, making this part of the defect the most critical area for avoiding injury to the conduction system.[39, 40]

The disposition of the branching bundle shows a slight variation in hearts with isolated perimembranous ventricular septal defects and those associated with tetralogy of Fallot. When the defect exists in isolation, the branching bundle is frequently found astride the septal crest. On the contrary, the bundle is more often to the left of the septal crest in hearts with tetralogy of Fallot.[41]

Defects with completely muscular borders, termed *muscular defects*, have varying relationships with the conduction axis depending on their location within the septum (Fig. 1–15). Those situated between the ventricular outlets are remote from the conduction axis, whereas defects in the apical trabecular part are in the environs of the ramifications of the bundle branches. Defects opening to the inlet part of the right ventricle need to be distinguished from those perimembranous defects that have an extensive posteroinferior incursion. The conduction axis runs in the anterosuperior quadrant of the

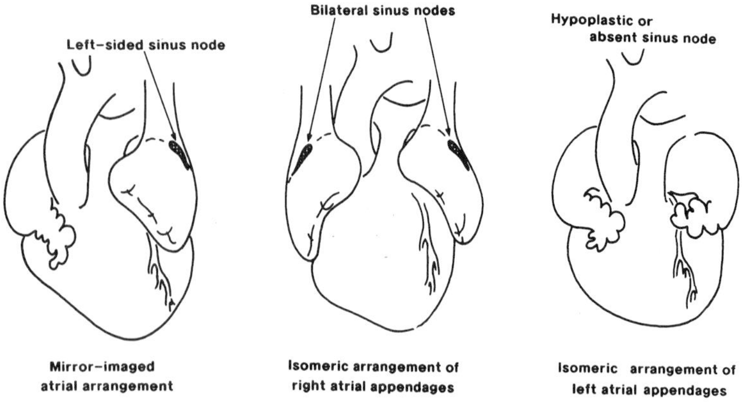

FIGURE 1–12. Locations of the sinus node in variations of arrangement of the atrial appendages.

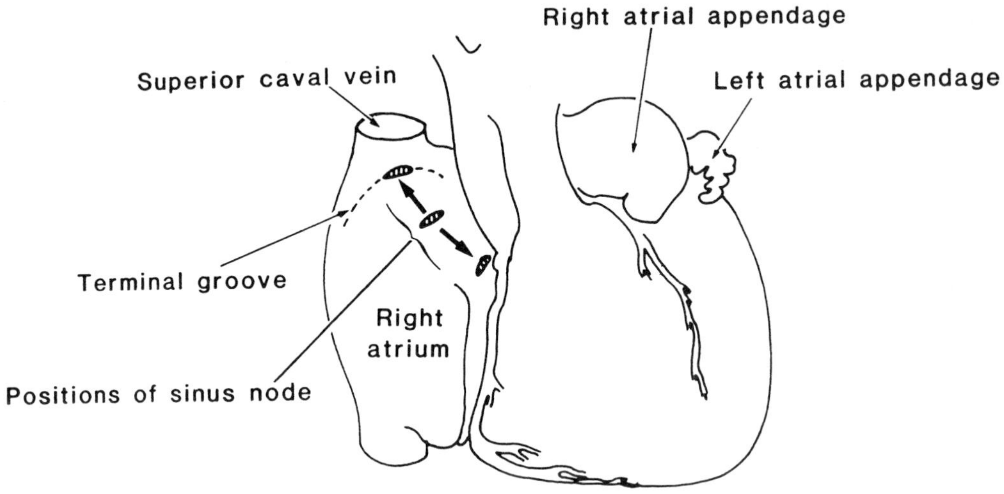

FIGURE 1–13. Variable locations of the sinus node in hearts with left juxtaposition of atrial appendages.

margin of a muscular inlet defect. This is in stark contrast to the posteroinferior location found with a perimembranous inlet defect (see Fig. 1–14). When both a perimembranous defect and a muscular inlet defect exist in the same heart, the conduction axis traverses the muscular bridge separating the defects (Fig. 1–16).

Defects situated immediately beneath both arterial valves *(doubly committed and juxta-arterial defects)* have a varying relationship to the conduction system depending on whether the posteroinferior margin is muscular or perimembranous. The conduction axis is protected within the muscular, posteroinferior rim, but is in the area of fibrous continuity between arterial and atrioventricular valves in the perimembranous type (Fig. 1–17).

Hearts with atrioventricular septal defect usually have a wide separation between atrial and ventricular septal structures. Consequently, the landmarks of the triangle of Koch no longer delineate the position of the connecting atrioventricular node (Fig. 1–18).[42] The connecting atrioventricular node is displaced posteroinferiorly at the atrial side of the junction between atrial and ventricular septa. The penetrating bundle pierces through the conjoined valvar attachment at the cardiac crux. The nonbranching bundle is long and runs on the crest of the ventricular septum. If there are separate valvar orifices (ostium primum defect), then both the nonbranching bundle and its continuation, the branching bundle, are covered over by the fusion of valvar tissues. In contrast, the branching bundle is "exposed" on the septal crest in those atrioventricular septal defects with a common valvar orifice.

HEART DEFECTS WITH MALALIGNMENT OF THE SEPTAL STRUCTURES

The atrial and ventricular septa are not in perfect alignment in several types of congenital cardiac malformations. The lesions considered here are hearts with straddling tricuspid valves, hearts with discordant atrioventricular connections in the setting of lateralized atrial arrangement, hearts with left-hand ventricular topology in the setting of isomeric arrangement of the atrial appendages, and some forms of hearts with univentricular atrioventricular connection.

The simplest hearts in this group are those with straddling of the tricuspid valve. In these, the posteroinferior part of the ventricular septum is deviated to the right of the cardiac crux. The connecting atrioventricular node is situated posteroinferiorly but is displaced to a position of the atrial wall that is nearest the point at which the ventricular septum rises to meet the tricuspid orifice at the atrioventricular junction (Fig. 1–19). The penetrating bundle burrows through the hinge of the tricuspid valve in this region and continues to a long nonbranching segment before dividing into the bundle branches.

Hearts with usual atrial arrangement and discordant atrioventricular connections have a ventricular arrangement similar to those with isomeric arrangement of the atrial appendages in association with left-hand ventricular topology. The distribution of the conduction system is also similar.[37, 43] In these hearts, the anterosuperior and right-sided ventricular chamber is morphologically a left ventricle. The connecting atrioven-

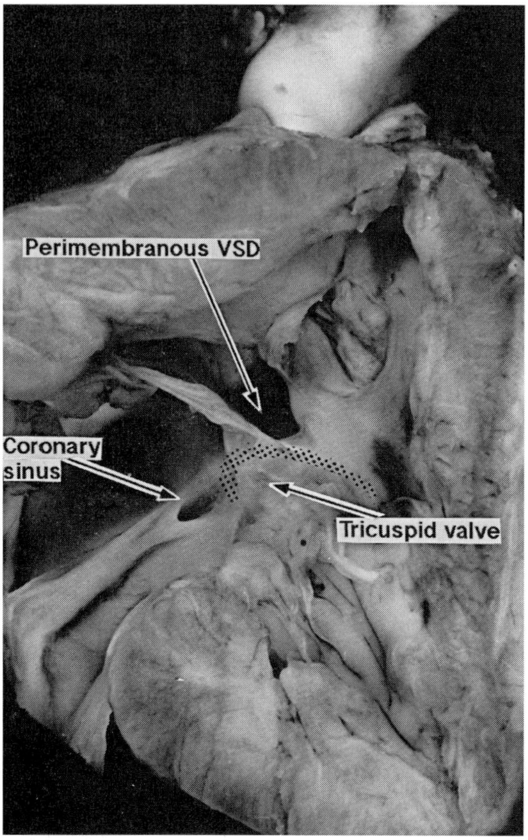

FIGURE 1–14. Right ventricular view of a specimen with a perimembranous ventricular septal defect (VSD). The conduction axis *(stippled area)* passes close to the posteroinferior margin of the defect.

tricular node is located in the atrial wall that is in the anterolateral quadrant of the mitral valve. The penetrating bundle runs in the region of fibrous continuity between the mitral valve and the valve of the posterior great artery. A long, nonbranching bundle then courses anterior to the outflow tract of the posterior great artery before descending along the anterosuperior margin of a ventricular septal defect (Fig. 1–20). The branching bundle gives origin to the left bundle branch, which descends down the right aspect of the ventricular septum, whereas the right bundle branch penetrates the septum to emerge on the left side. Occasionally, a second atrioventricular node is present. This is the regular node within the triangle of Koch. A sling of conduction tissues may sometimes be formed when the regular node also connects with the ventricular bundle branches. Rarely, only the regularly situated node makes the connection with the ventricles.

Hearts with univentricular atrioventricular connection include those with double-inlet connection, together with those having absence of either the right or left atrioventricular connections. Those that are significant in having an abnormal disposition of the conduction axis are hearts with the atria connected to a dominant left ventricle and those with a solitary indeterminate ventricle. Essentially, hearts with dominant left ventricle usually have an anteriorly located ventricular septum.[44] Those hearts with double-inlet connection have a connecting atrioventricular node at the acute marginal position of the right atrioventricular orifice.[45] From here, the bundle perforates the valvar attachment to enter the ventricular septum. The descending bundle passes to the border of the septal defect that is nearest the acute cardiac margin, irrespective of the location of the rudimentary right ventricle (Fig. 1–21).

When the right atrioventricular connection is absent and the dominant ventricle is of left morphology (tricuspid atresia), the atrioventricular node is found in the muscular floor of the right atrium. The ventricular course of the conduction axis is comparable to that described for double-inlet connection.[46, 47]

Hearts with a solitary ventricle of indeterminate morphology have been found to have an anterior or anterolaterally situated atrioventricular node. The bundle either penetrates directly into the ventricular wall or descends through a large free-running trabeculation to the ventricular apex. Bundle branches have not been identified.

ANATOMIC SUBSTRATES OF PRE-EXCITATION

Impulses may travel through several potential pathways to bypass the delay-producing areas of the specialized conduction system. These pathways are described in terms of accessory atrioventricular connections, accessory nodoventricular connections, accessory fasciculoventricular connections, accessory atrio-Hisian connections, and intranodal bypass tracts (Fig. 1–22).[22, 48]

Accessory atrioventricular connections have been located both in structurally normal hearts and in hearts with congenital malformations. These connect atrial with ventricular myocardium and can exist at any point around the atrioventricular junctions. As described previously, labels such as anterior and posterior septal areas obscure the true anatomic relationships of the cardiac structures in these parts. The majority of pathways identified histologically have been threads of working myocardium, although others

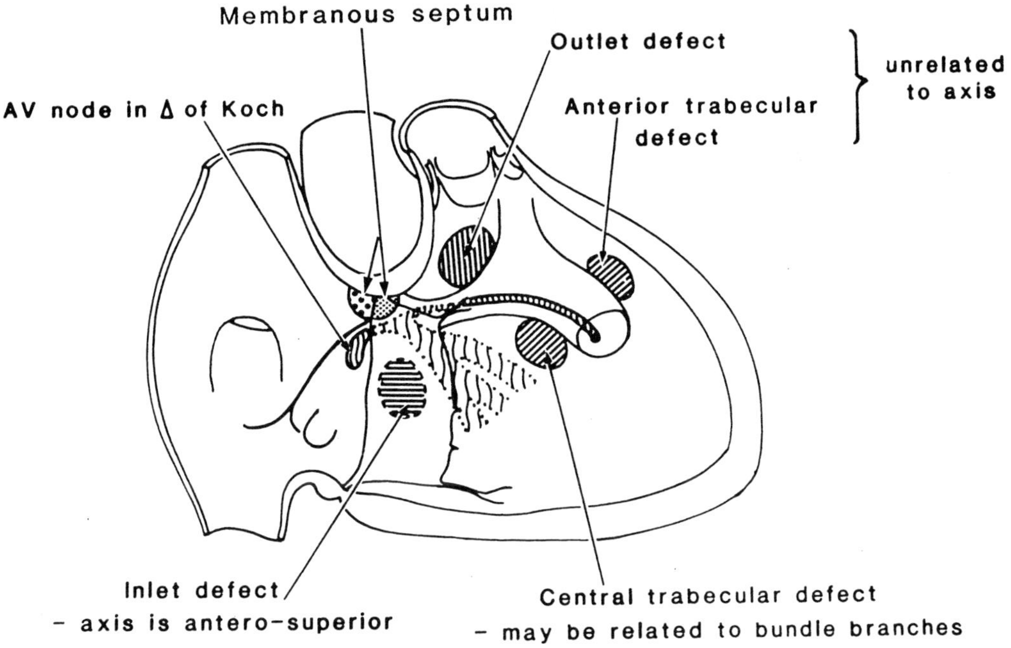

FIGURE 1–15. Diagram of the left side of the heart showing the relationship of the conduction axis to the various locations of defects that have completely muscular borders. (AV, atrioventricular).

are composed of histologically specialized tissues.[49] The majority of left-sided parietal pathways run close to the epicardial aspect of the fibrous hinge of the mitral valve. In contrast, accessory pathways along the right parietal junction either cross an area of deficiency in the fibrofatty tissues or traverse more peripherally through the fatty tissues of the atrioventricular groove. Some right-sided pathways may arise from a nodelike structure (node of Kent) at its atrial origin. In recent years, it has been recognized that "Mahaim physiology" can be produced by such histologically specialized right-sided pathways that connect with the atrioventricular conduction system via a bundle that descends in the right parietal wall. The pathways are hence described as "atriofascicular" connections. Such a sling of histologically specialized conduction tissue, with its various appellations,[50, 51] should be distinguished from the classic "Mahaim fiber," as described by Mahaim and Winston.[52, 53] These structures directly connect the atrioventricular node or bundle to the ventricular septum. Descriptively, these are better labeled nodoventricular and fasciculoventricular pathways (Fig. 1–23).

As described previously, the true septal area is very limited. True septal connections will be found between the offset attachments of the leaflets of the mitral and tricuspid valves (Fig. 1–24).[49] A further subset of accessory pathways has been described as being located close to the penetrating bundle ("intermediate septal"[54] or para-Hisian pathways). Procedures undertaken to destroy them risk damaging the specialized conduction axis, but can be achieved safely using catheter ablation at low levels of energy.[55] Another type of accessory pathway identified as the substrate for the "permanent form of junctional reciprocating tachycardia" has been located in the floor of the coronary sinus in a "posteroseptal" position,[56] but other locations have also been identified by electrophysiology.[57]

Instead of being related to the insertions of the atrioventricular valves, accessory atrioventricular connections can rarely be related to the coronary venous structures. Several cases have now been found in association with aneurysmal dilation of the coronary sinus.[58, 59] A further case was associated with aneurysmal formation of the anterior cardiac vein, where broad bands of accessory connections were found at the mouth of the aneurysm.[60]

As we have indicated, accessory pathways that extend from the underside of the nodal and fascicular components of the node-bundle conduction axis are described anatomically as nodoventricular and fasciculoventricular accessory connections, respectively (see Fig. 1–23). These fibers, initially labeled as paraspecific fibers by Mahaim and Winston,[52, 53] are regularly found

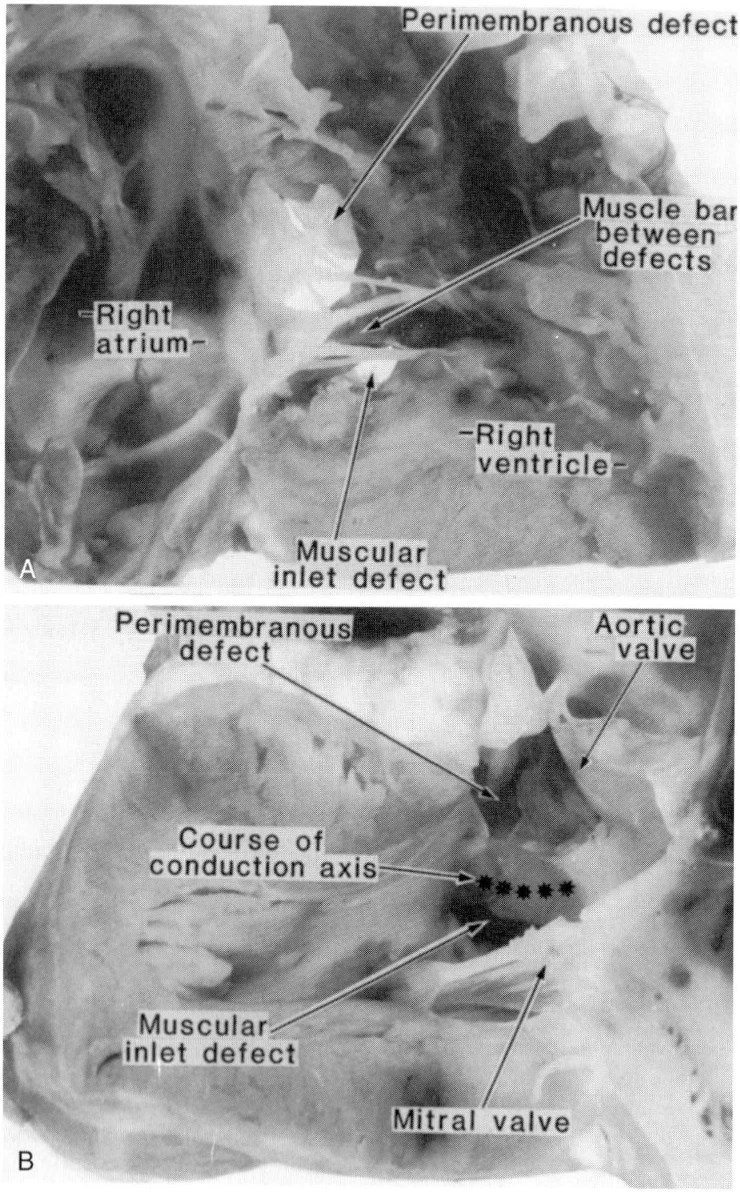

FIGURE 1–16. A heart with coexisting perimembranous inlet and muscular inlet defects. *A*, View of the right side of the heart. Reconstructions from serial histologic sections showed the course of the conduction axis in the muscle bar between the two defects. This course is marked in *B*, which shows the relationship of the defects as viewed from the left side of the heart.

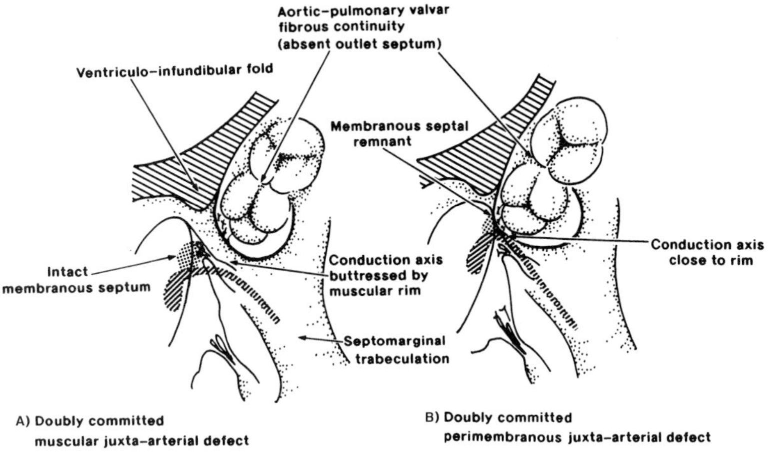

FIGURE 1–17. Proximity of the conduction axis to the posteroinferior rim of the defect in muscular *(A)* and perimembranous *(B)* defects. The defect shown is a doubly committed juxta-arterial type, but the relationship is equally relevant in those defects situated immediately underneath one arterial valve.

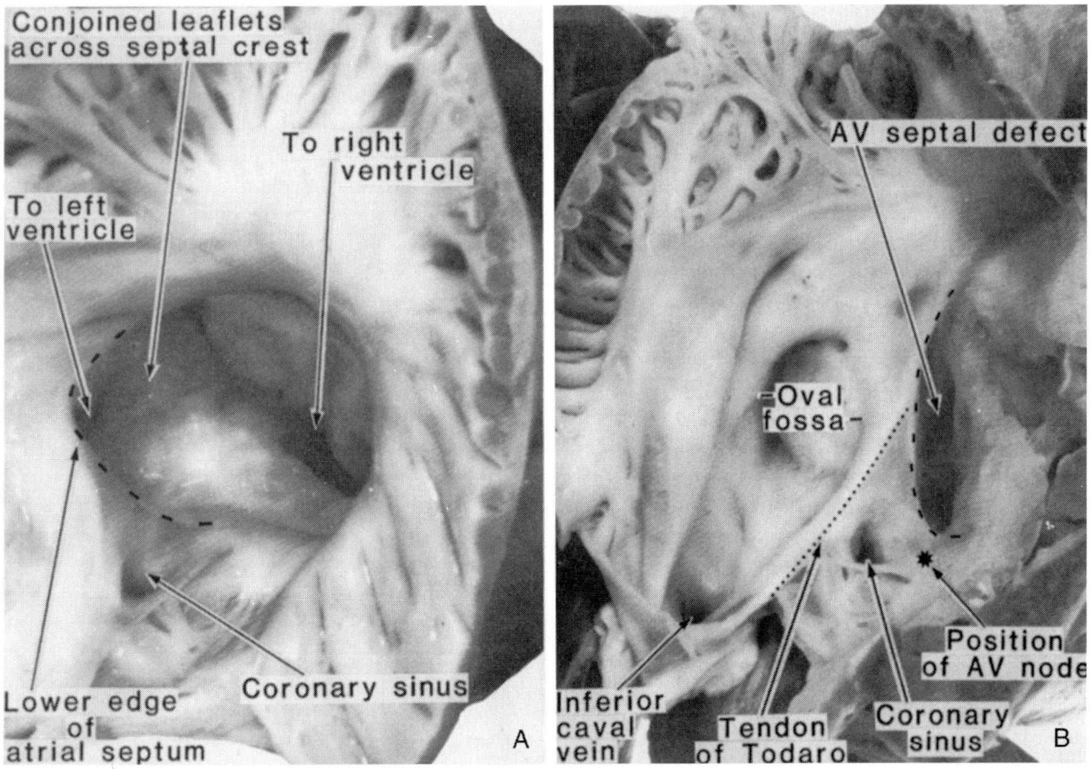

FIGURE 1–18. A heart with atrioventricular (AV) septal defect. The view from the right atrium toward the ventricular mass *(A)* shows the partition of the atrioventricular orifice by the conjoined leaflets. A lateral view of the right atrium *(B)* shows the posteriorly displaced position of the atrioventricular node. The angle between the tendon of Todaro *(dotted line)* and lower edge of the atrial septum *(dashed line)* does not contain the connecting node.

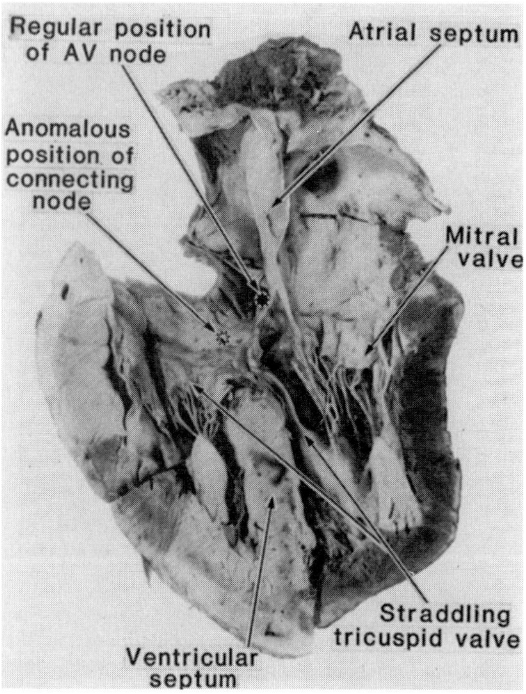

FIGURE 1–19. Four-chamber section through a heart with straddling tricuspid valve. The connecting node is deviated to the right. (AV, atrioventricular.)

in normal hearts, especially those in neonates.[26] Clinicopathologic correlations showing anomalous conduction across them, however, are scanty.[61] Current electrophysiologic investigations suggest that "Mahaim physiology" is more commonly produced by a conduction sling originating in a node of Kent (Fig. 1–23A).[50, 62]

Anatomically, atrio-Hisian connections (originally designated as "atriofascicular" by the European study group[48]) traverse through the central fibrous body, connecting atrial myocardium with the node-bundle axis distal to the nodal region. Such a bundle was identified by Brechenmacher[63] in a case known to have short PR interval and a normal QRS complex. These pathways should be distinguished from "last" fibers connecting the axis before penetration (see Fig. 1–10). Furthermore, they should also be distinguished from the specialized muscular connections originating in the node of Kent; these latter structures are now frequently described as atriofascicular tracts.[22, 51] The variety of pre-excitation with short PR interval and normal QRS complex, the Lown-Ganong-Levine syndrome, was also explained on the basis of a James fiber,[64] but the functional significance of these fibers, described by James himself as ubiquitous,[64] remains to be demonstrated.

The pathways that are possible candidates for intranodal bypass tracts must also be considered as substrates for dual nodal pathways and longitudinal dissociation. The fibers described by James[64] as extending from the eustachian ridge to insert at the junction of the atrioventricular node and bundle are such candidates for intranodal bypass tracts. Because they are found in normal hearts, it is difficult to implicate them as a

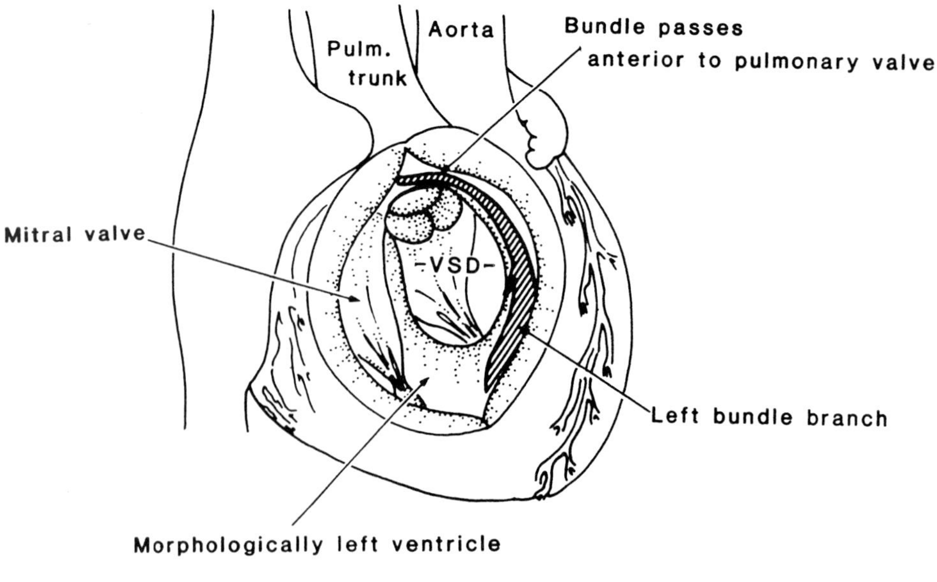

FIGURE 1–20. Course of the nonbranching bundle as viewed through an incision in the morphologically left ventricle in a heart with congenitally corrected transposition of the great arteries. (VSD, ventricular septal defect.)

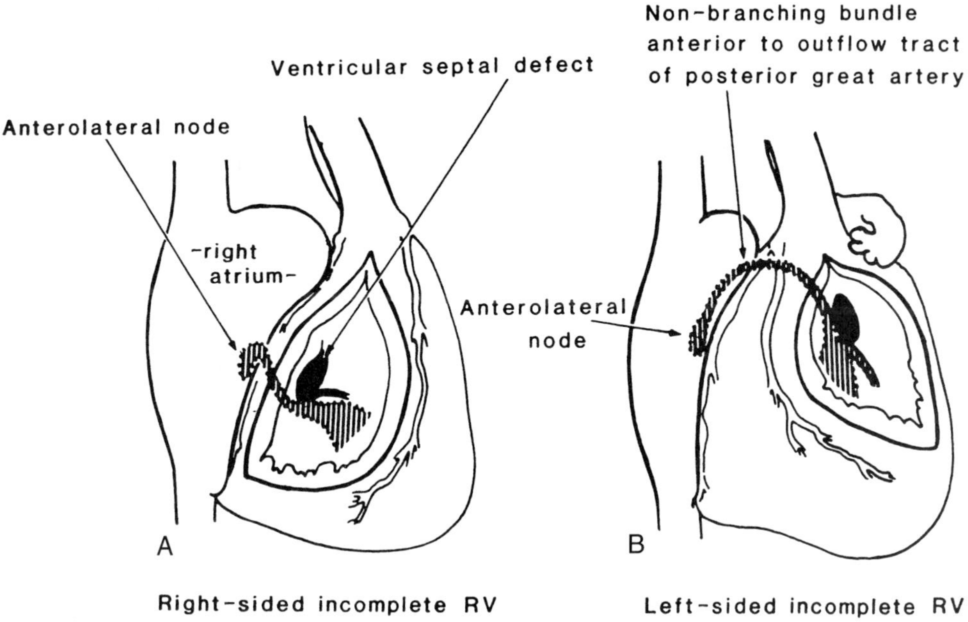

FIGURE 1–21. *A* and *B*, Course of the conduction axis as viewed through incisions in the incomplete right ventricle (RV) in hearts with double-inlet atrioventricular connection to a dominant left ventricle.

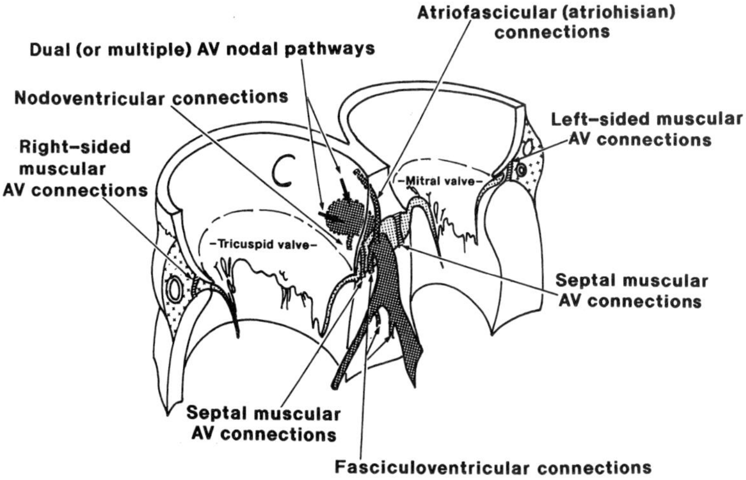

FIGURE 1–22. Potential anatomic substrates of pre-excitation. (AV, atrioventricular).

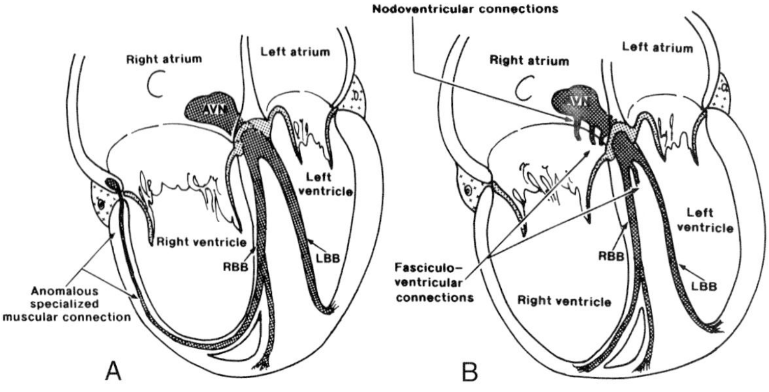

FIGURE 1–23. *A,* Configuration of the accessory pathway that produces Mahaim physiology. *B,* Locations of accessory nodoventricular and fasciculoventricular connections that are also described as Mahaim fibers. (RBB, right bundle branch; LBB, left bundle branch.)

source of pre-excitation without electrophysiologic correlations. Furthermore, there are numerous other possibilities for bypass within the atrial component of the specialized junctional area. For instance, there is considerable variation in the architecture of the "last" atrial fiber to make contact with the node-bundle axis before it becomes the penetrating bundle. Further variation exists with regard to the morphology of the compact node and its inferior extension. In some hearts, the inferior extension is predominantly to the left, whereas in others, the right extension is dominant. Within the compact node itself, the stratification (see Fig. 1–8) gives multiple possibilities for bypass pathways. As yet, none of these anatomic findings have been correlated with electrophysiologic investigations.

ATRIOVENTRICULAR NODAL RE-ENTRANT TACHYCARDIA

As previously described, the possible candidates for intranodal bypass tracts must also be those that could invoke dual-pathway physiology. There have been postulations that dual or multiple pathways are located within the atrioventricular node or involve the atrial tissues.[65, 66] The concept that the circuit was intranodal was challenged by Ross and colleagues.[67] They showed that this arrhythmia could be cured by dissections in the approaches to the atrioventricular node without disruption of atrioventricular nodal conduction. Transcatheter ablative procedures have also provided much evidence that the slow and fast pathways are outside the area of the histologically specialized conduction tissues. Our study of 10 hearts from patients who had electrophysiologic investigations before cardiac transplantation showed no discrete difference in the structure of the nodal area.[68] Extranodal tracts of specialized atrial tissues were not observed in any of the hearts, nine of which demonstrated dual- or multiple-pathway physiology. These pathways may be due to varying conduction properties of the perinodal tissues rather than a discrete anatomic entity. In this regard, the arrangement of the working atrial fibers themselves (see Fig. 1–4) is almost certainly of paramount importance (see prior discussion).[16]

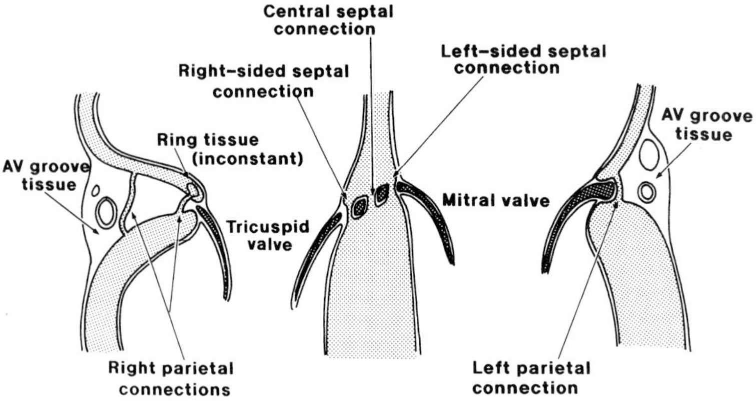

FIGURE 1–24. Locations of accessory atrioventricular (AV) connections and their relationship to the mitral and tricuspid valves and the septum.

ACKNOWLEDGMENT

This work was supported by the British Heart Foundation together with the Joseph Levy Foundation.

REFERENCES

1. His W Jr: Die Thätigkeit des embryonalen Herzens und deren Bedeutung für die Lehre von der Herzbewegung bein Erwachsenen. Arb Med Klinik Leipzig 1:14–49, 1893.
2. Kent AFS: Researches on the structure and function of the mammalian heart. J Physiol 14:233–254, 1893.
3. Keith A: An autobiography. New York, Philosophical Library, 1950, pp 254–259.
4. Tawara S: Das Reizleitungssystem des Saugetierherzens. Jena, Gustav Fischer, 1906.
5. Keith A, Flack MW: The auriculo-ventricular bundle of the human heart. Lancet 2:359–364, 1906.
6. Wenckebach KF: Beiträge zur Kenntnis der menschlichen Herztätigkeit. Arch Anat Physiol 2:1–14, 1907.
7. Thorel C: Verläufige Mitteilung über eine besondere Muskelverbindung zwischen der Cava superior und dem Hisschen Bundel. Münchener Med Wochenschr 56:2159, 1909.
8. James TN: The connecting pathways between the sinus node and the A-V node and between the right and the left atrium in the human heart. Am J Cardiol 66:498–508, 1963.
9. Mönckeberg JG: Zur Entwicklungsgeschichte des Atrioventrikularsystems. Verh Dtsch Ges Pathol 16:228–249, 1913.
10. Aschoff L: Referat über die Herzstörungen in ihren Beziehungen zu dem spezifischen Muskelsystem des Herzens. Verh Dtsch Ges Pathol 14:3–35, 1910.
11. Tranum-Jensen J, Janse MJ: Fine structural identification of individual cells subjected to microelectrode recording in perfused cardiac preparations. J Mol Cell Cardiol 14:233–240, 1982.
12. Hutchinson MC: A study of the atrial arteries in man. J Anat 125:39–54, 1978.
13. Busquet J, Fontan F, Anderson RH, et al: The surgical significance of the atrial branches of the coronary arteries. Int J Cardiol 6:223–234, 1985.
14. Janse MJ, Anderson RH: Specialized internodal atrial pathways—Fact or fiction? Eur J Cardiol 2:351–359, 1975.
15. Anderson RH, Ho SY, Smith A, et al: The internodal atrial myocardium. Anat Rec 201:75–82, 1981.
16. Sanchez-Quintana D, Davies DW, Ho SY, et al: Architecture of the atrial musculature in and around the triangle of Koch; its potential relevance to atrioventricular nodal reentry. J Cardiovasc Electrophysiol 8:1396–1407, 1997.
17. Koch W: Der funktionelle Bau des menschlichen Herzens. Berlin, Urban v. Schwarzenburg, 1922, p 92.
18. Hummel JD, Strickberger SA, Man KC, et al: A quantitative fluoroscopic comparison of the coronary sinus ostium in patients with and without atrioventricular nodal reentrant tachycardia. J Cardiovasc Electrophysiol 6:681–686, 1995.
19. Anderson RH, Latham RA: The cellular architecture of the human atrioventricular node, with a note on its morphology in the presence of a left superior caval vein. J Anat 109:443–455, 1971.
20. Dean JW, Ho SY, Rowland E, et al: Clinical anatomy of the atrioventricular junctions. J Am Coll Cardiol 7:1725–1731, 1994.
21. Anderson RH, Becker AE: Stanley Kent and accessory atrioventricular connections. J Thorac Cardiovasc Surg 81:649–658, 1981.
22. Anderson RH, Ho SY, Gillette PC, Becker AE: Review—Mahaim, Kent and abnormal atrioventricular conduction. Cardiovasc Res 31:480–491, 1996.
23. Truex RC, Smythe MQ: Reconstruction of the human atrioventricular node. Anat Rec 158:11–20, 1967.
24. Scherf D, Cohen J: The Atrioventricular Node and Selected Cardiac Arrhythmias. New York, Grune & Stratton, 1964, p 5.
25. James TN, Marshall ML: Subitaneas Mortibus 18. Persistent fetal dispersion of the atrioventricular node and His bundle within the central fibrous body. Circulation 53:1026–1034, 1976.
26. Ho SY, Anderson RH: Conduction system and SIDS. Ann NY Acad Sci 533:176–190, 1988.
27. Taussig HB: On the boundaries of the sino-auricular node and the atrioventricular node in the human heart. Bull Johns Hopkins Hosp 48:162–178, 1931.
28. Hecht H, Kossman CE, Childers RW, et al: Atrioventricular and intraventricular conduction. Revised nomenclature and concepts. Am J Cardiol 31:232–244, 1973.
29. Racker DK: Atrioventricular node and input pathways: A correlated gross anatomical and histological study of the canine atrioventricular junctional region. Anat Rec 224:336–354, 1989.
30. Lev M, Bharati S: Lesions of the conduction system and their functional significance. In Sommers SC (ed): Pathology Annual. New York, Appleton-Century-Crofts, 1974, pp 157–207.
31. Ho SY, Kilpatrick L, Kanai T, et al: The architecture of the atrioventricular conduction axis in dog compared to man: Its significance to ablation of the atrioventricular nodal approaches. J Cardiovasc Electrophysiol 6:26–39, 1995.
32. Spach MS, Lieberman M, Scott JG, et al: Excitation sequences of the atrial septum and AV node in isolated hearts of the dog and the rabbit. Circ Res 29:156–172, 1971.
33. Davis MJ, Anderson RH, Becker AE: The Conduction System of the Heart. London, Butterworths, 1983, p 37.
34. Kurosawa H, Becker AE: Dead end tract of the conduction axis. Int J Cardiol 7:13–18, 1985.
35. Ho SY, Anderson RH: Conduction tissue in congenital heart surgery. World J Surg 9:550–567, 1985.
36. Ho SY, Monro JL, Anderson RH: The disposition of the sinus node in left sided juxtaposition of the atrial appendages. Br Heart J 41:129–132, 1979.
37. Dickinson DF, Wilkinson JL, Anderson KR, et al: The cardiac conduction system in situs ambiguus. Circulation 59:879–885, 1979.
38. Ho SY, Seo JW, Brown NA, et al: Morphology of the sinus node in human and mouse hearts with isomerism of the atrial appendages. Br Heart J 74:437–442, 1995.
39. Titus JL, Daugherty GW, Edwards JE: Anatomy of the atrioventricular conduction system in ventricular septal defect. Circulation 28:72–81, 1963.
40. Anderson RH, Wilcox BR: The surgical anatomy of ventricular septal defect. J Card Surg 7:17–35, 1992.
41. Anderson RH, Monro JL, Ho SY, et al: Les voies de conduction auriculo-ventriculaires dans le tetralogie de Fallot. Coeur 8:793–807, 1977.
42. Ho SY, Gerlis LM, Toms J, et al: Morphology of the posterior junctional area in atrioventricular septal defects. Ann Thorac Surg 54:264–270, 1992.
43. Anderson RH, Becker AE, Arnold R, et al: The conduct-

ing tissues in congenitally corrected transposition. Circulation 50:911–923, 1974.
44. Ho SY, Zuberbuhler JR, Anderson RH: Pathology of hearts with univentricular atrioventricular connection. Perspect Pediatr Pathol 12:69–99, 1988.
45. Anderson RH, Arnold R, Thaper MK, et al: Cardiac specialized tissues in hearts with an apparently single ventricle chamber (double inlet left ventricle). Am J Cardiol 33:95–106, 1974.
46. Guller B, DuShane JW, Titus JL: The atrioventricular conduction system in 2 cases of tricuspid atresia. Circulation 40:217–226, 1969.
47. Dickinson DF, Wilkinson JL, Smith A, et al: Atrioventricular conduction tissues in univentricular hearts of left ventricular type with absent right atrioventricular connection ("tricuspid atresia"). Br Heart J 42:1–8, 1979.
48. Anderson RH, Becker AE, Brechenmacher C, et al: Ventricular pre-excitation. A proposed nomenclature for its substrates. Eur J Cardiol 3:27–36, 1975.
49. Becker AE, Anderson RH, Durrer D, et al: The anatomical substrates of Wolff-Parkinson-White syndrome: A clinico-pathologic correlation in seven patients. Circulation 57:870–879, 1978.
50. Klein GJ, Guiraudon GM, Ker CR, et al: "Nodoventricular" accessory pathway: Evidence for a distinct accessory atrioventricular pathway with atrioventricular node-like properties. J Am Coll Cardiol 11:1035–1040, 1988.
51. Tchou P, Lehman MH, Jazayeri M, et al: Atriofascicular connection or a nodoventricular Mahaim fibre? Electrophysiologic elucidation of the pathway and associated reentrant circuit. Circulation 77:837–848, 1988.
52. Mahaim I, Winston MR: Recherches d'anatomie comparie et de pathologie experimentale sur les connexions hautes des His-Tawara. Cardiologia 5:139–260, 1941.
53. Mahaim I: Kent's fiber in the A-V paraspecific conduction through the upper connection of the bundle of His-Tawara. Am Heart J 33:651–653, 1947.
54. Gallagher JJ, Selle JG, Svenson RH, et al: Surgical treatment of arrhythmias. Am J Cardiol 61:27a–44a, 1988.
55. Haissaguerre M, Fischer B, Marcus F, et al: Role of catheter ablation for treatment of supraventricular tachyarrhythmias. In Mandel WJ (ed): Cardiac Arrhythmias, 3rd ed. Philadelphia, JB Lippincott, 1995, p 945.
56. Critelli G, Gallagher JJ, Monda V, et al: Anatomic and electrophysiologic substrate of the permanent form of junctional reciprocating tachycardia. J Am Coll Cardiol 4:601–610, 1984.
57. Langberg JJ, Chin MC, Rosenquist M, et al: Catheter ablation of the atrioventricular junction with radiofrequency. Circulation 80:1527–1535, 1989.
58. Gerlis LM, Davies MJ, Boyle R, et al: Pre-excitation due to accessory sinoventricular connections associated with coronary sinus aneurysms. A report of two cases. Br Heart J 53:314–322, 1985.
59. Guiraudon GM, Guiraudon CM, Klein GJ, et al: The coronary sinus diverticulum a pathologic entity associated with the Wolff-Parkinson-White syndrome. Am J Cardiol 62:733–735, 1988.
60. Ho SY, Russell G, Rowland E: Coronary venous aneurysms and accessory atrioventricular connections. Br Heart J 60:348–351, 1988.
61. Gmeiner R, Ng CK, Hammer I, et al: Tachycardia caused by an accessory nodoventricular tract: A clinico-pathologic correlation. Eur Heart J 5:233–242, 1984.
62. Murdock CJ, Leitch JW, Klein JG, et al: Epicardial mapping in patients with "nodoventricular" accessory pathways. Am J Cardiol 68:208–214, 1991.
63. Brechenmacher C: Atrio-His bundle tracts. Br Heart J 37:853–855, 1975.
64. James TN: Morphology of the human atrioventricular node with remarks pertinent to its electrophysiology. Am Heart J 54:430–435, 1961.
65. Josephson ME, Kastor JA: Paroxysmal supraventricular tachycardia: Is the atrium a necessary link? Circulation 54:430–435, 1976.
66. Holman WL, Hackel DB, Lease JG, et al: Cryosurgical ablation of atrioventricular nodal reentry: Histologic localization of the proximal common pathway. Circulation 77:1356–1362, 1988.
67. Ross DZ, Johnson DC, Deniss AR, et al: Curative surgery for atrioventricular junctional ("AV nodal") re-entrant tachycardia. J Am Coll Cardiol 6:1383–1392, 1985.
68. Ho SY, McComb JM, Scott CD, et al: Morphology of the cardiac conduction system in patients with electrophysiologically proven dual atrioventricular nodal pathways. J Cardiovasc Electrophysiol 4:504–512, 1993.

CHAPTER 2

NONINVASIVE DIAGNOSTIC TECHNIQUES

Beth Bubolz and Christopher L. Case

Since the turn of the century, when Einthoven recorded an electrogram of the human heart using a string galvanometer,[1] scientists and physicians have sought to improve methods of recording rhythm patterns of the heart. Today electrocardiograms (ECGs) can be recorded and transmitted under almost any circumstances. Advanced methods of processing ECGs yield signals that are virtually free of motion artifact, even during treadmill exercise testing. Even more sophisticated methods of recording and transmission are being pursued.

The goal of arrhythmia evaluation is to establish a diagnosis, predict prognosis, implement appropriate therapy, and assess the effectiveness of treatment once it has been initiated. Many noninvasive tools are now available for this purpose. They are the mainstay of arrhythmia diagnosis and management because noninvasive recordings are made in a more physiologic state than invasive electrophysiologic studies. Often they are less costly, are associated with less morbidity, and are readily available to the general cardiologist.

This chapter addresses the historic and technical background of the noninvasive tests available today. Indications as well as the relative strengths and weaknesses for each test are discussed. Some comment is made on future developments of noninvasive techniques that are not currently in clinical use.

Holter monitoring, ambulatory blood pressure (ABP) monitoring, transtelephonic monitoring (TTM), event recorders, in-hospital telemetry, and signal-averaged electrocardiography (SAECG) are discussed.

HOLTER MONITORING

BACKGROUND

When Norman J. Holter presented his new technique for physiologic recording of an electrogram at a distance in 1948, the apparatus consisted of an 80-pound transmitter, which was carried in a backpack by the patient.[2] Electrograms were received at a distant station with an oscilloscope and an antenna on a cart, which could be positioned for optimal reception. Once he established that physiologic electric signals could indeed be transmitted over a distance, Holter went back to his laboratory behind the family hardware store in Helena, Montana to make the system practical for clinical use.[3] Encouraged by Dr. Paul D. White, he devised a portable (4-pound) recording system that could record 10 to 24 hours of ambulatory ECGs for later scanning and analysis. This system was commercially available in the 1970s and revolutionized noninvasive monitoring when the number of premature ventricular contractions (PVCs) was found to correlate with the risk of sudden death.[4]

Today recorders weigh less than half as much as the original devices. Five electrodes can produce two- or three-channel recordings. Scanning is aided by computer recognition and labeling of normal, ectopic, and premature beats. High-resolution recording can demonstrate subtle changes such as ST-segment depression. Computer storage and retrieval make this information easily accessible.

INDICATIONS

Suspected Arrhythmias

Arrhythmias may be suspected on the basis of symptoms (e.g., palpitations, dizziness, or syncope),[5] resting ECG (i.e., Wolff-Parkinson-White [WPW] pattern), or a history of congenital heart disease or surgery (Fig. 2–1).[6] Holter monitoring is best suited to record arrhythmias that occur daily. The Holter monitor is useful for both symptomatic and asymptomatic rhythm disturbances. Diaries of perceived events generally do not correlate closely with arrhythmias. Ambulatory ECG recordings can make a quantitative

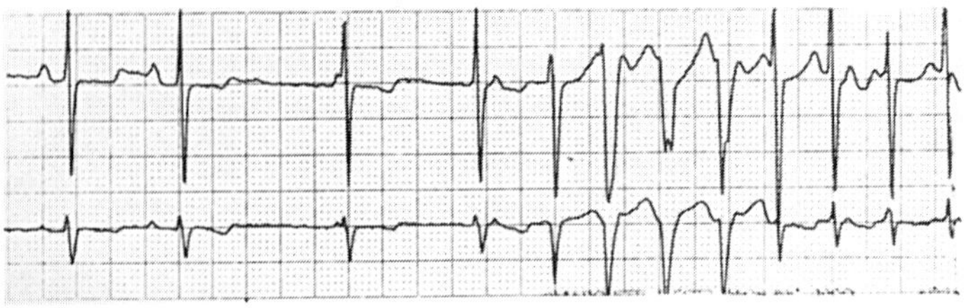

FIGURE 2–1. Surface electrocardiogram leads II and V_1 from a Holter monitor tracing exhibiting the onset of supraventricular tachycardia (SVT) as a result of atrioventricular dissociation caused by sinus slowing and a junctional escape. The sinus P wave merges into the QRS complex. The P wave in the fourth QRS complex conducts slowly to the fifth QRS complex. Four beats of SVT with left bundle branch block ensue, followed by narrow QRS SVT with no visible P waves.

assessment of the number of ectopic beats in 24 hours; high, low, and average heart rates; and length of pauses. Sensitivity of this test may be increased with 48 to 72 hours of recording. Holter monitors may be used in conjunction with transtelephonic monitors and recorders to document suspected arrhythmias. The latter are discussed later in this chapter.

Sinus Node Function

Twenty-four-hour Holter monitoring is useful in the evaluation of patients suspected of having sinus node dysfunction. Postoperative Mustard, Senning, and Fontan patients are at relatively high risk for sick sinus, or bradycardia-tachycardia syndrome.[7, 8] Less commonly, sinus node dysfunction occurs after secundum atrial septal defect or tetralogy of Fallot repair. Information obtained during sleep with regard to high and low heart rates can identify rhythm problems before they produce symptoms and thus guide further testing and therapy.

Atrioventricular Node Function

Atrioventricular (AV) node function can be assessed using ambulatory Holter monitoring. The identification of first-degree AV block and Mobitz type I (Wenckebach) second-degree AV block are considered normal. The discovery of Mobitz type II second-degree or third-degree AV block warrants further workup and possible treatment.

Congenital Complete Atrioventricular Block

Holter monitoring can measure many parameters that help the clinician decide when permanent pacing is required in a patient with congenital complete AV block (CCAVB). Serial Holter monitors are routinely performed in these patients. Minimum, maximum, and average heart rates as well as trends can be accurately documented. Junctional versus ventricular escape rhythm can be discerned and followed serially.

Traditionally, electrical parameters that suggest the need for permanent pacing include a resting heart rate of less than 55 bpm in infants or less than 50 bpm in older children, frequent ventricular ectopy, or a prolonged corrected QT interval. Other parameters that suggest that it is time to pace include fatigue, syncope, increased heart size on chest x-ray, atrial enlargement by 12-lead ECG, and congestive heart failure.[9]

One prospective study reports a 7- to 30-year follow-up on patients with CCAVB. We recommend prophylactic pacemaker implantation even for asymptomatic adults with CCAVB because of the high incidence of fatal first-time Stokes-Adams attacks, the inevitability of decreasing ventricular escape rates with increasing age, significant morbidity, and a high incidence of "acquired" mitral insufficiency.[10] In response, an editorial comment by a pediatric electrophysiologist debated the question of early intervention with pacing therapy in adolescents.[11]

Premature Ventricular Contractions

Benign PVCs of childhood may produce no symptoms and in general do not require treatment. Often they are discovered on routine physical examination. Holter monitoring can define the frequency (number per hour), timing (singles, couplets, triplets), and morphology (uniform or multiform) of PVCs. Benign PVCs occur as single uniform beats in children with a structurally normal heart. Couplets or multiform PVCs require further evaluation.

Postoperative Arrhythmias

Both supraventricular and ventricular arrhythmias contribute to sudden cardiac death in patients after congenital heart surgery.[12] Routine surveillance Holter monitoring in these patients should be performed on a regular basis. Particular postoperative attention should be given to patients who have undergone the Fontan, Mustard, or Senning procedures for atrial incisional tachycardia, atrial flutter, or atrial ectopic tachycardia. After surgical repair of tetralogy of Fallot, ventricular dysrhythmias predominate. Atrial flutter may also occur after atrial septal defect repair.

Preoperative Arrhythmias

Valvar aortic stenosis is an example of congenital heart disease that may lead to ventricular ectopy or ST-segment changes. These changes may be a sign that it is time to relieve the obstruction. Holter monitoring can identify these changes.[13]

Cardiomyopathy/Collagen Vascular Diseases

Many patients with dilated or hypertrophic cardiomyopathy, collagen vascular disease, and other systemic diseases may present with arrhythmias. Any part of the conduction system or myocardium may be affected; therefore, any rhythm disturbance may occur. Holter monitoring is useful in documenting baseline status as well as tracking the patient's response to therapy. Improvement may occur with treatment of the underlying disease or with treatment of the dysrhythmia using antiarrhythmic drugs.

Assessment of Pharmacologic and Nonpharmacologic Therapy

Holter monitoring helps assess the response of rhythm disturbances to pharmacologic therapy The number of PVCs or the presence of couplets or ventricular tachycardia (VT) may be quantified after drug therapy is initiated. With atrial ectopic tachycardia, an increase in the average heart rate during a 24-hour period compared with baseline values may indicate a proarrhythmic effect. Often the P waves of atrial tachycardia cannot be differentiated on Holter monitor from sinus P waves; therefore, the use of 24-hour average heart rates or the amount of time spent at the tachycardia rate is a practical way to maximize the use of this noninvasive test before invasive electrophysiologic testing.

Holter monitoring may also be utilized to assess the efficacy of nonpharmacologic treatment of arrhythmias. After radiofrequency catheter ablation, patients are often sensitive to premature atrial and ventricular contractions. When symptoms occur daily, Holter monitoring can distinguish sinus rhythm from single premature beats, brief tachycardia episodes, or sustained tachycardia. Holter monitoring may reveal the return of a delta wave after radiofrequency ablation of WPW syndrome. Lastly, it is helpful in assessing asymptomatic arrhythmias, quantifying incessant tachycardias, and identifying either tachyarrhythmias or bradyarrhythmias in patients too young to verbalize symptoms.

Pacemakers are another form of nonpharmacologic therapy for which Holter monitors can be used to evaluate. Although pacemakers today offer very advanced functions of memory and event recording, the 24-hour ambulatory ECG is sometimes the only way to assess the percentage of paced beats and the incidence of sinus rhythm. Holter monitoring may also demonstrate asymptomatic episodes of noncapture and over- or undersensing.

STRENGTHS

Holter monitoring is a readily available noninvasive mode of recording surface ECGs in a physiologic state. It is best employed to document events that occur daily, quantify ectopy, assess the extremes of heart rate, and evaluate the efficacy of pharmacologic and nonpharmacologic therapy. It also has applications in routine screening of patients at risk for arrhythmias on the basis of hemodynamic disturbances or prior open heart surgery.

WEAKNESSES

It is difficult to document sporadic events with a Holter monitor. Computer algorithms have difficulty distinguishing certain classes of normal beats from abnormal beats on select Holter recordings. For example, atrial ectopic tachycardias and junctional rhythms cannot be differentiated by automated scanning from normal sinus beats. Uneven tape speed during recording may lead to artifactual tachycardia. Batteries in the Holter recorder should be replaced every 24 hours to guard against this pitfall. Generally, accurate measurements of the QT interval cannot be made from Holter monitor tracings and must be confirmed by 12-lead ECG.

FUTURE

Shortly after the implementation of Holter monitoring in the clinical setting, PVCs were found to predict sudden cardiac death in certain clinical situations. Today much more sophisticated methods allow measurement of heart rate variability (HRV) from Holter recordings. HRV describes the variation of cycle length from one cardiac cycle to the next. Initially, HRV was measured as the standard deviation from a mean RR interval. With the development of power spectral analysis using fast Fourier transformation and autoregression, new methods of expressing HRV are evolving.[14]

Decreased HRV has been documented after acute myocardial infarction,[15] in diabetes,[16] and after heart transplantation.[17] Normal HRV is an indicator of increased survival after myocardial infarction.[15] Changes in HRV with advanced congestive heart failure have been graphically represented using Poincare plots.[18] Short-term changes in HRV have also been studied with regard to assessment of the autonomic nervous system.[19] Parasympathetic and sympathetic activity can be identified by characteristic power spectral frequencies. The relative roles of parasympathetic and sympathetic tone during maneuvers such as tilt testing[20] are being investigated, and clinical correlations are being sought.

AMBULATORY BLOOD PRESSURE MONITORING

BACKGROUND

ABP monitoring is available in conjunction with some ambulatory ECG recording systems. One method involves R-wave gating of auscultatory blood pressure measurements. Blood pressure is measured at scheduled intervals throughout the day. A limited number of additional recordings may be triggered by the patient when symptoms occur.

INDICATIONS

ABP monitoring is most useful to discern "white coat hypertension" from true hypertension.[21] If the diagnosis of hypertension has been made, ABP monitoring can be used to evaluate responses to therapy. It has been tried in patients with frequent syncope, but we have not found it to be a powerful tool.

STRENGTHS

The major strength of this modality lies in recording physiologic events (i.e., blood pressure) during normal daily activities and correlating it to the ECG.

WEAKNESSES

The added cost of ABP monitoring over Holter monitoring alone may not be justified for the few pediatric patients needing this type of monitoring. If this is used to document blood pressure in relation to symptoms, the patient must have a prodrome to trigger the blood pressure measurement. This modality is also limited by the finite number of readings that may be made in a 24-hour period.

TRANSTELEPHONIC ELECTROCARDIOGRAPHY

BACKGROUND

TTM has been in use since the 1970s. It has a small transmitter, which senses the ECG and transmits it via telephone to a receiver in the hospital or office setting (Fig. 2–2).

Transmitters

Three types of transmitters are employed in our center. The simplest and most frequently used is a Pacer Tracer (Fig. 2–3). This transmitter sends a live recording of the heart rhythm over the telephone to the receiving center. Chil-

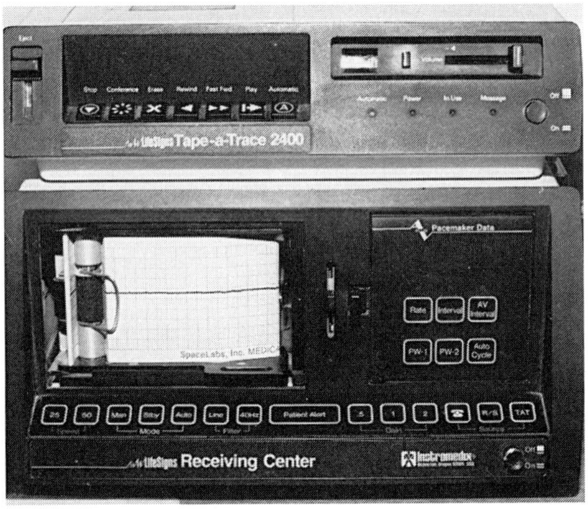

FIGURE 2–2. Transtelephonic receiving station with answering machine. This is a standard office system that allows sound-activated recording 24 hours a day. The receiving center takes the sound signal transmitted over the telephone wire and decodes it into a filtered electrocardiogram recording.

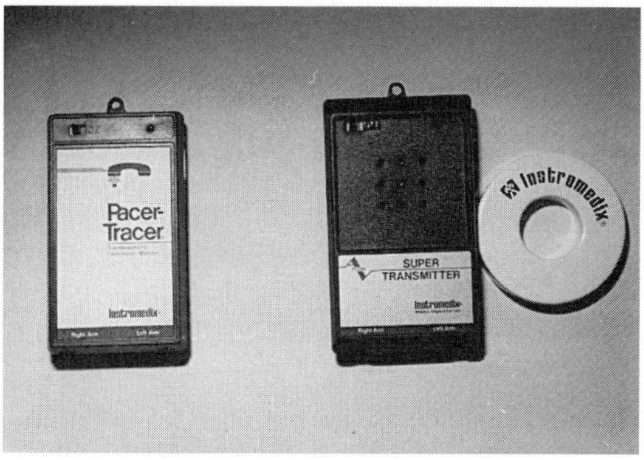

FIGURE 2–3. The transtelephonic monitor on the left is routinely used for patients with known or suspected arrhythmias. The four electrodes located on the back of the transmitter make direct contact with the chest while the mouthpiece of the telephone is placed over the hole on the upper one third of the device. The right arm and left arm receptacles allow the use of finger or wrist electrodes. The monitor on the right functions in the aforementioned manner but was made specifically for patients with pacemakers. The doughnut-shaped magnet is standardly used for testing in patients with implanted pacemakers.

dren as young as 7 years have been trained to use these successfully. It is most helpful in routine transmissions (i.e., pacemaker follow-up), but has a role in the documentation of episodes of palpitations that last 10 to 20 minutes.

The Heart Card is an event monitor. This transmitter is about the size of a credit card. When the patient has symptoms, the transmitter must be placed firmly against the skin of the chest. When the record button is pressed, a 30-second event is recorded. The device can store three events. The ECGs are stored for transmission via telephone at a later time. This particular transmitter works well for transient, short-lived events that may occur when a telephone is not handy. Unlike some of the other transmitters that are unwieldy and conspicuous, this one is probably the best accepted in the adolescent age group.

The King of Hearts Express monitor is a loop recorder (Fig. 2–4). It consists of a system of two leads, which attach to the chest and connect to a small "beeper-sized" recorder. When activated, it records the electrogram for the specified amount of time preceding activation and continues to record for a specified amount of time after activation. A total of 300 seconds worth of ECGs can be stored. The loop recorder is particularly helpful in evaluating rhythms or symptoms that are very transient and that have a prodrome. Patients as young as 6 years of age have successfully used this transmitter to record events. This transmitter is better accepted in the preadolescent age group. It must be worn continuously to capture the onset of symptoms.

Receivers

The receiver that we use has single-channel recording capability. A pacemaker data module that prints out pacemaker pulse rate, atrial and ventricular pulse widths, and AV intervals for permanent pacemaker patients is available but does not add much to the interpretation in arrhythmia cases. The receiver may be attached to an acoustic coupler or an answering machine.

INDICATIONS

A transtelephonic system may be employed for routine pacemaker follow-up, to document arrhythmias, and to assess heart rhythm during symptoms of chest pain, palpitations, or syncope.[22–24] The usefulness and cost effectiveness of TTM has been compared with that of Holter monitoring,[25–27] but the two methods of monitoring should be considered complementary[28] with some overlap but, occasionally, very different indications. To maximize the cost effectiveness of memory and loop-type TTMs, they should be issued for approximately 1 month.

Pacemaker Follow-Up

For pacemaker follow-up, a single-channel transmitter powered by a 9-V battery is needed, similar to the Pacer Tracer (see Fig. 2–3). Wrist electrodes, sticker electrodes, or the four metal

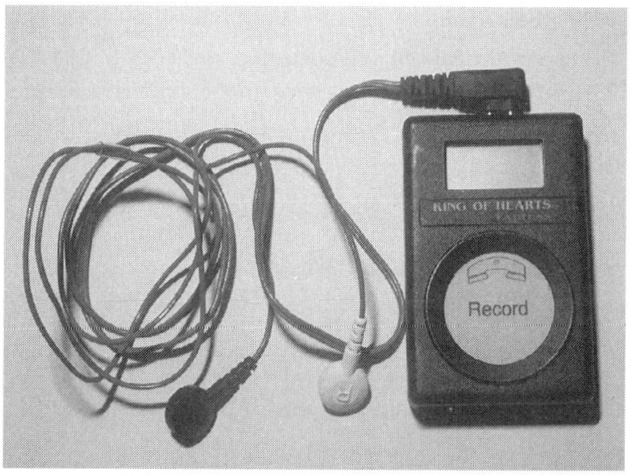

FIGURE 2–4. Standard loop recorder with two lead wires that attach to skin electrodes. When the patient experiences a symptom, a single push of the button stores electrocardiograms before, during, and after the event.

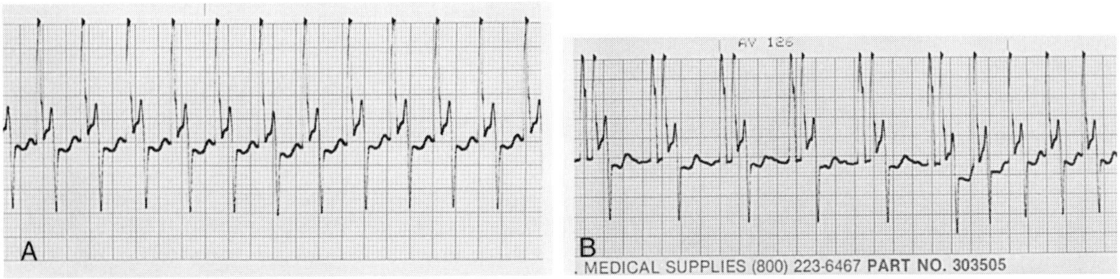

FIGURE 2–5. *A*, Transtelephonic electrocardiographic (ECG) recording of a patient with a dual-chamber atrial synchronous pacemaker. The patient was known to be recovering from a Mustard repair, and he presented with complaints of palpitations. Differential diagnosis of this strip is appropriate atrial sensing of an atrial re-entry versus pacemaker-mediated tachycardia. *B*, Transtelephonic ECG recording of the same patient with magnet application. At the left side of the strip, the magnet has been applied with appropriate pacemaker function. At the right side, when the magnet is removed, the pacemaker immediately reverts back to the rapid ventricular paced rhythm at the upper rate limit, suggesting an atrial tachycardia.

electrodes on the back of the transmitter sense the ECG. The patient or parent dials a specific number, which can be answered by an automated recorder at the hospital or a technician or nurse. After stating the patient's name and telephone number, the patient places the mouthpiece over the transmitter and a 30-second tracing is recorded. Next the magnet is applied, and an additional 30 seconds are recorded. All ECGs are printed and screened by a nurse or technician who is familiar with pacemakers and arrhythmias (Fig. 2–5A and B). They are read daily by a physician, and the patient is called if any abnormality is seen or if the tracing cannot be read because of artifact.

When issuing a transmitter, either for arrhythmia evaluation or pacemaker follow-up, approximately 45 minutes are spent with the family teaching the use of the transmitter (Fig. 2–6). It is essential to send a practice tracing. This practice builds confidence, increases compliance, and gives a baseline recording to compare with future tracings.

The transmission without the magnet gives information about pacemaker function at that time. Application of the magnet gives a sequence of pulses at a rate specified by the pacemaker manufacturer. There may be a reduction in output on the last pulse. This is called a *threshold margin test* and shows whether an adequate safety margin exists at the programmed pacemaker output.

The pediatric pacemaker TTM follow-up schedule after initial implant is as follows:

1 to 6 weeks: weekly transmissions
1 to 12 months: monthly
13 to 48 months: every third month
Near elective replacement: monthly

In conjunction with routine transmissions, additional recordings may be sent if symptoms occur. Pacemaker-mediated tachycardia, lead dysfunction, and sensing or capture problems can be detected by these transmissions. Patients can then receive a hands-on evaluation if necessary for device reprogramming. This system helps to avoid unnecessary office visits and reassures patients when all is working well. In this way, it is a very cost-effective technique.

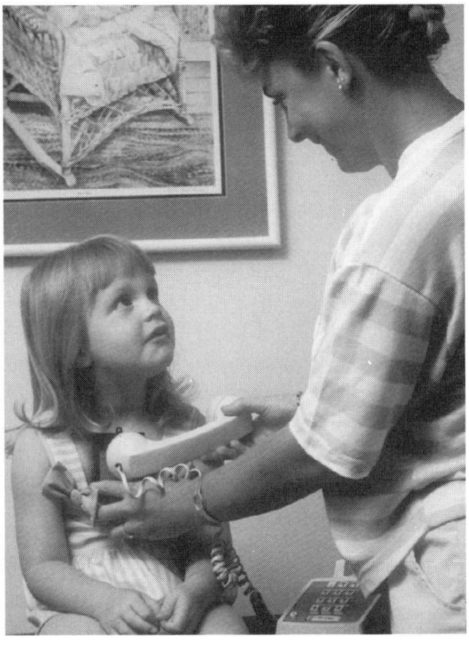

FIGURE 2–6. The telephone transmitter is easily placed over the heart, even in small children. With proper training, the patient or parent can determine when the recorder is properly positioned by listening to the tones emitted from the transmitter.

Suspected Arrhythmias: Symptomatic

TTM may be used for monitoring the rhythm of patients complaining of palpitations, dizziness, syncope, or chest pain. This method of monitoring is especially well suited for the documentation of symptomatic events that occur sporadically and last long enough to be documented by one of the monitors previously mentioned. Pediatric patients whose chief complaint is chest pain rarely have a cardiac cause, but the documentation of normal sinus rhythm during these events may be reassuring to the patient and family (Fig. 2–7A and B).

Suspected Arrhythmias: Asymptomatic

Another way in which TTM may be helpful is for scheduled, routine documentation of a rhythm not associated with symptoms. The patient is instructed to transmit an ECG daily, weekly, and so on to document rhythm. This method may be good in patients with asymptomatic rhythm disturbances or rhythm abnormalities in children too young to communicate their symptoms. Rhythms that are incessant, such as atrial ectopic tachycardia, permanent junctional reciprocating tachycardia, and some cases of atrial flutter, lend themselves to this method.

STRENGTHS

The advantages of TTM include portability and cost effectiveness. When issued for approximately 1 month, TTM is better suited and more cost effective for documentation of sporadic, symptomatic events than the Holter monitor.[29] It is excellent for routine follow-up of pacemakers, helps avoid unnecessary office visits, and identifies problems that need prompt attention. Careful selection of the proper type of monitor is necessary to optimize diagnosis.

WEAKNESSES

In our experience, simple Pacer Tracers and loop recorders are the most reliable transmitters. Minor problems have been encountered with the event recorders, related to electronic malfunction or user difficulties. It is possible that symptomatic patients may delay seeking medical care with the TTM. This problem can be avoided by carefully counseling the patients regarding when to use the TTM versus when to seek medical care.

FUTURE

With the popularity of cellular telephones, transmission is possible from almost any place at any time. Some cellular telephones have been noted to have magnets, which could reprogram pacemakers.[30] A cellular telephone is not recommended for the transmission of pacemaker TTM recordings. Excessive artifact has been found with cordless telephones. If cellular telephones are used for conversations (not TTM) by patients with pacemakers, it is recommended that the telephone be held on the opposite side of the pacemaker pocket location.

EVENT AND LOOP RECORDERS

STRENGTHS AND WEAKNESSES

Event and loop recorders are extremely helpful to document sporadic events that are too short to be transmitted live via simple real-time (e.g., Pacer Tracer) TTMs and when access to a telephone is limited. The major drawback for the loop recorders (e.g., King of Hearts Express) is that it must be worn constantly until the event is documented. This limits the acceptance in adolescents. The initial investment for the pur-

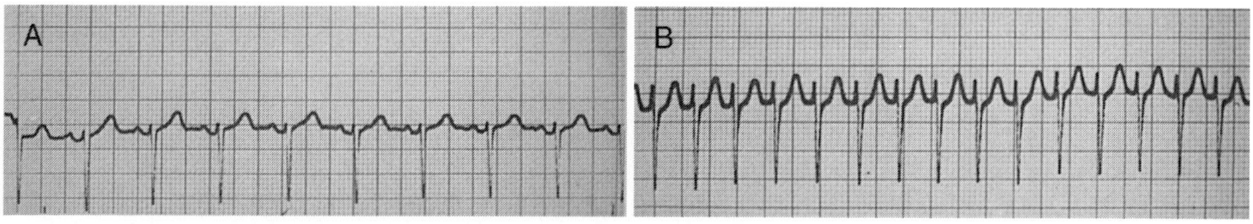

FIGURE 2–7. *A*, This transtelephonic recording shows sinus rhythm during an episode of chest pain and shortness of breath in a 15-year-old girl. This documents that these symptoms are not a result of tachycardia. *B*, This recording shows supraventricular tachycardia at 214 bpm in the same patient. Her only symptom at this time was the sensation of palpitations. Transtelephonic ECGs helped differentiate two types of episodes in this patient: one related to an arrhythmia and one not related to a rhythm disturbance.

chase of such recorders is greater than that of event recorders and that of simple real-time transmitters. The event recorders (e.g., Heart Card) are smaller but carry doubt regarding reliability of the unit, although they are more easily accepted by the adolescent age group.

TELEMETRY

BACKGROUND

Telemetry consists of continuous radio transmissions of cardiac rhythm in hospitalized children or children requiring short-term monitoring after certain procedures (Fig. 2–8). Battery-operated transmitters that are attached to the patient with leads and electrodes send a signal to an antenna, which displays the incoming signal on an oscilloscope for continuous rhythm monitoring. The system can print out multiple standard ECG leads. Holter monitoring can be performed through the same system without the need for additional leads or recorders with select equipment. Upper and lower rate limits are predetermined, and rhythm strips are automatically printed out when these limits are exceeded. Multiple leads may be viewed and printed if desired. Even without an arrhythmia or aberrant beats, telemetry technicians print out a representative rhythm strip for each 8-hour time frame. These are reviewed daily by the cardiologist with prompt notification of any abnormalities or changes.

There is very little information in the literature concerning the role of telemetry monitoring in the non-intensive care unit (ICU). Most reports pertain to adults with coronary artery disease and cannot be extrapolated to the pediatric population.[31] Physicians who routinely employ telemetry believe that it dramatically reduces the incidence of cardiac arrests on pediatric cardiac inpatient units because precipitating events that affect the cardiac rate and rhythm can be delineated earlier.

INDICATIONS

Postoperative Monitoring

After transfer from the ICU to the floor following open heart surgery, some patients are at risk for rhythm disturbances. Patients with arrhythmias before surgery might benefit from telemetry monitoring before discharge. Because bradycardia follows apnea in a very few seconds, cardiac monitoring is an effective method of apnea monitoring in weak infants. Aside from the immediate postoperative period, there are patients, mentioned earlier (e.g., those who have undergone Fontan, Mustard, and Senning procedures), who are at risk for rhythm disturbances. When these patients are hospitalized for other reasons, it may be a good time to screen for arrhythmias.

Assessment of Antiarrhythmic Therapy

In-hospital monitoring via telemetry is mandatory when initiating and possibly when increasing the dose of some antiarrhythmic drugs, such as amiodarone, flecainide, or sotalol. Such monitoring should be done during any drug treatment of patients with ventricular arrhythmias. Telemetry monitoring during antiarrhythmic drug therapy is helpful in assessing the drug's potential proarrhythmic effects as well as efficacy.

Syncope

In certain situations, syncope must be evaluated in the hospital setting. These situations include syncope associated with exercise, WPW syndrome, or long QT interval on the surface

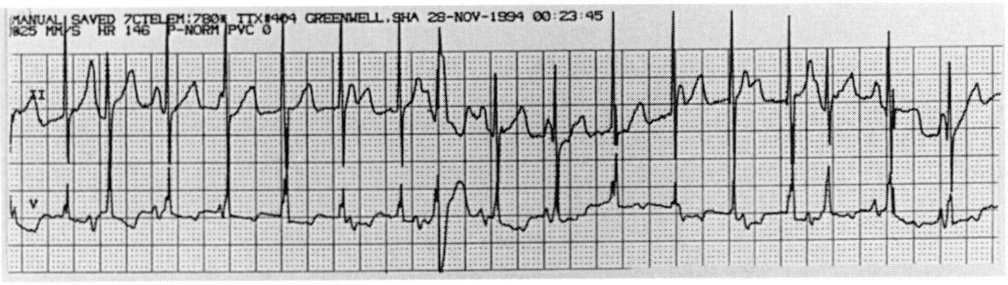

FIGURE 2–8. Inpatient telemetric recording of surface leads II and V_1 in a patient with congenital junctional ectopic tachycardia, retrograde block, and antegrade conduction from sinus atrial beats. Note that one of the conducted beats is aberrantly conducted.

ECG. Telemetry provides physiologic monitoring, which may assist in correlating symptoms to ECG findings in these situations.

Noncardiac Problems

Telemetric monitoring is useful for assessing patients with electrolyte disturbances, overdoses, and other noncardiac problems that may affect the conduction system. It is good for monitoring postoperative patients with feeding problems at risk for bradycardia or aspiration.

Postpacemaker Implantation

When patients are hospitalized for intravenous antibiotics after pacemaker implantation, telemetry provides immediate information about lead dislodgment, pacemaker malfunction, and underlying rhythm. It is extremely helpful when observing a patient with postoperative complete heart block while determining whether permanent pacing is necessary.

STRENGTHS

Physiologic monitoring can allow immediate assessment of activity and symptoms if arrhythmias are noted. When patients do not need intensive care but still have unresolved rhythm disturbances, it is not necessary to prolong the ICU stay at added expense and patient discomfort. These issues can be resolved on a telemetry unit, which allows more patient mobility at a decreased cost. Full-disclosure monitoring gives very complete information.[32]

WEAKNESSES

Educating nurses or technicians to staff a telemetry unit is a challenge. Creative scheduling[33] and transmission of telemetry to remote ICUs has been effective in some settings.[34] The potential for the technician or nursing staff to over- or underreact to events is a weakness. Appropriate identification of rhythms can be facilitated by facsimile transmission to a cardiologist on call. Nonetheless, unidentified abnormalities can have severe results. Alarms must be set to age-appropriate and diagnosis-specific limits. Careful attention must be paid to patients with leads off and out of the range of the antenna.

Although debated in other centers,[35] we consider it mandatory to have a dedicated telemetry technician to watch the monitor.

EXERCISE STRESS TESTING ELECTROCARDIOGRAPHY

BACKGROUND

Exercise testing may be used to provoke rhythm disturbances in children (Fig. 2–9). This modality adds another dimension in the noninvasive workup of an arrhythmia patient. Our center employs a Bruce protocol. Metabolic exhaled gas analysis is available, but is generally not necessary for a rhythm evaluation that is not associated with any other disease state, cardiac or otherwise.

INDICATIONS

Sinus Node Function

Abnormal sinus node function can be discerned from sinus bradycardia because the patient with sinus node dysfunction will have an abnormal chronotropic response to exercise. In normal children and adolescents, a maximum heart rate of less than 180 bpm at maximal effort[36] or an exaggerated decrease in heart rate after exercise is indicative of sinus node dysfunc-

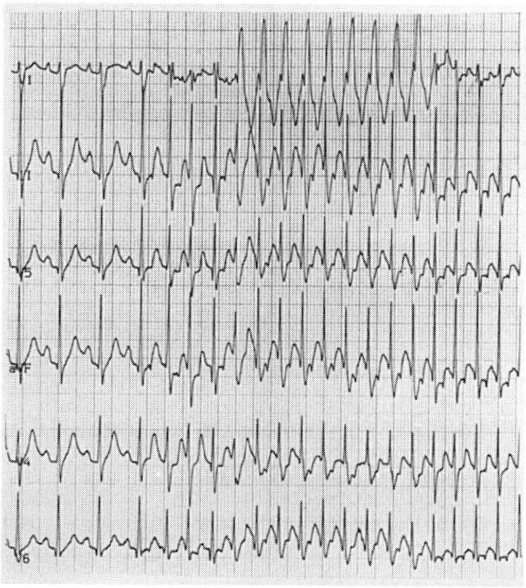

FIGURE 2–9. Onset of supraventricular tachycardia during an exercise stress test. Leads V_1 to V_6 reveal that the first several beats are sinus without a delta wave. A retrograde P wave is seen in the ST segment of the fourth sinus beat followed by four narrow QRS tachycardia beats, nine wide QRS tachycardia beats, and finally a narrow QRS tachycardia beat. The patient was known to have exercise-induced palpitations. He underwent a successful radiofrequency ablation of a concealed left posterior pathway.

tion. Insignificant sinus bradycardia will exhibit the normal reproducible response to the stress of exercise. Exercise testing should be considered periodically in patients after Fontan, Mustard, or Senning procedures, in whom the incidence of sinus node dysfunction is high.

Supraventricular Tachycardia/Syncope

Exercise testing rarely precipitates supraventricular tachycardia (SVT), but occasionally it is helpful when there is a history of tachycardia or syncope during or after exercise. In patients with WPW syndrome on ECG, the sudden loss of the delta wave during exercise correlates relatively well with a long antegrade effective refractory period of the accessory connection. This is not generally regarded as reliable documentation of a clinically insignificant pathway, which requires invasive electrophysiologic testing.

Ventricular Ectopy

Any patient with ventricular ectopy should undergo exercise testing. PVCs that are extinguished with exercise in patients with structurally normal hearts are considered benign and may not require further workup. Ventricular ectopy that worsens on the treadmill is abnormal and requires further invasive and noninvasive investigation.[37]

Exercise-induced VT after surgery for tetralogy of Fallot has been shown to correlate with poor hemodynamics and is considered to be a marker for sudden death.[38] This condition warrants treatment to improve hemodynamics if possible and with antiarrhythmic therapy if tachycardia persists thereafter. Exercise testing is not considered an adequate test of efficacy of therapy in this situation, and invasive electrophysiologic testing is required.

Exercise testing has been shown to precipitate T-wave alternans in patients with long QT syndrome. It may help assess the adequacy of beta blockade. We look for a 30% reduction in maximum heart rate to determine adequate blockade. Exhaled gas analysis can ensure that maximum exercise is achieved.

Pacemaker Programming

Programming pacemaker rate response parameters can be facilitated by exercise testing. The rate of response to activity may be programmed to a more or less aggressive slope. Upper rate behaviors can be optimized to avoid causing 2:1 block at the upper rate limit. This is done by ensuring that the postventricular atrial refractory period (PVARP) plus the AV delay does not exceed the cycle length of the programmed upper rate limit. Ideally, Wenckebach block will occur before 2:1 block at rates of 180 to 200 bpm.

Most of the data on sinus node function are based on studies of adults, with little application to the pediatric population. Nonetheless, rate responsive pacing is more physiologic than fixed rate pacing, and exercise testing may help optimize programming of these parameters.[39]

STRENGTHS AND WEAKNESSES

Stress testing has the advantage of being readily available in most hospital and office settings. It has the disadvantage of low yield for provoking SVT and limited use in patients younger than 5 years.

SIGNAL-AVERAGED ELECTROCARDIOGRAMS

BACKGROUND

SAECG is a method of recording high-resolution ECGs. Multiple PQRS complexes are recorded from three sets of orthogonal electrodes in the X, Y, and Z axes. Signals are digitized, summed, and filtered. Random noise is canceled out, but low-voltage signals are additive and become visible.[40]

This technique was first utilized in the early 1970s by Simson. It was hoped that SAECGs could monitor the HV interval serially and in lieu of invasive electrophysiology. Although this application has not gained widespread clinical use, Simson published technical advances for the Butterworth filter; the X, Y, and Z axes for recording; and "normal" values.[41] He identified late potentials and suggested that they might be a marker for VT. Late potentials represent very low-amplitude electrical activity, which continues to conduct in the scar tissue surrounding an infarction, after the normal end point of the QRS complex on the traditional surface ECG.

INDICATIONS

SAECGs are obtained in symptomatic patients with ventricular ectopy when evaluating for arrhythmias after congenital heart surgery and in the evaluation of survivors of sudden cardiac death (Fig. 2–10). The presence of late potentials may predict inducibility of VT on invasive electrophysiologic study, but this is not the sole criterion.

In general, three parameters are measured with SAECG. These include filtered QRS duration, the amplitude of the terminal 40 milliseconds of the filtered QRS complex, and the root mean square of the terminal 40 milliseconds of the QRS complex.[42]

Research in adults has shown that the combination of SAECG with Holter monitoring allows increased sensitivity and specificity to predictions. It is thought that PVCs seen on the surface ECG are a trigger for ventricular arrhythmias, whereas the late potentials represent the substrate for VT.

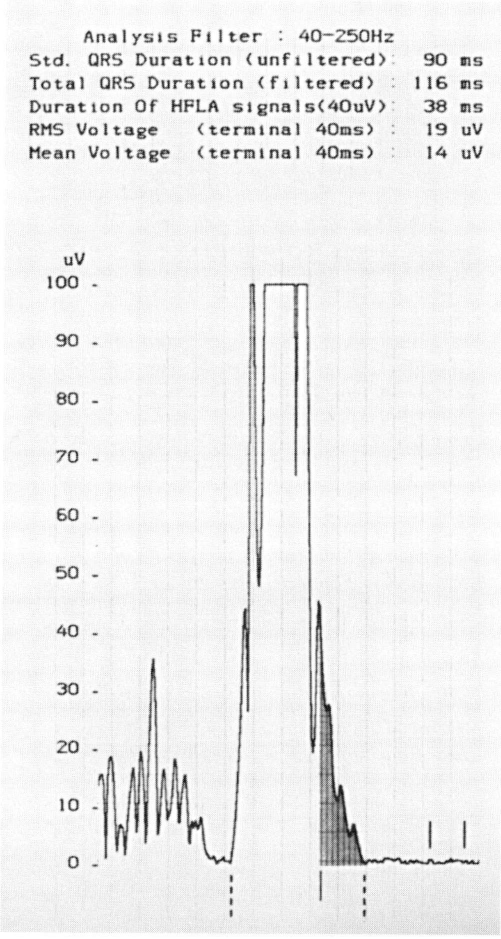

FIGURE 2–10. Signal-averaged electrocardiogram in a postoperative patient without bundle branch block. Abnormal late potentials are highlighted at the end of the QRS complex. (HFLA, high frequency, low amplitude; RMS, route mean square.)

STRENGTHS

SAECGs can noninvasively provide high-resolution analysis of myocardial depolarization characteristics. There may be some correlation with information obtained invasively. SAECGs are obtained with a traditional ECG machine and three extra pairs of electrodes. There is a relatively short recording time, and the information is stored and processed quickly.

WEAKNESSES

The weaknesses of SAECGs perhaps outweigh the strengths at this time. The cost of the software necessary, without any clear-cut clinical applications, is a problem. Currently, in the managed care environment, this test is not reimbursable. More research is needed to establish clinical conditions that will benefit from this technique. Substantial variation exists between the various commercial systems available.[43]

Unfortunately, the drawbacks previously published still persist. Although sudden cardiac death risk stratification in adults after myocardial infarction is a generally accepted use for SAECG, other uses have yet to be firmly established.

FUTURE

Investigation of SAECG as a diagnostic tool is ongoing in arrhythmogenic right ventricular dysplasia,[44] transplant rejection,[45] and congestive heart failure,[46] to name a few.

With regard to pediatrics and congenital heart disease, many are trying to discern the connection between late potentials and the risk of ventricular arrhythmias after surgical repair of congenital heart disease. Although guidelines for SAECG in adults have been published,[42] the lack of established guidelines for the interpretation of results is limited in pediatrics and congenital heart disease. Some studies have provided recommendations pertinent to pediatrics and congenital heart disease.[47–49]

Stelling et al[50] cited a correlation between inducibility of VT on invasive electrophysiology study and the presence of 100-μV or less terminal root-mean-square voltage in pediatric patients with surgically repaired heart disease. Zimmermann et al[51] found late potentials to have a sensitivity of 100% and specificity of 75% to predict inducibility of VT by programmed electrical stimulation. Vaksmann et al[52] examined the influence of clinical and hemodynamic characteristics on the SAECG in postoperative tetralogy of Fallot patients. They reported the opposite of Stelling, with an amplitude of greater than 170 μV in the terminal 40 milliseconds of the filtered QRS to correlate with spontaneous ventricular arrhythmias as well as right ventricular systolic hypertension. They attributed the difference in findings to adjustment of signal-average parameters for age and body size. Obviously, many variables are yet to be accounted for with SAECG.

Signal averaging of the P wave is being explored as a test to assess the risk of atrial arrhythmias.[53] Perhaps in time it will shed light on atrial flutter in postoperative congenital heart patients.

In summary, SAECG is a method of analysis that is easy to obtain, is noninvasive, and has the power of high resolution, but has not yet found its clinical niche.

SUMMARY

Noninvasive diagnostic techniques are a valuable adjunct in caring for patients with known or suspected cardiac rhythm disturbances. Each technique has its own unique set of advantages and disadvantages that should be taken into consideration in each individual patient's clinical situation.

ACKNOWLEDGMENTS

I would like to acknowledge Paul Gillette for teaching me and helping me take care of patients. (BB)

REFERENCES

1. Fye WB: Disorders of the heartbeat: A historical overview from antiquity to the mid-20th century. Am J Cardiol 72:1055–1070, 1993.
2. Holter NJ, Gengerelli JA: Remote recording of physiological data by radio. Rocky Mountain Med J 46:747–751, 1949.
3. Roberts WC, Silver MA: Norman Jefferis Holter and ECG monitoring. Am J Cardiol 52:903–906, 1983.
4. Lown B: Cardiovascular collapse and sudden death. In Braunwald E (ed): Heart Disease: A Textbook of Cardiovascular Medicine. Philadelphia, WB Saunders, 1984, p 774.
5. Ehlers K: Ambulatory electrocardiographic monitoring. Pediatr Ann 16:535–545, 1987.
6. Ringel RE, Kennedy HL, Brenner JI, et al: Detection of cardiac dysrhythmias by continuous electrocardiographic recording in children undergoing cardiac surgery. J Electrocardiol 17:1–6, 1984.
7. Gillette PC, El-Said GM, Sivarajan N, et al: Electrophysiological abnormalities after Mustard's operation for transposition of the great arteries. Br Heart J 36:186–191, 1974.
8. Silka MJ, Manwill JR, Kron J, et al: Bradycardia-mediated tachyarrhythmias in congenital heart disease and response to chronic pacing at physiologic rates. Am J Cardiol 65:488–493, 1990.
9. Scholler GF, Walsh EP: Congenital complete heart block in patients without anatomic cardiac defects. Am Heart J 118:1193–1198, 1989.
10. Michaelsson M, Jonzon A, Riesenfeld T: Isolated congenital complete atrioventricular block in adult life—A prospective study. Circulation 92:442–449, 1995.
11. Friedman R: Congenital atrioventricular block. Pace me now or pace me later? (Editorial) Circulation 92:283–285, 1995.
12. Garson A Jr, Randall DC, Gillette PC, et al: Prevention of sudden death after repair of tetralogy of Fallot: Treatment of ventricular arrhythmias. J Am Coll Cardiol 6:221–227, 1985.
13. Fyler DC: Aortic outflow abnormalities. In Nadas A (ed.): Nadas' Pediatric Cardiology. St. Louis, Mosby-Year Book, 1992, pp 493–512.
14. Malik M, Camm J: Heart rate variability and clinical cardiology. Br Heart J 71:3–6, 1994.
15. Dougherty CM, Burr RL: Comparison of heart rate variability in survivors and nonsurvivors of sudden cardiac arrest. Am J Cardiol 70:441–448, 1992.
16. Rollins MD, Jenkins JG, Carson DJ, et al: Power spectral analysis of the ECG in diabetic children. Diabetologia 35:452–455, 1992.
17. Constant I, Girard A, Le Bidois J, et al: Spectral analysis of systolic blood pressure and heart rate after heart transplantation in children. Clin Sci 88:95–102, 1995.
18. Woo MA, Stevenson WG, Moser DK, et al: Patterns of beat-to-beat heart rate variability in advanced heart failure. Am Heart J 123:704–710, 1992.
19. Lippman N, Stein KM, Lerman BB: Failure to decrease parasympathetic tone during upright tilt predicts a positive tilt-table test. Am J Cardiol 75:591–595, 1995.
20. Malliani A, Lombardi F, Pagani M: Power spectral analysis of heart rate variability: A tool to explore neural regulatory mechanisms. Br Heart J 71:1–2, 1994.
21. Hohn AH: Blood pressure measurements and normal pressure values. In Hohn AH (ed): Guidebook for Pediatric Hypertension. Armonk, New York: Futura, 1994, pp 45–46.
22. Linzer M, Comegno A: Long-term ambulatory ECG monitoring in syncope: The state of the art. Cardiovascular Reviews and Reports 14:11–29, 1993.
23. Houyel L, Fournier A, Centazzo S: Use of transtelephonic electrocardiographic monitoring in children with suspected arrhythmias. Can J Cardiol 8:741–744, 1992.
24. Cumbee SR, Pryor RE, Linzer M: Cardiac loop ECG recording: A new noninvasive diagnostic test in recurrent syncope. South Med J 83:39–43, 1990.
25. Kinlay S, Leitch JW, Neil A, et al: Cardiac event recorders yield more diagnoses and are more cost-effective than 48 hour Holter monitoring in patients with palpitations: A controlled clinical trial. Ann Intern Med 124:16–20, 1996.
26. Grodman RS, Capone RJ, Most AS: Arrhythmia surveillance by transtelephonic monitoring: Comparison with Holter monitoring in symptomatic ambulatory patients. Am Heart J 98:459–464, 1979.
27. Karpawich PP, Cavitt DL, Sugalski JS: Ambulatory arrhythmia screening in symptomatic children and young adults: Comparative effectiveness of Holter and telephone event recordings. Pediatr Cardiol 14:147–150, 1993.

28. Brown AP, Dawkins KD, Davies JG: Detection of arrhythmias: Use of a patient-activated ambulatory electrocardiogram device with a solid-state memory loop. Br Heart J 58:251–253, 1987.
29. Wu J, Kessler DK, Chakko S: A cost-effectiveness strategy for transtelephonic arrhythmia monitoring. Am J Cardiol 75:184–185, 1995.
30. Chen WH, Lau CP, Leung MB, et al: Interference of cellular phones with implanted permanent pacemakers. Clin Cardiol 19:881–886, 1996.
31. Estrada CA, Rosman HS, Prasad NK, et al: Role of telemetry monitoring in the non-intensive care unit. Am J Cardiol 76:960–965, 1995.
32. Kotar SL, Gessler JE: Full disclosure monitoring: A concept that will change the way arrhythmias are detected and interpreted in the hospitalized patient. Heart Lung 22:482–489, 1993.
33. Gresk KD: Twelve-hour shifts on a new telemetry unit. Nurs Manage 22:40–42, 1991.
34. Capuano TA, Molchany C, Peters C, et al: Remote telemetry: New twists for old technology. Nurs Manage 26:26, 28, 30–32, 1995.
35. Hitchens M: Telemetry: Who's watching the monitor? Critical Care Nurse 12:100–102, 1992.
36. Hesslein PS: Noninvasive diagnosis of dysrhythmias. In Gillette PC, Garson A Jr (eds): Pediatric Cardiac Dysrhythmias. New York, Grune & Stratton, 1981, p 59.
37. Rosansky JJ, Dimich I, Steinfeld L, et al: Maximal exercise stress testing in evaluation of arrhythmias in children: Results and reproducibility. Am J Cardiol 45:951–956, 1979.
38. Garson A, Gillette PC, Guttgessel HP, et al: Stress induced ventricular arrhythmias after repair of tetralogy of Fallot. Am J Cardiol 46:1006–1012, 1980.
39. Wienecke, MM. Hemodynamics of pacing. In Gillette PC, Zeigler VL (eds): Pediatric Cardiac Pacing. Armonk, NY, Futura, 1995, pp 89–91.
40. Gomes JA, Winters SL, Ip J, et al: Identification of patients with high risk of arrhythmic mortality. Role of ambulatory monitoring, signal-averaged ECG, and heart rate variability. Cardiol Clin 11:55–63, 1993.
41. Simson MB: Use of signals in the terminal QRS complex to identify patients with ventricular tachycardia after myocardial infarction. Circulation 64:235–242, 1981.
42. Breithardt G, Cain ME, El-Sherif N, et al: Standards for analysis of ventricular potentials using high-resolution or signal averaged electrocardiography: A statement by a task force committee of the European Society of Cardiology, the American Heart Association, and the American College of Cardiology. J Am Coll Cardiol 17:999–1006, 1991.
43. Moreno FL, Karagounis LA, Villanueva T, et al: Comparison of signal-averaging electrocardiographic systems using device specific criteria in 104 normal subjects. Pacing Clin Electrophysiol 17:2178–2182, 1994.
44. Oselladore L, Nava A, Buja G, et al: Signal-averaged electrocardiography in familial form of arrhythmogenic right ventricular cardiomyopathy. Am J Cardiol 75:1038–1041, 1995.
45. Graceffo MA, O'Rourke RA: Cardiac transplant rejection is associated with a decrease in the high frequency components of the high-resolution, signal-averaged electrocardiogram. Am Heart J 132:820–826, 1996.
46. Middlekauff HR, Stevenson WG, Woo MA, et al: Comparison of frequency of late potentials in idiopathic dilated cardiomyopathy and ischemic cardiomyopathy with advanced congestive heart failure and their usefulness in predicting sudden death. Am J Cardiol 66:1113–1117, 1990.
47. Fallah-Najmabadi H, Dahdah NS, Palcko M, et al: Normal values and methodologic recommendations for signal-averaged electrocardiography in children and adolescents. Am J Cardiol 77:408–412, 1996.
48. Moser DK, Stevenson WG, Woo MA: Optimal late potential criteria for reducing false positive signal averaged electrocardiograms. Am Heart J 123:412–416, 1992.
49. Lander P, Berbari EJ, Lazzara R: Optimal filtering and quality control of the signal-averaged ECG: High fidelity 1 minute recordings. Circulation 91:1495–1505, 1995.
50. Stelling JA, Danford DA, Kugler JD, et al: Late potentials and inducible ventricular tachycardia in surgically repaired congenital heart disease. Circulation 82:1690–1696, 1990.
51. Zimmermann M, Freidli B, Adamec R, et al: Ventricular late potentials and induced ventricular arrhythmias after surgical repair of tetralogy of Fallot. Am J Cardiol 67:873–878, 1991.
52. Vaksmann G, Kohen ME, Lacroix D, et al: Influence of clinical and hemodynamic characteristics on signal-averaged electrogram in postoperative tetralogy of Fallot. Am J Cardiol 71:317–321, 1993.
53. Ehlert FA, Steinberg JS: The P-wave signal-averaged electrocardiogram. Prim Cardiol 20:43–48, 1994.

CHAPTER 3

INTRACARDIAC ELECTROPHYSIOLOGY STUDIES

Paul C. Gillette and Henry L. Blair

Intracardiac electrophysiology studies (ICEPS) have changed a great deal since they were first published.[1] They are still used when unique information is needed to care for the patient that cannot be obtained otherwise. The knowledge we have gained from ICEPS now allows us to care for some patients without ICEPS. Various forms of noninvasive electrical tests, together with histories and physical examinations, suffice to make treatment decisions. In some cases, transesophageal electrophysiology studies (EPSs) can be substituted. These currently allow recording and stimulation of the atria only. In most cases, when an EPS is needed, a multicatheter intracardiac study is indicated. Many EPSs now also include an intervention, such as a radiofrequency catheter ablation, which is performed in an attempt to cure the arrhythmia.

INDICATIONS

The indications for ICEPS can be classified as diagnostic or therapeutic.[2] An ICEPS is absolutely needed to perform catheter ablation, and this is the most frequent, current indication in the majority of laboratories.

The ICEPS associated with a catheter ablation of narrow QRS tachycardia may be very limited and directed. For example, in a patient with manifest Wolff-Parkinson-White (WPW) syndrome who has a history of atrial fibrillation and syncope, the most pressing indication is to eliminate antegrade conduction through the accessory connection. Localization of the earliest ventricular activation is of paramount importance (Fig. 3–1). Recording of a short, local atrioventricular (AV) interval with a possible pathway potential confirms the site for ablation, although it is not always possible to record pathway potentials. A detailed, functional study of the sinoatrial node, the AV node, and the accessory pathway is not necessary at this point, but delineation of retrograde conduction is important. An important, secondary objective in this type of patient is prevention of supraventricular tachycardia. Thus, elimination of all abnormal retrograde conduction is necessary. In 10 to 30% of patients, abnormal retrograde conduction is anatomically separate from abnormal antegrade conduction.

A second common indication for ICEPS is wide QRS tachycardia. This type of study is more complex because the causes are more diffuse. Most wide QRS tachycardias are ventricular, but a significant minority are supraventricular with antidromic conduction over an accessory pathway or wide because of aberrant conduction, either pre-existing or secondary to the rapid rate. Although many pediatric ventricular tachycardias may be focal in nature or have well-defined reentry circuits, others are diffuse, possibly because of myocarditis or repolarization abnormalities.

Delineation of the potential risk of sudden death is an important indication, although the number of instances in which this is necessary is diminishing. Most patients with WPW syndrome have enough symptoms to warrant ablation, but those who do not should have their risk of sudden death assessed by induction of atrial fibrillation at approximately school age. In our institution, it is preferable to do this with an ICEPS rather than a transesophageal study. The substrate is then ablated during the same procedure when indicated. Ablation is also performed if supraventricular tachycardia can be induced. An RR interval during atrial fibrillation of 220 milliseconds (shortest) on isoproterenol is used as an ablation indication. If atrial fibrillation cannot be induced, an antegrade effective refractory period of less than 220 milliseconds or less than 200 milliseconds on isoproterenol are indications. Using these indications, the majority of WPW syndrome patients will require ablation. We do not believe that noninvasive testing, such as ambulatory monitoring or treadmill testing, adequately predicts the potential risk for sudden death in pediatric patients. The pediatric patient must be considered separately from the adult, because all adults have "survived" adolescence.

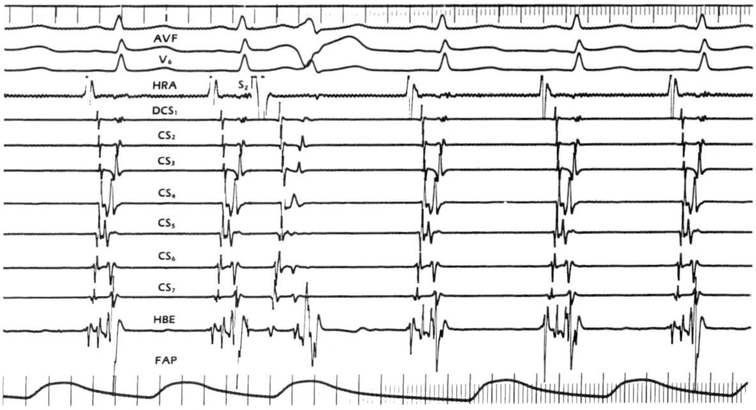

FIGURE 3–1. Demonstration of mapping of an accessory pathway with antegrade conduction. From top to bottom are surface leads I, aVF, V_6, high right atrial (HRA) electrogram, seven pairs of coronary sinus (CS) electrograms, His bundle electrograms (HBE), and femoral artery blood pressure (FAP). At CS pair 5, the shortest A to V time can be seen as the earliest ventricular activation. The delta wave is not very apparent on the surface electrocardiogram. When a premature beat is introduced into the high right atrium, the widening of the QRS is more evident. The earliest point of activation is still on pair 5 of the CS catheter.

Invasive risk stratification for postoperative patients is also becoming less needed. Surface electrocardiographic (ECG) criteria are becoming more accepted as indications for ICEPS. Extreme QRS prolongation on the surface ECG correlates well with the incidence of ventricular arrhythmias and sudden death and the inducibility of ventricular arrhythmias.[3, 4]

Risk stratification in patients with cardiomyopathy continues to be controversial. Definitive treatment is usually not available, but device therapy may be employed palliatively. Tachycardia-induced cardiomyopathy remains a strong indication for ICEPS, usually in conjunction with catheter ablation.

Atrioventricular block (congenital or acquired) or sick sinus syndrome are not usually indications for ICEPS because pacemaker indications are based on noninvasive criteria. The association of tachyarrhythmias may be an indication for ICEPS.

Repolarization abnormalities are not an indication for ICEPS because programmed stimulation does not induce the dysrhythmia in these patients. Recording of monophasic action potentials is not yet clinically useful.

EPSs are required in the evaluation of patients for implantable antitachycardia pacemakers and cardioverter defibrillators. Because of the increasing reliability of the devices, they are capable of terminating most tachyarrhythmias. Increasingly, the ICEPS is performed at the time of device implantation. The device is then programmed specifically for each patient. Fine tuning is done with the implanted device and a device programmer; noninvasive EPS can then be performed, with reprogramming of the device as necessary.

EQUIPMENT AND PERSONNEL

Pediatric ICEPS should be performed in pediatric electrophysiology laboratories. Very few centers perform enough electrophysiology and hemodynamic cardiac catheterizations to support separate electrophysiology and hemodynamic laboratories. It is feasible to use one laboratory for both purposes without losing quality for either study. Considering the length for pediatric procedures, optimally 400 studies can be performed in one room per year. This requires the room to operate 8 to 10 hours per day with enough staff to absorb the workload. An occasional day should be allowed for preventive maintenance or troubleshooting.

The radiographic equipment for an electrophysiology laboratory should be a modern, digital system capable of pulsed fluoroscopy and zoom acquisition to minimize radiation exposure. Biplane fluoroscopy is imperative. Proper placement of physiologic monitoring screens to accommodate ICEPS, hemodynamic cases, and device implants is also necessary. Adequate lighting for all procedures is important.

Consideration must be given to the necessity for general anesthesia and transesophageal echocardiography for some procedures. The monitoring team should be in an x-ray–shielded room with excellent visual and audio communication to the procedure room. For device implantation, operating room standards of sterility, including air handling and traffic flow, are required.

The pediatric ICEPS should be led by a qualified pediatric cardiac electrophysiologist. A scrubbed assistant is necessary for catheter ablation procedures. One to two nurses are required, depending on the presence of an anesthesiologist and at least one monitoring technician. Either an anesthesiologist or a trained nurse anesthetist must anesthetize or sedate the patient, respectively. Relatively short diagnostic procedures may be done with a nurse performing conscious sedation. It is optimal to perform longer procedures, such as catheter ablation, under general anesthesia or anesthesia-monitored deep sedation.

The effect of anesthetics on the electrophysiology and hemodynamics of the cardiovascular and autonomic nervous systems is an important consideration. Some arrhythmias are very sensitive to many anesthetic and sedative agents. This is particularly true for automatic focus arrhythmias and AV node re-entry tachycardias. The use of short-acting agents and agents that are thought to have few cardiac effects is optimal. Midazolam and remifentanil are often given in our institution. Sometimes proarrhythmic agents, such as ketamine, halothane, or isoflurane, are also used.

Adequate presedation sets the stage for a smooth procedure. Intravenous midazolam mixed with liquid acetaminophen is provided orally for younger children. For older children, oral diazepam is given and is much less expensive. These agents should be given 30 to 45 minutes before the procedure and are probably preferable to intravenous presedation for psychological reasons. They are certainly preferable to intramuscular presedation.[5]

When an intravenous catheter is to be started while the patient is even partially awake, a topical EMLA (eutectic mixture of local anesthetics) cream[6] should be applied over prospective insertion sites. For sedation cases, either midazolam, fentanyl, or a combination may be given intravenously under careful monitoring. The combination of ketamine and midazolam is also useful, although ketamine results in unpleasant emergence reactions, particularly in older children.[5]

When general anesthesia is provided, fentanyl is a good agent. Newer, shorter acting derivatives may be even better. Narcotics often lead to postprocedure nausea and vomiting. Halothane or isoflurane may be considered in patients with relatively normal cardiac function.

Continuous monitoring of ECG, pulse oximetry, and indwelling arterial blood pressure is mandatory. End-tidal carbon dioxide (CO_2) measurement is very helpful, as is intermittent measurement of arterial blood gases. The ability to measure central venous pressure intermittently through the side arm of a sheath is often helpful for lengthy cases and in patients with coexisting heart disease.

For pulse oximetry without end-tidal CO_2 when conscious sedation is used, it may be better not to provide supplemental oxygen (O_2) because a very high carbon dioxide level (P_{CO_2}) with a normal O_2 saturation could result. It has been our experience that pulse oximetry predicts hypercapnia in the absence of supplemental, inhaled O_2.

Adequate suctioning equipment is an absolute must. It is probably wise to place a nasogastric tube initially for all but the shortest procedures. Observation of the nasogastric and endotracheal tube by fluoroscopy helps document placement as well as effectiveness. All necessary emergency equipment and drugs must be available, and a team member must assess all monitored parameters at all times. One person, besides the operator, should be assigned to this task to allow the operator to focus on the technicalities of the procedure.

The capability for rapid defibrillation or external pacing requires specific radiolucent pads to be applied over the cardiac apex and the right scapula at the beginning of the procedure. These are attached to a device capable of defibrillation, cardioversion, and external pacing. The device must be tested frequently, and all personnel must be familiar with its operation. The device may also serve as a back-up ECG. A second defibrillator must also be in the room.

The electrophysiologic recording system is attached to the patient using extremity and chest radiolucent pads and wires. It is best not to make the synchronization of the cardioverter dependent on the monitoring system. A standard 12-lead ECG should be possible on the physiologic monitor. A total of 25 to 30 simultaneous channels is optimal, including two pressure channels. Simultaneous displays of other monitoring parameters, such as O_2 saturation and numeric arterial and venous pressure, are helpful, as are parameters from the ablation system itself. All channels should be presented on a screen visible by the operator.

A second or split screen should be "freezable" so data can be examined and manipulated with electronic calipers. Real-time monitoring data must not be lost at any time. Computer measurement of data is desirable, but not always practical. A hard copy of the data is also necessary. Continuous recording of the data on tape or disk is important, as is instant review capability. Integration of the electrophysiologic data with the radiographic data is desirable. Presenting all of the data to the operator in a useful format is a challenge but is possible. Certain data should also be available to all team members inside the laboratory itself as well as the control room.

Electrical stimulation of the heart in a programmed manner is integral to ICEPS. Two separate channels on a programmable stimulator are necessary. These must be electrically isolated and controllable by a physician or technician. We use a custom digital system based on a personal computer. This system also measures, plots, presents, and stores selected data in a data base format.

A second, simple, battery-powered stimulator must be available in the laboratory for emergencies. Linking the monitoring and stimulating systems to the patient by fiberoptic cable has eliminated a large amount of electrical interfacing. Preprocessing the digitized electrical signal closer to the patient also appears to help signal quality. Frequent testing of all equipment and cables is necessary to optimize signal quality as well as to provide electrical safety. The more ancillary equipment linked to the monitoring equipment, the greater the challenge.

CATHETER INSERTION AND POSITIONING

The goal of catheter insertion and positioning is to derive the greatest amount of useful data in the least invasive manner possible, because catheter insertion into a vessel can cause thrombosis or bleeding.[7] Great improvements have become available. Preplanning of the likely studies and interventions can ensure a smooth procedure. The most important recent advance is the ability to insert multiple electrode catheters through a single sheath (Figs. 3–2 and 3–3).

To insert three catheters with one venipuncture, a 14-French, a 12-French, and a 7-French sheath have become available. The 7-French system or catheter can be inserted through a standard 7-French sheath with an introducer long enough to reach the diaphragm. Three 2-French, quadripolar catheters with different curves can be inserted. This system is used from the left leg to position the high right atrial, His bundle, and right ventricular apex catheters. A 5-mm or 2-5-2-mm interelectrode spacing works best. A 10-mm interelectrode distance may be better for His bundle recording in larger patients. In addition to the three preformed curves, different curves can be prepared by the operator. Excellent control of the catheter is possible, and these catheters (i.e., the 2-French catheters) provide superior electrograms and have superior stability. The visibility of these smaller catheters is fair to good; they are more difficult to see in larger patients. If more complex or larger catheters are desired, 12- or 14-French sheaths will accept three standard catheters of various sizes.

For recording left-sided activations or stimulating the left atrium, a coronary sinus catheter is optimal (see Fig. 3–3). It accomplishes the

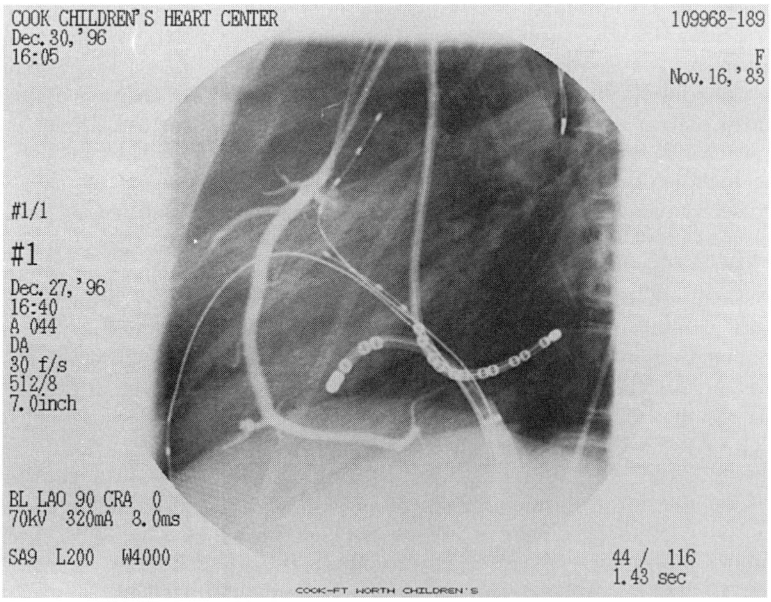

FIGURE 3–2. Lateral projection of catheter courses and right coronary angiogram in a patient with a right posterior accessory pathway. Seen are three 2-French catheters positioned in the high right atrium, the His bundle area, and the right ventricular apex. A 6-French, 12-polar catheter is positioned in the coronary sinus and a 7-French quadripolar, 4-mm tip ablation catheter is positioned at the site of the right posterior accessory pathway. Visualizing the right coronary artery, it is easier to determine the site of the tricuspid valve annulus and, therefore, the optimal ablation target.

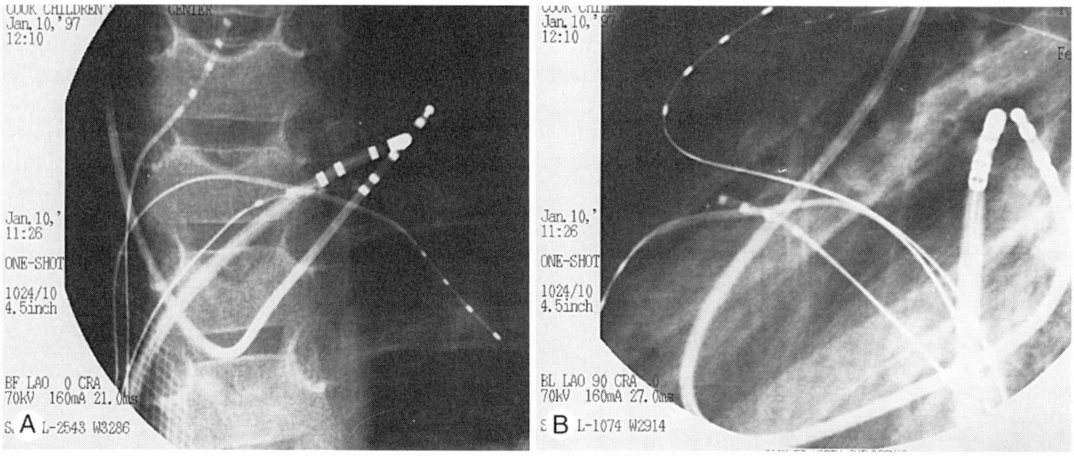

FIGURE 3–3. *A,* Radiograph of a patient with a normal heart using minimally invasive catheters for ablation of a left posterior pathway. Seen are three 2-French quadripolar catheters positioned at the high right atrium, the His bundle area, and the right ventricular apex. A 5-French hexipolar catheter is positioned in the coronary sinus, and a 5-French 4-mm tip ablation catheter is positioned through the atrial septum to the accessory pathway. *B,* Lateral catheter projection of the same patient. Note the proximity of the distal ablation electrode to the coronary sinus catheter.

aforementioned goals at the AV groove without the danger of systemic emboli. The coronary sinus is most easily accessed from a superior approach, particularly if one wishes to enter the coronary sinus deeply to record left lateral activity. We prefer the left brachial vein because of the decreased incidence of complications rather than the subclavian or jugular veins. We achieve entry into the brachial vein greater than 95% of the time in infants and children older than 6 months. The cephalic vein can also be utilized, but the nearly right-angle transition between the cephalic and subclavian veins can be difficult in regard to catheter manipulation. Use of the brachial vein may result in brachial plexus nerve injuries because the arm must be positioned cephalad when the lateral x-ray tube is used. Left anterior oblique x-ray tube positioning allows lowering of the left arm. Frequent passive range of motion of the affected extremity also minimizes adverse events, as does careful positioning. Placement of a 10- to 12-polar, 5- or 6-French catheter into the coronary sinus allows excellent mapping of the left AV groove. Short (i.e., 2 mm or alternating 2 and 5 mm) interelectrode distances are necessary for pediatric applications. Entry into the coronary sinus from the right atrium necessitates posterior and medial direction of the catheter. When the catheter reaches the tricuspid valve annulus, it begins to move in an up-and-down direction with the heartbeat. Coronary sinus entry can usually be done at this time. Confirmation by lateral fluoroscopy is useful. Characteristic electrograms of nearly equal atrial and ventricular size also validate catheter position. Coronary sinus entry may be facilitated by catheters with small, sharp curves at their tips or by deflectable catheters. Coronary sinus catheters with a lumen are also available to facilitate angiography to demonstrate abnormalities of the coronary venous system that may be related to accessory pathways.

For further mapping of the left atrium and catheter ablation in the left atrium, placement of a transseptal sheath is helpful.[6] This is performed by standard technique, employing standard transseptal sheaths in most cases. Sheaths with several curves are available. Previous placement of the coronary sinus catheter gives additional landmarks for transseptal puncture (Fig. 3–4). The coronary sinus itself is at the back of the heart, whereas the catheter shaft in the superior vena cava (SVC) delineates the usual position of the aorta in the lateral view. If puncture of the left atrium is made inside the "J" of the coronary sinus catheter in both planes, the left atrium should be entered.

Transseptal puncture should be performed by adequately trained teams using optimal equipment. The fluoroscopy tubes should be in the posteroanterior (PA) and lateral projections. The right femoral vein should be entered and a long, straight wire positioned into the SVC through the right atrium. A transseptal sheath and dilator set is advanced over the wire after the vein is dilated. The wire is removed when the tip of the dilator is in the SVC. The tip of the dilator is sharp and should never be moved without a wire

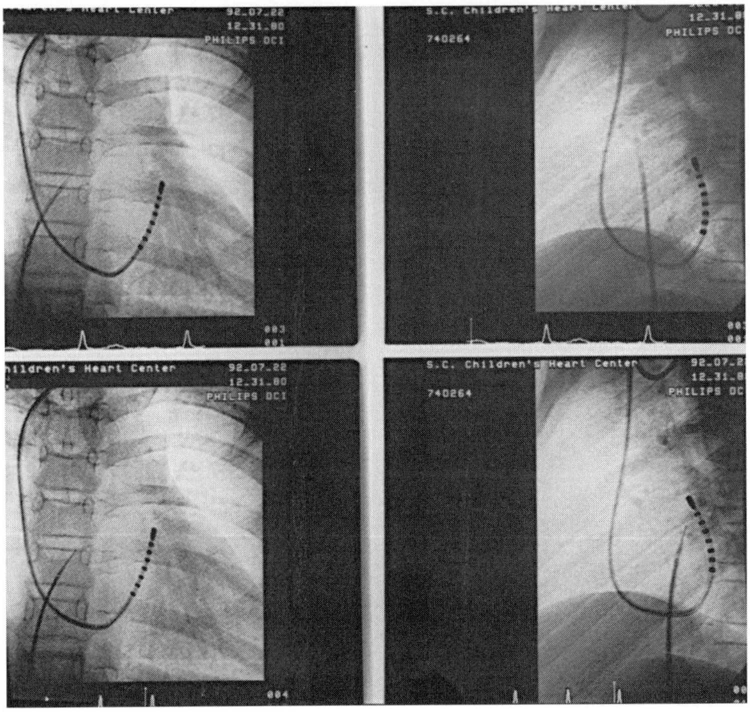

FIGURE 3–4. Posteroanterior and lateral catheter course positions demonstrating the usefulness of prepositioning a coronary sinus catheter before transseptal puncture during an intracardiac electrophysiology study. The transseptal puncture should be made in the "J" area both on the PA and the lateral projections. The top two frames indicate the sheath dilation set with the needle still inside the dilator positioned slightly anterior for puncture. The bottom two frames indicate that the dilator has been slightly withdrawn and turned slightly posterior with the needle extended from the dilator.

in it. The sheath-dilator-needle set should be tested for fit and distances before insertion into the body. Once the dilator is positioned and flushed, the needle is advanced close to the tip. Pressure monitoring is established. The sheath-dilator-needle complex is then retracted with the tip pointing left and cephalad until the foramen ovale is reached. A "bump" in the feel of the needle may help indicate this. A slight, further withdrawal is preferred and, after the PA and lateral positions are checked, as well as the needle pressure, the needle is advanced (Fig. 3–5). Pressure is felt by the operator and the pressure curve from the needle tip damps, then there is a "give," and left atrial pressure may be visualized. If it is not, flushing the needle with radiographic contrast will help confirm a left atrial position and restore pressure recording. The entire assembly can now be slightly advanced, taking care not to puncture the roof or the back wall of the left atrium. Damping of the pressure curve of the needle tip indicates contact with an atrial wall and requires retraction and redirection.

Next, the dilator is advanced slightly off of the needle, and finally the sheath is advanced well off of the dilator. The dilator and needle are then withdrawn slowly as a unit to minimize the chance of creating negative pressure and an air bubble. The sheath is then carefully flushed with heparinized saline after withdrawal of blood. Heparin must be given at a dose to produce an activated clotting time (ACT) of 320 seconds or greater. The dose is usually 100 to 150 units per kilogram of body weight and is manufacturer specific. The ACT should be performed in the catheterization laboratory for expedited results. The initial measurement is performed 5 to 10 minutes after the first dose of heparin and is repeated every 10–30 minutes until the sheath is removed from the left atrium. The ACT is kept high the entire time the sheath remains in the left atrium. The heparin is not reversed. Flushing the entire sheath dilator needle assembly before its use with undiluted heparin may prevent some clots.

The deflectable catheter is then positioned well into the left atrium through the transseptal sheath before positioning the other catheters. The length of sheath remaining outside the femoral vein, with the tip of the sheath just inside the left atrium, is a helpful number to record because the sheath may be partially withdrawn to facilitate other catheters' positions. Sheaths with variable shapes to facilitate access to pathways at various sites around the mitral annulus are available, but we have little experience with them at this time.

A 7-French catheter in a 7-French sheath that has been well flushed minimizes clot formation. This combination does not require periodic withdrawal and flushing of blood. A sheath larger than the catheter itself requires withdrawal and

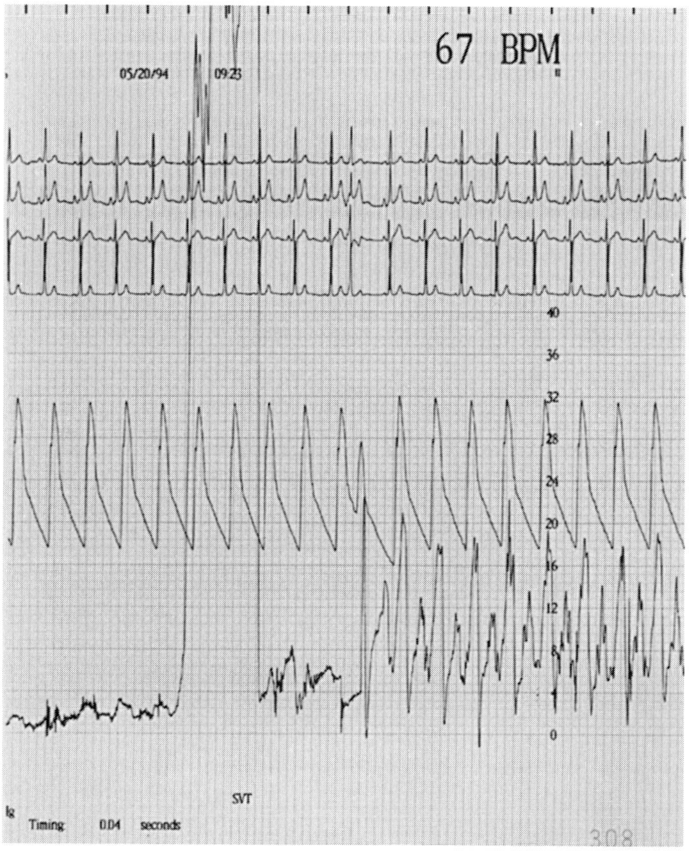

FIGURE 3–5. Demonstration of the transseptal puncture. Recordings include surface electrocardiogram leads I, aVF, V_1, and V_6, femoral artery blood pressure, and the pressure from the tip of the transseptal needle. From left to right, an initial right atrial pressure of approximately 5 mm Hg is seen. When the tip touches the atrial septum and advances through it, a large upward deflection is noted followed by a higher pressure in the left atrial chamber.

flushing with the increased possibility of air entry into the left atrium. If this approach is required, it should be done by the operator with careful visualization to minimize the chance of air embolism. No energy applications should be made in the left side of the heart until the ACT is documented to be greater than 320 seconds. Left-sided pathways can also be reached by a retrograde technique (Fig. 3–6).

A modern protocol for patients with narrow QRS tachycardia without known pre-excitation is to utilize fewer catheters. The coronary sinus and right ventricular apex catheters are positioned, and mapping of left atrial activation during ventricular pacing with premature ventricular stimulation helps to determine the presence or absence of a left-sided concealed accessory pathway. If this protocol is carried out before additional catheter or ablation catheter sheath insertion, time and equipment can be minimized.

ELECTROGRAMS

At the beginning of the procedure, surface ECG leads are placed on the patient to obtain a 12-lead ECG. The 12 lead is displayed and recorded and a hard copy printed. For the remainder of the procedure, four surface ECG leads are continuously displayed, usually leads I, aVF, V_1, and V_6. Alternate leads may be added or substituted to elucidate certain important ECG patterns. Our protocol is to position all four ECG leads at the top of the paper or screen. Next, a bipolar right atrial electrogram is displayed from the proximal electrodes of a quadripolar catheter. Next, five to six bipolar coronary sinus electrograms, starting distal to proximal, are displayed. A space is then left for two bipolar electrograms from the ablation catheter, followed by two or three bipolar His bundle electrograms and a bipolar right ventricular electrogram. The arterial blood pressure waveform is continuously displayed at the bottom. Several physiologic parameters can be numerically displayed on the same screen. This screen should be easily visualized by the operator and his or her assistant, the anesthesiologist, and the control room staff. Electrograms should be limited electrically in order not to cross over each other and interfere with interpretation (Fig. 3–7).

The gains may then be adjusted to display the

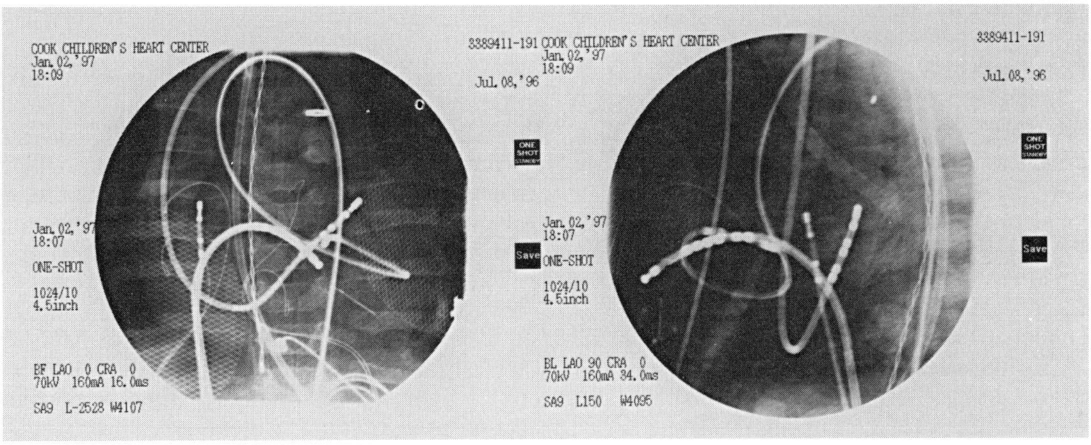

FIGURE 3–6. Catheter course in a patient with complex congenital heart disease and multiple accessory pathways. Wolff-Parkinson-White syndrome was diagnosed before surgery but was not corrected. Incessant tachycardia ensued, and an attempt at surgical ablation of a right anterior pathway was unsuccessful. A hexipolar 5-French catheter is positioned into the coronary sinus from the left arm. A 4-French quadripolar catheter is placed in the high right atrium. A 6-French catheter is placed in the HBE position, and a 5-French quadripolar 4-mm tip ablation catheter is positioned retrograde through the aortic valve on the left posterior septal pathway. Multiple burns using this catheter eventually eliminated the tachycardia, but damage did occur to the aortic valve.

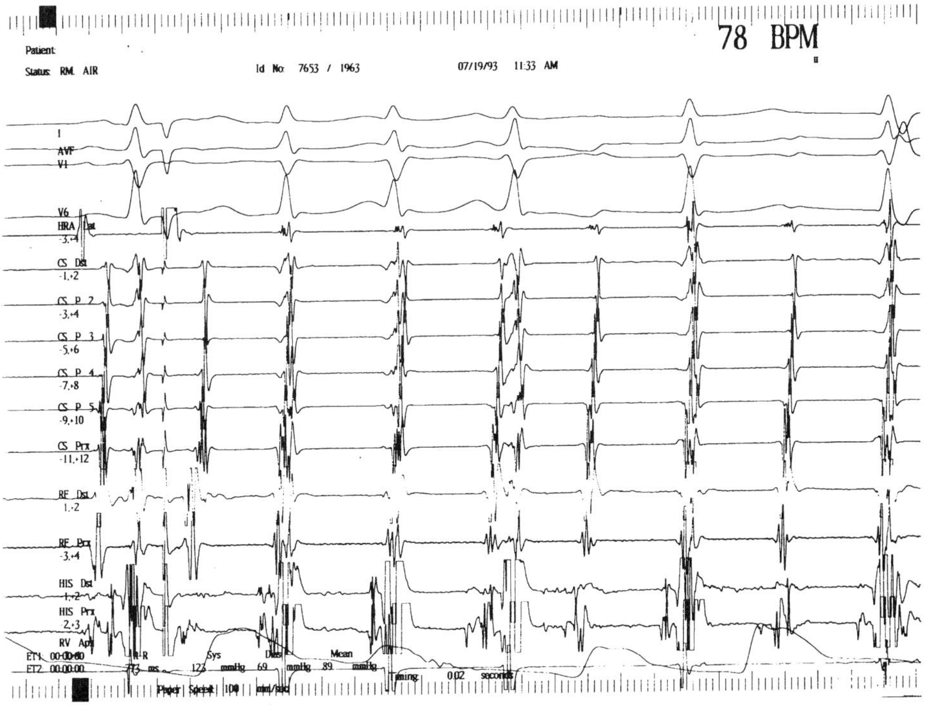

FIGURE 3–7. Demonstration of atrioventricular (AV) nodal re-entry tachycardia induced by a single premature atrial stimulus with 1:1 and 2:1 conduction. Shown from top to bottom are surface leads I, aVF, V_1, V_6, high right atrium (HRA), six pairs of coronary sinus (CS) electrograms, two of the potential ablation electrograms, two His bundle electrograms, and femoral artery pressure. The first sinus beat at the left shows normal AH and HV conduction. A premature stimulus introduced in the high right atrium results in a large delay in conduction through the AV node with retrograde reactivation of the atrium by the fast pathway. Antegrade conduction occurs over the slow pathway, and this is repeated twice until the antegrade conduction fails to reach the ventricles in a 2:1 pattern. This is a frequent finding in AV node re-entry tachycardia in children with block below the His bundle and is often misconstrued as atrial flutter.

needed details. High gain facilitates measuring the earliest onset of activity, whereas lower gain allows observation of the details of the electrogram. Bandpass filter settings between 30 to 50 and 250 to 1000 Hz improve electrogram quality as well as stability and are commonly used in ICEPS.

Electrogram timing is measured from the beginning of each depolarization to the next. The "beginning" is defined as the first depolarization at an angle of 45° or more. Obviously, this is influenced by gain setting. Other criteria for measuring electrograms have been used, but these appear to be a good compromise.

MEASURING CONDUCTION TIMES

Conduction times are measured as described previously.[8] Intra-atrial conduction time from the area near the sinus node (high right atrium [HRA]) to the area near the bundle of His (low septal right atrium [LSRA]) is measured from the onset of the HRA electrogram to the beginning of the LSRA electrogram on the His bundle electrogram. This measurement represents right atrial conduction time. It is normally 15 to 40 milliseconds. It is prolonged in atrioventricular septal defects and less commonly in secundum atrial septal defects.[9] It is rarely prolonged in postoperative atrial surgery.[10] Conduction to other parts of the atria (i.e., low lateral right atrium or left atrium) can also be measured. The low lateral right atrium is usually activated rapidly (i.e., 15–20 milliseconds after the HRA). It is frequently delayed after intra-atrial surgery, such as Mustard and Senning operations.[10]

AV node conduction time is measured by the LSRA to His bundle conduction time (LSRA-H).[11] It is normally 70 to 120 milliseconds and is prolonged with AV node disease. This interval is the one most commonly prolonged in first-degree AV block seen on the surface ECG. The LSRA-H interval is also prolonged during type I (Wenckebach) second-degree AV block. The AV node is also the usual site of block in congenital complete AV block. Hence, one will observe LSRA depolarizations not followed by His bundle depolarization and a His bundle depolarization preceding each ventricular depolarization.

The conduction time through the His bundle, the bundle branches, and the Purkinje system to the ventricular myocardium is represented by the HV interval, which usually measures 30 to 55 milliseconds. It is measured from the beginning of the His potential to the earliest ventricular depolarization on the surface ECG. The HV interval is prolonged if the bundle branches are damaged, which can occur during ventricular surgery. It is short in WPW syndrome because it is bypassed by the accessory pathway, and the ventricles are activated prematurely. Intra-Hisian block can also be delineated with the recording of proximal and distal His bundle electrograms. Intra-Hisian block may be first, second, or third degree and may be seen in some cases of congenital complete AV block.

Conduction times across accessory pathways may also be measured to discover the insertions of the pathway.[12] For pathways with bidirectional conduction, conduction times can be measured both in the antegrade (atrium to ventricle) and retrograde (ventricle to atrium) direction. These conduction times are often very short and difficult to measure (Figs. 3–8 and 3–9). Potentials of the accessory pathway may lie between ventricular and atrial depolarizations and further complicate measurement. The concept of fusion must be constantly considered because in patients with two pathways any area may be activated from both directions. Conditions of pure conduction must be sought, such as during a re-entry tachycardia in which each pathway is used in a different direction. In addition, physiologic differences, such as decremental conduction through the AV node during very premature stimulation, may help purify conduction patterns. A common situation is the patient with a left-sided, unidirectional pathway and rapid antegrade and retrograde AV node conduction. These two conditions seem to be statistically and probably physiologically related and are a common finding in young patients with narrow QRS tachycardias.[13] Another factor that often complicates measurement of conduction time across accessory pathways is that the exact site of depolarization often has a low amplitude depolarization (see Fig. 3–1). This, however, can be used as a qualitative marker of pathway insertion.

In certain clinical situations, alternate catheter locations and different measurements of conduction intervals are necessary. Primary atrial tachycardias, such as atrial automatic tachycardias and atrial re-entry tachycardias, require more catheters and electrodes in the affected atrium.[14] We frequently have two or more 12-polar catheters. Occasionally, one 24-polar "halo" catheter is helpful. Angiography of the right coronary artery may help define the tricuspid valve annulus (see Fig. 3–2).

In ventricular tachycardias, sufficient catheters and electrodes must be placed in the affected ventricle to localize the automatic focus or re-

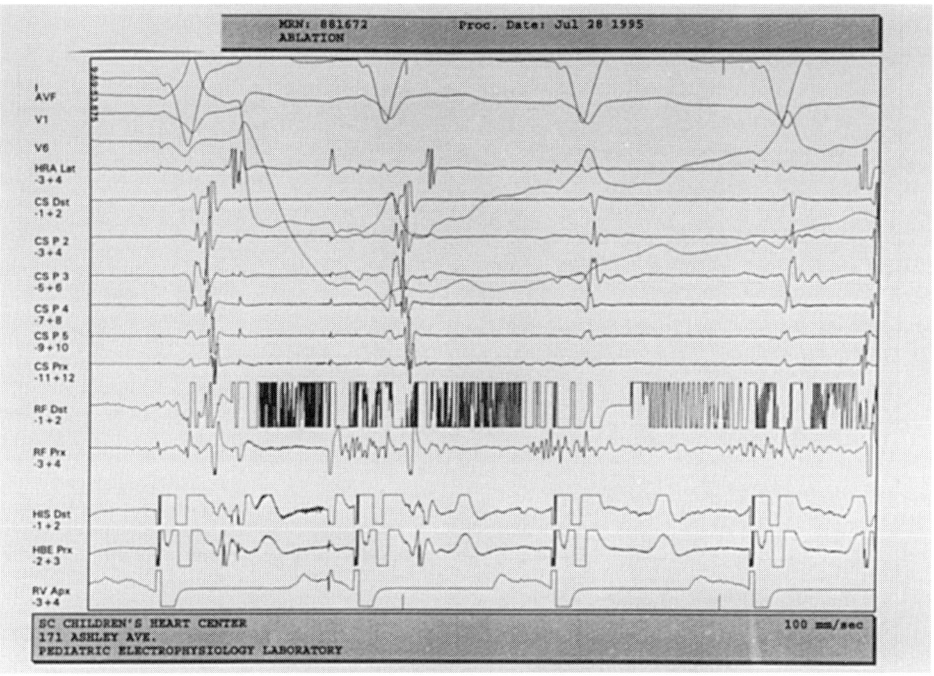

FIGURE 3–8. Demonstration of ablation of a left posterior accessory pathway during ventricular pacing. From top to bottom are surface leads I, aVF, V_1, V_6, high right atrial (HRA) electrogram, six coronary sinus (CS) electrograms, two ablation electrograms, two His bundle electrograms, and a right ventricular apex electrogram. The first beat shows rapid retrograde conduction earliest at CS pair 2 during ventricular pacing. The radiofrequency current is then applied, causing a loss of signal on the distal ablation catheter. The retrograde conduction persists for the next beat but is then absent for the next two beats, and a sinus escape beat is seen at the extreme right-hand side of the figure. This rapid loss of retrograde conduction is indicative of a likely permanent, successful burn. Applying the energy during ventricular pacing rather than supraventricular tachycardia results in an increased degree of catheter stability, because the rate does not change at the time of the energy application. During ventricular pacing, care must be taken not to confuse fusion conduction from atrioventricular node conduction.

entry circuit. In the frequently encountered, right ventricular outflow tract tachycardia, one vertical multipolar catheter complements one horizontal multipolar catheter.[15] A His bundle catheter and an ablation catheter complete the necessary catheters. Right ventricular outflow tract tachycardias are mostly automatic, so the earliest site of activation identifies the point for ablation.[15]

STIMULATION PROTOCOLS

The objective of most ICEPS is the induction of tachycardia to determine its mechanism and the anatomic site of the arrhythmogenic substrate. Because most tachycardias are re-entrant, the requirements for re-entry must be considered. The requirements are an anatomically or physiologically isolated re-entry circuit, unidirectional conduction, and slow conduction in one limb. The AV node–His bundle axis and an accessory connection may fulfill these criteria. Premature stimulation may induce both unidirectional conduction and slow conduction in the other limb.

The most common type of tachycardia in children is orthodromic with antegrade slow conduction over the AV node and retrograde unidirectional conduction over an accessory pathway. Induction of AV node re-entrant tachycardia with antegrade conduction over the slow perinodal pathway and retrograde conduction over the fast perinodal pathway requires a delicate balance of conduction properties, which is heavily influenced by the autonomic nervous system. Frequently, SVT can be induced by pacing the atrium at a cycle length that results in slow enough AV antegrade conduction to place the atrial pacing spike in the preceding QRS in an eight-beat burst. Single and double premature stimuli into sinus rhythm or into an eight-beat drive cycle may also be effective.

Stimulation protocols may also be used to test the function of the various parts of the conduction system. The sinus node is tested in two ways.

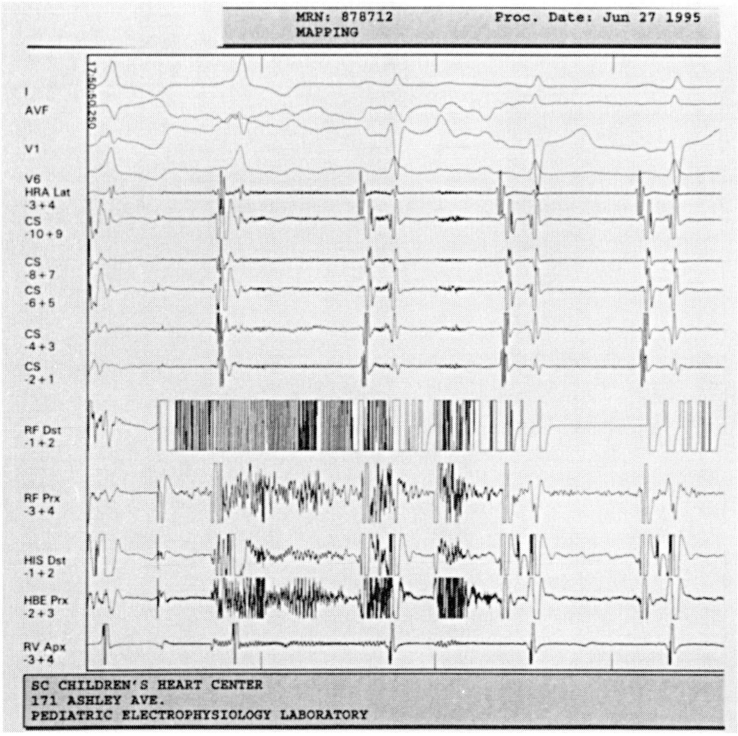

FIGURE 3–9. Demonstration of mapping and ablation of a left posterior accessory pathway during sinus rhythm. A wide QRS complex and short PR interval are noted on the surface electrocardiogram, with earliest activation occurring at coronary sinus (CS) pair 1, which has been moved down for easier comparison to the ablation electrograms. After the initiation of energy delivery through the radiofrequency electrode, the delta wave persists for one more beat and then disappears with normalization of atrial and ventricular intervals.

Automaticity is tested by 30 seconds of overdrive pacing followed by measurement of the first escape interval, which is then subtracted from the nonpaced sinus cycle length. This corrected sinus node recovery time (CSNRT) is normally less than 300 milliseconds in the sedated patient and less than 525 milliseconds in the unsedated adult.[10] The conduction time into and out of the sinus node is tested by introducing single premature stimuli into sinus rhythm and is described more fully in Chapter 4 on the sinus node.

These stimulation protocols also address the AV node and His-Purkinje system, particularly the AV node. Normal values are available for the degree of prolongation of the components of the AV conduction system with certain degrees of premature stimulation.[16] These parameters are rarely used to make clinical decisions because surface ECG and clinical criteria are available to determine the need for intervention in patients with bradycardia.

For induction of ventricular tachycardia, several stimulation protocols are used. Single premature ventricular contractions into a paced ventricular rhythm define the ventricular effective refractory period. Double premature ventricular extrasystoles using a toggle technique will induce some ventricular tachycardias. Stimulation using triple premature ventricular extrasystoles is used only when a clinical ventricular tachycardia has been recorded, because this protocol is more likely to induce nonclinical ventricular tachycardias. Eight-beat burst pacing to 2:1 stimulus to ventricle block is also useful. These protocols are repeated under isoproterenol stimulation. These protocols (single, double, and burst extrasystoles) at one site and with one cycle length induce most ventricular tachycardias and do not produce nonclinical dysrhythmias in patients with normal hearts.

In summary, the value of ICEPS cannot be understated in certain clinical situations. Although today's ICEPS are generally associated with an intervention (i.e., radiofrequency catheter ablation or rhythm control device placement), they can still be used when unique information pertinent to patient care is needed that cannot be obtained otherwise.

REFERENCES

1. Scherlag BJ, Lau SH, Helfant RH, et al: Catheter techniques for recording His bundle activity in man. Circulation 39:13–19, 1969.
2. Zipes DP, DiMarco JP, Gillette PC, et al: ACC/AHA Task Force report. Guidelines for clinical intracardiac

electrophysiological and catheter ablation procedures. Circulation 92:673–691, 1995.
3. Balaji S, Lau Y, Case C, et al: Ventricular tachycardia in tetralogy of Fallot. Am J Cardiol 80:160–163, 1997.
4. Gatzoulis MA, Till JA, Somerville J, et al: Mechanoelectrical interaction in tetralogy of Fallot. QRS prolongation relates to right ventricular size and predicts malignant ventricular arrhythmias and sudden death. Circulation 92:231–237, 1995.
5. Zeigler VL, Brown LE: Conscious sedation in the pediatric population: Special considerations. Crit Care Nurs Clin North Am 9:381–394, 1997.
6. Gillette PC, Zeigler VL, Case CL: Pediatric arrhythmias: Are they different? In Zipes DP, Jalife J (eds): Cardiac Electrophysiology—From Cell to Bedside, 2nd ed. Philadelphia, WB Saunders, 1995, pp 1265–1268.
7. Miga DE, McKellar LF, Denslow S, et al: Incidence of femoral vein occlusion following catheter ablation in children: Evaluation with magnetic resonance angiography. Pediatr Cardiol 18:204–207, 1997.
8. Gillette PC, Reitman MJ, Gutgesell HP, et al: Intracardiac electrography in children and young adults. Am Heart J 89:36–44, 1975.
9. Jacobsen JR, Gillette PC, Corbett BN, et al: Intracardiac electrography in endocardial cushion defects. Circulation 54:559–603, 1976.
10. Kugler JD, Gillette PC, Mullins CE, et al: Sinoatrial conduction in children: An index of sinoatrial node function. Circulation 59:1266–1277, 1979.
11. Roberts NK, Gillette PC: Electrophysiologic study of the conduction system in normal children. Pediatrics 60:858–863, 1977.
12. Gillette PC: The mechanisms of supraventricular tachycardia in children. Circulation 54:133–139, 1976.
13. Henglein D, Gillette PC, Garson A Jr, et al: Antegrade conduction and AV node function in patients with unidirectional retrograde accessory pathways (URAP). Am Heart J 107:411–417, 1984.
14. Gillette PC, Wampler DG, Garson A Jr, et al: Treatment of atrial automatic tachycardia by ablation procedures. J Am Coll Cardiol 6:405–409, 1985.
15. O'Connor BK, Case CL, Sokoloski MC, et al: Radiofrequency catheter ablation of right ventricular outflow tachycardia in children and adolescents. J Am Coll Cardiol 27(4):869–874, 1996.
16. Thapar MK, Gillette PC: Dual atrioventricular nodal pathways: A common electrophysiologic response in children. Circulation 60:1369–1374, 1979.

SECTION II

Arrhythmias

CHAPTER 4

SINUS NODE DYSFUNCTION

Ameeta B. Martin and John D. Kugler

Sinus node dysfunction (SND) constitutes a spectrum of cardiac arrhythmias, including sinus bradycardia, sinus pause-arrest, sinoatrial (SA) block, slow escape rhythms, bradyarrhythmias and tachyarrhythmias, and atrial muscle re-entry tachycardias. SND is relatively uncommon in children. The exact incidence is unknown because diagnostic criteria are not uniform in studies and most children with SND, in general, are asymptomatic. SND may be primary (from organic sinus node disease) or secondary (from autonomic imbalance, drug effect, or postsurgical). The term *sick sinus syndrome* is avoided because its implications are imprecise.[1–5] Therefore, to avoid confusion, any disorder of the sinus node in this chapter is described as SND.

The diagnosis of SND is established when one or more abnormal findings are found by noninvasive or invasive procedures. Invasive testing is now seldom required because noninvasive testing allows correlation of clinical symptoms with abnormal findings of SND and thus a better assessment of severity of SND.[6, 7]

CLINICAL PRESENTATION

The clinical presentation of the patient with SND is variable and depends on many factors. The patient's age (and ability to verbalize symptoms), underlying hemodynamic status (threshold for symptoms), presence and severity of associated underlying conduction system disease (associated arrhythmias), as well as follow-up and monitoring practices of physicians (frequency of detection) impact on the ultimate clinical presentation.

SYMPTOMS

Most children with SND are asymptomatic. In two reports, Yabek et al[8, 9] showed that 74% of 30 children were asymptomatic with SND. In a Holter survey study of 624 healthy children, Roifman et al[10] found 12 children with electrocardiographic (ECG) evidence of SND.[10] The most common arrhythmia (10 patients) was sinus arrest, but no symptoms were present and no patient had a history of symptoms. Because most children are asymptomatic, SND is usually detected incidentally or on routine monitoring of high-risk patients.

Of children with SND who are symptomatic, the most common symptoms appear to be fatigue and exercise intolerance or dizziness/syncope. These symptoms are difficult to document and even more difficult to correlate with specific evidence of SND. The manifestations of fatigue and exercise intolerance are related to the age of the patient. In infants, poor feeding, lethargy, or signs and symptoms of congestive heart failure exist; in older children, inability to maintain the same level of activity as peers, tiredness in the absence of activity, and frequent naps may be the only signs of fatigue.

Dizziness secondary to SND is probably more common than syncope. Although syncope usually attracts more attention as a potentially life-threatening problem, dizziness or near syncope also should prompt further investigation. Syncope sometimes is difficult to detect in infants and young children. In infants as well as children, seizures may be a secondary problem to unwitnessed syncope. It is imperative to evaluate the patient's rhythm when the presenting symptom is unexplained seizures. This is especially indicated when the patient has an underlying disorder with an associated risk of SND (or risk of any other arrhythmia that causes syncope).[11]

Sudden death is an uncommon presentation, and its true incidence relative to SND is impossible to determine. Differentiating whether sudden death was secondary to SND or to other life-threatening arrhythmias (e.g., atrial or ventricular tachyarrhythmia) in the same patient is often impossible to ascertain.[12–16] For example, the incidence of sudden death was 2.5% in 372 patients with postoperative Mustard repair for transposition of the great arteries, and the only risk factor identified (weakly) was the presence of atrial tachyarrhythmia (atrial flutter). Although many of the 372 patients had SND, sudden death was not associated with the presence of bradycardia.[12] In a 1997 article by Gelatt,[17] 31 of 478 (6.5%) postoperative Mustard patients died suddenly. Although sudden death was presumed to be arrhythmogenic, the circumstances surrounding the deaths are unclear. Although SND was frequently seen in this population with loss of sinus rhythm in 60% of 448 operative survivors 20 years postoperatively, SND was not a significant independent risk factor for death.

The clinical manifestations of SND are directly related to the function of the remaining conduction system and the underlying hemodynamic state. In patients with significant SND (e.g., sinus arrest) at any age, symptoms of dizziness and syncope usually are uncommon when there is adequate atrioventricular (AV) nodal/His-Purkinje or even ventricular escape rate and no underlying hemodynamic disorder. This is particularly true in infants, who usually are recumbent and are, therefore, not as susceptible to the posture-related effects of relative hypotension, as seen in older children. Regardless of age and status of underlying disease, symptoms of dizziness and syncope are less likely (or if present, less severe) if SND occurs when the patient is supine or sitting. However, children who have undergone surgical repair of congenital heart disease have a greater chance of associated conduction system dysfunction; therefore, if syncope is present, they may have more severe symptoms, even in recumbent positions. In addition, any patient with compromised hemodynamic function may have exacerbation during times of SND. Patients who have decreased or marginal cardiac output have a lower threshold for symptoms of dizziness/syncope during times of SND. The incidence and prevalence of the causes of SND as well as the associated severity are unknown, but most children with SND have less than severe SND.

CAUSES OF SND

Multiple causes of SND exist. Previous reviews have extensively listed and referenced these causes. Because SND from cardiac surgery comprises much of SND in children and adolescents, the causes of SND are best classified as either surgical or nonsurgical.[18, 19] However, it must be emphasized that more than one cause may exist in an individual patient and the effects may be additive. This is particularly important with antiarrhythmic drugs but is also true of endocrine-metabolic and hypervagotonia causes.

DIAGNOSIS OF SINUS NODE FUNCTION

NONINVASIVE DIAGNOSIS

Noninvasive testing is commonly used to establish the diagnosis of SND and assist in determining its severity. Noninvasive testing carries a potentially greater value than invasive testing because it allows a greater chance of documenting symptoms with the associated SND arrhythmia, and the specificity and sensitivity of invasive sinus node evaluation has been disappointing.[20–24] Noninvasive evaluation of SND utilizes the surface standard ECG, ambulatory ECG, ECG event recorder, and exercise testing. Transesophageal atrial recording and pacing is a minimally invasive technique used to evaluate SND. It is important to re-emphasize that, although SND may be detected by one or more of these tests (either intentionally or incidentally), the clinical significance of the dysfunction is a separate issue.

Surface Standard ECG and Ambulatory ECG

Sinus node function is assessed by inferring from the atrial depolarization (P wave). The sinus node is relatively constant in its location at the high right atrial (HRA)–superior vena caval junction and may extend inferiorly in the lateral right atrial wall to nearly the inferior vena cava.[25] The dominant pacemaker cell normally may be anywhere within the node; therefore, the P-wave axis may range from 0° to +90°. Several limb leads (preferably leads I and aVF) are necessary to establish the P-wave axis and, therefore, to infer whether the rhythm is originating within the sinus node or elsewhere in the atria. Ambulatory 24-hour ECG (Holter) monitoring systems used to assess sinus node function ideally should use two perpendicular limb leads to optimize P-wave evaluation.[5]

The arrhythmias listed in Table 4–1, alone or in combination, are characteristic of SND. Only one of these criteria is necessary for the diagnosis, although frequently more than one of the findings exist.

Sinus bradycardia is present when the sinus

Table 4–1. Surface Electrocardiographic Criteria for Sinus Node Dysfunction

Sinus bradycardia
Severe sinus arrhythmia
Sinus pause or arrest
Slow escape rhythms
Sinoatrial exit block (second-degree type I and II)
Bradyarrhythmias and tachyarrhythmias
Sinus node re-entry tachycardia*
Atrial muscle re-entry tachycardia* (e.g., atrial flutter-fibrillation)

*May be found in some patients without sinus node dysfunction.

Reprinted with permission from Kugler JD: Sinus node dysfunction. In: Gillette P, Garson A, Jr (eds): Pediatric Arrhythmias: Electrophysiology and Pacing. Philadelphia, WB Saunders, 1990, pp 250–300.

Table 4–2. Low Heart Rate by 24-Hour Ambulatory (Holter) Electrocardiography in Normal Infants, Children, and Young Adults

INVESTIGATOR	N	PATIENT AGE	LOWEST HEART RATE BY HOLTER (bpm ± SD)
Montague et al.[28]	29	3.5 days	107 ± 15 (awake)
			92 ± 11 (asleep)
Southall et al.[26]	134	<1 month	93 ± 12 (asleep)
Southall et al.[27]	92	7–11 years	56 ± 6
Viitasalo et al.[29]	35	23 ± 6.1 years (endurance athletes)	37.7 ± 4.3 (asleep)
	35	23 ± 5.8 years	45.4 ± 6.3 (asleep)

Reprinted with permission in part from Kugler JD: Sinus node dysfunction. In Gillette P, Garson A Jr (eds): Pediatric Arrhythmias: Electrophysiology and Pacing. Philadelphia, WB Saunders, 1990, pp 250–300.

rate slows below what is expected for the patient's age. It is important to remember that heart rate on standard ECG is often different than on Holter monitor. Therefore, when evaluating whether a heart rate is abnormal, one needs to first know how and when (if on Holter, the time of day) it was recorded. Table 4–2 lists four Holter studies in normal children and young adults in which a mean low heart rate was calculated as well as a standard deviation.[26–29] From these data (see the last column in Table 4–2), it seems reasonable to suggest the following guidelines for the Holter diagnosis of sinus bradycardia relative to age:

Neonates (< 1 month) and infants (1 month–1 year):	< 60 bpm sleeping and < 80 bpm during waking hours
Children age 1 to 6 years:	< 60 bpm
Children age 7 to 11 years:	< 45 bpm
Adolescents and young adults:	< 40 bpm
Endurance and other highly trained athletes:	< 30 bpm

It must be emphasized that these guidelines are derived from Holter studies and that most of the reports did not distinguish between sleeping and waking heart rates. It is, therefore, practical to assume that these guidelines should be increased somewhat for heart rate determined by standard ECG. The following guidelines appear reasonable for the diagnosis of sinus bradycardia by surface standard ECG[23]:

Infants and children to 3 years of age:	< 100 bpm
Children age 3 to 9 years:	< 60 bpm
Children age 9 to 16 years:	< 50 bpm
Children older than 16 years:	< 40 bpm

The differential diagnosis of sinus bradycardia should be considered each time the disorder is suspected. First, as with any arrhythmia, artifact should be considered. Fast recordings by Holter tape or by paper speed are confirmed when all intervals appear prolonged and when other recordings from the same patient show normal intervals.

Severe sinus arrhythmia may suggest the presence of SND. It is defined by a variation in RR interval of 100% or more.[30] This arrhythmia usually is found in association with sinus bradycardia and is difficult to distinguish from SA exit block (see following discussion).

Sinus pause or arrest occurs when the sinus node fails to generate an impulse. If the sinus arrest is prolonged and sinus rhythm does not resume, an escape focus may act as the pacemaker of the heart for variable periods of time until the sinus node recovers and fires at a rate faster than the subsidiary pacemaker focus. Escape beats or rhythm may originate from the right or left atrium, AV junction, or fascicles or ventricles. When more than several consecutive escape beats from a focus other than the sinus node are found, the escape rhythm is referred to as atrial, junctional, or ventricular rhythm. The term *by default* may be added, implying that the rhythm exists in default of the sinus node. The interval from the sinus arrest to escape beats depends on the automaticity characteristics and function of the escape pacemaker focus. The presence of long periods without a junctional beat may also imply an abnormality of AV nodal or His bundle (junctional) automaticity. Junctional escape rhythms may be normal at any age and most commonly are found during sinus arrhythmia. The "normal" junctional escape rate is unknown for humans but probably relates to age. The mean maximum duration of sinus pause, plus two standard deviations, is 1.82 seconds for children and 2.02 seconds for young adults.[26, 31]

Escape rhythms at slow rates are signs of SND. Sometimes the onset of sinus arrest is not recorded, and the escape rhythm is the only suggestion of SND. However, it is important to distinguish escape rhythms (i.e., by default) from rhythms that result from abnormally increased automaticity (i.e., usurpation). Rhythms of usurpation exist when a rate greater than the sinus rate is present from a focus other than the sinus node. Therefore, SND is not necessarily present when usurpation is present. The problem in differentiating between usurpation and default rhythms is maximized when the rate of the nonsinus focus is only slightly faster or slightly slower than the lower limit of sinus rate for age. In these borderline cases, it is often impossible to determine the site of disease unless the transition from rhythm to rhythm is recorded. Usurpation or default rhythm then can be differentiated: if the sinus node slows, the rhythm is a default rhythm; if the secondary focus increases, the rhythm is a usurpation rhythm.

Arrhythmias that should be considered in the differential diagnosis of sinus pause or arrest include intermittent nonconducted premature atrial beats. Another possible cause of an erroneous diagnosis of sinus pause or arrest includes problems associated with recording equipment. The opportunity for artifactual pauses is high when Holter monitoring is carried out in active children. Holter monitor leads can malfunction (e.g., separate from skin), as shown by the recording in Figure 4–1.

SA exit block, also known as SA block, varies in severity (first, second, or third degree). *First-degree SA block* is present when there is prolonged conduction out of the sinus node through the perinodal fibers (SA junction) to the high right atrium. Although the word *block* traditionally is used, first-degree SA block means that only prolonged conduction is present, but there is no interruption of the impulse (i.e., normal P wave is generated). Because the sinus nodal impulse is not recordable by surface ECG, first-degree SA block is not directly evident. It is possible to diagnose first-degree SA block by electrophysiologic testing; however, this is not commonly done.

Second-degree SA block may be either type I or type II. Type I SA exit block is synonymously known as SA Wenckebach block. In second-degree SA block, as in second-degree AV block, only some of the impulses (SA) are blocked and not conducted.

Third-degree (complete) SA exit block implies normal sinus node impulse generation, but none of the impulses are conducted to the right atrium. This cannot be distinguished on the ECG from sinus arrest caused by automaticity dysfunction. As with complete sinus arrest, an escape rhythm is present on the ECG (either atrial, junctional, or ventricular).

Bradyarrhythmias and *tachyarrhythmias* encompass all arrhythmias that have variable peri-

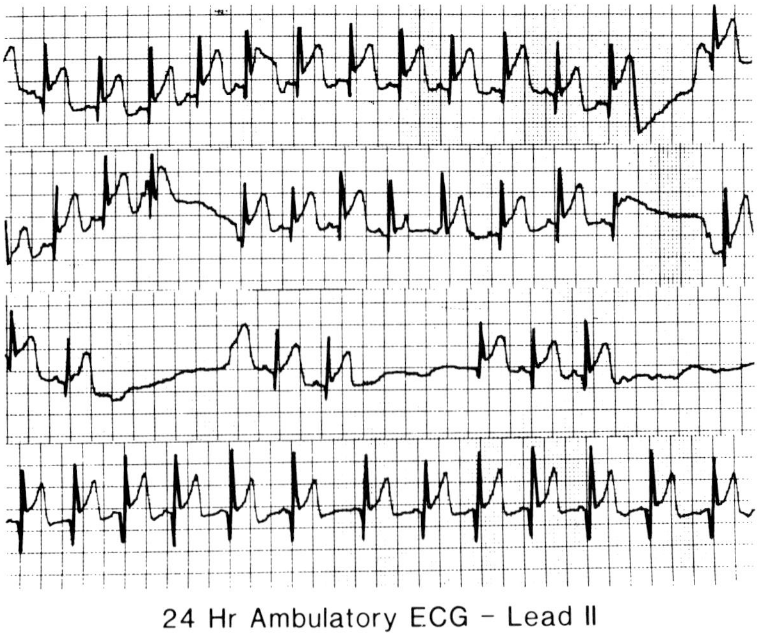

FIGURE 4–1. Electrocardiographic (ECG) recordings by a Holter monitor in an infant demonstrate that sinus arrest can be simulated by intermittent lead malfunction. In this example, the third complex in the third strip shows a T wave without preceding QRS, thus supporting the interpretation that the other pauses were artifactual. The ECG leads were found to be intermittently malfunctioning. Paper speed was 25 mm/s.

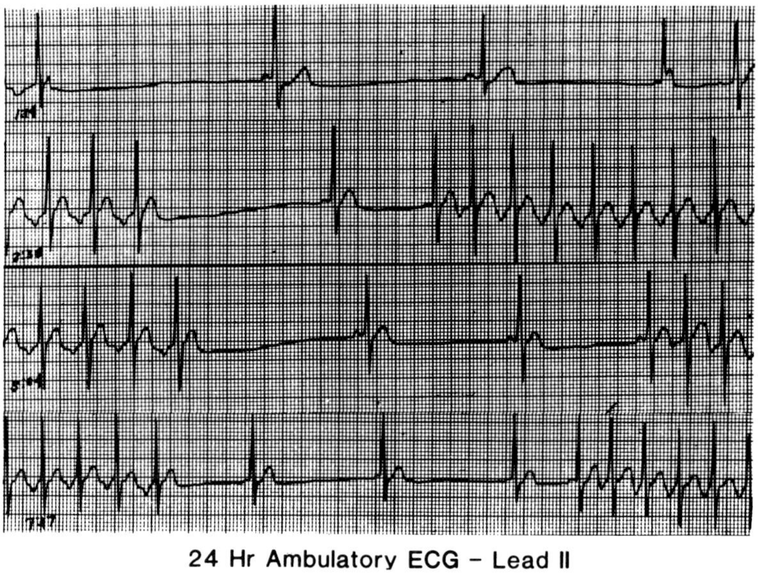

FIGURE 4–2. Bradyarrhythmia-tachyarrhythmia was recorded by Holter monitor in a patient who had undergone atrial septal defect closure. Sinoatrial bradycardia is present in the top recording. In each of the other recordings, pauses were interrupted by paroxysmal atrial tachycardia. The atrial tachycardia probably consisted of an atrial rate of 270 to 300 bpm, and the ventricular rate was 135 to 150 bpm. Paper speed was 25 mm/s. (ECG, electrocardiogram.)

ods of alternating bradycardia and tachycardia (Figs. 4–2 and 4–3). The slow heart rate may be of sinus, atrial, junctional, or even ventricular origin if junctional disease coexists. Most young patients with bradyarrhythmias or tachyarrhythmias previously have undergone an intracardiac operation of one or more of the following types: atrial septal defect repair, atrial repair of transposition of the great arteries, partial or total anomalous pulmonary venous connection, or repair of any defect requiring extensive atrial surgery (e.g., Fontan). Operated or nonoperated patients with right atrial (e.g., Ebstein's anomaly) or left atrial (e.g., mitral regurgitation or stenosis) volume/pressure overload also are at risk for these arrhythmias.

The mechanism of the tachyarrhythmia typically is atrial muscle re-entry. For each patient, the atrial rate is relatively constant, but the ventricular rate ranges from 150 bpm to 350 bpm among patients of different ages. The most common atrial/ventricular rate ratio is 2:1, but with excellent AV conduction or slower atrial rates, 1:1 conduction is relatively common. Atrial flutter usually is considered a type of atrial muscle re-entry tachycardia.[32] Although the term *atrial flutter* often is used loosely to describe any atrial muscle re-entry tachycardia with an atrial rate of 200 bpm to 350 bpm, classic atrial flutter by ECG shows typical sawtooth "flutter" waves. Atrial fibrillation is uncommon in infants, children, and adolescents.

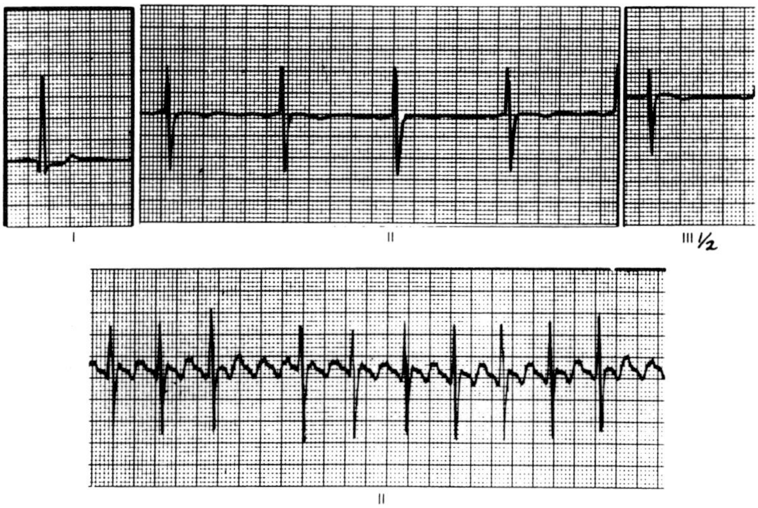

FIGURE 4–3. Rhythm was recorded by electrocardiogram at different times and shows bradyarrhythmia-tachyarrhythmias in a 5-year-old girl who recently had undergone repair of ostium primum atrial septal defect. In the top recording, low right atrial rhythm at 53 bpm depicts bradycardia, and in the bottom recording, typical atrial flutter with variable atrioventricular block depicts the tachyarrhythmia. During electrophysiology study, corrected sinus node recovery time measured more than 4000 ms. Paper speed was 25 mm/s.

Sinus nodal re-entry tachycardia is thought to involve re-entry within the sinus node as part of the micro-re-entry circuit.[33–35] Atrial muscle re-entry tachycardia within the HRA muscle would be expected to produce a P-wave axis and morphology identical to that produced by sinus nodal re-entry. Therefore, these two types of tachycardias are virtually indistinguishable by electrophysiologic study (EPS). Atrial muscle re-entry in other parts of the atrium causes P waves with a different morphology.

Automatic ectopic focus atrial tachycardia from the high right atrium also may be indistinguishable by surface ECG from the various atrial muscle re-entry tachycardias and from sinus nodal re-entry tachycardia. This is especially true if the onset and termination are not available for review. The onset and termination of re-entry atrial tachycardias (including atrial flutter) are paroxysmal, whereas the automatic ectopic tachycardias typically show a gradual shortening of atrial cycle length during onset and a gradual lengthening during termination.[36]

The mechanism of the bradycardia, regardless of the tachycardia, has been thought by some to be a result of "overdrive suppression" of an abnormal sinus node.[2] Although no data have been reported in children, there are conflicting data in adults. Some investigators have found that abnormal sinus node automaticity is independent of the tachycardia episodes. Often the atrial tachycardia is incessant, and the underlying bradycardia is not evident until measures are taken to control the tachycardia. When tachycardia stops, if sinus node automaticity is abnormal, pauses and bradycardia prevail. The type of bradycardia is dependent on the function and automaticity of the sinus node, atria, and AV node-His bundle.

Bradycardia predisposes to the development of ectopy, because longer sinus cycle lengths provide the opportunity for increased automaticity of subsidiary foci (e.g., premature atrial beats). Moreover, these patients often have coexisting atrial muscle disease that provides the substrate for abnormal atrial electrical function. Areas of abnormal atrial conduction and automaticity thus provide the opportunity for spontaneous induction and maintenance of atrial muscle or sinus node re-entry tachycardia.

Differential diagnosis of bradyarrhythmias or tachyarrhythmias is primarily made from studying the tachycardias. One of the most overlooked tachyarrhythmias is an atrial muscle tachycardia (discussed previously) with 2:1 AV conduction. Most commonly, the diagnosis of "sinus tachycardia" is made erroneously. A P wave is detected before each QRS, but another P wave is often missed because it is "buried" in the T wave of the preceding QRS. Another helpful clue is to note that the ventricular rate with this tachyarrhythmia varies little with activity or sleep (most commonly, heart rate is approximately 150 bpm). A high index of suspicion is essential to the diagnosis of this subtle tachyarrhythmia. Confirmation in most patients is necessary by either transesophageal or intracardiac recordings.

Exercise Testing

Exercise testing is a valuable noninvasive technique to evaluate sinus node function in patients older than 4 to 5 years. The major objective during exercise evaluation of sinus node function is to determine the maximum heart rate response. Therefore, it is imperative that the test is carried out to exhaustion. This is generally only possible in older children who are cooperative and motivated to perform. Measurement of aerobic capacity is valuable in determining whether maximal exercise has been achieved. Both bicycle ergometer and treadmill are accepted methods of exercise testing. It is important to record simultaneous limb leads. In this manner, the P-wave axis is determined, and sinus rhythm is confirmed before, during, and after exercise.

Exercise testing is most valuable in (1) patients with sinus bradycardia, (2) patients without sinus bradycardia in whom the diagnosis of SND is suspected for other reasons, and (3) patients in whom SND is known, but severity or clinical significance is unknown.

In patients with sinus bradycardia or decreased maximal heart rate response, the following question often arises: is this a sign of SND, or is it merely a clinically insignificant finding? The maximum heart rate response of normal children and adolescents during treadmill testing is frequently greater than 190 bpm and virtually always greater than 180 bpm.[37] Therefore, if maximum heart rate is less than 180 bpm during exercise to exhaustion, SND is present. Exercise testing also may be helpful in identifying patients with SND by noting an exaggerated decrease in heart rate after exercise, especially when symptoms correlate.

In patients who have underlying heart disease with a relatively high incidence of associated SND (e.g., atrial repair of transposition of the great arteries), SND may only become evident during exercise testing. This finding was noted by Hesslein et al in their study of 29 pediatric patients who had previously undergone Mustard repair for transposition of the great arteries.[24]

Only 2 patients had a resting heart rate less than two standard deviations from normal, but 22 had subnormal heart rate response during maximal treadmill testing. These investigators also found that in these patients treadmill exercise testing was a more sensitive indicator of SND than electrophysiologic testing. This conclusion was based on the finding that of 16 patients having an abnormal exercise heart rate response, only 9 were identified by electrophysiologic testing as having SND.

Moreover, in patients complaining of excessive "fatigue," exercise testing is valuable in differentiating between decreased exercise tolerance, decreased heart rate response, decreased motivation, and decreased conditioning.[38, 39]

Transesophageal Atrial Recording and Pacing

Transesophageal atrial recording and pacing is a minimally invasive technique whose utility is greatest with the tachyarrhythmias of SND. Often the question arises as to whether atrial tachycardia with 2:1 block is present. With this arrhythmia, the atrial electrogram recorded by transesophageal technique is diagnostic. The technique also is valuable because the atrial tachycardia can be converted by overdrive transesophageal atrial pacing. Although the technique also can be used to determine sinus node recovery time after atrial pacing, this is not often done. Blomstrom-Lundqvist and Edvardsson[40] found no statistical difference in either the sinus node recovery times or the SA conduction times between the transesophageal technique and the intracardiac technique. The specific methodology of transesophageal atrial recording and stimulation has been reviewed by Benson et al.[41]

Atrial Recording and Pacing Using Temporary Epicardial Electrodes

Like transesophageal atrial pacing, atrial recording and pacing using temporary epicardial electrodes is not strictly noninvasive. The epicardial wires are placed during intracardiac operation, but later, when these leads are used for recording and pacing, only a noninvasive technique is used.

Similar to transesophageal atrial pacing, this technique is valuable in detecting atrial activity when the surface ECG does not show distinct P waves and when there is a high index of suspicion that "buried" P waves may be present. Sinus node function is assessable with this technique by connecting a pacing stimulator to the temporary leads and then carrying out the same pacing protocol used for intracardiac electrophysiology testing. Other than establishing a baseline, however, the interpretation and clinical significance of SND immediately postoperatively is unknown.

INVASIVE DIAGNOSIS

Intracardiac Electrophysiology Study

Although intracardiac EPS has been considered the "gold standard," it is now virtually never used as a primary indicated test. During intracardiac EPS, sinus node activity is assessed directly by recording the sinus node electrogram or indirectly by recording the HRA electrogram. The sinus node electrogram can be recorded by special techniques as well and can be used to directly assess sinus node automaticity. By measuring the time from the onset of the sinus node electrogram to the onset of the HRA electrogram, a direct measurement of the SA conduction time can be obtained but is rarely performed. The indirect technique, whether during measurement of sinus node recovery or during calculation of SA conduction time, always includes the unknown atriosinus conduction time.

The vast majority of electrophysiology laboratories use indirect methods. The indirect techniques, although associated with many confirmed limitations, have compared favorably to the direct technique in several studies. These results are important, because the direct technique requires more time and effort in the electrophysiology laboratory. The details of electrophysiologic evaluation of sinus node function, which consist of determining the sinus node recovery time (SNRT) or the total SA conduction time (SACT), with or without autonomic blockade,[42] are not reviewed here. A detailed description of intracardiac electrophysiologic testing of sinus node function has been given previously.[6]

Indications

The lack of high sensitivity and specificity of sinus node function testing during intracardiac EPS has resulted in fewer patients undergoing these invasive studies. Although it was common practice several years ago to study children only for evaluation of sinus node function, it is now uncommon because of the evidence that shows noninvasive testing is often as good as or better than invasive EPS.[23, 24] Clinical decisions and recommendations are based predominantly on symptoms documented with noninvasive testing.

TREATMENT

PREVENTION

The surgeon may affect the incidence of SND after operation with attention to three principles during surgery. First, it is imperative that the anatomy of the sinus node and sinus node artery is known. Anderson, Ho, and Anderson studied 25 infant hearts at necropsy and found that the sinus node location was relatively constant, but the sinus node artery supply was considerably variable.[43] In 22 of the 25 hearts, the sinus node was located in the lateral area of the superior vena caval–HRA junction. In the other three, it was located at the summit of the crest of the right atrial appendage. The caudal extension of the sinus node was more variable, and in some hearts the border extended inferiorly to the inferior vena caval orifice. The sinus node artery approached the sinus node posteriorly in 40% of the hearts, anteriorly in 40% of the hearts, and by both directions in an anastomotic ring in 16% of the hearts. Second, the surgeon's attention to superior vena caval cannulation is important because SND may result from superior vena caval cannulation via the orifice to the high right atrium.[44] After cannulation was changed from low to high superior vena cava, the incidence of SND decreased.[45] Third, myocardial preservation during surgery is an important factor. Bink-Boelkens et al found that lack of cardioplegia and long ischemic time were associated with postoperative SND.[46]

SND arrhythmias can also be prevented by other efforts. Age at operation appears to be an important factor. For example, the optimum age for surgery appears to be between 3 and 12 months for atrial repair for transposition of the great arteries. Also, closure of atrial septal defect in early childhood is associated with a decreased incidence of SND and atrial arrhythmias compared with closure during adolescence or adulthood.[47]

Prevention of SND and atrial arrhythmias has been a major impetus to change the type of surgical repair for transposition of the great arteries. The arterial switch repair pioneered by Jatene has now become the procedure of choice. The Senning repair previously gained popularity over the Mustard procedure because the technique appeared to offer less potential damage to the sinus node and atrium. However, a prospective study by Deanfield et al revealed no differences in clinical SND after the Senning procedure compared with the Mustard operation.[48]

INDICATIONS

The decision to recommend treatment is straightforward when symptoms of syncope or near syncope occur during documented arrhythmias of SND. It is also not difficult to recommend treatment for patients with symptoms of congestive heart failure or severe fatigue that are direct results of SND. However, treatment decisions are complicated when symptoms are not present or are difficult to document during SND, especially in high-risk patients. For these reasons, recommendations for asymptomatic patients and for symptomatic patients with undocumentable SND are somewhat controversial.

One of the most arbitrary recommendations concerns the lower limit of accepted asymptomatic bradycardia.[6] A "safe" lower heart rate limit is unknown. Controlled studies have not been performed comparing nontreated asymptomatic patients who have very low heart rates with those who undergo permanent pacemaker implantation. There are no data to show that sleeping sinus or junctional bradycardia is more life threatening at rates between 20 bpm and 30 bpm than at rates between 30 bpm and 40 bpm. Moreover, it is unknown what the difference is between sleeping and awake heart rates when considering permanent pacemaker implantation. In a prospective study of congenital complete AV block by Dewey et al,[49] mean awake heart rate less than 50 bpm was associated with symptoms.

Many variable associated factors and the extent of underlying disease are important. In a multicenter study of 372 patients who had undergone Mustard repair, pacemaker implantation was carried out in all 7 patients with rates less than 30 bpm, and each survived.[12] Because the study did not include an equal number of patients who did not undergo pacemaker implantation and data regarding symptoms (it is implied that they were asymptomatic), it is not known whether pacemakers are truly necessary in similar patients. However, it appears prudent to recommend treatment for such patients, because each of the 7 patients survived. It also is important to point out that 11 asymptomatic patients (average age, 6 years) with heart rates between 30 bpm and 40 bpm did not receive a permanent pacemaker, and each survived (average follow-up, 4.5 years). More controlled studies are needed before specific treatment recommendations can be made for asymptomatic patients on the basis of age and heart rate.

Another recommendation concerns permanent pacemaker implantation when starting antiarrhythmic drugs in patients with known SND or patients at high risk for SND. An association was made between the use of quinidine and sudden death in patients who had previously undergone Mustard repair for transposition of the great arteries.[50] The decision to recommend prophylactic permanent pacemaker implantation in these patients was based on quinidine's known adverse effects on sinus node function and the known high incidence of SND in these patients. Since then, other causes for sudden death in these patients have been proposed, specifically, quinidine-induced torsades de pointes. Subsequently, the recommendation to prophylactically implant a permanent pacemaker with any antiarrhythmic drug was modified, and pacemaker implantation may not be necessary in all patients.[51] From available data and with the knowledge that torsades de pointes is highly associated with sinus pauses, it seems prudent to strongly consider prophylactic pacemaker implantation for patients with SND (to prevent sinus pauses) who are treated with antiarrhythmic drugs that prolong the QT interval (classes IA, IC, and III).

Further caution is emphasized when using quinidine. Torsades de pointes occurs only rarely and usually during onset of treatment or during hypokalemia.[52, 53] Hospitalization with ECG telemetry is indicated during the first few days of starting quinidine therapy.[54] Monitoring of serum quinidine and potassium is advised during acute and chronic treatment to decrease the chance of torsades de pointes. Similarly, other type IA, IC, and III drugs are known to cause torsades de pointes, and similar caution and monitoring are advised during therapy with these drugs.

The risk of sudden death does not appear to be great for the asymptomatic patient older than 6 years with sinus or junctional bradycardia at rates greater than 30 bpm.[12] There are no data to show that sudden death is prevented by pacemaker implantation in these patients, including those who have undergone atrial baffle repair for transposition of the great arteries.[12] However, the long-term effects of bradycardia-induced or bradycardia-associated cardiomegaly are possibly related to adverse outcomes, but no data exist.

The last category of patients is the patient with syncope but in whom only mild SND is found during evaluation. Frequently, the event ECG is valuable, because symptoms of dizziness are not associated with an arrhythmia severe enough to cause the reported symptoms.[5] These patients do not require treatment. However, the decision for treatment is complicated in patients with only mild SND who have a syncope history compatible with an arrhythmogenic cause but in whom correlation with SND cannot be documented. It is imperative that complete EPS be carried out to search for other arrhythmic causes of syncope. If none are found, the clinician is faced with a treatment dilemma. Usually the best plan is to make additional efforts to document correlation of symptoms with arrhythmia. However, in some patients, circumstances may warrant treatment if further delay is considered dangerous.

MEDICAL TREATMENT

Acute emergency medical treatment is indicated when severe sinus or junctional bradycardia or frequent sinus arrest results in loss of consciousness. Regardless of cause, intravenous atropine (0.04 mg/kg) or isoproterenol (0.05–0.5 μg/kg/min), or both, usually is effective. A temporary transvenous pacemaker should be placed if these drugs are unsuccessful in increasing heart rate to a satisfactory level.

Chronic medical treatment has not been acceptable as standard treatment for SND. Several pharmacologic agents are available, but success has been variable and side effects have been prevalent. The patients with the greatest chance of benefit appear to be those with vagotonia-related causes (i.e., those with neurocardiogenic mechanisms and symptoms). Successful treatment has been achieved with one or more of the following agents: fludrocortisone acetate (Florinef)–scopolamine patches, atropine derivatives (propantheline bromide), adrenergic stimulatory drugs (sublingual isoproterenol, prenalterol, xamoterol), theophylline, hydralazine, ephedrine, disopyramide, and, surprisingly, beta blockers have been successful in selected patients.

The early data show promise for only a few selected patients. The patients who appear to have the greatest chance of benefit from medical treatment are those who have mild to moderate symptoms (e.g., dizziness, fatigue), with hypervagotonia as the major underlying mechanism for SND. Furthermore, hypervagotonia is self-limited in many patients, because symptoms have disappeared in follow-up. It must be emphasized, however, that these agents are contraindicated in patients with bradyarrhythmias who also have (or are likely to experience) tachyarrhythmias.

PERMANENT PACEMAKER IMPLANTATION

Bradycardia remains the most frequent indication for implantation of pacemakers in children.[55] When treatment is indicated for infants, children, and adolescents with SND, the accepted mode is permanent pacemaker implantation. The pacemaker choices for SND treatment include the following types of multiprogrammable generators: atrial demand (AAI), dual-chambered demand or triggered (DDD), and ventricular demand (VVI); rate response may be added to any mode. The type of pacemaker system recommended depends on the underlying arrhythmias, AV conduction function, underlying heart disease (ventricular function), age and body size, and patient preference for location of the pacemaker generator (scar).

In patients with normal AV conduction, atrial demand with rate response (AAIR) is often the ideal choice because it offers the advantage of the atrial contribution to cardiac output. The AAIR is best suited for transvenous leads, although the subxiphoid approach and the thoracotomy approach are available.

Choosing the type of pacemaker is somewhat more complex when tachyarrhythmias are also a part of the patient's SND bradyarrhythmias. Data in adult and pediatric patients have suggested that improved hemodynamics from atrial or dual-chamber pacemakers may, in fact, decrease the incidence of atrial tachyarrhythmias.[56–58] Automatic antitachycardia pacemaker systems are useful in selected patients with SND who have tachyarrhythmias as a major clinical problem.

FOLLOW-UP OF PACEMAKER IMPLANTATION

Follow-up data are readily available because SND is a relatively common indication for pacemaker implantation in children and young adults.[55] Gillette et al found that 45 of 49 symptomatic children (92%) had relief of symptoms after pacemaker implantation.[59] No early deaths occurred, but 2 patients died later of causes unrelated to SND. In those with coexisting tachyarrhythmias, symptoms are more difficult to eliminate. Gillette et al found that only 11 of 18 patients (61%) with SND and concomitant tachyarrhythmia were free of symptoms after pacemaker implantation, suggesting that simple bradycardia pacemaker implantation does not prevent tachyarrhythmias in these children. Exercise testing has proven valuable in the follow-up of patients who have a DDD or activity-detecting rate-variable pacemaker.[60] In this manner, the high rate performance can be checked to verify optimum programmed indexes.

When atrial pacemakers were initially implanted for SND in patients who had normal AV conduction, investigators were uncertain as to whether late AV conduction dysfunction would appear. Follow-up studies in adults have shown an insignificant incidence of AV conduction disorders.[61, 62] Although similar studies have not been carried out in children, the adult data are supportive of the use of atrial pacemakers in patients with SND without AV conduction dysfunction.

REFERENCES

1. Mandel WJ, Obayashi K, Laks MM: Overview of the sick sinus syndrome. Chest 66:223–224, 1974.
2. Kaplan BM, Langendorf R, Lev M, et al: Tachycardia-bradycardia syndrome (so-called "sick sinus syndrome"). Am J Cardiol 31:497–508, 1973.
3. Ferrer IM: The Sick Sinus Syndrome. Mt Kisco, NY, Futura, 1974, p 37.
4. Dhingra RC: Sinus node dysfunction. Pacing Clin Electrophysiol 6:1062–1069, 1983.
5. Kugler JD, Yabek SM: Sick sinus syndrome: Clinical features and noninvasive evaluation. In Yabek SM, Gillette PC, Kugler JD (eds): The Sinus Node in Pediatrics. London, Churchill Livingstone, 1984, p 48.
6. Kugler JD: Sinus node dysfunction. In Gillette P, Garson A Jr (ed): Pediatric Arrhythmias: Electrophysiology and Pacing. Philadelphia, WB Saunders, 1990, pp 250–300.
7. Kugler JD: Sinus node dysfunction. Prog Pediatr Cardiol 3:226–235, 1994.
8. Yabek SM, Swensson RE, Jarmakani JM: Electrocardiographic recognition of sinus node dysfunction in children and young adults. Circulation 56:235–239, 1977.
9. Yabek SM, Jarmakani JM: Sinus node dysfunction in children, adolescents, and young adults. Pediatrics 61:593–598, 1978.
10. Roifman C, Dembo L, Grenadier E, et al: Sinus node dysfunction in a healthy pediatric population. Isr J Med Sci 20:497–500, 1984.
11. Bricker JT, Garson A Jr, Gillette PC: A family history of seizures associated with sudden cardiac deaths. Am J Dis Child 138:866–868, 1984.
12. Flinn CJ, Wolff GS, Dick M II, et al: Cardiac rhythm after the Mustard operation for complete transposition of the great arteries. N Engl J Med 310:1635–1638, 1984.
13. Hayes CJ, Gersony WM: Arrhythmias after the Mustard operation for transposition of the great arteries: A long-term study. J Am Coll Cardiol 7:133–138, 1986.
14. Beerman LB, Neches WH, Fricker FJ, et al: Arrhythmias in transposition of the great arteries after the Mustard operation. Am J Cardiol 51:1530–1534, 1983.
15. Scagliotti D, Strasberg B, Duffy CE, et al: Inducible polymorphous ventricular tachycardia following Mustard operation for transposition of the great arteries. Pediatr Cardiol 5:39–43, 1984.
16. Kugler JD: Sinus node dysfunction in young patients with congenital long QT syndrome. Am Heart J 121:1132–1136, 1991.

17. Gelatt MD, Hamilton RM, McCrindle BW, et al. Arrhythmia and mortality after the Mustard procedure: A 30-year single-center experience. J Am Coll Cardiol 29:194–201, 1997.
18. Kugler JD: The sinoatrial node and its dysfunction. In Liebman J, Plonsey R, Rudy Y (eds): New Directions in Pediatric and Fundamental Electrocardiography. The Hague, The Netherlands, Martinus Nijhoff, 1987, pp 107–135.
19. Beder SD, Gillette PC: Non-surgical etiologies of sick sinus syndrome. In Yabek SM, Gillette PC, Kugler JK (eds): The Sinus Node in Pediatrics. London, Churchill Livingstone, 1984, p 121.
20. Pop T, Fleischman D: Measurement of sinus node recovery time after atrial pacing. In Bonke FIM (ed): The Sinus Node: Structure, Function and Clinical Relevance. The Hague, The Netherlands, Martinus Nijhoff, 1978, p 23.
21. Reiffel JA, Bigger JT Jr, Cramer M, et al: Ability of Holter electrocardiographic recording and atrial stimulation to detect sinus nodal dysfunction in symptomatic and asymptomatic patients with sinus bradycardia. Am J Cardiol 40:189–194, 1977.
22. Thormann J, Schlepper M, Kramer W: Diurnal changes and reproducibility of corrected sinus node recovery time. Cathet Cardiovasc Diag 9:439–451, 1983.
23. Fournier A, Smith RT, Moak JP, et al: Sinus bradycardia in children. Proceedings from the XXII Annual Meeting of the Association of European Paediatric Cardiologists, Dubrovnik, Yugoslavia, May 5–9, 1986 (abstract).
24. Hesslein PS, Gutgesell HP, Gillette PC, et al: Exercise assessment of sinoatrial node function following the Mustard operation. Am Heart J 103:351–357, 1982.
25. Anderson RH, Yen HS, Becker AE, et al: The development of the sinoatrial node. In Bonke FIM (ed): The Sinus Node. The Hague, The Netherlands, Martinus Nijhoff, 1978, p 166.
26. Southall DP, Richards J, Mitchell P, et al: Study of cardiac rhythm in healthy newborn infants. Br Heart J 43:14–20, 1980.
27. Southall DP, Johnston F, Shinebourne EA, et al: Twenty-four-hour electrocardiographic study of heart rate and rhythm patterns in population of healthy children. Br Heart J 45:281–291, 1981.
28. Montague TJ, Taylor PG, Stockton R, et al: The spectrum of cardiac rate and rhythm in normal newborns. Pediatr Cardiol 2:33–38, 1982.
29. Viitasalo MT, Kala R, Eisalo A: Ambulatory electrocardiographic recording in endurance athletes. Br Heart J 47:213–220, 1982.
30. Garson A Jr, Gillette PC, McNamara DG (eds): A Guide to Cardiac Dysrhythmias in Children. New York, Grune & Stratton, 1980, p 117.
31. Brodsky M, Wu D, Denes P, et al: Arrhythmias documented by 24 hour continuous electrocardiographic monitoring in 50 male medical students without apparent heart disease. Am J Cardiol 39:390–395, 1977.
32. Disertori M, Inama G, Vergara G, et al: Evidence of a reentry circuit in the common type of atrial flutter in man. Circulation 67:434–440, 1983.
33. Wu D, Amat-Y-Leon F, Denes P, et al: Demonstration of sustained sinus and atrial reentry as a mechanism of paroxysmal supraventricular tachycardia. Circulation 51:234–243, 1975.
34. Jazayeri MR, Massumi A, Mihalick MJ, et al: Sinus node reentry: Case report and review of electrocardiographic and electrophysiologic features. Texas Heart Inst J 12:249, 1985.
35. Gomes JA, Hariman RJ, Kang PS, et al: Sustained symptomatic sinus node reentrant tachycardia: Incidence, clinical significance, electrophysiologic observations and the effects of antiarrhythmic agents. J Am Coll Cardiol 5:45–57, 1985.
36. Gillette PC, Garson A Jr: Electrophysiologic and pharmacologic characteristics of automatic ectopic atrial tachycardia. Circulation 56:571–575, 1977.
37. Hesslein PS: Noninvasive diagnosis of dysrhythmias. In Gillette PC, Garson A Jr (eds): Pediatric Cardiac Dysrhythmias. New York, Grune & Stratton, 1981, p 59.
38. Paridon SM, Humes RA, Pinsky WW: The role of chronotropic impairment during exercise after the Mustard operation. J Am Coll Cardiol 17:729–732, 1991.
39. Washington RL, VanGundy GC, Cohen C, et al: Normal aerobic and anaerobic exercise data for North American school-age children. J Pediatr 112:223–233, 1988.
40. Blomstrom-Lundqvist C, Edvardsson N: Transesophageal versus intracardiac atrial stimulation in assessing electrophysiologic parameters of the sinus and AV nodes and of the atrial myocardium. Pacing Clin Electrophysiol 10:1081–1095, 1987.
41. Benson DW Jr, Dunnigan A, Benditt DG, et al: Transesophageal cardiac pacing: History, application, technique. Clin Prog Pacing Electrophysiol 2:360, 1984.
42. Marcus B, Gillette PC, Garson A Jr: Intrinsic heart rate following autonomic blockade in children and young adults: An index of sinus node function isolated from autonomic control. Am Heart J 119:911–915, 1990.
43. Anderson KR, Ho SY, Anderson RH: Location and vascular supply of sinus node in human heart. Br Heart J 41:28–32, 1979.
44. Smith PK, Buhrman WC, Levett JM, et al: Supraventricular conduction abnormalities following cardiac operations. J Thorac Cardiovasc Surg 85:105–115, 1983.
45. El-Said GM, Gillette PC, Cooley DA, et al: Protection of the sinus node in Mustard's operation. Circulation 53:788–791, 1976.
46. Bink-Boelkens M, Velvis H, Homan van der Heide JJ, et al: Dysrhythmias after atrial surgery in children. Am Heart J 106:125–130, 1983.
47. Brandenburg RO Jr, Holmes DR Jr, Brandenburg RO, et al: Clinical follow-up study of paroxysmal supraventricular tachyarrhythmias after operative repair of secundum type atrial septal defect in adults. Am J Cardiol 51:273–276, 1983.
48. Deanfield JE, Macartney FJ, Bull C, et al: Arrhythmia and late mortality after Mustard and Senning operations for transposition: A 7-year prospective study. Circulation 74(suppl II):50, 1986 (abstract).
49. Dewey RC, Capeless MA, Levy AM: Use of ambulatory electrocardiographic monitoring to identify high-risk patients with congenital complete heart block. N Engl J Med 316:835–839, 1987.
50. Kugler JD: Sinoatrial node dysfunction. In Gillette PC, Garson A Jr (eds): Pediatric Cardiac Dysrhythmias. New York, Grune & Stratton, 1981, p 265.
51. Dreifus LS, Fisch C, Griffin JC, et al: Guidelines for implantation of cardiac pacemakers and antiarrhythmia devices. Circulation 18:1–13, 1991.
52. Webb CL, Dick M, Rocchini AP, et al: Quinidine syncope in children. J Am Coll Cardiol 9:1031–1037, 1987.
53. Roden DM, Thompson KA, Hoffman BF, et al: Clinical features and basic mechanisms of quinidine-induced arrhythmias. J Am Coll Cardiol 8:73A, 1986.
54. Garson A Jr: Medicolegal problems in the management of cardiac arrhythmias in children. Pediatrics 79:84–88, 1987.
55. Friedman RA, Collins E, Fenrich AL: Pacing in children: Indications and techniques. Prog Pediatr Cardiol 4:21–29, 1995.

56. Rosenqvist M, Brandt J, Schuller H: Atrial versus ventricular pacing in sinus node disease: A treatment comparison study. Am Heart J 111:292–297, 1986.
57. Stone JM, Bhakta RD, Lutgen J: Dual chamber sequential pacing management of sinus node dysfunction: Advantages over single chamber pacing. Am Heart J 104:1319–1327, 1982.
58. Silka MJ, Manwill JR, Kron J, McAnulty JH: Bradycardia-mediated tachyarrhythmias in congenital heart disease and responses to chronic pacing at physiologic rates. Am J Cardiol 65:488–493, 1990.
59. Gillette PC, Shannon C, Garson A Jr, et al: Pacemaker treatment of sick sinus syndrome in children. J Am Coll Cardiol 1:1325–1329, 1983.
60. Bricker JT, Garson A Jr, Traweek MS, et al: The use of exercise testing in children to evaluate abnormalities of pacemaker function not apparent at rest. Pacing Clin Electrophysiol 8:656, 1985.
61. Hayes DL, Furman S: Stability of AV conduction in sick sinus node syndrome patients with implanted atrial pacemakers. Am Heart J 107:644–647, 1984.
62. Rosenqvist M, Vallin H, Edhag O: Clinical and electrophysiologic course of sinus node disease: Five-year follow-up study. Am Heart J 109:513–522, 1985.

CHAPTER 5

ATRIOVENTRICULAR BLOCK AND BUNDLE BRANCH BLOCK

Bertrand A. Ross and Paul C. Gillette

This chapter deals with the definition and clinical features of atrioventricular (AV) block. The varying degrees (i.e., first, second, and third degree), although sharing a common feature (conduction changes from sinus node activation to ventricular activation), may be much different in cause and clinical significance. Additionally, bundle branch block, including right and left bundle branch block (LBBB), as well as fascicular blocks are also addressed.

FIRST-DEGREE AV BLOCK

First-degree AV block is defined as a PR interval greater than established norms. This interval is more age dependent than rate dependent, so normal intervals have been determined based on the age of the patient. A number of causes or associations between first-degree AV block and disease states have been reported (Table 5–1). It has generally been proposed that those structural heart lesions that produce first-degree AV block do so by stretching the atria in the area of the AV node. First-degree AV block has also been reported to occur in up to 6% of neonates.[1] Narula et al[2] found that the delay occurs at more than one site in adults, but the AV node was the dominant site, occurring in 83% of patients. There is little clinical significance of first-degree AV block when it is found.

Table 5–1. Disease States Associated with First-Degree Atrioventricular Block

Rheumatic fever
Diphtheria
Trichinosis
Chagas' disease
Rubella
Mumps
Lyme disease
Hypothermia
Increased parasympathetic tone
Electrolyte abnormalities: hypokalemia, hyperkalemia; hypocalcemia, hypercalcemia; hypoglycemia; hypomagnesemia
Congenital heart disease: PDA, ASD (primum and secundum), Ebstein's anomaly, TAPVC, LTGA
Duchenne's muscular dystrophy
Myotonic dystrophy
Viral myocarditis
Kearns-Sayre syndrome

PDA, patent ductus arteriosus; ASD, atrial septal defect; TAPVC, total anomalous pulmonary venous connection; LTGA, levotransposition of the great arteries.

SECOND-DEGREE AV BLOCK

Second-degree AV block was first described by Wenckebach in 1899 and again in 1906 when he timed jugular venous pulsations and associated atrial beats with blocked ventricular beats.[3, 4] Hay also reported the same findings in 1906.[5] Later Wenckebach described one type of periodicity in which the A-C interval gradually prolonged, with the eventual dropping out of the C wave (thought to be a result of impaired AV conduction) and a second type consisting of dropped beats not associated with A-C lengthening, but instead resulting from decreased ventricular excitability. After the introduction of electrocardiography, Mobitz described these two types of conduction abnormalities as type I (progressive prolongation of the PR interval until a dropped ventricular beat occurs) and type II (a constant PR interval with dropped ventricular beats).[6] Wenckebach and Winterburg were suggesting by 1927 that there were frequent variations from the typical periodicity.[7] Mobitz then called attention to the association of Adams-Stokes syndrome with type II block.[8]

MOBITZ TYPE I (WENCKEBACH) BLOCK

Wenckebach described type I block as (1) progressive PR lengthening, (2) the greatest increase in the PR occurring between the first and second

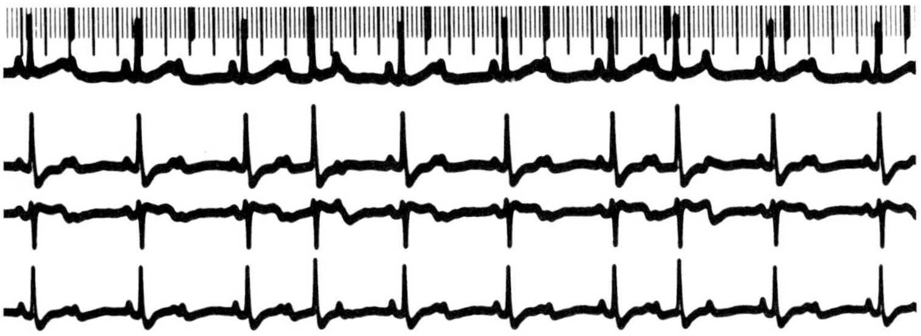

FIGURE 5–1. Wenckebach (Mobitz Type I) atrioventricular block in a 3:2 and 2:1 pattern. The initial P wave after the blocked P waves has a shorter PR interval than the last conducted P wave.

conducted beats, (3) progressive shortening of the RR intervals, and (4) a pause equal to less than twice the preceding PP interval.[7] The incidence of type I second-degree AV block appears to be low for both adults and children, although there is much more information available about adults (Fig. 5–1).

The periodicity that meets the four criteria originally described by Wenckebach has been labeled *typical Wenckebach*. However, there are numerous cases of *atypical Wenckebach* in which one or more of these criteria are not met, but the general pattern of a lengthening PR interval followed by a nonconducted P wave occurs.[9–14] Denes et al[15] determined the frequency of typical and atypical Wenckebach (both spontaneous and pacing induced) in a group of adults. In naturally occurring Wenckebach, 86% was atypical and 14% typical.[15] In addition, the incidence of atypical Wenckebach was 100% when the Wenckebach ratio increased to greater than 4:3. (The 4:3 ratio was the most common spontaneous ratio.) It should be noted that the spontaneous Wenckebach periods were secondary to myocardial infarction or digitalis excess. However, even in those patients who had Wenckebach block periods produced by atrial pacing during routine electrophysiology testing, the atypical type was more common (66% vs. 34%). Once again, the atypical form was more common with the higher ratios. Five types of atypical Wenckebach have been described and are listed in Table 5–2. Kinoshita and Konishi in the early 1980s showed other variants as well.[16] Wenckebach periodicity has been reported to occur at an increased incidence in highly trained athletes, in which the atypical form also appears to be predominant.[16, 17] El-Sherif and colleagues[18] described a type of atypical Wenckebach that appeared to mimic Mobitz type II block. However, this has less relevance in pediatric patients because this entity was associated with an acute inferior myocardial infarction. Autonomic tone probably plays a role in the variances of type I second-degree block.

The exact pathophysiologic mechanism of type I second-degree AV block is unknown, but there are numerous theories (Table 5–3). All of the presented theories are affected by hemodynamics and variations in autonomic nervous system tone as well as by the very complex anatomic and electrophysiologic characteristics of the AV node. Clearly, the association of Wenckebach periodicity with individuals with a predominance of vagal tone implicates the autonomic nervous system at least at some point in the production of Wenckebach periodicity. However, the exact interaction between autonomic tone and cellular mechanisms is unknown and may not be the same for all Wenckebach periodicity.

MOBITZ TYPE II AV BLOCK

Second-degree Mobitz type II AV block is defined as the intermittent loss of AV conduction without a preceding lengthening of the PR interval. In addition, the first PR interval after the dropped beat should be no shorter than the PR interval of the last conducted P wave. It has

Table 5–2. Types of Atypical Wenckebach Block

Last increment increased from the previous increment
Last increment was the largest increment
PR interval repeated at least once during the period
PR interval decreasing at least once during the cycle
Incremental increase in the PR interval not the greatest between the first and second conducted P waves

Table 5–3. Theories of Wenckebach Block

Increased vagal tone (absolute or relative)
Increase in conduction time
Longitudinal dissociation
Concealed dissociation
Concealed re-entry
Fatigue
Accumulation of extracellular potassium ions
Encroachment of succeeding impulses
Electrotonus

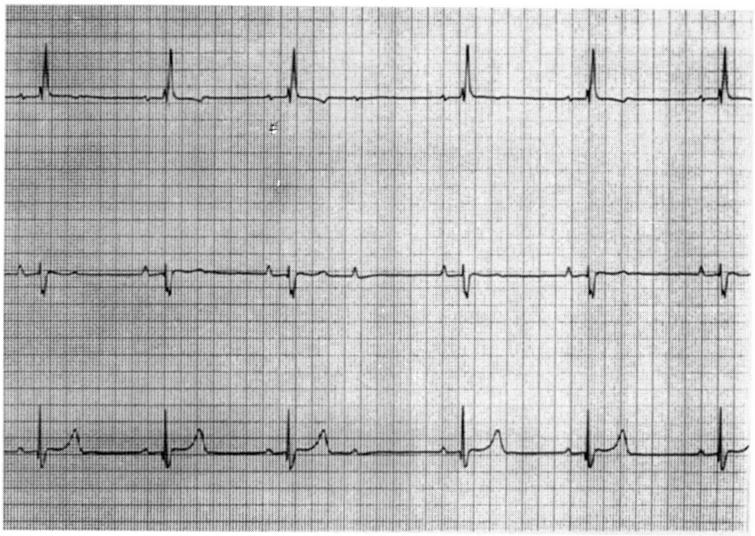

FIGURE 5–2. Surface electrocardiogram leads V_1, II, and V_6 show right bundle branch block, left axis deviation, first-degree atrioventricular (AV) block, and Mobitz type II second-degree AV block in a 5-year-old patient who presented with syncope.

been stated that a shortening of greater than 20 milliseconds in the first PR interval after the dropped beat is more likely to be indicative of Wenckebach block.[19] However, as Zipes pointed out, this approach may be too simplistic (Fig. 5–2).[20] Type II AV block is uncommon and, if present, usually implies an abnormal conduction system. In children it may be found in normally structured hearts or in patients with a damaged conduction system from surgery for structural congenital heart disease. In both cases, there is usually progression to complete heart block. In adults it most commonly occurs after an anterior myocardial infarction. The concern regarding type II AV block is its association with Adams-Stokes attacks and sudden death.[21–23]

TWO-TO-ONE AV BLOCK

The inability of alternating atrial impulses to conduct to the ventricles is termed *2:1 AV block.* This can be caused by block either in the AV node or the proximal His-Purkinje system (Fig. 5–3). However, 2:1 block cannot be classified as type I or type II, because the surface electrocardiogram (ECG) cannot determine whether there is any degree of PR lengthening before the dropped beat. Therefore, a variation must be found in the conduction pattern from 2:1 to be certain of the true nature of the block (see Fig. 5–2).

ADVANCED SECOND-DEGREE AV BLOCK

Advanced second-degree AV block is the loss of AV conduction for several consecutive P waves. When one atrial impulse is conducted to the ventricle, followed by two nonconducted impulses, it is termed 3:1 conduction; conduction of one out of four atrial impulses is 4:1 conduc-

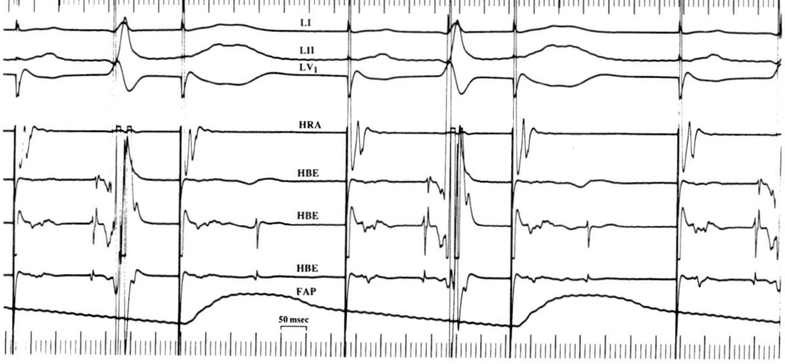

FIGURE 5–3. Two-to-one (2:1) atrioventricular (AV) block below the His bundle recording site during atrial pacing in a syncopal but otherwise normal infant.

tion. This type of block generally progresses to complete heart block.

CLINICAL SIGNIFICANCE

The concern regarding any type of heart block centers around the symptoms it produces and the likelihood of sudden death. Mobitz type II is associated with Adams-Stokes attacks, sudden death, and progression to complete heart block, whereas Mobitz type I is, for the most part, an incidental finding of little long-term significance.

The clinical significance of Mobitz type I or II block may also be dependent on whether it is associated with a wide QRS complex. Second-degree AV block in the presence of intraventricular conduction delay is usually associated with Mobitz type II AV block and may have a more ominous prognosis.[24] Therefore, differentiating Mobitz type I from Mobitz type II is clinically important. Mobitz type I has, for the most part, been localized to the AV node, whereas Mobitz type II occurs more distally in the His bundle or bundle branches.

The association of symptoms (i.e., syncope) with Mobitz type II AV block is primarily based on studies of adult patients after myocardial infarction. However, Kelly, Brodsky, and Krovetz documented two pediatric cases of Mobitz type II AV block that progressed to complete heart block.[25] One patient had undergone surgery to repair tetralogy of Fallot, and the other patient was without structural heart disease. Both patients also had associated right bundle branch block (RBBB). In these two patients, Mobitz type II block preceded the development of complete heart block. One patient had symptoms while suffering from Mobitz type II block, and one had no symptoms until the development of complete heart block. Because Mobitz type II block is uncommon in children, its natural history is unclear; however, available information indicates that Mobitz type II block that is produced by surgery or that develops as an idiopathic abnormality of the conduction system mirrors the experience in adults, progressing to high-grade second-degree block and complete AV block.

TREATMENT

Treatment of second-degree AV block consists of an implantable pacemaker and is generally necessary only for those patients with Mobitz type II AV block. However, the timing of the intervention depends on the clinical situation and must be individualized for each patient. We recommend treatment for the postoperative patient with Mobitz type II block if it continues for more than 7 days. In a child with a structurally normal heart, development of Mobitz type II AV block probably indicates advancing conduction system disease. Permanent pacing is indicated at the time Mobitz type II AV block is diagnosed.

THIRD-DEGREE (COMPLETE) AV BLOCK

Third-degree (complete) AV block is defined as the inability of an atrial impulse to be propagated to the ventricles. The diagnosis is, therefore, dependent on electrocardiographic proof that no atrial impulse that should conduct to the ventricles actually does conduct. Care must be taken to ensure that the AV dissociation seen on ECG is caused by complete AV block and not by a junctional or ventricular rate faster than the atria, as that seen in accelerated junctional rhythm or severe sinus bradycardia with an appropriate junctional rate. Generally, a long rhythm strip will be helpful in making this distinction (Fig. 5–4).

CONGENITAL COMPLETE AV BLOCK

INCIDENCE

The incidence of congenital complete AV block has generally been reported to be between 1/15,000 and 1/25,000 live births, with most estimates at 1/22,000 live births.[26–30] In addition, congenital complete AV block may present as familial clusters. The cooperative study of Michaelsson and Engle showed 14 families in which two siblings were affected and in which examples of congenital complete AV block in more than one generation were evident.[27] Congenital complete AV block spanning three generations has also been reported by Winkler, Nora, and Nora.[31] Approximately 25 to 33% of the cases of congenital complete AV block will have associated structural heart disease. By far, the most commonly associated lesion is L-transposition of the great arteries with ventricular inversion. However, congenital complete AV block is also frequently seen in abnormalities of atrial and ventricular septum formation as well as in isolated cases with other cardiac abnormalities.

ETIOLOGY

The cause of congenital complete AV block is not fully understood at this time but appears to

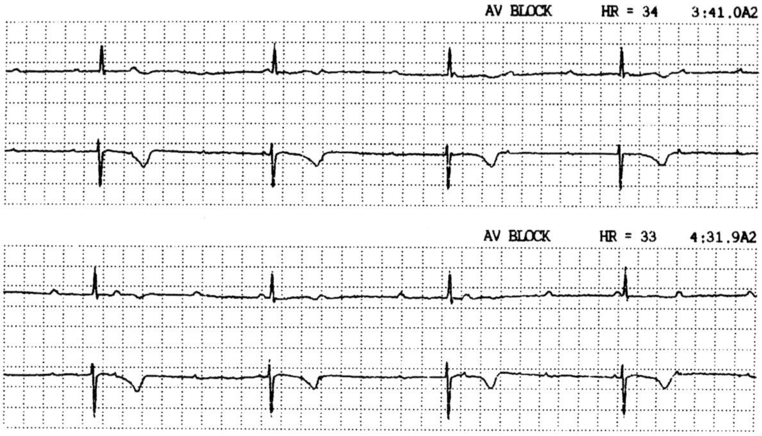

FIGURE 5–4. Ambulatory monitor electrocardiogram strips showing a patient with congenital complete atrioventricular (AV) block and a narrow QRS complex.

involve two concepts. The first is the association of collagen vascular abnormalities (either overt or subclinical) in the mothers of children with congenital complete AV block. The majority of these patients have structurally normal hearts. This association was first commented on by Hull, Binns, and Joyce in 1966, but no causality was investigated.[32] Chameides and McCue and their colleagues, in separate 1977 reports, appear to be the first to have reported a demonstrable association between congenital complete AV block in infants and clinical or laboratory evidence of connective tissue disease in the mothers.[33, 34] However, not all of the cases listed in the aforementioned studies were complete AV block. Nonetheless, this area has seen a large amount of study lending further credence to this association.

There now appears to be a clear association between SS-A/Ro or SS-B/La autoantibodies in the mother and the development of congenital complete AV block in the child.[35–38] The antibodies are of the immunoglobulin (Ig) G class and can, therefore, cross the placental barrier and enter the fetal circulation. The timing of the antibody transfer is unknown, although the onset has been reported as early as the 16th and 23rd weeks of gestation.[39, 40] The antibodies continue to be present in the neonatal circulation for up to 3 months after birth. Scott et al[41] found that 75% of asymptomatic mothers who had infants with congenital complete AV block had anti-Ro (SS-A) antibodies, more than 600 times the expected incidence. However, not all anti-Ro–positive mothers had children with congenital complete AV block.[41] Litsey et al[42] demonstrated IgG deposits only in the conduction system of a fetus with congenital complete AV block. Singsen et al[43] and, more recently, Taylor et al[44] could not demonstrate any antibody specific for the conduction system. Taylor et al demonstrated (via immunofluorescence staining) deposition of Ig and complement components in all cardiac tissues of fetal specimens. Reactivity of maternal antibody to fetal cardiac tissue was positive in 51% of mothers of infants with congenital complete AV block versus only 10% for controls.[44]

Although these studies show a correlation between immunologic abnormalities and congenital complete AV block, and the description of the disorder of the AV node in these patients is similar to the changes seen in the AV node of adults with connective disease, the causality has yet to be shown; that is, the proof of the cytotoxic nature of the antibodies on the AV node has not been demonstrated. Not all mothers with immunologic abnormalities have children with congenital complete AV block. Some other factor such as human leukocyte antigen (HLA) type, in utero environment, or timing of antibody transfer to the fetus may be necessary.

On these same lines, some work indicates that there may be an association between certain HLA types (HLA-DR3, B8, DRw52, DQw2) in the mother or the fetus that increases the likelihood of neonatal lupus, whose sole manifestation may be congenital complete AV block.[45, 46] More research needs to be done in this area before any definitive statements can be made.

The second possible cause of congenital complete AV block is abnormal embryonic development of the AV node from AV canal musculature. Lev[47] postulated that the various types of disorders seen in congenital complete AV block may be a result of abnormal development of the central fibrous body, lack of union between the AV node and AV bundle (assuming separate development), or formation of conduction system from anterior endocardial tissue (L-transposition of the great arteries with ventricular inversion).

CLINICAL FEATURES

The symptoms of patients with a structurally normal heart and congenital complete AV block range from a total lack of symptoms to syncope, exercise intolerance, and congestive heart failure. This great diversity in symptoms is directly related to the baseline junctional or ventricular escape rate of each patient. Those with a faster underlying rate will generally demonstrate less fatigue or exercise intolerance. However, the baseline heart rate is only one factor. A second is the ability of the underlying pacemaker to increase its rate in response to various physiologic demands (i.e., exercise). Normally, the increase in cardiac output with exercise is produced by an increase in both stroke volume and heart rate; however, heart rate is the main component of the cardiac output increase. There are significant differences among various patients with congenital complete AV block in their ability to increase their heart rate with exercise. This ability does not seem to be related to resting heart rate, atrial rate, or heart size. Clearly, those individuals who can increase their ventricular rates are better able to handle the oxygen delivery demands that are produced by an increase in activity than those who cannot. Patients with complete AV block compensate for reduced resting heart rates by an increase in stroke volume and left ventricular end-diastolic volume.[48] Even though heart rate increases vary among these patients, there is evidence that the cardiac output response to exercise is blunted in all of them.[48] One of the difficulties in determining symptomatology in a child is that he or she has never experienced any other situation for comparison and may have no complaints. Once pacemaker therapy has been implemented, the child usually feels much better, presumably because of improved cardiac output or decreased atrial pressures.

In addition to ventricular rate, the incidence of premature ventricular contractions (PVCs) in patients with complete AV block has been a clinical feature of some concern. However, the clinical implications of this finding are still unclear. Winkler, Freed, and Nadas[49] as well as Chawla et al[50] presented differing opinions regarding the incidence of ventricular ectopy. Chawla et al found an association between lower resting heart rates and ventricular ectopy during exercise, whereas Winkler, Freed, and Nadas found an association between increasing age of the patient and premature ventricular beats.

The infant with isolated congenital complete heart block may be asymptomatic or may present with varying degrees of decreased cardiac output or even congestive heart failure. The age of presentation is important when considering the clinical features in this group of patients. The newborn infant with congestive heart failure requires intense medical support and treatment. These neonates may have significant anasarca, hepatomegaly, and lactic acidosis. Clearly, more severe symptoms indicate a more critical need for emergent pacing. Neonates who are clinically asymptomatic do not require immediate treatment, but instead can be monitored clinically in an intensive care unit as long as the baseline heart rate is above the rate considered to place one at risk for sudden death (i.e., 50–55 bpm).

The child with a structurally normal heart or a physiologically insignificant structural defect will have symptoms based on the ventricular or junctional escape rate. Symptoms will usually present as fatigue or exercise intolerance. Syncope may also occur. However, the child with congenital complete AV block may be asymptomatic, and the block may only be discovered on a routine well-child evaluation.

The infant or child with structural heart disease and congenital complete AV block is in a much different situation than the patients previously described. This group of patients requires the highest and most responsive cardiac output, yet has the least ability to respond appropriately. For this reason, this group presents the earliest in life (three times more likely to present in the first week of life compared to those with isolated complete AV block) and is in the most need of care and treatment.[27] Even with appropriate therapy, a number of these patients die in infancy.

In summary, the clinical features of patients with congenital complete heart block primarily involve the effect of the heart rate on cardiac output and the risk of sudden death. Treatment is based on the ability of pacing to improve symptoms or prevent sudden death.

DIAGNOSTIC TECHNIQUES

Prenatal

Until the 1970s, fetal monitoring for arrhythmias had consisted mostly of auscultation of the fetal heart rate. This, obviously, left much unknown, not the least of which was the type of rhythm. Fetal electrocardiography, which consisted of trying to obtain a fetal ECG through the maternal abdomen, was cumbersome and inaccurate until shortly before birth, when electrodes could be placed on the fetal scalp. Even with this method, the type of rhythm was still uncertain.[51] However, with the advent of fetal echocardiography, a method became available to determine the heart rate and the relationship of atrial and ventricular contractions by timing mitral valve opening and ventricular contraction.

Postnatal

Electrocardiogram and Holter Monitor

A surface ECG is all that is needed to make the diagnosis of congenital complete AV block. However, because the ECG represents an isolated event in time, it does not give enough information to determine the junctional or ventricular escape rate. A 24-hour Holter monitor is ideal for this, because the heart rate can be monitored over a spectrum of times and conditions, and the incidence and severity of ectopy can be evaluated. Because there may be an association between increasing age and ventricular ectopy in patients with congenital complete AV block, the ability to monitor the rhythm for 24 hours, encompassing a variety of situations and activities, is invaluable.[49]

Intracardiac Electrophysiology

Evaluation by invasive electrophysiologic testing has been used in the past to determine the site of block. It was thought that the site of block could help predict stability of the cellular pacemaker. This however, has not proven to be the case.[52] Benson et al[53] presented evidence that evaluating the automaticity of the pacemaker by using pacemaker recovery times may be helpful.[53] A junctional or ventricular recovery time of greater than 3 seconds in children may be correlated with clinical symptoms or sudden death.

Exercise Testing

Exercise testing is an important adjunct in the evaluation of the seemingly asymptomatic child with congenital complete AV block. Using this diagnostic tool, some objective criteria can be used to help document symptomatology and to determine whether any ectopy is present. Although the significance of exercise-induced ventricular ectopy has not been proven, it has been suggested that ventricular ectopy may increase the risk of sudden death in some patients with congenital complete AV block.[49]

TREATMENT

Treatment of patients with congenital complete AV block falls into two main categories: treatment of the patient with low cardiac output and treatment of those patients thought to be at risk of sudden death. Treatment for the most part involves permanent pacing, because chronotropic drugs appear to have only modest success at best.[54] However, if the patient is in extremis, chronotropic agents such as isoproterenol or atropine may be used while arrangements are being made for pacing. The use of external transcutaneous pacing may be appropriate in emergency situations.

The fetus with severe congestive heart failure and congenital complete AV block should be delivered as soon as is considered safe from an obstetric viewpoint. Transuterine pacing of a fetus in extremis but too young to deliver has been tried; however, after a short period of capture, pacing capability was lost, and the fetus died.[55] Infants with congenital complete AV block seem to tolerate vaginal delivery fairly well unless they are in distress or in congestive heart failure; in these cases, a cesarean section is indicated. Arrangements should be made before delivery for treatment of the congestive heart failure soon after birth with inotropic agents and diuretics as well as with temporary or permanent pacing. Placement of some type of pacing modality should have the highest priority.

The fetus or newborn with asymptomatic congenital complete AV block should be placed in an intensive care setting with the heart rate monitored very closely. The decision to pace this group of patients depends on the baseline ventricular rate and the likelihood of sudden death. Michaelsson and Engle showed only one death in patients who had a ventricular rate greater than 55 bpm and an atrial rate less than 140 bpm.[27] It should also be noted that there were no deaths in those with a ventricular rate greater than 60 bpm and an atrial rate less than 140 bpm, but there were also fewer patients who met these criteria. Karpawich et al found similar data in an older age group, with no infant or child with a heart rate greater than 50 bpm having syncope.[52] In the past, the need for a permanent pacemaker in an infant was reason for grave concern and implantation of a pacing system occasionally resulted in the patient's demise. However, current thought is that any patient considered to be at risk of sudden death from congenital complete AV block should have a pacemaker implanted. In the asymptomatic infant, this would include an infant with a persistent ventricular rate less than 50–55 bpm. As confidence in pacemakers rises, the cut-off rate may be raised to 60 bpm, as only one child in the collaborative study died with a ventricular rate greater than 60 bpm, regardless of the atrial rate.

The newborn with congenital heart disease and complete heart block, regardless of symptoms, should probably be paced, as the incidence of death in infancy in this group is exceedingly high (29% compared with 8% in those without congenital heart disease in the Michaelsson and Engle series and only an 80% first-year survival rate in patients in the Pinsky et al series).[56]

The child (compared with the infant) with congenital complete AV block presents a slightly different set of circumstances. The decision whether and when to pace these patients is much less clear. Generally, the older child is monitored with exercise testing and Holter monitoring to look for increasing exercise intolerance, arrhythmias, and very low baseline heart rate. Individual patients whose activity level is impaired because of decreased exercise tolerance should be paced. Exercise testing is helpful in determining tolerance as well as eliciting ventricular arrhythmias. This is important because syncope and sudden death in children with congenital complete AV block may be caused by ventricular arrhythmias as well as by severe bradycardia. Molthen et al[57] reported patients with congenital complete AV block having Adams-Stokes attacks and ventricular tachycardia. Studies of patients with congenital complete AV block undergoing exercise testing have shown an increased rate of ectopy.[50, 52, 58] There is disagreement as to the cause, whether it is increased age of the patient or an inadequate chronotropic response; however, it is unclear whether ventricular ectopy increases the risk of sudden death in these patients or whether permanent pacing is protective. It may be that the increase in heart size in these patients (a compensatory mechanism for decreased heart rate) may, through the years, predispose them to the development of ventricular arrhythmias, just as atrial dilatation predisposes to atrial flutter. Holter and ECG monitoring in children with congenital complete AV block has been used not only to determine the low heart rate but also to help guide therapy. The consensus is that average awake heart rates in children of less than 50 bpm are an indication for pacing. A random rate of less than 45 bpm is also considered an indication for a pacemaker. A sleeping heart rate less than 30 bpm is considered a pacemaker indication. Infants with congenital complete AV block must have their ventricular function evaluated closely because a small percentage of these patients will experience severe cardiomyopathy despite physiologic pacing. It has been suggested that all children with congenital complete AV block be paced.[59] Infants and children who receive cardiac pacemakers for congenital complete AV block require intense follow-up for other signs of congenital connective tissue disorders.[60, 61] It has been demonstrated that even cardiac pacing on the day of birth with a dual-chamber system does not always prevent the development of subsequent cardiomyopathy.

SURGICAL COMPLETE AV BLOCK

One of the complications of surgical correction of congenital heart defects is postsurgical complete AV block. This may be transient or permanent or may be transient in the immediate postoperative period, only to reappear in a permanent form later. Transient postsurgical AV block may last as long as 10 days to 2 weeks. As in congenital complete AV block, diagnosis requires proof that atrial impulses that should conduct to the ventricle do not. This may be somewhat complicated in postoperative patients, because many have a markedly accelerated junctional rhythm. If temporary atrial pacing wires are present, intact conduction can be proven by pacing the atria at a rate sufficiently faster than the existing junctional rate.

Because of an increased awareness of the location of the AV node and the His bundle, the incidence of postsurgical AV block is much lower than that of even 10 years ago. Any surgery involving the AV node area (e.g., surgical repair of ventricular septal defect, AV canal, or L-transposition of the great arteries with or without a ventricular septal defect, or a Fontan procedure requiring oversewing of the tricuspid valve) is still a risk for producing complete AV block.

TREATMENT

Once it has been ascertained that AV block has occurred, it is advisable to have both atrial and ventricular wires placed. This will aid in distinguishing complete AV block from an accelerated junctional rhythm and will allow for AV synchrony in the immediate recovery period. In addition, any patient suspected of having postsurgical block should be monitored closely; back-up pacing should be readily available if the junctional ectopic focus suddenly slows without a sufficient ventricular escape rhythm. We have had at least one patient suffer a cardiac arrest in a similar situation. The patient should be monitored closely for any sign of intact AV conduction, and the thresholds of the temporary pacing wires should be evaluated each day. This is especially important if the patient is pacemaker dependent with an inadequate ventricular escape rate. The ventricular output should be kept at twice the capture threshold.

Unless forced to implant a permanent pacemaker because of markedly elevated ventricular thresholds in a postoperative pacemaker-dependent patient, any decision regarding a permanent pacemaker should be delayed for 7 days, because sinus rhythm may return. Lillehei et al[62] reported a 60% mortality rate in postsurgical AV block patients during the first postoperative year alone. However, Hurwitz et al[63] reported a much lower incidence of death in postoperative AV block patients. In the latter series, only one of every three patients who had a pacemaker implanted died.

In the past 5 to 10 years, the capability to pace children effectively has improved markedly, as evidenced by the reports of Waelkens,[64] Beder et al,[65] and Gillette et al.[66] We generally implant a permanent pacemaker in any postsurgical AV block patient who has complete AV block lasting 7 days without performing electrophysiologic testing to determine the site of block.

BUNDLE BRANCH BLOCK

The bundle branch system takes its origin from the common or penetrating bundles. The anatomic landmark for this is generally the membranous septum. The bundle branches generally arise in the area between the membranous and muscular septum. On the right ventricular aspect, the right bundle originates as a continuation of the common bundle. The anatomic marker for it is the medial papillary muscle. At this level it is just subendocardial and histologically is a cordlike structure within a fibrous sheath. The right bundle reaches its end point at the apex of the right ventricle by passing intramyocardially through the septomarginal trabeculation. At the right ventricular apex, the right bundle then ramifies in the subendocardium.

The left bundle branch is significantly different from the right. The left system originates at an acute angle from the common bundle in an almost sheetlike series of conduction fibers. The anatomic location of these subendocardial fibers is in the left ventricular outflow tract below the noncoronary and right coronary cusp intersection. Whether the left bundle then forms into two or three fascicles is unclear.[67–72] The left anterior fascicle courses across the left ventricular outflow tract toward the anterior papillary muscle, whereas the left posterior fascicle winds its way toward the posterior papillary muscle. These then ramify distally.

RIGHT BUNDLE BRANCH BLOCK

With RBBB, activation proceeds through the left bundle branch then intramyocardially to the right ventricle and conceivably retrograde up the functioning portion of the right bundle branch that is distal to the point of conduction block (Fig. 5–5). The initial ventricular activation is normal because the electrical activation of the superior aspect of the interventricular septum is supplied first by the left bundle branch. These two facts account for the initial rapid ECG deflections followed by much slower deflections that are seen on "right-sided" ECG lead re-

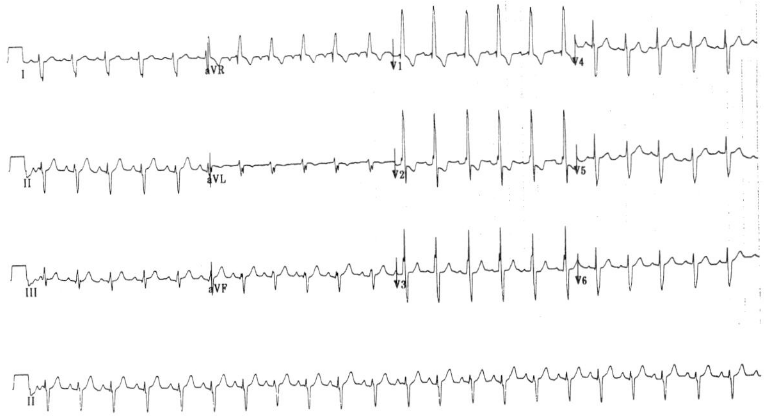

FIGURE 5–5. Right bundle branch block with right axis deviation in an 8-year-old patient after ventricular septal defect repair. The widened R′ in leads aVR & V_1 as well as the widened S waves in I and V_6 differentiate this tracing from right ventricular hypertrophy.

cordings. All the criteria used to make the diagnosis of RBBB originate from these electrophysiologic events.

ECG FINDINGS

Lead V_1 ECGs exhibit an initial rapid positive deflection owing to the initial superior and rightward activation originating from the left bundle. This is followed by an S wave as a result of unopposed left ventricular activation. The final part of the QRS is transcribed by a broad R wave as a result of the delayed right-sided activation via intramyocardial activation. Conversely, left-sided lead recordings (i.e., I and V_6) show a late S wave that is broad because of the delayed right-sided intramyocardial activation.[73] Rather than any particular pattern (i.e., rsR′), it is the discrepancy between the timing of the initial and terminal forces that is the key to the diagnosis of RBBB. For this reason, the diagnosis of incomplete RBBB is a misnomer, because, although there is an rsR′ pattern, there is no terminal conduction delay. The axis in RBBB should be computed using the fast portion of the QRS complex. This generally is the first 40 milliseconds of the QRS complex[74] and is identified by a breakpoint, which is the origin of the slow conduction. Because of the abnormalities of the depolarization vectors, ventricular hypertrophy cannot be diagnosed in the presence of RBBB.[75, 76]

ETIOLOGY

In children and adolescents, the most common cause of RBBB is cardiac surgery involving a right ventriculotomy such as a ventricular septal defect repair[77, 78] or subpulmonary excision of tissue.[79] In repaired tetralogy of Fallot patients, half of the RBBB is due to central damage to the bundle and half is due to peripheral damage.[80] Inflammation of the conduction system from myocarditis or endocarditis has also been reported as a cause of RBBB.[81] Congenital RBBB may be seen in rare, autosomal dominant, familial conduction system disease. Although patients with this disease may progress to complete heart block, this does not appear to be the case in those patients manifesting only RBBB.[82] Rate-related bundle branch block has been reported to occur during tachycardia in 2% of children with supraventricular tachycardia.[83]

INCOMPLETE RIGHT BUNDLE BRANCH BLOCK

Incomplete RBBB is generally used to describe an rsR′ pattern in ECG lead V_1 in which there is minimal if any QRS prolongation and no terminal conduction delay. The pattern is common in infants and is seen in 7% of normal children older than 6 months.[84] The significance of this ECG finding is its association with defects producing right ventricular volume overload. This is said to occur in more than 90% of patients with an atrial septal defect[85] and appears to be due to stretching of the right bundle peripherally or right ventricular hypertrophy.[86, 87]

LEFT BUNDLE BRANCH BLOCK

In LBBB, activation proceeds from the common bundle through the right bundle branch system. The left ventricle is then depolarized as electrical activation spreads from the right ventricular myocardium to the left. Unlike RBBB, in which the initial parts of the QRS configuration are normal, the entire QRS is affected in LBBB. This then leads to an abnormal initial vector followed by slower late depolarization of the left ventricle. Criteria used to make the diagnosis of LBBB are based on these electrophysiologic principles.

Electrocardiographic Findings

The majority of patients with LBBB exhibit a QS ECG pattern inscribed in lead V_1 because of the posterior spread of electrical forces. In the minority of cases, lead V_1 shows a small positive initial deflection followed by a large negative deflection, producing a small sharp R wave followed by a deep, wide S wave. Left-sided ECG leads (V_6) reflect the absence of the appropriate septal depolarization with an absence of Q waves. The delayed depolarization is characterized by a broad-notched R wave.

Etiology

The finding of LBBB is rare in children and adolescents and is most commonly caused by surgery involving the aortic valve or subvalve area.[88] It is caused less commonly by endocarditis, hypertrophic cardiomyopathy, hemochromatosis, or myocardial infarction.[89–91] Progressive conduction system disease associated with LBBB and syncope has been reported in three siblings who also had subtle findings of a cardiomyopathy.[92]

RATE-DEPENDENT BUNDLE BRANCH BLOCK

Bundle branch block can be precipitated by either an acceleration or a deceleration in the intrinsic heart rate of a patient. Rate acceleration–producing bundle branch block, although much more common in children than deceleration bundle branch block, is said to occur in less than 10% of children when they experience an episode of supraventricular tachycardia.[93] The bundle branch block can be either intermittent or persistent. Persistent rate-accelerated bundle branch block has been thought to be due to either (1) repetitive transseptal retrograde conduction from the nonblocked bundle into a more nonrefractory distal segment of the blocked bundle[94] or (2) prolongation of the bundle branch action potential (Fig. 5–6). Prolongation of the bundle branch action potential cannot account for all cases because block can occur at relatively slow rates in adults, which would imply an excessively long action potential duration. The transient block associated with rate acceleration may be due to the relative action potential duration prolongation. Deceleration bundle branch block is likely due to enhanced phase four depolarization in the affected bundle.[95–99]

EXERCISE-INDUCED BUNDLE BRANCH BLOCK

Exercise-induced bundle branch block is an uncommon finding in children. In a study of 2761 subjects who underwent treadmill exercise testing, the incidence was 0.2% with no occurrence in the 264 normal children who were tested. The most common abnormality associated with the exercise-induced bundle branch block was aortic stenosis.[100]

LEFT ANTERIOR HEMIBLOCK

Block in the anterior fascicle produces a shift in the QRS axis superiorly and to the left (between −30° and −90°).

LEFT POSTERIOR HEMIBLOCK

Electrocardiographic criteria for left posterior hemiblock are features that can be found in normal ECG findings in children. These are essentially diagnostic features for adult ECG interpretations.

BIFASCICULAR BLOCK

Block in any two fascicles of the conduction system can be rightfully called *bifascicular block,* but the term is usually used to implicate RBBB and either left anterior hemiblock or left posterior hemiblock (Fig. 5–7).

The combination of RBBB and left anterior hemiblock is frequently seen in children after surgical correction of tetralogy of Fallot (8–23%).[101–103] This combination may[104–106] or may not[103, 107, 108] be associated with progression to complete AV block in postoperative patients. However, the real predictor may be transient postoperative complete heart block because only those postoperative patients with RBBB plus left anterior hemiblock and transient postoperative complete heart block experienced permanent complete atrioventricular block.[109]

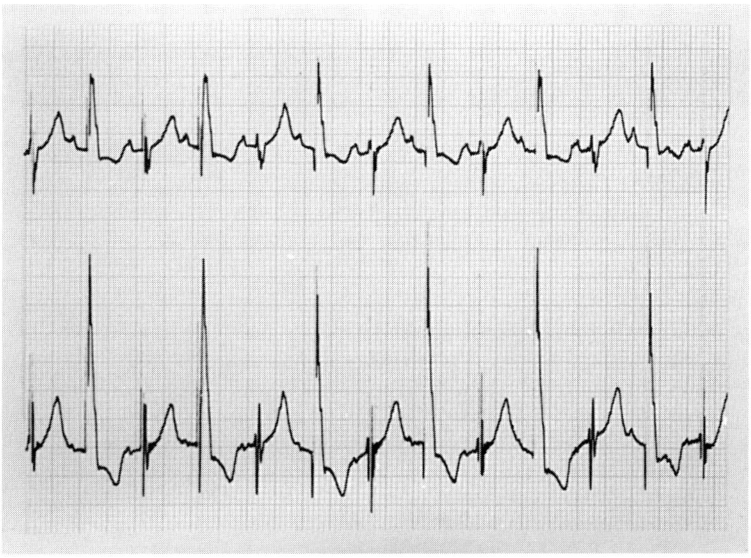

FIGURE 5–6. Variable bundle branch block caused by prolonged repolarization in an infant with congenital prolonged QT interval. Both pacing and propranolol were used in her successful treatment.

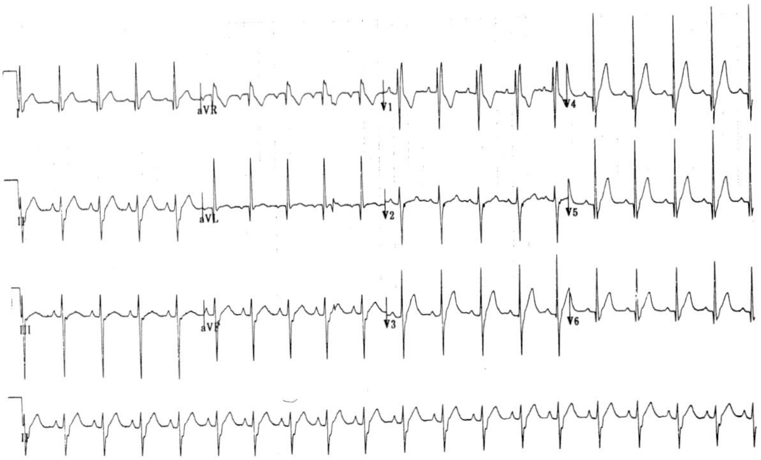

FIGURE 5–7. Right bundle branch block (RBBB) and left anterior fascicular block pattern. In addition to the RBBB and the frontal plane QRS axis (left and superior), there are Q waves in I and aVL.

TRIFASCICULAR BLOCK

Delay in all three fascicles is termed *trifascicular block*. This can only be determined by intracardiac electrophysiologic study showing a prolonged HV interval. This is seen more often in adults with ischemic heart disease and is rarely seen in children. The treatment with permanent pacing is dependent on the clinical situation.

Treatment

No specific treatment is required for RBBB (complete or incomplete), LBBB, rate-dependent or exercise-induced bundle branch block, or fascicular blocks. Pediatric patients with muscular dystrophy or cardiomyopathy and LBBB should be monitored closely with pacemaker implantation should syncope or near syncope develop. Although most patients with bifascicular block do not require treatment, those with Kearns-Sayre syndrome may require permanent pacemaker implantation after progressing from bifascicular to complete AV block.

Summary

Bundle branch blocks and fascicular blocks are rare in the pediatric population and are most often seen in patients after surgery for congenital heart disease. Although there are reports of congenital bundle branch block in children with anatomically normal hearts, their real significance (either acquired or congenital) remains unknown.

REFERENCES

1. Ferrer PL: Arrhythmias in the neonate, infant, and child. In Roberts NK, Gelband H (eds): Arrhythmias in the Neonate. New York, Appleton-Century-Crofts, 1977, pp 265–316.
2. Narula OS, Scherlag BJ, Samet P, et al: Atrioventricular block: Localization and classification by His bundle recordings. Am J Med 50:146–165, 1971.
3. Wenckebach KF: Zur Analyse des unregel massigen Pulses. Z Klin Med 37:475–488, 1899.
4. Wenckebach KF: Beitrage zur Kenntnis der menschlichen Herztatigkeit. Arch Anat Physiol (Physiol Abth) 1–2:1–10, 1907.
5. Hay J: Bradycardia and cardiac arrhythmia produced by depression of certain functions of the heart. Lancet 1:139, 1906.
6. Mobitz W: Uber die unvollstandige storung der erregungsuberleitung zwischen Vorhof und Kammer des menschlichen Herzens. Z Ges Exp Med 41:180, 1924.
7. Wenckebach KF, Winterberg H: Die unregelmassige Herztatigkeit. Leipzig, W Engelmann, 1927, pp 313–320.
8. Mobitz W: Uber den partiellen Herzblock. Z Klin Med 107:449, 1928.
9. Katz LN, Pick A: Clinical electrocardiography, part I. In The Arrhythmias. Philadelphia, Lea & Febiger, 1956.
10. Dressler W, Swiller SL: Atypical Wenckebach periods with dropped atrial beats. Am J Cardiol 2:575, 1958.
11. Watanabe Y, Dreifus LS: Second degree atrioventricular block. Cardiovasc Res 1:150–158, 1967.
12. Castillo C, Maytin O, Castellanos A Jr: His bundle recordings in atypical A-V nodal Wenckebach block during cardiac pacing. Am J Cardiol 27:570–574, 1971.
13. Gambetta M, Denes P, Childers RW: Vagally induced second degree A-V block, Mobitz type I, and the hyperactive S-A node. Chest 62:152–154, 1972.
14. Friedman HS, Gomes JAC, Haft JI: An analysis of Wenckebach periodicity. J Electrocardiol 8:307–314, 1975.
15. Denes P, Levy L, Pick A, et al: The incidence of typical and atypical A-V Wenckebach periodicity. Am Heart J 89:26–31, 1975.
16. Kinoshita S, Konishi G: Atrioventricular Wenckebach periodicity in athletes: Influence of increased vagal tone on the occurrence of atypical periods. J Electrocardiol 20:272–279, 1987.
17. Meytes I, Kaplinsky E, Yahini JH, et al: Wenckebach A-V block: A frequent feature following heavy physical training. Am Heart J 90:426–430, 1975.
18. El-Sherif N, Aranda J, Befeler B, et al: Atypical Wenckebach periodicity simulating Mobitz II AV block. Br Heart J 40:1376–1383, 1978.

19. Langendorf R, Cohen H, Gozo EG Jr: Observations on second degree atrioventricular block, including new criteria for the differential diagnosis between type I and type II block. Am J Cardiol 29:111–118, 1972.
20. Zipes DP: Second-degree atrioventricular block. Circulation 60:465–472, 1979.
21. Johansson B: Adams-Stokes syndrome: A review and follow-up of forty-two cases. Am J Cardiol 8:76–93, 1961.
22. Donoso E, Adler L, Friedberg C: Unusual forms of second degree atrioventricular block, including Mobitz type II block, associated with the Morgagni-Adams-Stokes syndrome. Am Heart J 67:150–157, 1967.
23. Kaufman J, Wachtel F, Rothfield E, et al: The association of complete heart block and Adams-Stokes syndrome in two cases of Mobitz type of block. Circulation 23:253–256, 1961.
24. Watanabe Y, Dreifus L: Atrioventricular block: Basic concepts. In Mandel W (ed): Cardiac Arrhythmias: Their Mechanisms, Diagnosis, and Management. Philadelphia, JB Lippincott, 1987, pp 297–320.
25. Kelly DT, Brodsky SJ, Krovetz LJ: Mobitz type II atrioventricular block in children. J Pediatr 79:972–976, 1971.
26. Gochberg SH: Congenital heart block. Am J Obstet Gynecol 88:238–241, 1964.
27. Michaelsson M, Engle MA: Congenital complete heart block: An international study of the natural history. In Brest AN, Engle MA (eds): Cardiovascular Clinics. Philadelphia, FA Davis, 1972, pp 85–101.
28. Landtmann B, Linder E, Hjelt L, et al: Congenital complete heart block: I. A clinical study of 37 cases. Ann Paediatr Fenn 10:99–104, 1964.
29. Linton D, Human D: Peri-operative management and administration of anesthesia in children with congenital complete heart block. A case report and review. S Afr Med J 66:875–876, 1984.
30. Camm AJ, Bexten RS: Congenital heart block. Eur Heart J Suppl A, 5:115–117, 1984.
31. Winkler RB, Nora AH, Nora JJ: Familial congenital complete heart block and maternal systemic lupus erythematosus. Circulation 56:1103–1106, 1977.
32. Hull D, Binns BAO, Joyce D: Congenital heart block and widespread fibrosis due to maternal lupus erythematosus. Arch Dis Child 41:688–690, 1966.
33. Chameides L, Truex RC, Vetter V, et al: Association of maternal systemic lupus erythematosus with congenital complete heart block. N Engl J Med 297:1204–1207, 1977.
34. McCue CM, Mantakas ME, Tinglestad JB, et al: Congenital heart block in newborns of mothers with connective tissue disease. Circulation 56:82–90, 1977.
35. Reed BR, Lee LA, Harmon C, et al: Autoantibodies to SS-A/Ro in infants with congenital heart block. J Pediatr 103:889–891, 1983.
36. Parke A, Rothfield NF: Congenital heart block, systemic lupus erythematosus and anti-Ro antibodies [letter]. Arthritis Rheum 28:1077–1078, 1985.
37. Harley JB, Kaine JL, Fox OF, et al: Ro (SS-A) antibody and antigen in a patient with congenital complete heart block. Arthritis Rheum 28:1321–1325, 1985.
38. Franco HL, Weston WL, Peebles C, et al: Autoantibodies directed against Sicca syndrome antigens in the neonatal lupus syndrome. Am Acad Dermatol 4:67–72, 1981.
39. Lee LA, Weston WL: New findings in neonatal lupus syndrome. Am J Dis Child 138:233–236, 1984.
40. Herreman G, Betous F, Batisse P, et al: Intra-uterine detection of atrioventricular block in two children whose mother had Sjögren's syndrome. Nouv Presse Med 11:657–660, 1982.
41. Scott JS, Maddison PJ, Taylor PV, et al: Connective tissue disease, antibodies to ribonucleoprotein, and congenital heart block. N Engl J Med 309:209–212, 1983.
42. Litsey SE, Noonan JA, O'Connor WN, et al: Maternal connective tissue disease and congenital heart block. Demonstration of immunoglobulin in cardiac tissue. N Engl J Med 312:98–100, 1985.
43. Singsen BH, Akhter JE, Weinstein MM, et al: Congenital complete heart block and SSA antibodies: Obstetric implications. Am J Obstet Gynecol 152:655–658, 1985.
44. Taylor PV, Scott JS, Gerlis LM, et al: Maternal antibodies against fetal cardiac antigens in congenital complete heart block. N Engl J Med 315:667–672, 1986.
45. Lee LA, Bias WB, Arnett FC, et al: Immunogenetics of the neonatal lupus syndrome. Ann Intern Med 95:592–596, 1983.
46. Watson RM, Lane AT, Barnett NK, et al: Neonatal lupus erythematosus. A clinical, serological and immunogenetic study with review of the literature. Medicine 63:362–378, 1984.
47. Lev M: Pathogenesis of congenital atrioventricular block. Prog Cardiovasc Dis 25:145–162, 1972.
48. Manno BV, Hakki AH, Eshaghpour E, et al: Left ventricular function at rest and during exercise in congenital complete heart block: A radionuclide angiographic evaluation. Am J Cardiol 52:92–94, 1983.
49. Winkler RB, Freed MD, Nadas AS: Exercise-induced ventricular ectopy in children and young adults with complete heart block. Am Heart J 99:87–92, 1980.
50. Chawla K, Serratto M, Cruz J, et al: Response to maximal and submaximal exercise testing in patients with congenital complete heart block. Circulation 56:171, 1977.
51. Shenker L: Fetal cardiac arrhythmias. Obstet Gynecol Surv 34:561–572, 1979.
52. Karpawich PP, Gillette PC, Garson A Jr, et al: Congenital complete atrioventricular block: Clinical and electrophysiologic predictors of need for pacemaker insertion. Am J Cardiol 48:1098–1102, 1981.
53. Benson DW, Edwards SB, Serwer GA, et al: Heart block in children: Evaluating pacemaker recording times. Circulation 60:11–114, 1979.
54. Nakamura F, Nadas A: Complete heart block in infants and children. N Engl J Med 270:1261–1268, 1964.
55. Carpenter RJ Jr, Strasburger JF, Garson A Jr, et al: Fetal ventricular pacing for hydrops secondary to complete atrioventricular block. J Am Coll Card 8:1434–1436, 1986.
56. Pinsky WW, Gillette PC, Garson A Jr, et al: Diagnosis, management and long-term results of patients with complete atrioventricular block. Pediatrics 69:728–733, 1982.
57. Molthen ME, Miller RA, Hastreiter AR, et al: Congenital heart block with fetal Adams-Stokes attacks in childhood. Pediatrics 30:32–41, 1962.
58. Ikkos D, Hanson JS: Response to exercise in congenital complete atrioventricular block. Circulation 22:583–590, 1960.
59. Michaelsson M, Riesenfeld T, Jonzon A: Natural history of congenital complete atrioventricular block. Pacing Clin Electrophysiol 20:98–101, 1997.
60. Taylor-Albert E, Reichlin M, Toews WH, et al: Delayed dilated cardiomyopathy as a manifestation of neonatal lupus: Case reports, autoantibody analysis, and management. Pediatrics 99:733–735, 1997.
61. Hubscher O, Carrillo D, Reichlin M: Congenital heart block and subsequent connective tissue disorder in adolescence. Lupus 6:283–284, 1997.

62. Lillehei C, Sellers RD, Bonnabeau RC, et al: Chronic post-surgical complete heart block. J Cardiovasc Surg 46:436–456, 1973.
63. Hurwitz RA, Riemenschneider TA, Moss AJ, et al: Chronic postoperative heart block in children. Am J Cardiol 21:185–189, 1968.
64. Waelkens JJJ: Cardiac pacemakers in infants and children. Pediatr Cardiol 3:337–340, 1982.
65. Beder SD, Hanisch DG, Cohen MH, et al: Cardiac pacing on children: A 15 year experience. Am Heart J 109:152–156, 1985.
66. Gillette PC, Shannon C, Blair H, et al: Transvenous pacing in pediatric patients. Am Heart J 105:843–847, 1983.
67. Anderson KR, Ho SY, Anderson RH: The location and vascular supply of the sinus node in the human heart. Br Heart J 41:28–32, 1979.
68. Demoulin JC, Kulbertus HE: Histopathological examination of concept of left hemiblock. Br Heart J 34:807–814, 1972.
69. Massing GK, James TN: Anatomical configuration of the His bundle and bundle branches in the human heart. Circulation 53:609–621, 1976.
70. Rossi L: Sistema di conduzione trifascicolare ed emiblocchi di branca sinistra. Considerazioni anatomiche ed istopatologiche. G Ital Cardiol 1:55–62, 1971.
71. Rossi L: Histopathology of conducting system in left anterior hemiblock. Br Heart J 38:1304–1311, 1976
72. Rosenbaum MB, Elizari MV, Lazzari JO: The hemiblocks. Tampa Tracings, FL, Oldsman, 1970.
73. Cooksey JD, Dunn M, Massie E: Clinical vectorcardiography and electrocardiography, 2nd ed. Chicago, Yearbook Medical, 1977, pp 89–112.
74. Garson A Jr: The Electrocardiogram in Infants and Children: A Systematic Approach. Philadelphia, Lea & Febiger, 1983, p 123.
75. Brohet CR, Styns M, Arraud P, et al: Vectorcardiographic diagnosis of right ventricular hypertrophy in the presence of right bundle branch block in young subjects. Am J Cardiol 42:602–612, 1978.
76. Wasserburger RH, Young WP, Siebecker K, et al: Further electrocardiographic observations on direct epicardial potentials in congenital heart lesions. Differential features of right ventricular preponderance and right bundle branch block. Circulation 26:561–573, 1962.
77. Coggin CJ, Wareham EE, Selvester RH: Post ventriculotomy right bundle branch block: Its etiology. Circulation 22:734, 1960.
78. Gelband H, Waldo AL, Kaiser GA, et al: Etiology of right bundle branch block in patients undergoing total correction of tetralogy of Fallot. Circulation 44:1022–1033, 1971.
79. Horowitz LN, Simson MB, Spear JF, et al: The mechanism of apparent right bundle branch block after transatrial repair of tetralogy of Fallot. Circulation 59:1241–1246, 1979.
80. Garson A Jr, Porter CJ, Gillette PC, et al: Ventricular tachycardia induction during electrophysiologic study after repair of tetralogy of Fallot. J Am Coll Card 1:1493–1502, 1983.
81. Gumbiner CH: Bundle branch and fascicular block. In Gillette PC, Garson A Jr (eds): Pediatric Cardiac Dysrhythmias. New York, Grune & Stratton, 1981, pp 405–419.
82. Husson GS, Blackman MS, Rogers MC, et al: Familial congenital bundle branch system disease. Am J Cardiol 32:365–369, 1973.
83. Garson A Jr: Supraventricular tachycardia. In Gillette PC, Garson A Jr (eds): Pediatric Cardiac Dysrhythmias. New York, Grune & Stratton, 1981, pp 177–254.
84. Burch GE, DePasquale NP: Electrocardiography in the diagnosis of congenital heart disease. In Electrocardiography. Philadelphia, Lea & Febiger, 1967, pp 30–105.
85. Gillette PC: Interpretation of conduction abnormalities in pediatric electrocardiography. In Liebman J, Plonsey R, Gillette PC (eds): Pediatric Electrocardiography. Baltimore, Williams & Wilkins, 1985, pp 172–191.
86. Garson A Jr: Interventricular conduction disturbances. In Garson A Jr: The Electrocardiogram in Infants and Children. Philadelphia, Lea & Febiger, 1983, pp 119–142.
87. Moore EN, Boineau JP, Patterson DF: Incomplete right bundle branch block: An electrocardiographic enigma and possible misnomer. Circulation 44:678–687, 1971.
88. Garson A Jr: The Electrocardiogram in Infants and Children: A Systematic Approach. Philadelphia, Lea & Febiger, 1983, p 127.
89. Josephson ME: Intraventricular conduction disturbances. In Josephson ME: Clinical Cardiac Electrophysiology. Philadelphia, Lea & Febiger, 1979, pp 103–118.
90. Barson WJ, Craenem J, Hosier DM, et al: Survival following myocarditis and myocardial calcification associated with infection by Coxsackie virus B-4. Pediatrics 68:79–82, 1981.
91. Cohen HC, Singer DH: Bundle branch block and other forms of aberrant intraventricular conduction: Clinical aspects. In Mandel, WJ (ed): Cardiac Arrhythmias. Philadelphia, JB Lippincott, 1987, pp 413–451.
92. Fuhrman BP, Bass JL, Laurence C, et al: Progressive cardiac conduction defect and cardiomyopathy in siblings with syncope. Pediatr Cardiol 2:57–62, 1982.
93. Gumbiner CH: Bundle branch and fascicular block. In Gillette PC, Garson A Jr (eds): Pediatric Cardiac Dysrhythmias. New York, Grune & Stratton, 1981, p 410.
94. Moe GK, Mendez C, Han J: Aberrant A-V impulse propagation in the dog heart: A study of functional bundle branch block. Circ Res 16:261, 1965.
95. Okoroma EO, Guller B, Maloney JD, et al: Etiology of right bundle branch block pattern after surgical closure of ventricular septal defects. Am Heart J 90:14–18, 1975.
96. Massumi RA: Bradycardia-dependent bundle branch block: A critique and proposed criteria. Circulation 38:1066–1073, 1968.
97. Rosenbaum MB, Elizari MV, Lazzari JO, et al: The mechanism of intermittent bundle branch block: Relationship to prolonged recovery, hypopolarization and spontaneous diastolic depolarization. Chest 63:666–677, 1973.
98. Singer DH, Lazzara R, Hoffman BF: Interrelationships between automaticity and conduction in Purkinje fibers. Circ Res 21:537–558, 1967.
99. El-Sherif R, Scherlag BJ, Lazarra R, et al: Pathophysiology of tachycardia- and bradycardia-dependent block in the canine proximal His-Purkinje system after acute myocardial ischemia. Am J Cardiol 33:529–540, 1974.
100. Bricker JT, Traweek MS, Danford DA, et al: Exercise related bundle branch block in children. Am J Cardiol 56:796–797, 1985.
101. Krongrad E: Postoperative arrhythmias in patients with congenital heart disease. Chest 85:107–113, 1984.
102. Vetter VL, Horowitz LN: Electrophysiologic residua and sequelae of surgery for congenital heart defects. Am J Cardiol 50:588–604, 1982.
103. Friedli B, Bolens M: Intraventricular conduction disturbance after correction of tetralogy of Fallot: Can bifascicular and trifascicular block be diagnosed from the surface ECG? Pediatr Cardiol 6:133–136, 1985.
104. Downing JW, Kaplan S, Bove KE: Postsurgical left ante-

rior hemiblock and right bundle branch block. Br Heart J 34:263–270, 1972.
105. Gillette PC, Yeoman MA, Mullins CE, et al: Sudden death after repair of tetralogy of Fallot: Electrocardiographic and electrophysiologic abnormalities. Circulation 57:566–577, 1977.
106. Stegg CN, Krongrad E, Davachi F, et al: Postoperative left anterior hemiblock and right bundle branch block following repair of tetralogy of Fallot: Clinical and etiologic considerations. Circulation 51:1026–1029, 1975.
107. Wolff GS, Rowland TW, Ellison RC: Surgically induced right bundle branch block with left anterior hemiblock: An ominous sign in postoperative tetralogy of Fallot. Circulation 46:587–594, 1972.
108. Lasser RP, Haft JI, Friedberg CK: Relationship of right bundle branch block and marked left axis deviation (with left parietal or periinfarction block) to complete heart block and syncope. Circulation 37:429–434, 1968.
109. Sondheimer HM, Izukawa T, Olley PM, et al: Conduction disturbances after total correction of tetralogy of Fallot. Am Heart J 92:278–282, 1976.

CHAPTER 6

TACHYARRHYTHMIAS CONFINED TO THE ATRIUM

Mary C. Sokoloski

Several of the important supraventricular tachycardias originate in the atria and can continue without the participation of the bundle of His or ventricles. These have been termed *primary atrial tachycardias*. They remain the most challenging supraventricular tachycardias to treat successfully, medically, with catheters, or with surgical ablation. These atrial tachycardias may be of either an automatic or a re-entry mechanism. Some, such as chaotic atrial tachycardia and atrial fibrillation, have at least partially undefined mechanisms. Primary atrial tachycardias can be either paroxysmal or incessant. Patients can present at any age with or without structural heart disease.

Tachyarrhythmias confined to the atria are not important so much for their frequency of occurrence as for their relative risk of morbidity and mortality as well as the difficulty in controlling them both medically and nonpharmacologically. Several factors make their treatment much more difficult: they occur in patients with congenital heart disease who may or may not have undergone surgical procedures, they are associated with a lack of reserve, and they have a propensity to adverse effects.

The tachyarrhythmias that are discussed in this chapter include atrial ectopic-automatic tachycardia, atrial flutter, atrial fibrillation, chaotic atrial tachycardia, and sinus node re-entry tachycardia. The order in which they are discussed is based on their relative frequency of occurrence in the pediatric population.

ATRIAL ECTOPIC-AUTOMATIC TACHYCARDIA

Atrial ectopic-automatic tachycardia (AET) is a tachycardia that arises from a microfocus within the atrial wall itself. There appear to be two distinct forms of AET: one arising from an ectopic focus and one from a micro–re-entry circuit. The most common form of AET in children is that which is caused by an automatic focus. Because the electrophysiologic and clinical characteristics of the two forms vary, they are discussed separately, with an emphasis on the former.

AUTOMATIC FOCUS: ATRIAL ECTOPIC TACHYCARDIA

Electrophysiologic Features

As implied by its definition, an AET arises from a focus in the atria separate from the sinus node at a faster rate than that expected for the autonomic state of the patient (Fig. 6–1). A wide range of atrial rates are seen during AET (e.g., 90–330 bpm); rates vary widely among patients and within the same patient.[1–4] One marker for clinically significant AET is a higher than normal average heart rate seen on 24-hour ambulatory monitor. AET is often an incessant rhythm. Garson et al[3] reported their experience in 54 pediatric patients with AET. Tachycardia was present 100% of the time in 76% of patients, 50 to 99% of the time in 13%, and 10 to 19% of the time in 11%.

As in any rhythm confined to the atria, the atrioventricular (AV) node and ventricles are not needed for the maintenance of the rhythm, and the rhythm persists in the presence of AV block. In fact, AV block is commonly seen (Fig. 6–2). Garson et al reported that on routine electrocardiogram (ECG) first-degree AV block was seen in 91% and second-degree AV block in 24% of their patients with AET.[3] In Von Bernuth et al's series, 76% of the patients had second-degree AV block documented at least once during tachycardia.[4] AET is considered to be in the group of long RP tachycardias; however, if first-degree AV block is present at higher rates, a short RP relationship may be present.

Distinct P waves are usually seen during the tachycardia. In the 50 patients mapped in Garson's series of young patients (aged 2 days to 31

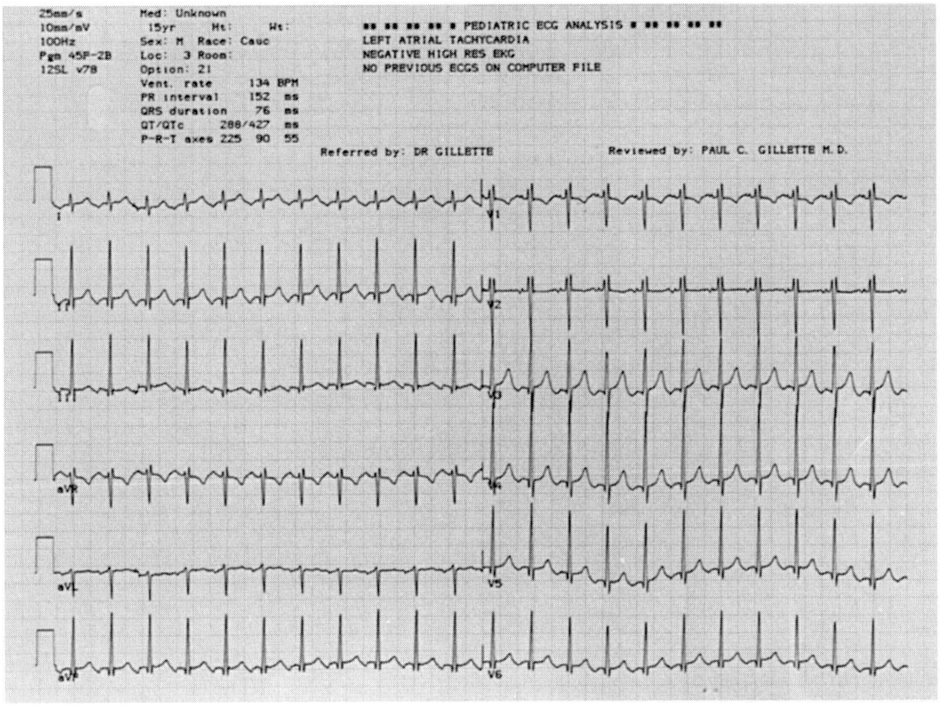

FIGURE 6–1. Twelve-lead electrocardiogram; limb leads are depicted on the left and chest leads on the right. The patient is having a left atrial ectopic-automatic tachycardia, as evidenced by the negative P waves in the chest leads and lead I. Because leads II and III also have initial negative forces, the tachycardia probably originates low in the left atrium. Characteristic of an atrial ectopic-automatic tachycardia, the rate is only moderately increased and the PR interval is normal to slightly prolonged.

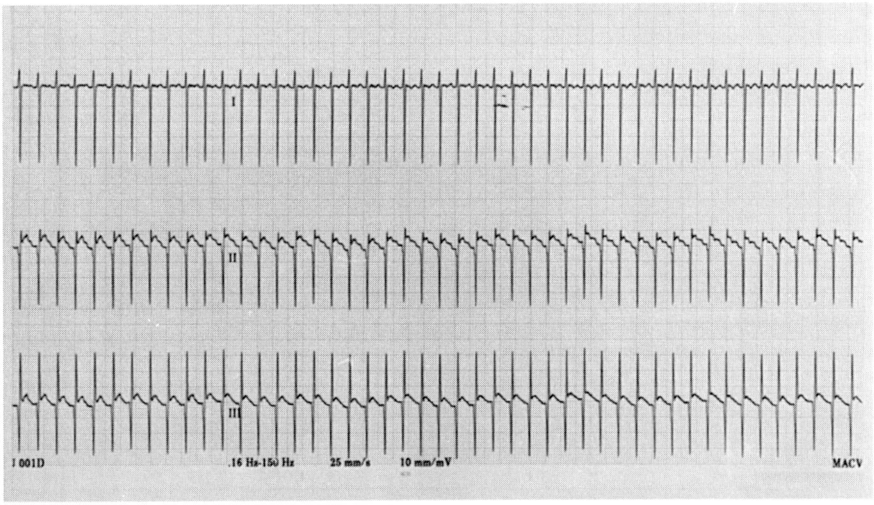

FIGURE 6–2. Surface electrocardiogram leads I, II, and III in a patient with atrial ectopic-automatic tachycardia. There is 1:1 atrioventricular (AV) conduction with first-degree AV block. At this fast rate, the P wave is difficult to separate from the T wave to determine the site of the focus (i.e., right atrial or left atrial).

years), the location of the automatic focus was the right atrial appendage (44%), the base of the left atrial appendage (26%), the midposterior right atrium (14%), the right side of the atrial septum (6%), the high lateral right atrium (6%), the mouth of the coronary sinus (2%), and the posterior left atrium (2%).[3] Of Walsh et al's 12 patients who underwent radiofrequency catheter ablation, 7 had left atrial foci; the majority (5) were near the orifices of the pulmonary veins.[5] In the 28 patients who underwent surgical ablation in Garson et al's series, half had multiple foci.[3]

All patients with multiple foci had right AET, and all had only one P-wave morphology apparent before the surgical procedure.[3] As one would surmise from the location of foci, some patients with AET have a P-wave axis consistent with sinus rhythm (Fig. 6–3). The documentation of two P-wave morphologies may help in the diagnosis (an AET focus and a sinus focus). Characteristic of an automatic focus, warm-up on initiation and cool-down on termination are seen (Fig. 6–4). The first P wave of tachycardia is the same as subsequent P waves, and the tachycardia is not initiated or terminated by pacing. The usual response seen with premature atrial beats given into tachycardia is reset of the tachycardia. Synchronized direct current cardioversion does not terminate the tachycardia.

Clinical Features

AET was present in 18% of the 178 pediatric patients who underwent an electrophysiologic study for supraventricular tachycardia.[6] It is the most common form of chronic supraventricular tachycardia in children. Onset of the tachycardia can be seen prenatally and continues throughout childhood and adolescence.[1, 2, 4] In various studies, 33 to 100% of patients present with symptoms, the majority of which are those of congestive heart failure (CHF). In the one series that mentioned palpitations, only 1 of 8 patients had this symptom.[1] The majority of patients with AET have structurally normal hearts, although cases have been seen in patients with repaired and unrepaired congenital heart disease. One case of an atrial rhabdomyoma[7] and one case of multiple atrial aneurysms have been reported.[8] At least half the patients have evidence of a dilated cardiomyopathy. Reports suggest that the development of cardiomyopathy is related to higher heart rate[3, 4] and the fact that the tachycardia is incessant.[4] In adults, AET has been associated with hypoxia, myocarditis, myocardial infarction, alcohol ingestion, electrolyte disturbances, acute catecholamine release, and stimulant medications. These causes do not appear to play a major role in AET in pediatric patients. Atrial tissue surgically removed for treatment of AET in 28 patients showed no pathologic abnormalities.

In those patients who present with cardiomyopathy, the cardiomyopathy resolved with abolition of the AET. Up to 33% of patients presenting with AET may have resolution of the tachycardia after a period of successful medical therapy once the antiarrhythmic medications

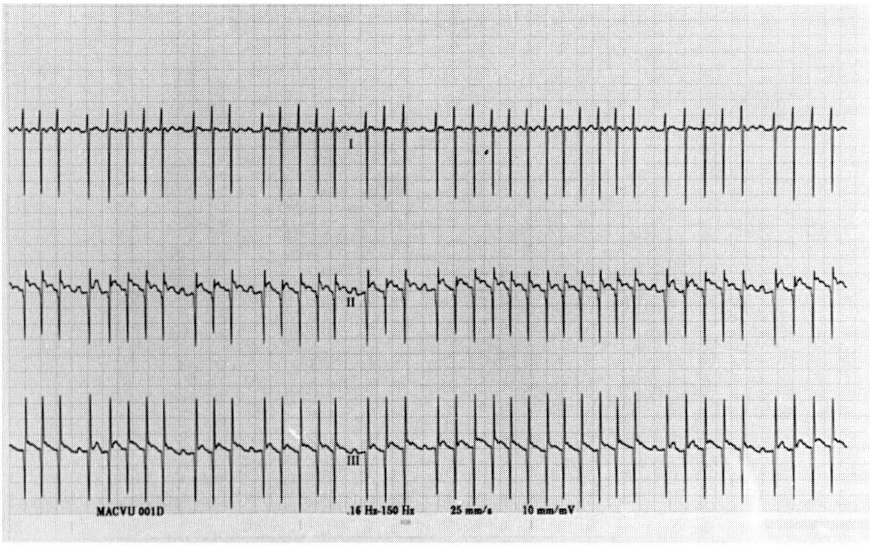

FIGURE 6–3. Surface electrocardiogram leads I, II, and III in the same patient as Figure 6–2. With variable degrees of atrioventricular block, the P waves can now be distinguished as being positive, suggesting a high right atrial ectopic-automatic focus.

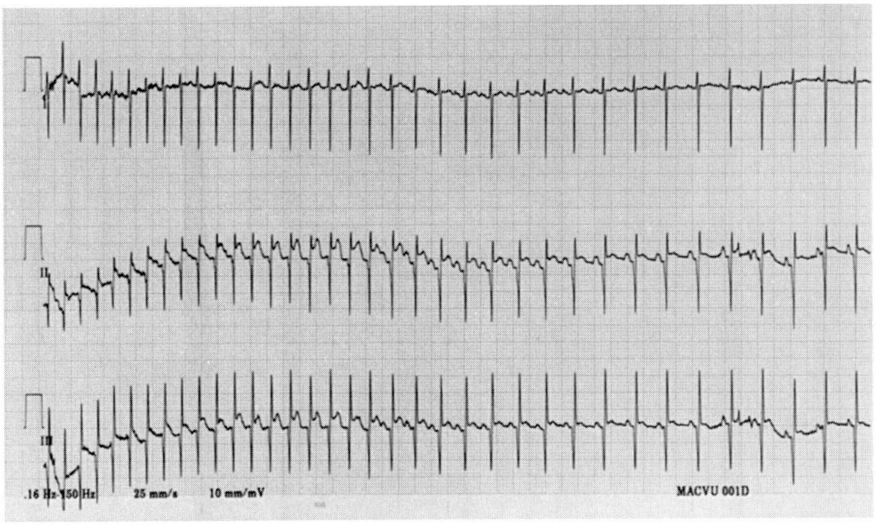

FIGURE 6–4. Surface electrocardiogram leads I, II, and III in the same patient in Figures 6–2 and 6–3. The tachycardia "warms down" to an apparent sinus rhythm, although a slower version of the tachycardia is also a possibility, because the P waves have the same morphology. This tachycardia can be differentiated from sinus tachycardia because of the rapidity of the rate at its peak.

have been stopped.[1, 2, 4] This is particularly true for infants, although late recurrences have also been noted.

Therapy

The patient with AET is often resistant to medical management and does not respond to direct current cardioversion. Two responses to adenosine may be seen; neither affords more than brief termination of the tachycardia. One response is no change in the atrial tachycardia with transient AV block. The second response is termination of atrial tachycardia followed quickly by reinitiation of AET (i.e., warm-up is typically seen). Close examination of the post-termination period to identify sinus P waves confirms the diagnosis of AET. Acute management consists of ventricular rate control and support of cardiac output. Although digoxin, verapamil, and beta blockers do not afford a high success rate for AET control, they may improve hemodynamics by decreasing the ventricular rate. Intravenous verapamil should not be used in children because of its propensity to cause profound hypotension. Because verapamil and beta blockers have negative inotropic effects, they may not be suitable for use in patients with cardiomyopathy. Intravenous amiodarone has resulted in rapid control in a high percentage of patients needing emergent tachycardia control. Rapid atrial pacing at rates faster than the atrial tachycardia rate may result in AV block, thus providing a slower ventricular response.

The efficacy of antiarrhythmic agents in pediatric patients with AET is difficult to assess in that no large series with a constant treatment strategy has been reported. In general, class IA antiarrhythmic agents and digoxin are ineffective as sole agents for the treatment of AET. Some success has been seen with beta blockers as single agents. In general, better control was achieved with amiodarone[3, 4, 9] and flecainide,[3, 4, 10] although results are variable and medication combinations were often needed. A high percentage of patients treated with moricizine have tachycardia control; however, this report consists of only a small number of patients with AET.[11] Variable control has been achieved with sotalol[2, 9, 12] and propafenone.[4, 13]

Nonpharmacologic therapy has been used in patients who remain resistant to antiarrhythmic drug therapy and those who have cardiomyopathy.[14] Surgical techniques utilized in the past[15] have been replaced by radiofrequency catheter ablation.[5] This potentially curative procedure has resulted in an 80% success rate according to a report of the pediatric radiofrequency catheter ablation registry; AET had the highest recurrence rate.[16]

MICRO–RE-ENTRANT FOCUS: ATRIAL ECTOPIC TACHYCARDIA

Little information is available on the few pediatric patients who have an AET resulting from a micro re-entrant focus. In the study of Ludomirsky and Garson,[6] a series of 178 patients undergoing electrophysiologic studies for supraventricular tachycardia, only 2 patients had what the authors termed atrial muscle re-entry. Tachycardia can be initiated or terminated with pacing; initiation is dependent on a critical A_1-A_2 interval. Intracardiac electrophysiologic mapping reveals a site of origin separate from the sinoatrial node.[6]

ATRIAL FLUTTER

CRITERIA

Atrial flutter can be defined as a re-entrant atrial tachycardia with beat-to-beat uniformity of cycle length and morphology of the surface ECG P waves and intracardiac electrograms. Atrial flutter possesses the characteristics of a re-entrant rhythm that is confined to the atria but is not sinus node re-entry. The characteristics of re-entry typical of atrial flutter include sudden onset or termination, initiation or termination by pacing, and termination by direct current shock. Some have reserved the term *atrial flutter* for such a rhythm with classic "sawtooth" flutter waves on the surface ECG, labeling other tachycardias that fulfill the prior criteria without sawtooth flutter waves intra-atrial re-entry.

In 1956, Puech et al distinguished between typical atrial flutter, which has negative sawtooth flutter waves in ECG leads II, III, and aVF, and atypical flutter, which has positive flutter waves in leads II, III, and aVF.[17] Wells et al[18] labeled this typical flutter as type I atrial flutter and a more rapid atrial flutter that was not pace terminable as type II atrial flutter (Fig. 6–5). These subclassifications of atrial flutter are often not applicable in pediatric patients, especially those who have undergone surgery for congenital heart disease. Such young patients with atrial flutter can have a wide range of atrial rates and P-wave morphologies on the surface ECG.

MECHANISM

Atrial flutter is believed to be a macro–re-entrant rhythm confined to the atria. The three classic requisites for re-entry are a pathway, slow conduction, and unidirectional block. Investigators have mapped the circuits involved in "typical" atrial flutter in adult patients to identify targets for radiofrequency catheter ablation.[19] The circuits are confined to the right atrium. The wave of activation courses from the area of the coronary sinus superiorly around the foramen ovale, posteriorly to reach the high lateral right atrial free wall, inferiorly on the free wall toward the tricuspid valve, and medially across the isth-

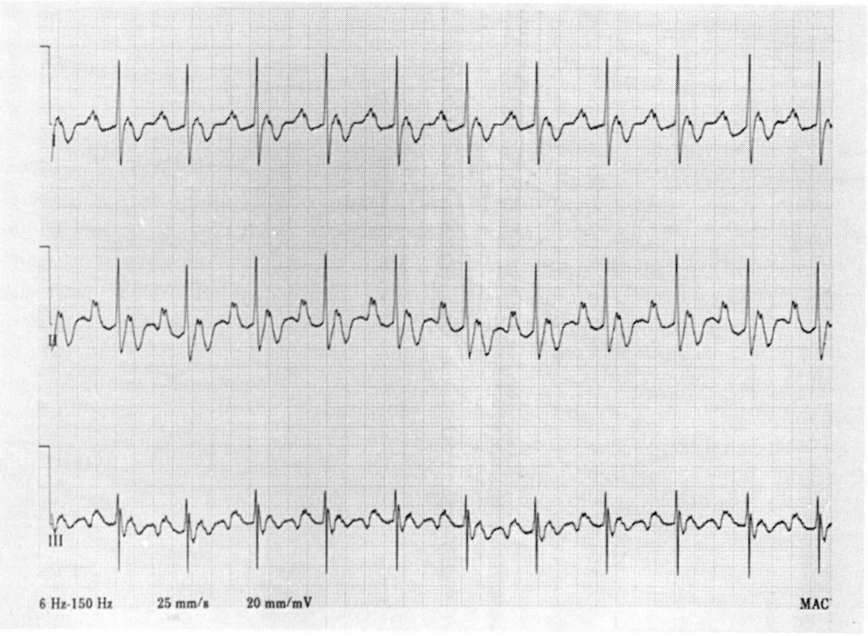

FIGURE 6–5. Surface electrocardiogram leads I, II, and III in a patient with atrial flutter with large P waves and 2:1 atrioventricular block. The P waves are positive in leads I, II, and III, indicative of atypical atrial flutter.

mus between the inferior vena cava (IVC) and tricuspid valve in the area of the coronary sinus.[19] An area of slow conduction is typically found in the region of this isthmus of tissue.

Animal models have given insight into possible atrial flutter circuits in young patients, and electrophysiologic studies and ablation in young patients have supported the conclusions of these models.[20] Cronin et al performed multielectrode mapping studies in a canine Mustard model.[21] As with any animal model, there are differences between these animals and patients who have undergone the Mustard operation. Because the animals had structurally normal hearts, they could not totally mimic the heart after a true Mustard procedure. An atriotomy was performed, an atrial septal defect (ASD) created, and Mustard suture lines were placed without the baffle; however, unlike many of the patients who experience atrial flutter after the Mustard procedure, the atrial flutter was induced and mapped at the time of the Mustard surgery. Although there are obvious differences in the animal models and actual patients, this model has given valuable insight into the atrial flutter circuits in patients who have undergone intra-atrial switch operations.

In Cronin et al's study, the investigators mapped atrial flutter in one animal that had undergone only an atriotomy, and this circuit coursed around the tricuspid valve annulus.[21] Two animals were mapped that had undergone an atriotomy and the creation of an ASD, both of which had flutter circuits that coursed around the atriotomy suture line. Animals that had undergone the "complete" Mustard operation primarily had one of these two circuits. In one animal the flutter coursed around both atria, and in another it coursed around the mitral valve. In six animals, an incision was made connecting the atriotomy to the tricuspid valve ring, eliminating all of the right atrial circuits.[21]

Rodefeld et al[22] reported a canine model of atrial flutter after a simulated lateral tunnel Fontan operation. Again, these animals had normal hearts and had undergone arrhythmia induction at the surgical procedure. In this model, the lateral tunnel suture line was found to be a critical component of the atrial flutter circuit.[22] Boyden described a model of right atrial enlargement in dogs in which multiple atrial flutter circuits were identified.[23] These animals had undergone creation of tricuspid insufficiency, and pulmonary stenosis was produced by an occluder. Multiple episodes of atrial flutter involving different circuits were induced in each of four animals. All episodes were due to re-entrant circuits in the right atrium, and anatomic block played a role in some cases. Functional block was defined as an area across which there was normal conduction during sinus rhythm, but during atrial flutter there was no conduction or no effective conduction because of extremely slow conduction.[23] One could postulate that atrial flutter circuits in pediatric patients could involve any of these mechanisms. This has been supported by the work that has been done to date in ablation patients who have undergone previous surgery for congenital heart disease.[20, 24–26]

Kalman et al[25] described in detail intra-atrial re-entrant circuits in their patients who underwent ASD closure and one patient who underwent Rastelli repair. In these patients, circuits coursed around the atriotomy scar or around the ASD patch. Other barriers or areas of block included the tricuspid valve annulus, the IVC or superior vena cava (SVC), the base of a Fontan conduit, or an atrioseptal baffle. Successful radiofrequency catheter ablation was accomplished by bridging the barriers critical to the circuit with lesions, creating block to prevent electrical conduction around the pathway of the circuit.[25]

ELECTROPHYSIOLOGIC CHARACTERISTICS

In the pediatric population, the atrial rates during atrial flutter can vary between 200 and 600 bpm. Slower rates may occur in patients who are taking antiarrhythmic medications. There may be cycle length variability at the onset and termination of atrial flutter. Otherwise, there is beat-to-beat uniformity of cycle length and morphology of the atrial flutter waves on ECG and on intracardiac electrograms. Classic flutter waves may be seen but not often in pediatric patients with atrial flutter (Fig. 6–6). Atrial morphologies range from very low-amplitude P waves to large-amplitude, long-duration P waves. However, for any one episode of atrial flutter, there is uniformity of rate and P-wave morphology. A patient who has undergone surgery for congenital heart disease may have more than one atrial rate and P-wave morphology during different episodes. In some patients, electrograms obtained from transesophageal or intracardiac electrodes are necessary to discern the diagnosis due to P wave morphology or 2:1 AV block.

Atrial flutter is generally paroxysmal but can become incessant. The AV node and the ventricles are not part of the re-entrant circuit (Fig. 6–7). All levels of AV block can be seen, including very fast ventricular rates with 1:1 AV con-

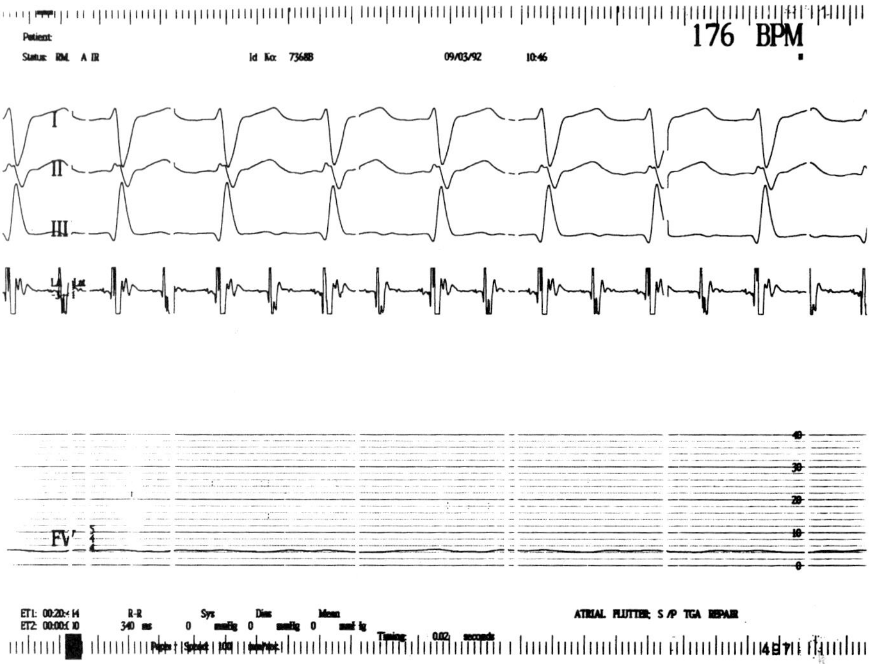

FIGURE 6–6. Surface leads I, II, and III and an atrial electrogram recorded from a bipolar transesophageal pacing catheter. The rhythm is atrial flutter with 2:1 atrioventricular block. The P waves are relatively inapparent on the surface electrocardiographic leads, which is typical in patients who experience atrial flutter after Mustard or Senning operations.

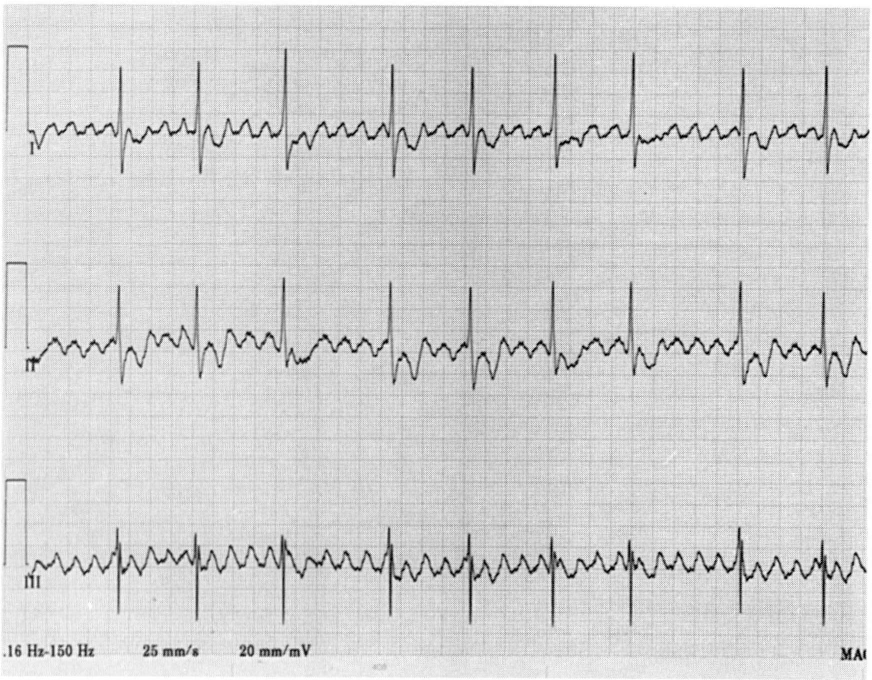

FIGURE 6–7. Surface electrocardiogram leads I, II, and III in the same patient in Figure 6–5. The atrial rate has greatly accelerated with subsequent 4:1 and 5:1 atrioventricular block. Although the P waves remain organized for the most part, there is some variation in the morphology, suggesting incipient atrial fibrillation.

duction. Adenosine administration during tachycardia typically creates high-grade AV block, often aiding in the diagnosis (Fig. 6–8); however, adenosine may uncommonly terminate atrial flutter. Atrial flutter can be induced with premature atrial extrastimuli or with rapid atrial pacing. The initiating cycle length has no effect on the tachycardia cycle length. Premature atrial beats given into atrial flutter can advance or reset the tachycardia but do not typically terminate it. Atrial pacing performed during atrial flutter may entrain or terminate the re-entry circuit. Termination can also be accomplished using direct current shock.

CLINICAL CHARACTERISTICS

Intrauterine (Fetal) and Infancy

Although most likely of the same mechanism, atrial flutter in the fetus or infant generally has a different clinical course than that later in childhood. Sweeping statements regarding this entity should be made with caution given the few number of cases reported. In Southall et al's[27] review of 3383 apparently healthy newborns, only one case of atrial flutter was identified. All 9 patients reported by Lundberg[28] had structurally normal hearts, and all did well with rare recurrences. Dunnigan et al[29] reported on 8 infants who presented with atrial flutter at or before 8 weeks of age: 1 converted to sinus rhythm after initiation of digoxin, 5 were converted with transesophageal pacing, 1 with transvenous pacing, and 1 with direct current cardioversion. Four of the patients had structurally normal hearts, 1 had systemic hypertension, 1 had d-TGA/status after balloon atrial septostomy, 1 had cardiomyopathy, and 1 had Ebstein's malformation of the tricuspid valve. Three patients had central venous pressure catheters in place. Classic flutter waves were seen in only 2 of the 8 patients, and the diagnosis was confirmed by transesophageal recording in the remaining 6. Three of the 8 patients had CHF. Only 2 patients received antiarrhythmic drugs (digoxin in 1, procainamide in 1), and only one had a single recurrence.[29]

In earlier reviews, the diagnosis of atrial flutter was made only if classic flutter waves were present on the surface ECG; thus, atrial flutter in the infant may not be as rare as previously suspected. In general, the prognosis for infants with structurally normal hearts is good with successful initial attempts at conversion and the absence of recurrences after 1 year of age. This prognosis may not be so for those patients with structural

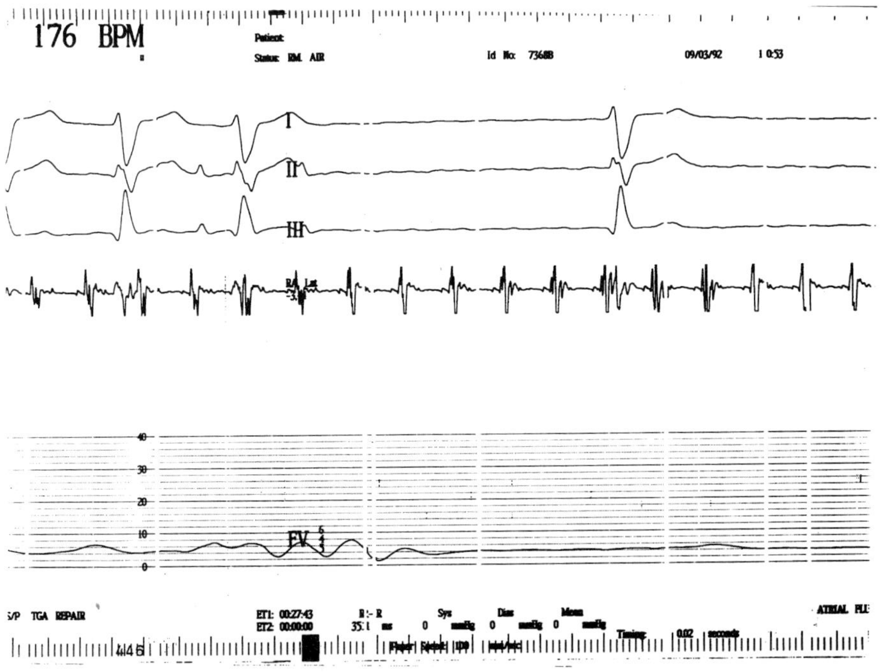

FIGURE 6–8. Surface electrocardiogram (ECG) leads I, II, and III in the same patient as Figure 6–6. Intravenous adenosine is administered with resultant atrioventricular block with a slow junctional escape rhythm. The atrial flutter persists, but once again the inapparent P waves on the surface ECG might lead one to believe that the tachycardia was momentarily terminated.

abnormalities or for those with mixed atrial arrhythmias.

Childhood

To characterize the clinical features and factors affecting the prognosis of atrial flutter, Garson and colleagues reported the collective experience of the Pediatric Electrophysiology Society in 1985.[30] Because of the large number of patients in this series and the subsequent clinical implications, this study is summarized next.[30]

Presentation. Three hundred eighty patients, aged 1 to 25 years, presented with at least one episode of atrial flutter. The mean age at onset was 10.3 ± 0.3 years. In patients who had undergone cardiac surgery, 23% had atrial flutter in the immediate postoperative period, whereas 37% experienced atrial flutter 1 to 5 years after surgery. The presenting symptoms included dyspnea/CHF (28%), palpitations (24%), syncope (9%), and presyncope (8%); 30% were asymptomatic. In 1% the atrial flutter was diagnosed after resuscitation from a sudden death episode. Of the patients being maintained on digoxin at presentation, only 6% had syncope with their first episode compared with 12% of those not maintained on digoxin, thus reinforcing the use of prophylactic digoxin.

Cardiac Diagnoses. The following diagnoses were present in 75% of the patients with atrial flutter: d-TGA (s/p Mustard or Senning), 20.4%; complex congenital lesions, 17.5%; ASD, 12.1%; tetralogy of Fallot, pulmonary atresia, or pulmonary stenosis, 7.9%; normal, 6.3%; congestive cardiomyopathy, 5.8%; and AV canal defect, 5%. The five most common operations (in the 75% of patients who had undergone previous cardiac surgery) included Mustard/Senning, 27.6%; Blalock-Hanlon, 16.1%; ASD repair, 11.1%; tetralogy of Fallot or pulmonary atresia repair, 7.9%; aorticopulmonary shunt, 6.6%. Of the patients with tetralogy of Fallot, pulmonary atresia, or pulmonary stenosis, 92% had tricuspid insufficiency, implying that these patients may be at higher risk for atrial flutter.

Follow-Up. Atrial flutter occurred only once in 33% of these patients; an additional 2% had episodes for less than 1 year. Spontaneous resolution occurred in approximately 20% of patients, which was more likely to occur if the left atrial size was normal. Medications were successful in eliminating atrial flutter in 58% of patients. In those who had undergone surgery after the onset of atrial flutter, the arrhythmia was easier to control in 52% but more difficult to control in 4%. Seventeen percent of patients died: 10% suddenly and 6% not suddenly. Risk factors for death included cardiomyopathy, complex congenital heart disease, increased left atrial size, and ineffective drug therapy. In patients in whom the atrial flutter could not be controlled with antiarrhythmic medications, there was a 20% rate of sudden and a 12% rate of nonsudden death. Successful antiarrhythmic drug therapy decreased the sudden death rate in both groups (sudden and nonsudden) to 5%. There were no deaths in patients with anatomically normal hearts. The conclusions of this study support the fact that the inability to control the atrial flutter is a risk factor for death.

Therapy

Acute Therapy

The hemodynamically unstable patient with atrial flutter should undergo synchronized, direct current cardioversion, unless overdrive pacing is immediately available. Rapid atrial pacing often terminates atrial flutter and can be used in select situations in which the patient is not hemodynamically compromised. Transesophageal pacing, temporary transvenous atrial pacing, temporary pacing with postoperative epicardial pacing wires, and atrial overdrive pacing through a permanently implanted device are additional modalities available for such conversion. If these maneuvers are not successful in terminating the atrial flutter, ventricular rate control can be acutely achieved with medication or with temporary atrial pacing fast enough to create 2:1 AV block. Conventional teaching is that antiarrhythmic medications are generally not effective in acutely converting atrial flutter; however, their use can increase the likelihood of a successful cardioversion with direct current or pacing and can prevent recurrent episodes in the future.

Direct Current Cardioversion. The energy used for direct current cardioversion of atrial flutter is 0.5 to 1 J/kg body weight. The defibrillation device must be set to synchronize to the patient's R wave. Although synchronization has greatly reduced the incidence of asynchronously induced ventricular arrhythmias, it has not totally eliminated this complication. There is evidence that toxic levels of digoxin may contribute to the induction of ventricular tachyarrhythmias; however, if the patient has no signs of digoxin toxicity and has a therapeutic serum concentration, withholding the digoxin or premedicating with lidocaine should offer no added safety.[31–33] Another risk of successful termination of atrial flutter is the development of transient bradycardia. Patients who are at risk for sinus node dysfunction apart from their atrial flutter, such as those who have undergone Fontan, Mustard, or Senning procedures, may be at high risk for bradycardia. In these patients, it would be prudent to have the capability to pace temporarily after the cardioversion. Many of the defibrillators that are currently commercially available have the capability to do this through the same pads or patches used for cardioversion and defibrillation. This may be especially prudent in patients undergoing their first cardioversion for atrial flutter because their response after flutter termination is unknown.

Feltes and Friedman performed transthoracic and transesophageal echocardiograms on 19 consecutive patients with nonfibrillatory atrial tachyarrhythmias and congenital heart disease.[34] Eight of these 19 patients had an atrial thrombus identified on transesophageal echocardiogram, yet these clots were detected by transthoracic echocardiogram in only 1 of the 8. There is currently no consensus on the identification and role of anticoagulation before cardioversion in this patient population.

Transvenous/Epicardial Temporary Overdrive Pacing. In a review of adult patients with atrial flutter, Waldo described the important principles of atrial overdrive pacing.[35] These principles include a critical overdrive pacing rate, a specific duration of atrial pacing, and a specific stimulus strength. When the termination was successful, there was a change in the P-wave morphology.[35] A reasonable algorithm for the termination of atrial flutter can be found in Table 6–1. Care should be taken not to subject the patient to prolonged periods of hypotension created by the rapid atrial pacing. The more aggressive the protocol, the more likely it is that the rhythm will progress into atrial fibrillation. Atrial fibrillation in these patients may convert spontaneously to sinus rhythm, may persist, or may convert back to atrial flutter. If the algorithm found in Table 6–1 is not useful at one specific pacing site, a repeat protocol at an alternative site, if possible, might prove useful.

Transesophageal Overdrive Pacing. Transesophageal pacing can terminate atrial flutter acutely.[36] The principles of transesophageal overdrive pacing are the same as those previously mentioned (see Table 6–1). Although this technique is minimally invasive, the actual pacing itself is painful and should be preceded by sedation with cardiorespiratory monitoring. In addition to ECG, blood pressure, and oxygen saturation monitoring, equipment for airway management and defibrillation should be readily available. The transesophageal pacing catheter is placed where the best possible atrial electrogram can be recorded. Because of the potential for discomfort to the patient, an attempt is made to use the lowest output and fewest number of stimuli to terminate this arrhythmia. Butto et al[37] described an algorithm that was successful in terminating 48 of 51 atrial flutter episodes in 14 patients who had undergone an atrial switch procedure. This algorithm uses high output, fewer stimuli, and a set cycle length versus a percentage of the tachycardia cycle length.[37]

Table 6–1. Atrial Flutter Termination Algorithm

1. Confirm that the chamber being paced is atrial and not ventricular.
2. Initiate pacing at 90% of the tachycardia cycle length for 8 beats.
3. Output may need to be adjusted three to four times higher than threshold to achieve 1:1 capture.
4. Decrease pacing cycle length by 10% and repeat 8-beat burst.
5. Continue to decrease pacing cycle length by 10% down to 60% until the tachycardia cycle length is reached.
6. If the tachycardia persists, repeat Steps 3 and 4 with 16 beats, 32 beats, 10 seconds, 20 seconds, and 30 seconds, respectively.
7. If tachycardia still persists, "ramping" of the paced cycle length from 90 to 60% can be attempted.

Adapted from Waldo AL: Some observations concerning atrial flutter in man. Pacing Clin Electrophysiol 6:1181–1189, 1983. Used with permission.

Long-term Therapy

Hemodynamic abnormalities can contribute to the occurrence of atrial flutter. Garson et al[30] reported that atrial flutter resolved or was easier to control in 52% of those patients who had undergone surgery after the onset of atrial flutter. There has been much discussion regarding the type of Fontan procedure and its association with the development of atrial flutter, although no clear consensus has been achieved. It is intuitive that patients who have undergone total cavopulmonary connections or external conduit Fontan procedures should be at less risk for atrial flutter.[38] Surgeons should be able to place cryothermia or radiofrequency lesions in critical positions to lessen the risk of atrial flutter development. The question has been raised as to whether or not conversion from a classic Fontan to a total cavopulmonary connection would help alleviate postoperative atrial flutter. It is hoped that these important issues will be resolved in the future.

Historically, the treatment method of choice for atrial flutter has been antiarrhythmic drug therapy. Despite this fact, there is little information about the efficacy of such medications for the treatment of atrial flutter in the pediatric population. The following drugs have been given for the treatment of atrial flutter in children and young adults: quinidine, procainamide, disopyramide, moricizine (Ethmozine), flecainide, propafenone, beta blockers, amiodarone, sotalol, and digoxin. Perry and Garson, in their review of the literature on flecainide for tachyarrhythmia treatment in children, reported that atrial flutter was eliminated in only 3 of 9 patients.[39] Proarrhythmia was observed in some patients, and one group that appeared to be at a higher risk for proarrhythmia were patients who had previously undergone surgery for congenital heart disease.[39] Guccione et al[40] found propafenone to be 50% effective in the 6 patients in their study being treated for atrial flutter. According to Moak et al,[41] amiodarone was effective in 94% of their reported 16 patients, whereas Guccione et al[42] found initial success in 32 of 33 patients receiving amiodarone. In the latter series, atrial flutter recurred in 7 of 33 patients within the first 6 months of therapy.[42] Sotalol was either completely or partially effective (84%) in 19 postoperative patients as reported by Pfammatter and colleagues.[43]

Beaufort-Krol and Bink-Boelkens reported conversion to sinus rhythm from atrial flutter in 11 of 13 (85%) of postoperative patients receiving oral sotalol.[44] Garson et al[30] reported atrial flutter elimination by antiarrhythmic medications in 58% of 380 patients. Digoxin had been used as a sole agent in 235 patients, successfully controlling atrial flutter in 44%. Amiodarone was the most effective drug in this series (78% control), but it was only used in 9 patients. The next most successful combination was digoxin and a type IA antiarrhythmic agent, yielding a 53% efficacy in 105 patients. The least effective medication was propranolol, with only a 33% efficacy.[30] Sotalol and propafenone were not being used for these tachyarrhythmias at the time of this study. A logical approach to treatment for the patient with atrial flutter starts with a trial of digoxin with progression to some of the other agents if digoxin fails. In patients with or at risk for sinus node dysfunction, particularly those who have undergone an intra-atrial baffle or Fontan procedure, any antiarrhythmic agent beyond digoxin may require the placement of a permanent cardiac pacemaker.

Radiofrequency catheter ablation has been successful in the management of atrial flutter.[20] Successful ablation can be accomplished in patients with anatomically normal hearts by targeting the isthmus of tissue between the inferior vena cava and the tricuspid valve.[45, 46] Success rates in the adult population have been reported as high as 90%.[47] Although technically more difficult, the ablation of critical isthmi in postoperative atrial flutter circuits has been somewhat successful in preventing atrial flutter.[20, 25, 26]

Permanent atrial antitachycardia pacing is yet another treatment modality for the long-term management of postoperative atrial flutter.[48, 49] Because most of the postoperative patients have concomitant sinus node dysfunction, which is thought to be associated with a higher incidence of atrial flutter,[50] the ability of the device to also provide bradycardia pacing makes it an attractive option. A device that provides these two features plus rate adaptive pacing is desirable to provide more heart rate variability in this patient population.

Surgical options for the treatment of postoperative atrial flutter in the young are being developed, but with the lack of long-term follow-up the efficacy of these modalities is yet to be seen. They include right atriectomy,[49] a right-sided Maze procedure,[51] a modification of the lateral tunnel operation,[52] and a combination of cryoablation and permanent antitachycardia pacing.[53]

ATRIAL FIBRILLATION

CRITERIA

On the surface ECG, atrial fibrillation is characterized by fine irregular undulations of the baseline. On intracardiac recordings, the electrograms are generally rapid and irregular in cycle length and morphology, although areas of the atria that appear more regular can be seen. The QRS complexes that result from atrial fibrillation are thus labeled as irregularly irregular in their timing (Fig. 6–9).

MECHANISM

Some maintain that the mechanism of clinical atrial fibrillation has not been shown. Despite this belief, a great deal of evidence supports the multiple-wavelet hypothesis of Moe (i.e., that atrial fibrillation is supported by the propagation

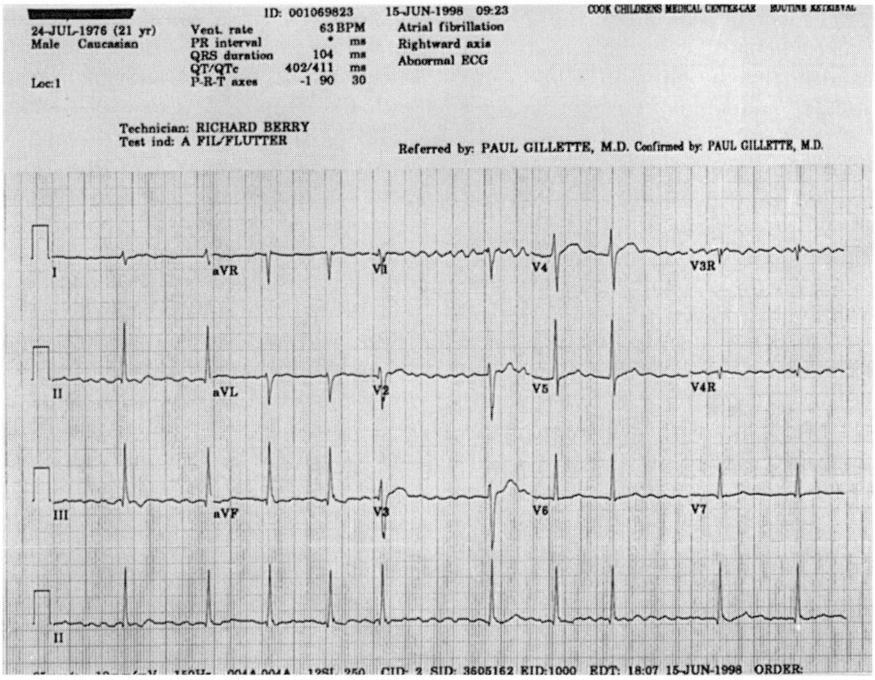

FIGURE 6–9. Twelve-lead electrocardiogram (ECG) with simultaneous lead II rhythm strip in a 21-year-old patient with an anatomically normal heart and atrial fibrillation. This rhythm is characterized by an irregular RR interval and a variable, undulating baseline.

of multiple wavelets within the atria).[54] Constantly changing and drifting re-entrant circuits can be seen within these wavelets.[55, 56]

ELECTROPHYSIOLOGIC CHARACTERISTICS

Atrial fibrillation can be induced with atrial burst pacing or extrastimuli or, less commonly, with ventricular stimulation that leads to atrial activation. A spectrum of atrial rates and intracardiac electrograms can be seen with atrial fibrillation. Some classify this spectrum into coarse versus fine atrial fibrillation or types of atrial fibrillation such as those described by Wells and colleagues.[57] Within their classification system, type I atrial fibrillation exhibits discrete electrograms of differing morphology separated by an isoelectric interval, whereas type II also exhibits discrete electrograms but with no isoelectric interval. Type III is characterized by fragmented electrograms without discreteness or isoelectric intervals. Type IV is the alternation of type III fibrillation with another type. The atrial rate increases from type I to type III.[57] In fact, some believe that atrial flutter is at one extreme of this same spectrum. With current techniques, pacing cannot terminate atrial fibrillation.

CLINICAL FEATURES

Although common in adults, atrial fibrillation is rare in children. The largest pediatric series was published in 1977 by Radford and Izukawa.[58] In this series, all young patients with the diagnosis of atrial fibrillation seen in the cardiology department of the Hospital for Sick Children in Toronto over a 22-year period were reviewed (N = 35, 23 males and 12 females). The age at onset was in utero to 19 years of age. Five of the patients had structurally normal hearts without evidence of ventricular pre-excitation. Four of these patients were infants, 1 of whom had an intrauterine diagnosis of atrial tachycardia. The other 3 infants presented with tachycardia at 3 months of age; 1 had supraventricular tachycardia in addition to atrial fibrillation and 2 presented with atrial flutter. The atrial flutter converted to atrial fibrillation with digoxin therapy. In these 4 patients, the arrhythmias resolved with digoxin therapy. In the remaining children, only 1 had a structurally normal heart, and no cause for the atrial fibrillation was found. Of those with congenital heart disease, 14 of the 17 had undergone cardiac surgery. One child with Ebstein's anomaly and the children with Eisenmenger's complex and single ventricle had not undergone surgery. At the time of the review, 18 patients were alive, 13 were known to have died, and 4 were lost to follow-up. Three children had cerebral emboli.[58]

Atrial fibrillation is often seen in conjunction with underlying disease, and it also has been associated with left atrial enlargement.[59] Hyperthyroidism and sinus node dysfunction have been reported in children,[60, 61] and atrial fibrillation in the early postoperative course is occasionally seen. In some patients, atrial fibrillation is autonomically mediated. Vagally mediated atrial fibrillation is more common in men than women. The typical age of occurrence is from 30 to 50 years. Episodes of this type of atrial fibrillation generally occur weekly and at night and usually alternate with atrial flutter. This type of atrial fibrillation does not occur with exercise but rather after exercise (in the resting state) or after alcohol ingestion. Digoxin or beta blockers may not be an effective treatment for vagally mediated atrial fibrillation and may actually aggravate the arrhythmia.

Sympathetically mediated atrial fibrillation is less common and has been associated with hyperthyroidism or pheochromocytoma. Episodes occur during the day during stressful periods or during exercise. Alternations with atrial flutter are not seen in this form of atrial fibrillation.[62] In their review of tachyarrhythmias in young athletes, Coelho et al[63] reported on 5 athletes younger than 35 years who presented with documented atrial fibrillation. One of these patients had manifest ventricular pre-excitation, whereas the other 4 had mitral valve prolapse.[63] Although rare, familial atrial fibrillation may present in childhood. Brugada et al[64] described a genetic locus associated with three families containing 43 family members, 19 of whom had atrial fibrillation. The age at diagnosis ranged between 2 and 46 years.[64]

Atrial fibrillation has been associated with Wolff-Parkinson-White (WPW) syndrome. It has been implicated in syncope and sudden death in patients with WPW syndrome. Rapid conduction to the ventricles results in ventricular fibrillation.[65] Some experts advocate that all patients with WPW syndrome undergo electrophysiologic testing to assess the risk of rapid AV conduction during atrial fibrillation. The effective refractory period of the accessory connection should be measured. The risk of sudden death is increased in those with refractory periods less than 250 milliseconds. Atrial fibrillation should also be induced while isoproterenol is infused and the shortest resulting RR interval measured. Those with RR intervals less than 250 milliseconds are at higher risk.

Atrial fibrillation is associated with hypertrophic cardiomyopathy[66] and has been implicated as a cause of sudden death in this patient population. Stafford et al[67] reported a case of a 15-year-old with this diagnosis in whom atrial fibrillation was believed to initiate clinical ventricular fibrillation. Other investigators have not found an increased incidence of death in patients with hypertrophic cardiomyopathy and atrial fibrillation compared with those without atrial fibrillation.[66]

THERAPY

Because few children have atrial fibrillation, no studies exist that examine antiarrhythmic drug use in this population. Current practices are based largely on the experience obtained in adults.

Initial Management

In the patient with significant hemodynamic compromise, synchronized direct current cardioversion may be necessary. If atrial fibrillation has been present for more than 48 hours, there is a risk of intra-atrial clot. If possible, the cardioversion should be delayed and the patient should undergo anticoagulation therapy for 3 weeks. Anticoagulation should be continued for 4 weeks after restoration of sinus rhythm.[68] If cardioversion cannot be delayed, heparin should be initiated with subsequent oral anticoagulation for 4 weeks. An alternative to anticoagulation is transesophageal echocardiography for clot visualization. If no clots are visualized, cardioversion should proceed; however, this approach may incur a small increase in the incidence of thromboembolism in the absence of anticoagulation. Additionally, the patient would still require anticoagulation after the procedure while the atria are regaining mechanical function. Class I antiarrhythmics (quinidine, procainamide, disopyramide, flecainide, and propafenone) and the class III agent amiodarone have been shown to be better than placebo in the pharmacologic conversion of atrial fibrillation.[68] If direct current cardioversion is delayed or if it does not restore sinus rhythm, ventricular rate control can be achieved with AV nodal blocking agents such as digoxin, beta blockers, or verapamil.

Long-term Management

The majority of data regarding the efficacy of long-term medical therapy for atrial fibrillation have been obtained in the adult population. The class IA antiarrhythmic agents have been found to be effective in controlling atrial fibrillation. Class IA agents may slow the atrial rate, allowing for more rapid conduction through the AV node and thus causing an increased ventricular rate. Because of this, when treating atrial fibrillation or atrial flutter, one should consider using AV nodal blocking agents in conjunction with class IA agents. The risk of proarrhythmia and potential adverse effects may outweigh the positive benefits. In adults, quinidine has been associated with a threefold increase in mortality.[69] There is some concern that quinidine will be proarrhythmic in the pediatric population, especially in those with structural heart disease. The high incidence of systemic side effects, including a lupus-like syndrome, makes the long-term use of procainamide difficult. Disopyramide has been shown to precipitate heart failure in 50% of patients with a history of heart failure.[70]

Class IC agents (flecainide, propafenone) have been shown to be efficacious in the treatment of atrial fibrillation[71]; however, in the Cardiac Arrhythmia Suppression Trial (CAST), there was increased mortality in postmyocardial infarction patients who received encainide or flecainide.[72] This trial raises the concern that all class IC agents may be significantly proarrhythmic in patients with heart disease. In a review of pediatric patients from 36 centers who received encainide (107 patients) and flecainide (472 patients), Fish et al[73] found the following percentages of cardiac arrest and death: encainide cardiac arrest, 7.5%; encainide death, 7.5%; flecainide cardiac arrest, 2.3%; flecainide death, 2.1%.[73] As expected, most of those with lethal or potentially lethal events had more serious underlying arrhythmia, decreased systemic ventricular function, or underlying heart disease or were otherwise known or suspected to be at high risk for sudden death. Interpretation of these data must incorporate the idea that the review is retrospective, and no comparisons to the risk profile of other antiarrhythmics were undertaken.[73] As suggested after their review of published articles on flecainide use in children, Perry and Garson described two situations in which the pharmacokinetics of flecainide may result in an increased risk of proarrhythmia: the child who requires high doses of flecainide but has low trough serum concentrations and the child whose diet changes to incorporate fewer dairy products.[39] They also found that most of the proarrhythmia occurred during the initiation of therapy and that those with structural heart disease were at a higher risk.[39]

Paul and Janousek[74] reported a 2% incidence of proarrhythmia in pediatric patients receiving propafenone. Because of the potential to slow the atrial arrhythmia with a resultant increase in the ventricular rate, AV nodal blocking agents should be considered when class IC agents are used. Class III agents, amiodarone and sotalol, have been given to treat atrial fibrillation. With amiodarone, there are several significant noncardiac side effects, as well as sinus node dysfunction and prolonged AV conduction. The risk of torsades de pointes is present, but appears to be low. With sotalol, there are significant beta-blocking effects. Pfammatter and colleagues[43] found proarrhythmia in 10% of patients receiving sotalol in their 1995 report. Their findings included bradycardia from sinoatrial block and high-grade AV block, increased ventricular ectopic activity, and in one patient torsades de pointes.[43] Chronic anticoagulation with warfarin should be considered in any patient with chronic or paroxysmal atrial fibrillation to lessen the incidence of thromboembolism.

The maze procedure is used in adults with atrial fibrillation and may have a role in the patient with congenital heart disease.[51] Investigative nonpharmacologic therapies for atrial fibrillation in adults currently include implanted transvenous defibrillators, with or without ventricular defibrillation capabilities, and catheter ablation for atrial fibrillation. In each patient, a strong effort to convert atrial fibrillation to sinus rhythm, even with surgical procedures to improve hemodynamics, should be included because of the likelihood of increased quantity and quality of life for the patient.

CHAOTIC ATRIAL TACHYCARDIA

CRITERIA

Chaotic atrial tachycardia, also known as multifocal atrial tachycardia and chaotic atrial rhythm, is characterized by five distinct criteria: a minimum of three P-wave morphologies; a lack of a dominant atrial rhythm; isoelectric intervals between P waves; varying PP, RR, and PR intervals; and average atrial rates greater than 100 bpm during tachycardia (Fig. 6–10).

MECHANISM

The mechanism of chaotic atrial tachycardia (CAT) is not known. The limited success that

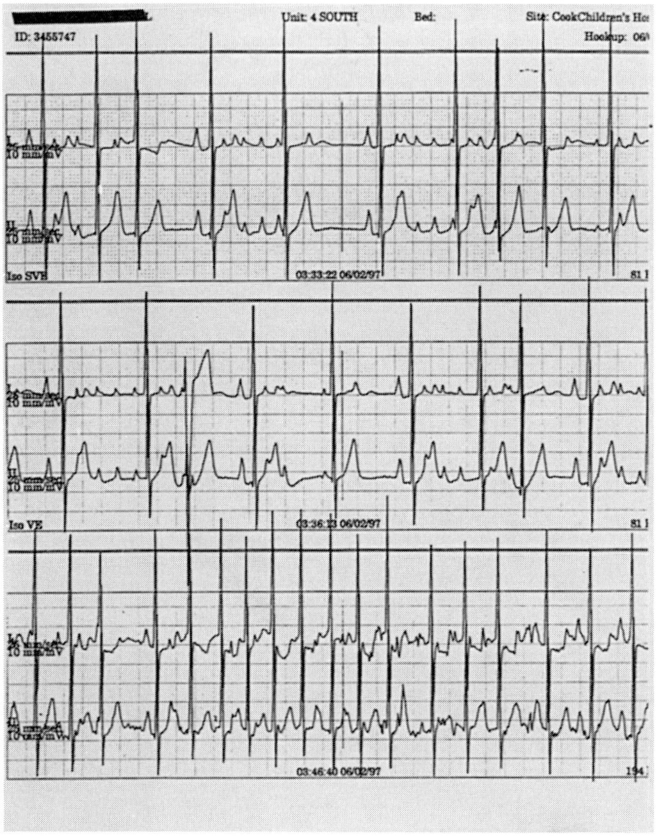

FIGURE 6–10. Ambulatory monitor electrocardiographic tracings from a 10-month-old with chaotic atrial tachycardia. Although not present in this recording, the child did have the classic three P-wave morphologies.

some cardiologists treating adults have had with verapamil supports a triggered rhythm. The presence of distinct, consistent P-wave morphologies and what appears to be AET would be consistent with increased automaticity. Patients with CAT can also exhibit atrial flutter; however, pacing, which typically initiates or terminates re-entrant rhythms, does not significantly affect CAT. Direct current cardioversion, which is useful in the termination of most re-entrant rhythms, is not effective for converting CAT. Increased levels of catecholamines have been implicated in the pathogenesis of CAT, as have methylxanthines.

ELECTROPHYSIOLOGIC FEATURES

CAT is usually an incessant, persistent tachycardia. In reported cases, the presenting atrial rates vary between 155 and 500 bpm with ventricular rates of 100 to 400 bpm. This tachycardia is not responsive to direct current cardioversion, vagal maneuvers, or intravenous antiarrhythmic medications. Patients with CAT often have other atrial arrhythmias, including atrial fibrillation, atrial flutter, AET, premature atrial contractions, periods of no atrial activity, or sinus bradycardia with a junctional escape.

CLINICAL FEATURES

CAT is an uncommon rhythm in both adults and children. The only estimate of the incidence in the pediatric population was made by Salim et al,[75] who diagnosed 5 patients with CAT of 1500 (0.2%) patients with new-onset arrhythmias who presented over a 7-year period.[75] Sixty-four cases of CAT in the pediatric population appear in the literature.[75–83] In these series, there were more males than females, with a ratio of 39:25. Ages ranged from in utero to 18 years; the majority were infants (ages: $<$ 1 week, 13 patients; 1 week–1 mo, 8; 1–6 mo, 27; 7–13 mo, 5; 1–2 years, 4; 2–5 years, 5; 5–10 years, 1; $>$ 10 years, 1). The majority of patients had structurally normal hearts, but 22 had structural heart disease (ASD, 6; ventricular septal defect (VSD), 5; hypertrophic cardiomyopathy, 5; signs of endocardial fibroelastosis, 4; postoperative congenital heart disease, 4; myocarditis, 3).

A large percentage of adults with CAT have

pulmonary disease. In reports of children, 24 of the patients had pulmonary disease, 19 of which were included in the series by Wu and colleagues.[76] Twenty-three patients had other medical diagnoses, among them prematurity (7) and infection (5). Seven of the patients are described as having features consistent with a genetic syndrome. Dodo et al[79] described three patients with identifiable syndromes—Simpson-Golabi-Behmel, Costello, and Noonan—in addition to hypertrophic cardiomyopathy. The only other evidence for possible genetic involvement in CAT are two siblings with structurally normal hearts, both of whom have CAT.

Most patients with CAT who are referred for cardiac evaluation are asymptomatic but have an irregularly irregular rhythm. Most of the patients continue to be asymptomatic throughout their treatment and follow-up. Twenty-one of the pediatric patients in the literature had respiratory symptoms, most likely resulting from pulmonary disease. Thirteen had CHF thought to be due to episodes of AET. In the majority of patients, CAT resolved, often before 1 year of age. Many of the patients received antiarrhythmic medications, but the relationship between drug therapy and tachycardia resolution is not always clear. Despite the seemingly benign nature of CAT, of the 64 patients reviewed, 10 died. Three of the 10 patients had structurally normal hearts. One had persistent CAT treated with digoxin, the dosage of which had been increased at the most recent outpatient visit. He presented with respiratory distress after a vomiting episode and a cardiac rhythm of CAT, followed by complete heart block, an idioventricular rhythm, and asystole.[77] One patient had resolution of CAT at 4 weeks of age, with documented sinus rhythm at the ages of 6 weeks, 4 months, and 6 months. He died suddenly in his crib at 7 months of age.[80] Another child had a single pulmonary lobe abnormality and bronchopneumonia and died of respiratory failure.[76] Two of the patients had hypertrophic cardiomyopathy: one died at the time of pacemaker placement after His ablation, and the other died of possible sepsis.[79] One patient had endocardial thickening and mitral valve prolapse. This patient presented with AET and at 3 months of age was found to have CAT. At 5 months of age, she presented to an emergency room with upper respiratory tract infection symptoms and suddenly became unresponsive. She was found to be in AET but died despite resuscitative efforts.[80] One patient had an ASD, and refractory CAT, and was believed to have died of respiratory failure and cardiac decompensation resulting from complications of therapy.[75] One patient had tetralogy of Fallot and chronic CAT. He died of severe respiratory distress after feeding.[80] The other two had ventricular septal defects and died at home.[76]

In general, CAT is believed to have a good prognosis if the child has a normal heart and no associated noncardiac disease. Thus, a careful investigation of the cardiac structure is prudent in the child's overall evaluation.

TREATMENT

The mainstay for adults with CAT is the treatment of any underlying conditions that may contribute to the arrhythmia, such as respiratory distress. Few of the pediatric patients in the literature had electrolyte abnormalities (hypocalcemia), correction of which did not affect the tachycardia. The use of antiarrhythmic medications in pediatric patients with CAT is controversial. Generally, antiarrhythmic medications are administered to patients with symptoms, incessant arrhythmias, high ventricular rates, presence of other arrhythmias warranting therapy, and structurally abnormal hearts. Multiple medications, including digoxin, beta blockers, amiodarone, flecainide, encainide, procainamide, and propafenone, have been used with inconsistent benefit. Digoxin is often given as an initial agent, but is usually not considered to be effective in either arrhythmia control or ventricular rate control.

Some consider combination therapy to be effective. Dodo et al[79] reported significant improvement (no CAT or occasional short runs with a slow ventricular response) in six of nine patients who received combination therapy, including amiodarone. Successful combinations were amiodarone and digoxin together or in combination with procainamide or propafenone.[79] Salim et al[75] reported tachycardia control in two of three patients who received digoxin and amiodarone alone or in combination with flecainide or encainide.[75] In our institution, digoxin is used first, followed by amiodarone and then flecainide for further control. Antiarrhythmic agents are withdrawn after at least a year of no tachycardia recurrences.

SINUS NODE RE-ENTRANT TACHYCARDIA

CRITERIA

Sinus node re-entrant tachycardia is characterized by four criteria: P-wave morphology similar or identical to sinus rhythm, intracardiac electrograms consistent with an origin at the sinus node, induction and termination with premature beats, and initiation independent of AV nodal conduction delay.[84–86]

MECHANISM

As the name implies, sinus node re-entrant tachycardia is believed to be a re-entrant rhythm. Unlike many of the other re-entrant rhythms, the exact pathway has not been definitively mapped in humans. It has been postulated that this rhythm involves micro–re-entry within the sinus node and its border zone or macro–re-entry, which travels circumferentially around the sinus node.[84]

ELECTROPHYSIOLOGIC CHARACTERISTICS

During sinus node re-entry tachycardia, the P waves are similar or identical to those during sinus rhythm. Sinus node re-entry tachycardia is initiated and terminated with premature impulses, and induction is not dependent on AV nodal conduction delay or dual AV nodal physiology. It can be terminated with burst pacing as well. The onset and termination are abrupt, without warm-up or cool-down, and cycle length variation is common.[84] Adenosine typically terminates sinus node re-entry tachycardia.[87]

CLINICAL FEATURES

In their review of 346 patients with supraventricular tachycardia, Ludomirsky and Garson identified 7% of the patients with sinus node re-entry tachycardia.[6] All patients were older than 2 years, and 5 of 12 had no predisposing factors. One had congenital heart disease but had not undergone an operation, and 4 had undergone surgery for congenital heart disease. Two of the 12 had CHF.[6] Sinus node re-entry tachycardia can be associated with palpitations, presyncope, and syncope.[88]

THERAPY

For acute termination, atrial pacing is effective, and termination with direct current cardioversion has been reported.[6] Although reports of medical therapy for sinus node re-entry tachycardia are small, digoxin and calcium channel blockers are suggested as first-line therapy.[6, 84]

In summary, although the incidence of tachyarrhythmias confined to the atria in children is low, those rare instances require astute arrhythmia recognition and aggressive management, either medically or nonpharmacologically. The patients who present with these arrhythmias have a somewhat higher risk of morbidity and mortality, especially those with structurally abnormal hearts.

REFERENCES

1. Garson A Jr, Gillette PC: Electrophysiologic studies of supraventricular tachycardia in children: I. Clinical-electrophysiologic correlations. Am Heart J 1981; 102:333–350, 1981.
2. Koike K, Hesslein PS, Findlay CD, et al: Atrial automatic tachycardia in children. Am J Cardiol 1988; 61:1127–1130, 1988.
3. Garson A Jr, Gillette PC, Moak JP, et al: Supraventricular tachycardia due to multiple atrial ectopic foci: A relatively common problem. J Cardiovasc Electrophysiol 1:132–138, 1990.
4. Von Bernuth G, Engerlhardt W, Kramer HH, et al: Atrial automatic tachycardia in infancy and childhood. European Heart J 13:1410–1415, 1992.
5. Walsh EP, Saul JP, Hulse E, et al: Transcatheter ablation of ectopic atrial tachycardia in young patients using radiofrequency current. Circulation 86:1138–1146, 1992.
6. Ludomirsky A, Garson A Jr: Supraventricular tachycardia in children. In Gillette PC, Garson A Jr (eds): Pediatric Arrhythmias: Electrophysiology and Pacing. Philadelphia: WB Saunders, 1990, pp 380–426.
7. Ross BA, Crawford FA, Whitman V, et al: Atrial automatic ectopic tachycardia due to an atrial tumor. Am Heart J 115:605–610, 1988.
8. Dhala AA, Case CL, Gillette PC: Evolving treatment strategies for managing atrial ectopic tachycardia in children. Am Heart J 74:283–286, 1994.
9. Naheed ZJ, Strasburger JF, Benson DW, et al: Natural history and management strategies of automatic atrial tachycardia in children. Am J Cardiol 1995; 75:405–407, 1995.
10. Perry JC, Garson A Jr: Flecainide acetate for treatment of tachyarrhythmias in children: Review of world literature on efficacy, safety, and dosing. Am Heart J 124:1614–1621, 1992.
11. Evans VL, Garson A Jr, Smith RT, et al: Ethmozine (moricizine HCl): A promising drug for "automatic" atrial ectopic tachycardia. Am J Cardiol 60:83F–9F, 1987.
12. Maragnes P, Tipple M, Fournier A: Effectiveness of oral sotalol for treatment of pediatric arrhythmias. Am J Cardiol 69:751–754, 1992.
13. Heusch A, Kramer HH, Krogmann ON, et al: Clinical experience with propafenone for cardiac arrhythmias in the young. Eur Heart J 15:1050–1056, 1994.
14. Gillette PC, Wampler DG, Garson A Jr, et al: Treatment of atrial automatic tachycardia by ablation procedures. J Am Coll Cardiol 6:404–409, 1985.
15. Crawford FA, Gillette PC: Surgical treatment of cardiac dysrhythmias in infants and children. Ann Thorac Surg 58:1262–1268, 1994.

16. Kugler JD, Danford DA, Deal BJ, et al: Radiofrequency catheter ablation for tachyarrhythmias in children and adolescents. The Pediatric Electrophysiology Society. N Engl J Med 330:1481–1487, 1994.
17. Puech P: L'Activite electrique auricularie normale et pathologique. Paris: Masson & Cie, 1956, p 214.
18. Wells JL Jr, MacLean WAH, James TN, et al: Characterization of atrial flutter. Studies in man after open heart surgery using fixed atrial electrodes. Circulation 60:665–673, 1979.
19. Feld GK, Fleck RP, Chen PS, et al: Radiofrequency catheter ablation for the treatment of human type 1 atrial flutter: Identification of a critical zone in the re-entrant circuit by endocardial mapping techniques. Circulation 86:1233–1240, 1992.
20. Triedman JK, Saul JP, Weindling SN, et al: Radiofrequency ablation of intra-atrial reentrant tachycardia after surgical palliation of congenital heart disease. Circulation 91:707–714, 1995.
21. Cronin CS, Nitta T, Mitsuno M, et al: Characterization and surgical ablation of acute atrial flutter following the Mustard procedure: A canine model. Circulation 88:461–471, 1993.
22. Rodefeld MD, Gandhi SK, Huddleston CB, et al: Anatomically based ablation of atrial flutter in an acute canine model of the modified Fontan operation. J Thorac Cardiovasc Surg 112:898–907, 1996.
23. Boyden PA: Activation sequence during atrial flutter in dogs with surgically induced right atrial enlargement: Observations during sustained rhythms. Circ Res 62:596–607, 1988.
24. Lesh MD, Van Hare GF: Status of ablation in patients with atrial tachycardia and flutter. Pacing Clin Electrophys 17:1026–1033, 1994.
25. Kalman JM, Van Hare GF, Olgin JE, et al: Ablation of "incisional" reentrant atrial tachycardia complicating surgery for congenital heart disease: Use of entrainment to define a critical isthmus of conduction. Circulation 93:502–512, 1996.
26. Van Hare GF, Lesh MD, Stanger P: Radiofrequency catheter ablation of supraventricular arrhythmias in patients with congenital heart disease: Results and technical considerations. J Am Coll Cardiol 22:883–890, 1993.
27. Southall DP, Johnson AM, Shinebourne EA, et al: Frequency and outcome of disorders of cardiac rhythm and conduction in a population of newborn infants. Pediatrics 68:58–66, 1981.
28. Lundberg A: Paroxysmal atrial tachycardia in infancy: Long term follow up study of 49 subjects. Pediatrics 70:638–642, 1982.
29. Dunnigan A, Benson DW, Benditt DG: Atrial flutter in infancy: Diagnosis, clinical features, and treatment. Pediatrics 1985; 75:725–729, 1985.
30. Garson A Jr, Bink-Boelkens M, Hesslein PS, et al: Atrial flutter in the young: A collaborative study of 380 cases. J Am Coll Cardiol 6:871–878, 1985.
31. Mann DL, Maisel AS, Atwood JE, et al: Absence of cardioversion-induced ventricular arrhythmias in patients with therapeutic digoxin levels. J Am Coll Cardiol 5:882–888, 1985.
32. Ditchey RV, Karliner JS: Safety of electrical cardioversion in patients without digitalis toxicity. Ann Intern Med 95:676–679, 1981.
33. Ditchey RV, Curtis GP: Effects of apparently nontoxic doses of digoxin on ventricular ectopy after direct-current electrical shocks in dogs. J Pharmacol Exp Ther 218:212–216, 1981.
34. Feltes TF, Friedman RA: Transesophageal echocardiographic detection of atrial thrombi in patients with nonfibrillation atrial tachyarrhythmias and congenital heart disease. J Am Coll Cardiol 24:1365–1370, 1994.
35. Waldo AL: Some observations concerning atrial flutter in man. Pacing Clin Electrophysiol 6:1181–1189, 1983.
36. Rhodes LA, Walsh EP, Saul JP: Conversion of atrial flutter in pediatric patients by transesophageal atrial pacing: A safe, effective, minimally invasive procedure. Am Heart J 130:323–327, 1995.
37. Butto F, Dunnigan A, Overholt ED, et al: Transesophageal study of recurrent atrial tachycardia after atrial baffle procedures for complete transposition of the great arteries. J Am Coll Cardiol 57:1356–1362, 1986.
38. Gelatt M, Hamilton RM, McCrindle BW, et al: Risk factors for atrial tachyarrhythmias after the Fontan operation. J Am Coll Cardiol 24:1735–1741, 1994.
39. Perry JC, Garson A Jr: Flecainide acetate for treatment of tachyarrhythmias in children: Review of world literature on efficacy, safety, and dosing. Am Heart J 124:1614–1621, 1992.
40. Guccione P, Drago F, DiDonato RM, et al: Oral propafenone therapy for children with arrhythmias: Efficacy and adverse effects in mid-term follow up. Am Heart J 122:1022–1027, 1991.
41. Moak JP, Smith RT, Garson A Jr: Newer antiarrhythmic drugs in children. Am Heart J 113:179–185, 1987.
42. Guccione P, Paul T, Garson A Jr: Long-term follow up of amiodarone therapy in the young: Continued efficacy, unimpaired growth, moderate side effects. J Am Coll Cardiol 1990; 15:1118–1124, 1990.
43. Pfammatter JP, Paul T, Lehmann C, et al: Efficacy and proarrhythmia of oral sotalol in pediatric patients. J Am Coll Cardiol 26:1002–1007, 1995.
44. Beaufort-Krol GC, Bink-Boelkens MT: Effectiveness of sotalol for atrial flutter in children after surgery for congenital heart disease. Am J Cardiol 79:92–94, 1997.
45. Feld GK, Fleck P, Chen PS, et al: Radiofrequency catheter ablation for the treatment of human type 1 atrial flutter. Circulation 86:1233–1240, 1992.
46. Cosio FG, Lopez-Gil M, Goicolea A, et al: Radiofrequency ablation of the inferior vena cava–tricuspid valve isthmus in common atrial flutter. Am J Cardiol 71:705–709, 1993.
47. Fischer B, Haissaguerre M, Garrigues S, et al: Radiofrequency catheter ablation of common atrial flutter in 80 patients. J Am Coll Cardiol 25:1365–1372, 1995.
48. Fukushige J, Porter CJ, Hayes DL, et al: Antitachycardia pacemaker treatment of postoperative arrhythmias in pediatric patients. Pacing Clin Electrophysiol 14:546–556, 1991.
49. Balaji S, Johnson TB, Sade RM, et al: Management of atrial flutter after the Fontan procedure. J Am Coll Cardiol 23:1209–1215, 1994.
50. Fishberger SB, Wernowsky G, Gentles TL, et al: Factors that influence the development of atrial flutter after the Fontan operation. J Thorac Cardiovasc Surg 113:80–86, 1997.
51. Theodoro DA, Danielson GK, Porter CJ, et al: Right-sided maze procedure for right atrial arrhythmias in congenital heart disease. Ann Thorac Surg 65:153–154, 1998.
52. Robotin MC, Serraf A, Houyel L, et al: Prevention of unbalanced lung perfusion and atrial arrhythmias after the lateral tunnel operation. Ann Thorac Surg 64:1389–1395, 1997.
53. Mavroudis C, Backer CL, Deal BJ, et al: Fontan conversion to cavopulmonary connection and arrhythmia circuit cryoablation. J Thorac Cardiovasc Surg 115:547–556, 1998.
54. Moe GK: On the multiple wavelet hypothesis of atrial fibrillation. Arch Int Pharmacodyn Ther 140:183–188, 1962.

55. Konings KTS, Kirchhof CJHJ, Smeets JRLM, et al: High density mapping of electrically induced atrial fibrillation in man. Circulation 89:1665–1680, 1994.
56. Allessie MA, Konings K, Kirchhof CJHJ, et al: Electrophysiologic mechanisms of perpetuation of atrial fibrillation. Am J Cardiol 77:10A–23A, 1996.
57. Wells JL, Karp RB, Kouchoukos NT, et al: Characterization of atrial fibrillation in man. Pacing Clin Electrophysiol 1:426–438, 1978.
58. Radford DJ, Izukawa T: Atrial fibrillation in children. Pediatrics 59:250–256, 1977.
59. Henry WL, Morganroth J, Pearlman AS, et al: Relation between echocardiographically determined left atrial size and atrial fibrillation. Circulation 53:273–279, 1976.
60. Perry LW, Hung W: Atrial fibrillation and hyperthyroidism in a 14-year-old boy. J Pediatr 79:668–671, 1971.
61. Radford DJ, Izukawa T: Sick sinus syndrome symptomatic cases in children. Arch Dis Child 50:879–885, 1975.
62. Coumel P: Paroxysmal atrial fibrillation: A disorder of autonomic tone? Eur Heart J 15:9–16, 1994.
63. Coelho A, Palileo E, Ashley W, et al: Tachyarrhythmias in young athletes. J Am Coll Cardiol 1986;7:237–243, 1986.
64. Brugada R, Tapscott T, Czernuszewicz GZ, et al: Identification of a genetic locus for familial atrial fibrillation. N Engl J Med 13:905–911, 1997.
65. Paul T, Guccione P, Garson A Jr: Relation of syncope in young patients with Wolff-Parkinson-White syndrome to rapid ventricular response during atrial fibrillation. Am J Cardiol 65:318–321, 1990.
66. Robinson K, Frenneaux MP, Stockins B, et al: Atrial fibrillation in cardiomyopathy: A longitudinal study. J Am Coll Cardiol 15:1279–1285, 1990.
67. Stafford WJ, Trohman RG, Bilsker M, et al: Cardiac arrest in an adolescent with atrial fibrillation and hypertrophic cardiomyopathy. J Am Coll Card 7:701–707, 1966.
68. Talajic M, MacDonald RG, Nattel S: Restoration of sinus rhythm in patients with atrial fibrillation. Can J Cardiol 12:29A–35A, 1996.
69. Coplen SE, Antman EM, Berlin JA, et al: Efficacy and safety of quinidine therapy for maintenance of sinus rhythm after cardioversion: A meta-analysis. Circulation 82:1106–1116, 1990.
70. Podrid PJ, Schoeneberger A, Lown B, et al: Congestive heart failure caused by oral disopyramide. N Engl J Med 302:614–617, 1980.
71. Newman D, Gillis A, Gilbert M, et al: Chronic drug therapy to prevent recurrence of atrial fibrillation. Can J Cardiol 12:24A–28A, 1996.
72. The Cardiac Arrhythmia Suppression Trial (CAST) Investigators: Preliminary report: Effect of encainide and flecainide on mortality in a randomized trial of arrhythmia suppression after myocardial infarction. N Engl J Med 321:406–412, 1989.
73. Fish FA, Gillette PC, Benson DW Jr: Proarrhythmia, cardiac arrest and death in young patients receiving encainide and flecainide. The Pediatric Electrophysiology Group. J Am Coll Cardiol 18:356–365, 1991.
74. Paul T, Jonousek J: New antiarrhythmic drugs in pediatric use: Propafenone. Pediatr Cardiol 15:190–197, 1994.
75. Salim MA, Case CL, Gillette PC: Chaotic atrial tachycardia in children. Am Heart J 129:831–833, 1995.
76. Wu MY, Wu ZF, Chen XY: Chaotic atrial tachycardia in 22 infants. Chinese Medical J 97:500–503, 1984.
77. Bisset GS, Seigal SF, Gaum WE, et al: Chaotic atrial tachycardia in childhood. Am Heart J 101:268–272, 1981.
78. Liberthson RR, Colan SD: Multifocal or chaotic atrial rhythm. Report of nine infants, delineation of clinical course and management, and review of the literature. Pediatr Cardiol 2:179–184, 1982.
79. Dodo H, Gow RM, Hamilton RM, et al: Chaotic atrial rhythm in children. Am Heart J 129:990–995, 1995.
80. Yeager SB, Hougen TJ, Levy AM: Sudden death in infants with chaotic atrial rhythm. Arch J Dis Child 138:689–692, 1984.
81. Houyel L, Fournier A, Davignon A: Successful treatment of chaotic atrial tachycardia with oral flecainide. Int J Cardiol 27:27–29, 1990.
82. Farooki ZQ, Green EW: Multifocal atrial tachycardia in two neonates. Br Heart J 39:872–874, 1977.
83. Zeevi B, Berant M, Sclarovsky S, et al: Treatment of multifocal atrial tachycardia with amiodarone in a child with congenital heart disease. Am J Card 57:344–345, 1986.
84. Gomes JA, Mehta D, Langan MN: Sinus node reentrant tachycardia. Pacing Clin Electrophysiol 1995; 18:1045–1057, 1995.
85. Narula OS: Sinus node reentry: Mechanism of supraventricular tachycardia (SVT) in man. Circulation 50:1114–1128, 1974.
86. Pauley KL, Baughese PJ, Damato AN: Atrial rhythms in response to early premature depolarization in man. Am Heart J 85:323–331, 1973.
87. Engelstein ED, Lippman N, Stein KM, et al: Mechanism-specific effects of adenosine on atrial tachycardia. Circulation 89:2645–2654, 1994.
88. Gomes AJ, Hariman RJ, Kang PS: Sustained symptomatic sinus node reentrant tachycardia: Incidence, clinical significance, electrophysiologic observations and the effects of antiarrhythmic agents. J Am Coll Cardiol 5:45–47, 1985.

CHAPTER 7

SUPRAVENTRICULAR TACHYCARDIA

George F. Van Hare

DEFINITIONS

The term *supraventricular tachycardia* (SVT) has been used to denote a condition in which there are attacks of abnormal tachycardia, generally with narrow or normal QRS duration during tachycardia. Various references define it broadly to include all forms of abnormal tachycardia other than ventricular tachycardia, whereas others define it more narrowly. For the purposes of this discussion, SVT is defined as all forms of re-entrant tachycardia, excluding ventricular tachycardia, that require participation of the atrioventricular (AV) junction for maintenance of tachycardia. This definition excludes atrial ectopic tachycardias as well as re-entrant tachycardias confined to the atrium that do not involve the AV junction in the circuit, namely atrial flutter, atrial fibrillation, sinus node re-entry, and intra-atrial re-entrant tachycardia. It also excludes sinus tachycardia. These mechanisms of tachycardia are covered elsewhere. SVT includes all tachycardias resulting from accessory pathways, either concealed or manifest, the various forms of AV node re-entrant tachycardia (AVNRT), and junctional ectopic tachycardia (JET).

INCIDENCE

SVT is clearly the most common form of abnormal tachycardia observed in children. This is in contrast to the situation in adults, in whom atrial fibrillation is much more common than SVT. In children, atrial fibrillation is a rare cause of tachycardia. The true incidence of SVT in children is unknown, but has been estimated from 1 per 25,000[1] to as high as 1 per 250 children.[2] The estimation of the true incidence is hampered by the difficulties in establishing a firm electrocardiographic diagnosis for paroxysmal episodes of tachycardia, which may disappear before an electrocardiogram (ECG) can be obtained. However, for one cause of SVT, Wolff-Parkinson-White (WPW) syndrome, the characteristic ECG findings of pre-excitation make a firm diagnosis possible. The WPW pattern on ECG is thought to occur with an incidence of 3 per 1000, a number derived from adult reports,[3] which has been confirmed in population-based pediatric studies.[4] In about half of these patients, the pathway is thought to be potentially symptomatic.

Within the category of SVT, the relative prevalence of AV node re-entry versus accessory pathway tachycardias is unknown in children. In adults, AVNRT is slightly more common than accessory pathway tachycardia, but there is a general impression that AVNRT is somewhat less common in children. The estimation of the true prevalence is hampered by the lack of invasive electrophysiologic data in small children. In a series from Houston of 121 children with SVT undergoing invasive electrophysiologic study, 29 (23%) had AVNRT, whereas the rest had various forms of accessory pathway tachycardia.[2] Only about half of children with possible SVT underwent electrophysiologic study, however. In a larger group of pediatric patients studied either invasively or via transesophageal electrophysiology, AVNRT, which accounted for only 13% of mechanisms, was found to be rare in those younger than 2 years, and accessory pathway–mediated SVT was found to be the most common diagnosis, accounting for 73% of mechanisms.[5]

The last 6 years have been a revolution in the care of children with all forms of abnormal tachycardia, with the advent of methods of radiofrequency ablation for definitive cure of these conditions.[6–11] These new techniques have not only changed the approach to pediatric patients with arrhythmias, but they have also provided a tool for better understanding of the underlying mechanisms of these tachycardias. The application of various therapies for SVT such as symptomatic treatment, suppressive therapy with antiarrhythmic agents, and ablation therapy depends on a detailed understanding of the natural history and clinical characteristics of each form of SVT as well as a knowledge of the potential risks and benefits of each type of therapy. In this chapter, we consider each mechanism in detail, including the natural history, electrocardiographic features, findings at electrophysiologic study, and methods for differentiating each mechanism from other forms of abnormal tachycardia. We discuss the possible treatments of each in the context of natural history of the conditions. Finally, we discuss the management of the new pediatric patient who presents with SVT without a previously diagnosed mechanism.

ACCESSORY PATHWAY TACHYCARDIA

ANATOMY

Several types of accessory pathways are generally recognized in the era after the introduction of radiofrequency ablation. The most common type of abnormal pathway is the AV accessory pathway (Fig. 7–1). Accessory pathways connect atrium to ventricle without the inclusion of any elements of the specialized conduction system such as AV node or bundle branches. These pathways may be capable of antegrade (AV) as well as retrograde (ventriculoatrial) conduction or may be unidirectional in the retrograde direction and incapable of antegrade conduction. Rarely, antegrade conduction only may be seen. When the pathway is capable of bidirectional or antegrade conduction, it is termed a *manifest accessory pathway*, because the presence of the pathway is manifest on a resting 12-lead ECG as a result of abnormal ventricular activation ("preexcitation") during sinus rhythm by the pathway (Fig. 7–2). If the pathway is capable only of retrograde conduction, it is termed a *concealed accessory pathway*, because the presence of the pathway is not manifest on the ECG in sinus rhythm. The diagnosis of WPW syndrome may be made when a patient has a manifest accessory pathway by ECG and also suffers from abnormal tachycardia because of the pathway. Note that patients with manifest accessory pathways who are asymptomatic are not strictly considered to have the WPW syndrome. Similarly, patients with tachycardia mediated by a concealed accessory pathway are also not considered to have WPW.

Accessory AV pathways may be located nearly anywhere along the right or left AV groove or in

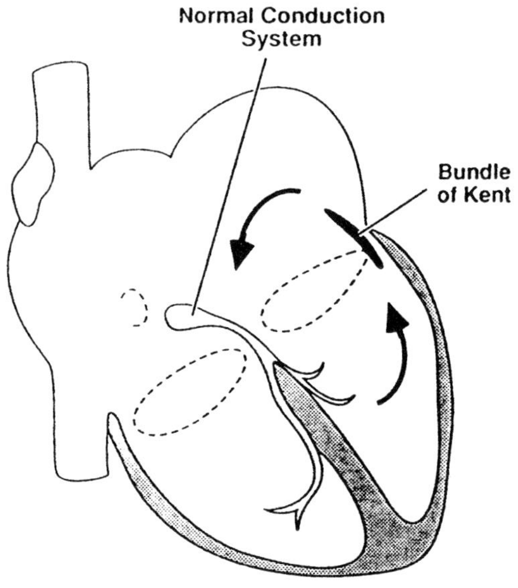

FIGURE 7–1. Diagram of the re-entrant circuit in Wolff-Parkinson-White syndrome. Impulses proceed down the normal conduction system to the ventricle and then retrograde up the bundle of Kent (accessory pathway) back to the atrium, where they may then re-enter the normal conduction system. From Van Hare GF. Circulation. In Rudolph AM, Kamei RK (eds.), Rudolph's Fundamentals of Pediatrics. Norwalk, CT, Appleton & Lange, 1994: 522, used with permission.

the septum. The most common sites are the left lateral AV groove and the posteroseptal region; right-sided locations and mid- and anterior paraseptal locations are less common.[11] One important exception to this rule is Ebstein's anomaly of the tricuspid valve, in which manifest right free wall accessory pathways are common.[12] In Ebstein's anomaly patients, multiple pathways are common.[13] Patients with L transposition of the great vessels (ventricular inversion) often have an associated Ebstein's anomaly of the tricuspid valve, which is the left-sided systemic AV valve in these patients. These patients may have WPW syndrome resulting from left-sided accessory pathways. Finally, there is an increased incidence of WPW syndrome with tricuspid atresia, double-outlet right ventricle, and hypertrophic cardiomyopathy.

These accessory pathway types are generally rapidly conducting pathways and exhibit nondecremental conduction (see following discussion). A special type of pathway is encountered with some frequency in children, which mediates persistent (or the permanent form of) junctional reciprocating tachycardia (PJRT). Patients with PJRT have a slowly conducting concealed accessory pathway with decremental conduction prop-

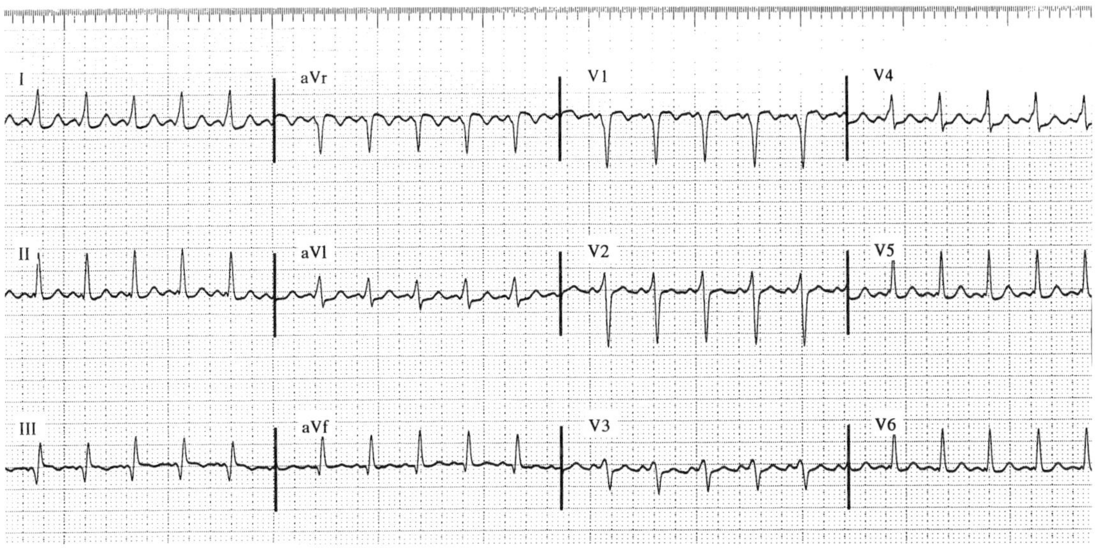

FIGURE 7–2. Twelve-lead electrocardiogram in a patient with Wolff-Parkinson-White syndrome. Note that the QRS complex is widened and there is a lack of the normal isoelectric interval between the end of the P wave and the onset of the QRS complex, which has a slurred upstroke.

erties, similar to the properties of the AV node.[14] This type of pathway leads to a slower but more incessant tachycardia. Such pathways generally have their atrial insertion in the posteroseptal right atrium near the mouth of the coronary sinus, although other locations, such as the midseptum or the left lateral AV annulus, have been occasionally reported.[15]

The term *Mahaim accessory pathway* refers to a group of accessory pathways that include elements of the specialized conducting system in their origins or insertions. Mahaim pathways are generally capable only of antegrade conduction, and they typically display nodelike electrophysiologic characteristics, with slow and decremental conduction. They are typically recognized by observing a characteristic pattern of pre-excitation with a normal PR interval. Views about the exact anatomy of such pathways have undergone a radical change in the last several years, largely because of the advent of radiofrequency ablation techniques.[16, 17] It is currently believed that the most common type of Mahaim accessory pathway is the *atriofascicular* pathway. Atriofascicular pathways connect the atrium to a portion of the right bundle branch, bypassing the AV node and bundle of His, and typically have their origins at the tricuspid annulus in an anteroseptal, anterior, or anterolateral location. A second type of Mahaim accessory pathway, the *nodofascicular pathway*, most likely exists and connects the AV node directly to the right bundle branch, bypassing the bundle of His. It was originally thought that nearly all Mahaim-type pathways were nodofascicular in type, with atriofascicular pathways being rare, but the ability to ablate selectively elements of the conducting system as well as to map and ablate along the tricuspid annulus has allowed investigators to delineate the true anatomic substrates of these conditions.[18] A third type of Mahaim pathway, the *fasciculoventricular pathway*, has been described and connects the more proximal right bundle branch directly to the right ventricular myocardium, bypassing only the more distal right bundle. This results in minimal pre-excitation but is not thought to mediate tachycardia.[19]

Older references have described the so-called James fiber, thought to be responsible for the syndrome known as Lown-Ganong-Levine (LGL) syndrome. This proposed pathway was thought to link the atrium directly to the distal AV node, bypassing parts of the AV node.[20] It is recognized as a short PR interval in sinus rhythm in a patient with a normal QRS (no delta wave) and episodes of SVT. The term is sometimes used interchangeably with "enhanced AV node conduction" because this proposed pathway has been thought to mediate rapid conduction of atrial fibrillation. It is difficult to separate the descriptions of such patients from characteristics of patients known to have dual AV node pathways and AVNRT. Since the advent of radiofrequency ablation, there are few reports of this diagnosis, and the term LGL syndrome may be falling into disuse.

CLINICAL PRESENTATION AND NATURAL HISTORY

Depending on the exact anatomy, patients may present at any age and may present with either paroxysmal or incessant tachycardia. With typical accessory pathway tachycardia, as is seen with WPW syndrome or a concealed nondecremental accessory pathway, episodes are paroxysmal. There is much individual variation in the inciting factors. Some patients have episodes without identifiable triggering events, whereas others only have episodes during exertion or stress. The degree of symptomatology present in any particular patient will depend on the rate and the duration of the tachycardia. In infants rates of 260 to 300 are typical, whereas in older children lower rates are seen. The typical adolescent experiences tachycardia rates of 160 to 200 beats per minute. It is rare for a patient with orthodromic AV reciprocating tachycardia to present with syncope. Syncope in a patient with WPW syndrome raises the possibility of atrial fibrillation with rapid AV conduction. More commonly, SVT is associated with lightheadedness, fatigue, and occasionally mild chest pain. Often the only complaint is the sensation of a rapid heart rate. In infants, if tachycardia is sustained for many hours, it is possible to present with signs of congestive heart failure, including pallor, tachypnea, retractions, diaphoresis, and hepatomegaly. For this to occur, tachycardia must be present for a substantial period of time, usually at least 12 to 24 hours. Infants may tolerate heart rates of 300 beats per minute for many hours before congestive heart failure intervenes.

Often patients have learned on their own to terminate episodes using various maneuvers, including the Valsalva maneuver, breath holding, and head stands. The history of effective use of such maneuvers helps to place a patient in the diagnostic category of SVT.

Patients with incessant tachycardia resulting from PJRT rarely present with symptoms related to the acute effects of rapid heart rate, because the heart rate in PJRT is lower than the typical rates seen with other forms of SVT at each age. Patients with PJRT may present after a pediatrician has recognized an accelerated heart rate on well-child care examination. Symptoms with which these patients present are usually those of congestive heart failure resulting from tachycardia cardiomyopathy. Such a presentation is sometimes seen in the fetus, in which fetal ultrasound examination shows hydrops fetalis.

Determination of the exact natural history of patients with accessory pathways is hampered by the difficulty in discriminating accessory pathway tachycardia from AV node re-entry in the patient without pre-excitation, because most infants with SVT do not undergo invasive electrophysiologic study. It is well known, however, that a substantial portion of infants presenting with SVT in the newborn period will be asymptomatic and not require antiarrhythmic medication by their first birthday. The situation in patients with manifest accessory pathways is somewhat more clear, although only 25% of children presenting with SVT have WPW syndrome on ECG.[2] Perry et al[21] showed that, of infants with WPW syndrome presenting before 2 months of age, 93% experienced disappearance of tachycardia, but 31% experienced reappearance at an average age of 8 years. If tachycardia was present after age 5 years, it persisted in 78% at long-term follow-up. Similarly, in patients with all forms of SVT, in a study from Taiwan, only 40% of patients presenting in infancy were still symptomatic by 5 years of age.[22]

One additional factor concerning the natural history of SVT is the risk of sudden death in patients who have WPW syndrome on ECG. There are no large prospective studies in children, but in adults the presence of WPW syndrome on ECG is associated with a risk of sudden death, almost certainly a result of atrial fibrillation with rapid conduction to the ventricles over the accessory pathway. In symptomatic patients (i.e., those with SVT or syncope), this risk is estimated to be 0.3 to 0.9% per patient year[23] and has been demonstrated to be dependent on the antegrade effective refractory period of the accessory pathway.[24] In asymptomatic patients, this risk is much lower and has been estimated to be about 0.1% per year.[25] Because sudden death depends on the occurrence of atrial fibrillation in this group, and because atrial fibrillation is rare in the pediatric population, it is believed that these risks are lower, but not absent, in children,[26] although they may increase in adolescence.

ELECTROCARDIOGRAPHIC RECOGNITION OF ACCESSORY PATHWAY–MEDIATED SVT

In patients with WPW syndrome, there is pre-excitation with a characteristic delta wave along with a short PR interval (see Fig. 7–2). Depending on the site of the pathway and the AV node conduction, pre-excitation may be subtle or obvious. The QRS is wider than normal and lacks a rapid initial deflection, but rather shows a slow "slurred" upstroke. The delta wave is due to slow cell-to-cell spread of ventricular activation from the accessory pathway, which starts before activation of the ventricle by the specialized conducting system. In most patients, the site of the pathway may be predicted based on the vector forces of the initial portion of the QRS. The principle involved is that, during pre-excitation, ventricular forces spread away from the site of the pathway. For example, in patients with posterior pathways, ventricular activation is spread in a superior direction, so that negative delta waves are inscribed in leads II, III, and aVF. Similarly, in patients with left lateral or anterolateral pathways, the spread of ventricular activation is directly to the right, so that negative delta waves are inscribed in leads I and aVL. Various algorithms have been developed for the rapid and reliable prediction of accessory pathway location in patients with WPW syndrome.[27–29]

During orthodromic AV reciprocating tachycardia (AVRT), in patients with accessory pathways, conduction proceeds down the AV node and bundle of His to activate the ventricles, then up the accessory pathway retrograde to activate the atrium, and so on. Because the accessory pathway conducts in the retrograde direction, there is no delta wave and the QRS is normal. Occasionally, sustained bundle branch aberration may be seen in children, but it is rare. Often, however, several beats of bundle branch aberration are seen at the onset of tachycardia as a result of Ashman's phenomenon. The tachycardia rate is typically about 300 bpm in infants and slower in older children. The P wave follows the preceding QRS complex in older children (Fig. 7–3). In infants, however, because of brisk AV conduction, P waves may fall halfway between the QRS complexes or may be difficult to discern on the T wave. There is little or no variation in the RR interval, and AV block always terminates the tachycardia, because the AV node is part of the re-entrant circuit. If bundle branch block develops during the tachycardia in the same ventricle as the accessory pathway, the ventriculoatrial (VA) time will lengthen and the tachycardia rate will frequently slow. In antidromic AVRT, conduction proceeds in the reverse direction from that in orthodromic AVRT; conduction proceeds antegrade down the accessory pathway to activate the ventricle, retrograde up the bundle of His and AV node to activate the atrium, and so on. Because the ventricle is activated entirely from the accessory pathway, the QRS complexes are wide. One may sometimes appreciate P waves just before the wide QRS complexes. Antidromic SVT may also occur with two accessory pathways: one antegrade and one retrograde.

In PJRT, conduction proceeds identically to that during orthodromic AVRT, except that the retrograde accessory pathway conduction is much slower than with the more common accessory pathways. This slow conduction is responsible for the relatively incessant nature of these

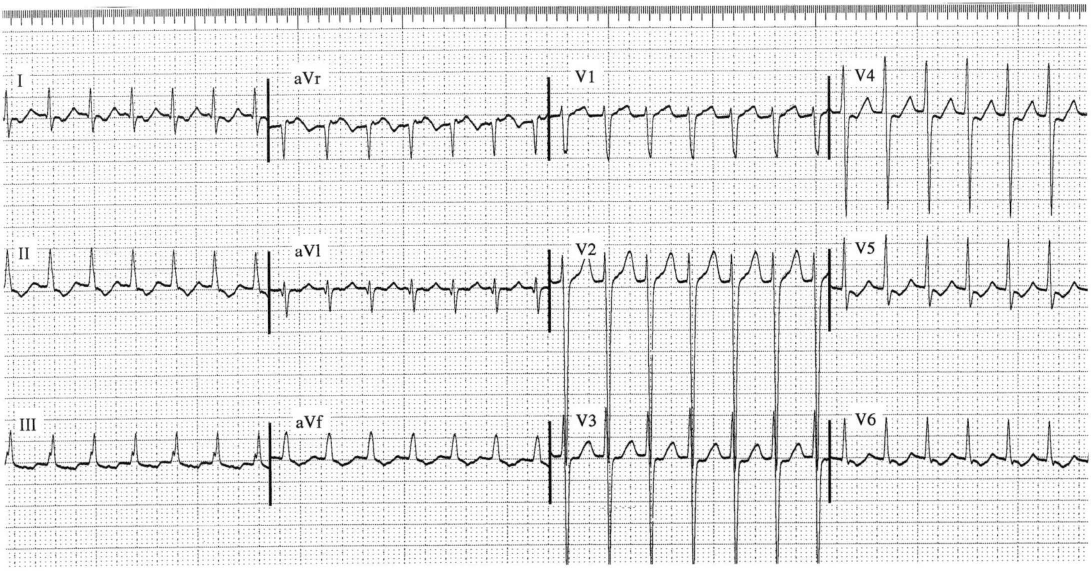

FIGURE 7–3. Twelve-lead electrocardiogram in a patient with an accessory pathway during atrioventricular reciprocating tachycardia. Note that the QRS is normal and P waves are visible on the upstroke of the T wave, best appreciated in leads I and III.

rhythms. The slow retrograde conduction allows enough time for the AV node and bundle of His to recover excitability. Likewise, the normally slow AV nodal antegrade conduction allows the pathway time to recover. The slow retrograde accessory pathway conduction causes the P wave to be located nearer the subsequent QRS complex than the previous one during tachycardia, and so they are easily appreciated (Fig. 7–4). Spontaneous terminations may occur with block in either the pathway or the AV node, so that these rhythms may end with either a QRS complex or a P wave. Because of the incessant nature of these rhythms and the location and morphology of the P wave, these are often misdiagnosed as incessant atrial tachycardia or even sinus tachycardia.

In patients with a *Mahaim* type of accessory pathway, the baseline ECG shows pre-excitation, which may be subtle, but with a normal PR interval. Two types of reciprocating tachycardia are recognized. In the first, best termed *Mahaim tachycardia*, conduction proceeds from the atrium down the atriofascicular pathway to excite the ventricle from the right bundle branch and subsequently retrograde up the bundle of His and AV node to activate the atrium. The abnormal ventricular activation gives rise to a wider-than-normal QRS complex, which has a left bundle branch block configuration and a horizontal or superior axis in the frontal plane. In the second type of reciprocating tachycardia, best termed *bystander Mahaim tachycardia*, tachycardia is actually mediated primarily by dual AV node pathways and is typical AVNRT (see later discussion). When a Mahaim pathway coexists with AVNRT, conduction proceeds up the fast pathway to activate the atrium retrograde and then conducts down both the slow AV node pathway as well as the Mahaim pathway. Because conduction down the Mahaim pathway reaches the ventricle before conduction down the slow AV node pathway, ventricular activation is abnormal, with the typical Mahaim configuration (see prior discussion). These two types of reciprocating tachycardia are difficult to differentiate on ECG. Bystander Mahaim tachycardia is recognized when one observes spontaneous loss of Mahaim QRS configuration, with normalization of the QRS and with continued tachycardia, indicating that the Mahaim pathway is not critical for maintenance of tachycardia. In both types, the occurrence of AV block should terminate the tachycardia, because the AV node is part of the re-entrant circuit in both. When the Mahaim fiber originates from the bundle of His, pre-excitation may never be lost, but the position of atrial depolarization simultaneous with ventricular depolarization is a clue.

ELECTROPHYSIOLOGIC STUDY

The diagnosis of accessory pathway–mediated tachycardia is made in the electrophysiology laboratory by the demonstration of the presence of

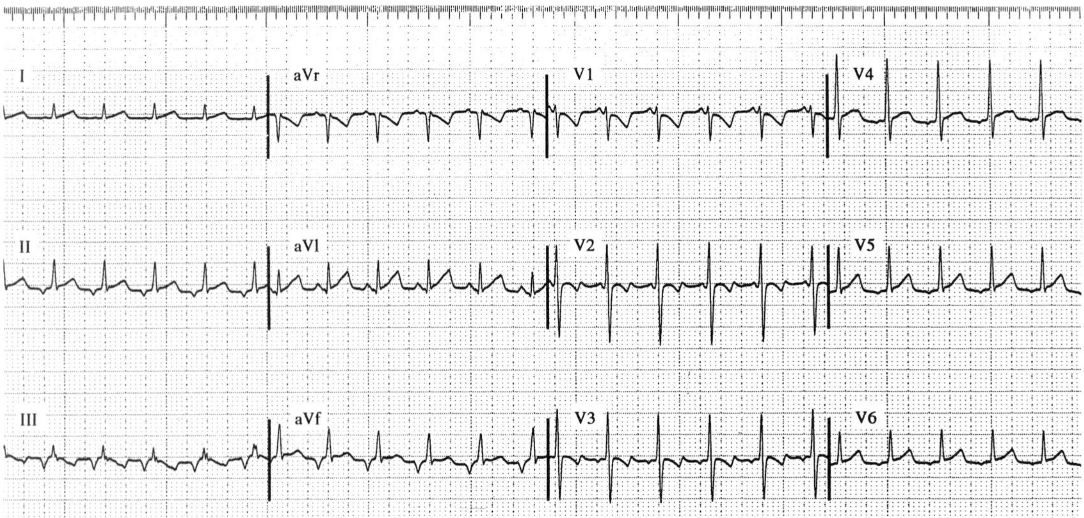

FIGURE 7–4. Twelve-lead electrocardiogram in a patient with permanent junctional reciprocating tachycardia. Note that P waves are closer to the subsequent QRS complex than the previous QRS and the P wave vector is superior, suggesting origin from the region of the mouth of the coronary sinus.

an accessory pathway and by the confirmation that tachycardia, when induced, is mediated by the accessory pathway.

In patients with WPW syndrome, pre-excitation is present in sinus rhythm but may not be obvious. This is particularly true in smaller children because AV nodal conduction times may be short enough that little of the ventricle is depolarized by the accessory pathway by the time normal activation is initiated by the His-Purkinje system. Pre-excitation can be brought out by several techniques. Simple atrial pacing at increasing rates will enhance pre-excitation, because antegrade accessory pathway conduction in WPW syndrome is nondecremental, whereas AV nodal conduction is decremental. That is, the AV node responds to increased rates and to prematurity by increasing conduction time, whereas accessory pathways in WPW syndrome respond to increasing prematurity with no increase in conduction time. Therefore, at faster rates, more of the ventricle is depolarized by the pathway by the time His-Purkinje activation arrives, until the antegrade block cycle length of the pathway is reached. Similarly, atrial extrastimulation will enhance pre-excitation until the antegrade accessory pathway effective refractory period (ERP) is reached. Finally, pacing the atrium near the location of the accessory pathway will also enhance pre-excitation by shortening the time from stimulus to accessory pathway activation and lengthening the time from stimulus to AV nodal activation. An example of this technique is in patients with left-sided accessory pathways, in whom coronary sinus pacing will bring out pre-excitation.

The degree of pre-excitation is assessed, as discussed previously, from the ECG and may also be assessed by the HV interval. Patients with pre-excitation caused by an accessory pathway will have shortening of the HV interval, measured from the occurrence of the His bundle potential to the earliest ventricular activation as seen on the surface ECG. The HV interval is short because, although the His activates normally, the earliest ventricular activation is dependent not on conduction from the His bundle to the distal conduction system and ventricle but rather on conduction from the atrium to the ventricle via the accessory pathway. In patients with minimal pre-excitation, atrial pacing will cause increased pre-excitation, as described previously, and the HV interval will further shorten. This shortening is due to His activation occurring later, as a result of decremental AV nodal conduction, with ventricular activation not occurring later as a result of nondecremental accessory pathway conduction. As the His bundle electrogram "moves into" the QRS in response to increasing atrial prematurity, the HV interval may shorten to 0 milliseconds and often becomes negative (i.e., the His bundle electrogram occurs after ventricular activation).

In patients with WPW syndrome and those with concealed accessory pathways, retrograde conduction is assessed. At least 50% of normal children without accessory pathways will have VA conduction mediated by the His-Purkinje system and AV node. This VA conduction normally is decremental, with longer VA times in response to shorter ventricular extrastimulation coupling intervals. Normal VA conduction is also "concentric"; the earliest retrograde atrial activation occurs in the region where the His bundle electrogram is recorded and with later activations in the coronary sinus mouth, distal coronary sinus, and right atrial sites. The presence of an accessory pathway is documented by observing nondecremental VA conduction and "eccentric" retrograde atrial activation; the earliest retrograde atrial activation occurs at the site of the accessory pathway. It must be remembered that the last criterion is problematic in patients with anteroseptal accessory pathways, in whom retrograde atrial activation via the accessory pathway happens to occur near the site of the His bundle electrogram but in whom VA conduction is nondecremental.

SVT may be inducible either from the atrium or the ventricle. Orthodromic tachycardia in patients with a concealed accessory pathway is usually easily inducible by atrial programmed stimulation of the atrium, but may not be inducible in patients with pre-excitation and a short antegrade effective refractory period of the accessory pathway. This is because, to induce tachycardia from the atrium, antegrade block in the pathway with continued conduction down the AV node must occur, allowing subsequent retrograde pathway conduction. Induction from the ventricle is more reliable, because retrograde His-Purkinje or AV node block must occur with continued pathway conduction, and pathway VA ERP is almost always shorter than AV junction VA ERP.

Once orthodromic AVRT is induced, rates are often faster in children than in adults because of shorter AV conduction times. However, the VA time during tachycardia is shorter than the AV time, because AV nodal conduction is slower than retrograde accessory pathway conduction. At the site of the pathway, the VA time, measured from the start of the surface QRS to the local atrial electrogram, may be as short as 60 milliseconds. Shorter VA times than this suggest a different mechanism of tachycardia, in particular AVNRT. During orthodromic AVRT, because there is no antegrade accessory pathway conduction, the QRS is usually normal, and pre-excitation is absent. Similarly, the HV interval is normal.

One additional common method of documenting the presence of an extranodal accessory pathway is the introduction of critically timed premature ventricular beats during tachycardia. The stimulator is set up to deliver premature beats to the ventricle, timed to the QRS, starting at a coupling interval of 10 milliseconds shorter than the tachycardia cycle length, and this extra beat is repeated, shortening the coupling interval by 10 milliseconds each time until tachycardia is terminated or the stimulus fails to capture the ventricle. Premature beats are sought that elicit a local ventricular activation in the His bundle channel that is early but later than or simultaneous with the expected His depolarization. If any so-timed PVC advances the next atrial depolarization at any site, an extranodal pathway must exist.[30] This is because such early atrial activation cannot be due to retrograde conduction up the His-Purkinje system and AV node because the timing of the PVC is such that these normal structures must be refractory. It should be noted that, although such a response rules in an accessory pathway, the lack of this response does not rule out an extranodal pathway, if such a pathway is distant from the stimulating electrode.[31]

Precise mapping of retrograde atrial activation during orthodromic tachycardia may be difficult in smaller hearts, but is possible using special catheters with close interelectrode spacing (Fig. 7–5). Mapping of retrograde atrial activation during ventricular overdrive pacing may be unreliable in children, particularly those with septal or paraseptal pathways, because VA conduction through the AV node is fast in most children, and it may be difficult to separate the respective contributions of accessory pathway and retrograde AV node activation of the atrium. Mapping atrial activation during tachycardia, therefore, is preferred.

Often one observes the spontaneous occurrence of sustained rate-dependent bundle branch block during orthodromic AVRT. Such aberration is often helpful in the initial mapping of accessory pathway location. For example, if a patient with a right free wall accessory pathway experiences right bundle branch block with continued tachycardia, this tachycardia will manifest longer VA times than in the absence of right bundle branch block (Fig. 7–6). This is because the wave of ventricular activation reaches the site of the right free wall pathway later than it would in the absence of right bundle branch block. Note that left bundle branch block would not have the same effect in the situation of a right free wall pathway, but would have a similar effect in the presence of a left free wall pathway. The prolongation of the VA time as a result of ipsilateral bundle branch block often, but not always, is accompanied by a slowing in the tachycardia rate. Although most tachycardias will slow under these circumstances, in some patients the later arrival of the retrograde impulse to the atrium leads to improved antegrade AV nodal conduction, essen-

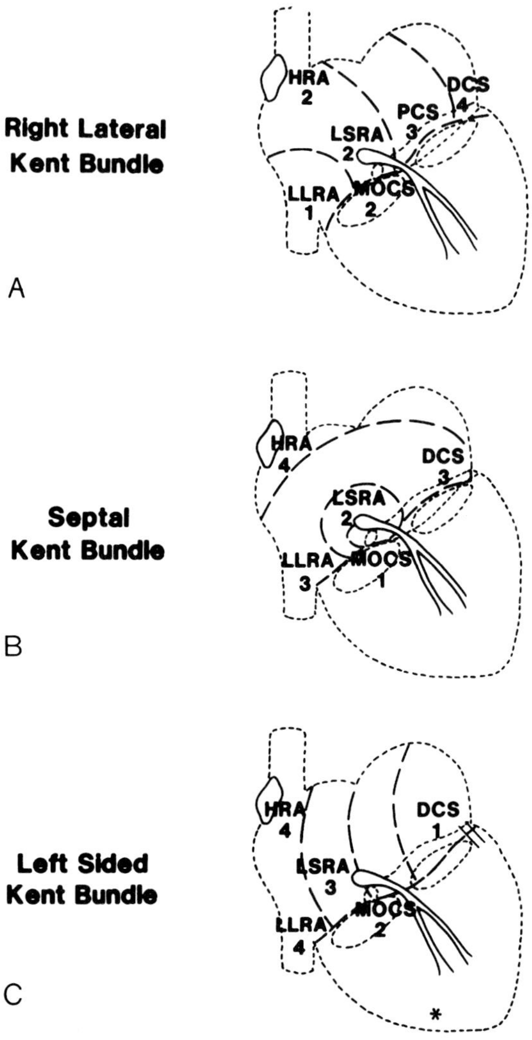

FIGURE 7–5. Atrial activation during orthodromic atrioventricular reciprocating tachycardia in three patients with accessory pathways. *A*, With a right lateral accessory pathway, the low lateral right atrium (LLRA) is activated first. *B*, With a septal pathway, the mouth of the coronary sinus (MOCS) is activated first and slightly in advance of the low septal right atrium (LSRA), where the bundle of His is recorded. *C*, With a far left-sided pathway, the distal coronary sinus (DCS) is activated first. (HRA, high right atrium; PCS, proximal coronary sinus.)

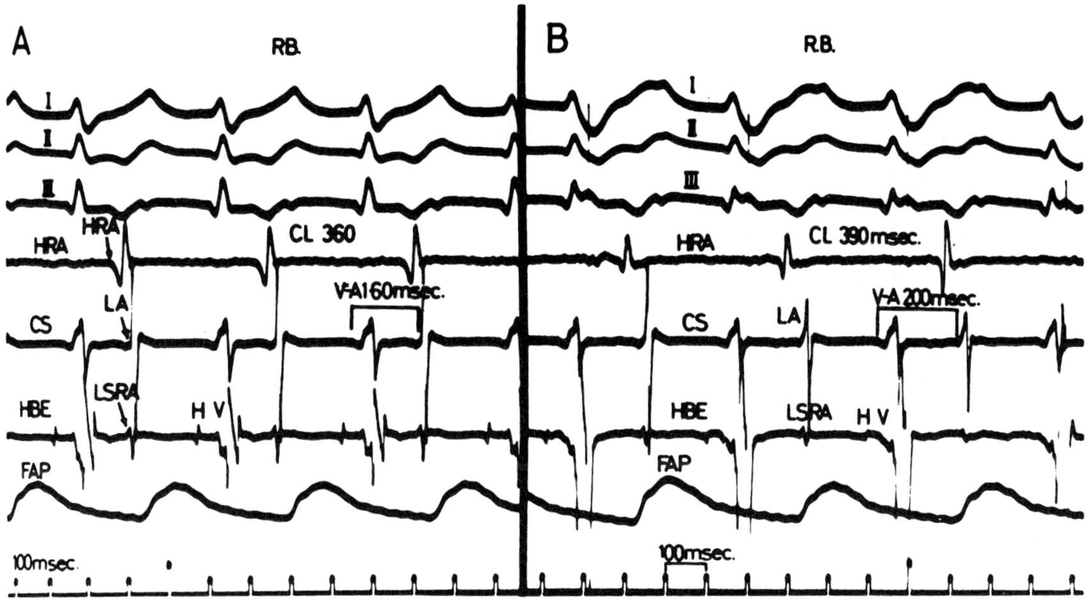

FIGURE 7–6. The effect of bundle branch block during supraventricular tachycardia is shown in a patient with a right freewall accessory pathway. *A,* With normal conduction, the ventriculoatrial (V-A) time is 160 ms measured in the coronary sinus (CS). *B,* After the development of sustained right bundle branch block, the V-A time increases to 200 ms, with a concomitant increase in tachycardia cycle length (CL) from 360 to 390 ms. The prolongation of the V-A time with sustained right bundle branch block proves that the pathway was located in the right freewall. (LSRA, low septal right atrium; LA, left atrium; HRA, high right atrium; HBE, His bundle electrogram; FAP, femoral artery pressure; HV, His-ventricle.)

tially canceling out the effect of the longer VA time on the tachycardia cycle length.

So-called accessory pathway potentials may be recorded from the AV annulus at the site of the pathway, and the recording of such potentials is perhaps the most accurate method of pathway mapping. The bipolar recording of such potentials is aided by the use of orthogonal electrodes (i.e., electrode pairs that run parallel to the course of the pathway).[32, 33] Such electrodes may be most conveniently used on a deflectable catheter with the tip positioned perpendicular to the annulus. Such potentials can be demonstrated to be separate from both the atrium and the ventricle by introducing critically timed PVCs or premature atrial contractions (PACs), which dissociate the ventricle or the atrium from the pathway.

In PJRT, retrograde atrial activation usually originates in the mouth of the coronary sinus (Fig. 7–7). Unlike other accessory pathways, retrograde conduction is usually decremental in the pathway, with prolongation in the VA time with prematurity. In PJRT, it may be difficult to demonstrate advancement of tachycardia in response to critically timed PVCs introduced into tachycardia, because such PVCs are usually conducted decrementally to the atrium over the accessory pathway, and the degree of delay resulting from decremental conduction may cancel the degree of prematurity resulting from the PVC.

Electrophysiologic features of *Mahaim accessory pathways* are somewhat complex, but can

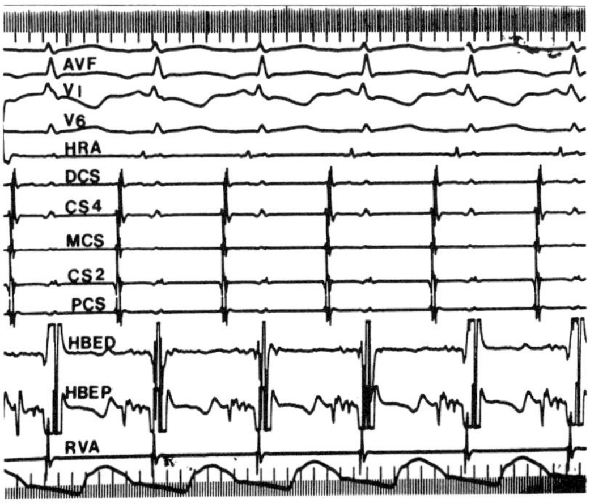

FIGURE 7–7. Typical intracardiac recordings in persistent junctional reciprocating tachycardia. The site of earliest retrograde atrial activation is the proximal coronary sinus (PCS). (HRA, high right atrium; DCS, distal coronary sinus; CS, coronary sinus; MCS, mouth of coronary sinus; HBED, His bundle electrogram distal; HBEP, His bundle electrogram proximal; RVA, right ventricular apex.)

be clearly separated from the features observed in accessory pathways. Similarly to the situation with WPW syndrome, atrial pacing and increasing atrial prematurity will lead to increased pre-excitation and to some shortening of the HV interval. However, because antegrade conduction in a Mahaim pathway is decremental, once maximum pre-excitation is reached, the HV interval stays relatively constant in response to increasing prematurity, whereas AH and PR intervals further increase. Mahaim pathways do not exhibit VA conduction, a point that further assists in the identification of these pathways. Finally, accessory pathway potentials may be recorded in patients with Mahaim pathways by placing deflectable catheters at the site of the pathway on either the atrial or ventricular side of the tricuspid valve annulus.[34] These potentials appear similar to His bundle electrograms, but are usually well separated physically from the site of recording of the His bundle electrogram.

DIFFERENTIAL DIAGNOSIS

Orthodromic AVRT is differentiated from AVNRT by the detection on the ECG of P waves superimposed on the upstroke of the T wave in the former but not the latter (Table 7–1). In the electrophysiologic laboratory, it is differentiated by measuring VA times greater than 60 milliseconds. It is also differentiated in patients with WPW syndrome by the demonstration of pre-excitation after termination of tachycardia, both

Table 7–1. Differential Diagnosis of Supraventricular Tachycardia

DIAGNOSIS	FINDINGS ON ELECTROCARDIOGRAM
Atrial and sinoatrial re-entry	P waves are present and precede next QRS complex. Tachycardia terminates with QRS rather than P wave. Variable AV conduction is possible. AV block does not terminate atrial rhythm. P-wave axis may be superior or inferior, depending on origin.
Atrial flutter	"Sawtooth" flutter waves are present. AV block does not terminate atrial rhythm. Atrial rate is up to 500 in newborns. Variable AV conduction is common.
Accessory pathway–mediated tachycardia (WPW syndrome, concealed accessory pathway)	P waves follow QRS on upstroke of T wave Superior or rightward P-wave axis AV block always terminates tachycardia. Tachycardia typically terminates with P wave After termination, patients with WPW syndrome have pre-excitation.
PJRT	Tachycardia is incessant. P waves precede QRS. There are inverted P waves in II, III, AVF. AV block always terminates tachycardia. May terminate with QRS or with P wave. There is no pre-excitation after termination.
Atrioventricular node re-entry	P waves usually are not visible on QRS. AV block usually terminates tachycardia.
Atrial fibrillation	Waves are irregularly irregular (no two RR intervals are exactly the same). P waves are difficult to see or are bizarre and chaotic.
Sinus tachycardia	There is a normal P-wave axis. P waves precede QRS. Tachycardia is due to extrinsic factors, such as heart failure, fever, anemia, catecholamine or theophylline infusion. Sinus tachycardia continues in presence of AV block.
Atrial ectopic tachycardia	Tachycardia is incessant. Abnormal P-wave axis predicts location of focus. P waves precede QRS. Tachycardia continues in presence of AV block.
Junctional ectopic tachycardia	Tachycardia is incessant. There is atrioventricular dissociation and slower atrial than ventricular rate. There are capture beats with no fusion.

AV, atrioventricular; WPW, Wolff-Parkinson-White; PJRT, permanent form of junctional reciprocating tachycardia.

on the ECG and by demonstrating the presence of a short HV interval, which further shortens during atrial pacing. It is differentiated from atrial tachycardia by observing the response to AV block, occurring either spontaneously or in response to adenosine infusion. If tachycardia continues in the face of AV block, orthodromic AVRT is excluded (Fig. 7–8). The response of tachycardia to PVCs timed to fall on the His bundle electrogram (see prior discussion) may rule in an accessory pathway. Furthermore, termination of tachycardia often occurs with this maneuver. If this occurs without advancement of the atrial electrogram, then atrial tachycardia is excluded.

Antidromic AVRT must be differentiated from ventricular tachycardia. As in orthodromic AVRT, if tachycardia continues in the face of AV block or if AV dissociation is observed, antidromic AVRT is excluded. Both forms of *Mahaim tachycardia* are differentiated from ventricular tachycardia in the same way. They are differentiated from antidromic AVRT with some difficulty, but in general, the QRS complex in Mahaim tachycardia is somewhat narrower with a sharper initial QRS deflection than in antidromic AVRT. Furthermore, the characteristic antegrade conduction characteristics are present with a Mahaim pathway, namely pre-excitation with decremental antegrade conduction and absent or concentric (nodal) VA conduction. Permanent form of junctional reciprocating tachycardia (PJRT) is differentiated from orthodromic AVRT by the timing of the P wave. In PJRT, the P wave is nearly always closer to the following QRS than the preceding QRS, whereas in orthodromic AVRT, the reverse relationship is present. PJRT must be differentiated from atrial tachycardia, and this may be difficult. The best method is to record as many spontaneous terminations as possible and search for spontaneous terminations in which a blocked P wave is the last event. Unfortunately, adenosine can block both the AV node and the pathway.

ACUTE TREATMENT

For all forms of accessory pathway–mediated tachycardia, acute treatment may be directed at either AV node conduction or accessory pathway conduction. Generally, the first choice for conversion of an episode of AVRT is adenosine, given intravenously. Vagal maneuvers or other drugs such as digoxin, verapamil, or propranolol may be used to affect the AV nodal limb of the re-entrant circuit. Accessory pathway conduction may be affected by intravenous procainamide. Esophageal pacing is very effective in terminating an episode, either by atrial overdrive or extrastimulation. DC cardioversion, of course, is also effective.

CHRONIC TREATMENT

Long-term management depends on the severity of the problem and frequency of the attacks. For children with rare, mildly symptomatic attacks of SVT that are easily terminated, it is reasonable to advise no treatment at all. Children with more frequent or symptomatic attacks are

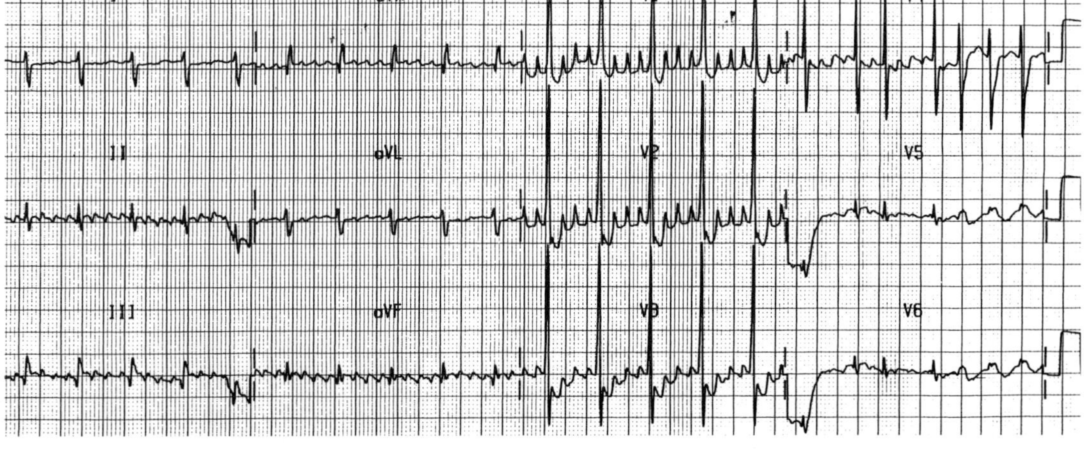

FIGURE 7–8. Twelve-lead electrocardiogram in a neonate with atrial flutter after administration of adenosine. The resulting second-degree atrioventricular block reveals the flutter waves and rules out atrioventricular reciprocating tachycardia caused by an accessory pathway.

treated initially with beta blockers or oral verapamil, or digoxin if there is no evidence of pre-excitation in sinus rhythm. Digoxin should probably be avoided in children with pre-excitation. It is known that about a third of adults and children with pre-excitation treated with cardiac glycosides will have a shortening of the antegrade effective refractory period of the accessory pathway, which may be dangerous if atrial fibrillation develops.[35, 36] Although atrial fibrillation is very uncommon in children and digoxin has been used for years in children with pre-excitation with few documented problems, some reports suggest that there may be the possibility of sudden death in infants treated with digoxin.[26] In patients who are refractory to these choices, chronic treatment with flecainide, sotalol, or amiodarone is often effective, but the risks of these medications are higher than those of the previously listed medications. Pharmacologic treatment of children with PJRT is often very challenging. In addition to these agents, success has been reported with flecainide.[37]

RADIOFREQUENCY ABLATION

Radiofrequency catheter ablation of the accessory pathway is recommended in several circumstances. Patients with frequent symptomatic attacks of tachycardia who have not responded to antiarrhythmic medications are the most frequent candidates. Ablation is often necessary for those with a short antegrade ERP of the accessory pathway, particularly if they have suffered an attack of syncope as a result of atrial fibrillation. Such patients, however, often respond to type IC agents such as flecainide, with a complete loss of antegrade accessory pathway conduction and loss of the delta wave. Finally, patients with serious congenital heart disease with an accessory pathway should have division of the pathway as part of their congenital heart surgery. This is particularly important because the postoperative course may be complicated by SVT or atrial tachycardia or fibrillation with rapid conduction, and these rhythms are very poorly tolerated in the immediate postoperative period.

The timing of ablation therapy depends on the degree of symptomatology in the particular patient and on the natural history of the condition. Catheter ablation has been quite effective, even in the youngest children.[38, 39] However, because most deaths and serious complications of pediatric catheter ablation reported to date have occurred in children in the first several years of life,[11, 40] this therapy is to be avoided when possible. In addition, patients in the first several years of life have a substantial chance of experiencing spontaneous loss of accessory pathway conduction or of improving clinically. Beyond the age of 6 years, however, this chance becomes very small,[21] whereas the risks of catheter ablation are much reduced. Therefore, it seems most reasonable to attempt treatment with antiarrhythmic medications, including flecainide and amiodarone, in the first several years of life and to offer catheter ablation only to those refractory to these medications. Beyond age 6, it is reasonable to offer ablation on a more elective basis. One exception to this guideline is the patient with PJRT. Such patients often do not respond to any antiarrhythmic agent, and incessant tachycardia can lead to congestive heart failure as a result of cardiomyopathy. PJRT pathways are usually quite accessible for catheter ablation, and earlier ablation in children younger than 6 years seems reasonable.

SURGICAL ABLATION

With the widespread availability and effectiveness of radiofrequency ablation, surgery is only rarely necessary. However, there are certainly patients who cannot be cured by radiofrequency ablation techniques, particularly those with multiple pathways. For these patients, surgery may offer the only hope of control of tachycardia.[27, 41]

ATRIOVENTRICULAR NODE RE-ENTRANT TACHYCARDIA

ANATOMY

It is now well accepted that AVNRT is mediated by the presence of dual AV nodal pathways: one "fast" pathway short conduction time but long ERP and one "slow" pathway with long conduction time but with a short ERP. During the "usual" form of AVNRT, conduction proceeds down the slow pathway and subsequently retrograde up the fast pathway to the atrium (Fig. 7–9). The bundle of His activates at about the time that retrograde fast pathway activation takes place. Initially, it was thought that these two pathways were functionally discrete but not anatomically distinct. Subsequently, it was recognized by Sung[42] and others that anatomically distinct fast and slow AV node pathways could be demonstrated in patients with AVNRT by demonstrating a shift in retrograde atrial activation with ventricular extrastimulation, with the fast

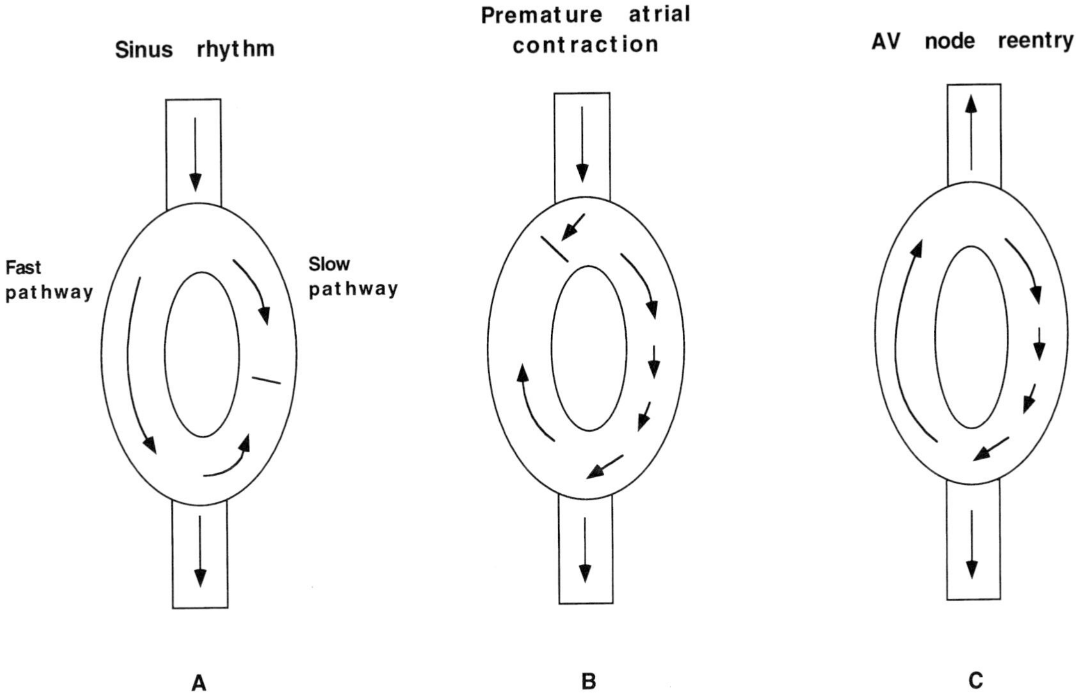

FIGURE 7–9. Simplified diagram of dual atrioventricular (AV) node pathways in patients with AV node re-entrant tachycardia (AVNRT). The diagram includes an upper common pathway, which may or may not exist (see text). *A*, Both "fast" and "slow" AV nodal pathways are present. The fast pathway has a short AH interval, but a long effective refractory period (ERP). The slow pathway has a long AH interval but a shorter ERP. During sinus rhythm, impulses reach the bundle of His and the ventricle over the fast pathway, and slow pathway conduction is not evident. *B*, After a critically timed premature atrial contraction, there is block in the fast pathway, with conduction down the slow pathway and a "jump" to a longer AH interval. *C*, AVNRT is established when subsequent retrograde conduction occurs in the fast pathway, which re-enters the slow pathway antegrade.

pathway activating the anterior septum near the site where the His bundle electrogram is recorded and the slow pathway activating the posterior septum near the mouth of the coronary sinus.

There is still controversy concerning the exact anatomy of the re-entrant circuit and whether or not it is limited to the AV node structures or involves the perinodal atrium as a critical part of the circuit. Convincing evidence has been presented to support both views,[43–45] and it seems most likely that the entity identified as AVNRT is somewhat heterogeneous. Thus far, it has not proved important to make this differentiation when considering treatment options.

CLINICAL PRESENTATION AND NATURAL HISTORY

As far as is known, the clinical presentation of AVNRT in children is similar to that of paroxysmal AVRT caused by accessory pathways (see prior discussion). However, tachycardia rates may be quite dependent on the adrenergic state; much faster rates are seen in children who have their episodes during exertion. It is also not rare for patients with AVNRT to experience more significant symptoms, including near syncope and syncope. This may be because the simultaneous timing of atrial and ventricular depolarizations means that the atrium will always be contracting against closed AV valves (see later discussion), and so the ventricle loses the atrial contribution to end-diastolic volume. By the same mechanism, patients with AVNRT will often be noted to have very prominent jugular venous pulsations during tachycardia. These are due to cannon waves, which occur with each heartbeat.

In children, the natural history of AVNRT is essentially unknown. One may assume that at least some if not most infants with AVNRT experience spontaneous resolution. However, the actual proportion who will go on to spontaneous resolution and how many will still later experience recurrence is completely unknown. This is because invasive electrophysiology studies are rare in infants, and invasive studies are required to establish firmly the presence of dual AV node pathways and AVNRT. A 1992 study of infants, children, and adolescents undergoing esophageal or invasive electrophysiologic study found an incidence of AVNRT of 14%.[5] However, AVNRT was extremely rare in the younger age groups and nearly absent in patients younger than 2 years.

ELECTROCARDIOGRAPHIC RECOGNITION OF AVNRT

These rhythms are due to re-entry involving dual pathways in the AV node: one fast pathway, usually with a long effective refractory period (ERP), and one slow pathway, with a shorter ERP. During normal sinus rhythm, conduction takes place down both pathways simultaneously, with the impulse from the fast pathway arriving in the bundle of His first, and the ECG is normal without evidence for pre-excitation. A minority of patients, however, will have a somewhat short PR interval. Two forms of tachycardia resulting from dual AV node pathways are recognized: the "usual" form of AVNRT and the "unusual" form. To initiate the usual form of AVNRT, a critically timed PAC can be blocked in the fast pathway and be conducted via the slow pathway, slowly enough that the fast pathway recovers and allows subsequent antegrade slow pathway conduction, establishing the re-entrant circuit. In children, tachycardia may also be induced by sudden sinus slowing followed by a junctional escape beat, as described by Levy et al.[46] Because transit from the distal node up the fast pathway to the atrium takes about as long as transit from the distal node to the ventricles, the P waves are buried on the QRS and are usually not discernible (Figs. 7–10 and 7–11). In some children, however, it may be visible slightly before or after the QRS complex. This may be because in children the fast AV node pathway is fast enough that it is traversed retrograde more rapidly than is the distal conduction system antegrade. There is little or no variability in RR intervals. The tachycardia starts with a premature beat and terminates suddenly. AV block, occurring spontaneously or induced by vagal maneuvers or medication, should with rare exceptions terminate the tachycardia. The rhythm may terminate with a P wave or QRS complex, depending on the site of block.

In the unusual form of AVNRT, a PVC is blocked in the fast pathway and is conducted up the slow pathway and down the fast pathway.[47, 48] Because conduction up the slow pathway to the atria takes longer than conduction to the ventricles, the P waves are discernible, usually closer to the subsequent QRS rather than the previous QRS (see Fig. 7–11). Because the P wave is retrograde and originates in the AV node, the P-wave axis is superior. In this regard, the unusual form of AVNRT may be indistinguishable from PJRT.

ELECTROPHYSIOLOGIC STUDY

AV conduction study classically demonstrates the presence of two pathways: one with a short AH interval and a long ERP and the other with a much longer AH interval but a shorter ERP. Tachycardia is induced at a critical atrial overdrive cycle length (the Wenckebach cycle length of the fast pathway) or at a critical A1-A2 coupling interval (less than or equal to the fast pathway ERP). The administration of low doses of isoproterenol may be necessary to elicit sustained tachycardia.

Unfortunately, evidence of dual AV node conduction curves is common in adults[49] and in normal children in the absence of inducible or clinical tachycardia.[50] In addition, AVNRT frequently exists without such a demonstrable discontinuity in conduction curves.[51] The order of retrograde atrial activation during tachycardia in both forms of AVNRT clearly suggests a nodal origin, with the low septal right atrial signal preceding all others. The VA time is usually very short ($<$ 10 milliseconds), and in children may even be negative, with P waves preceding the surface QRS deflection (see prior discussion).

DIFFERENTIAL DIAGNOSIS

On ECG, AVNRT may be difficult to distinguish from orthodromic AVRT. The complete lack of discernible P waves superimposed on the T waves or, better, the identification of P waves slightly in advance of the QRS makes AVRT much less likely (see Table 7–1). In the electrophysiologic laboratory, pre-excitation is absent, and retrograde conduction is concentric and decremental rather than eccentric and nondecremental, as in the presence of an accessory pathway. PVCs introduced into tachycardia when the His bundle is refractory fail to advance the next atrial depolarization, making the presence of extranodal accessory pathways less likely. The differentiation from atrial tachycardia may be challenging. Clearly, if one observes continuation of tachycardia in the presence of AV block, AVNRT is very unlikely but not impossible. Occasionally,

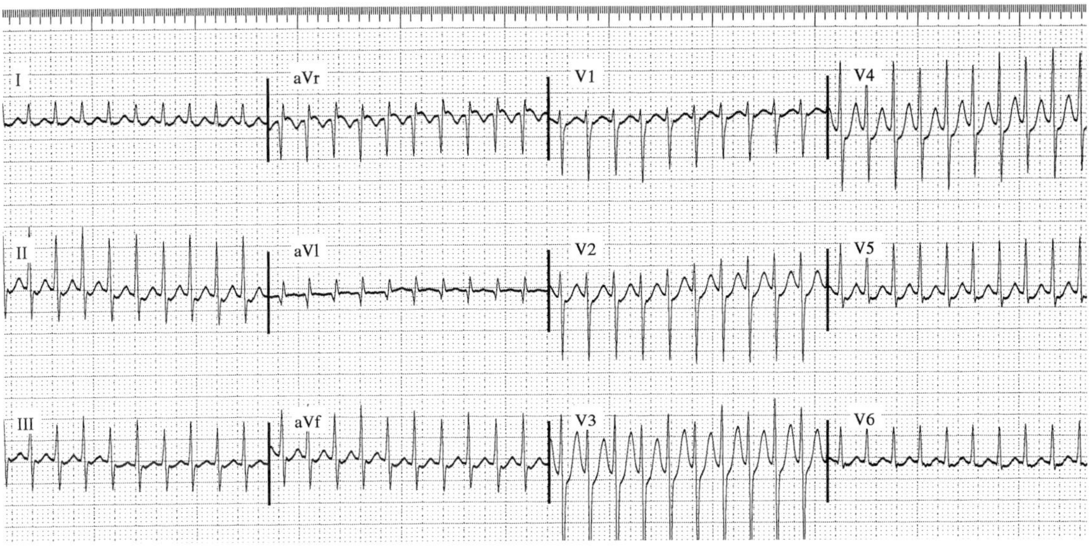

FIGURE 7–10. Twelve-lead electrocardiogram in a patient with atrioventricular node re-entrant tachycardia. Note that P waves are not discernible, because they are buried in the QRS complex.

very fast AVNRT rates may be associated with second-degree AV block in the distal conducting system or elements of the AV node.[52] If a spontaneous termination occurs with simultaneous atrial and ventricular signals, then atrial tachycardia is very unlikely. Very early PVCs introduced into tachycardia, in advance of the His bundle electrogram, may advance the tachycardia via ret-

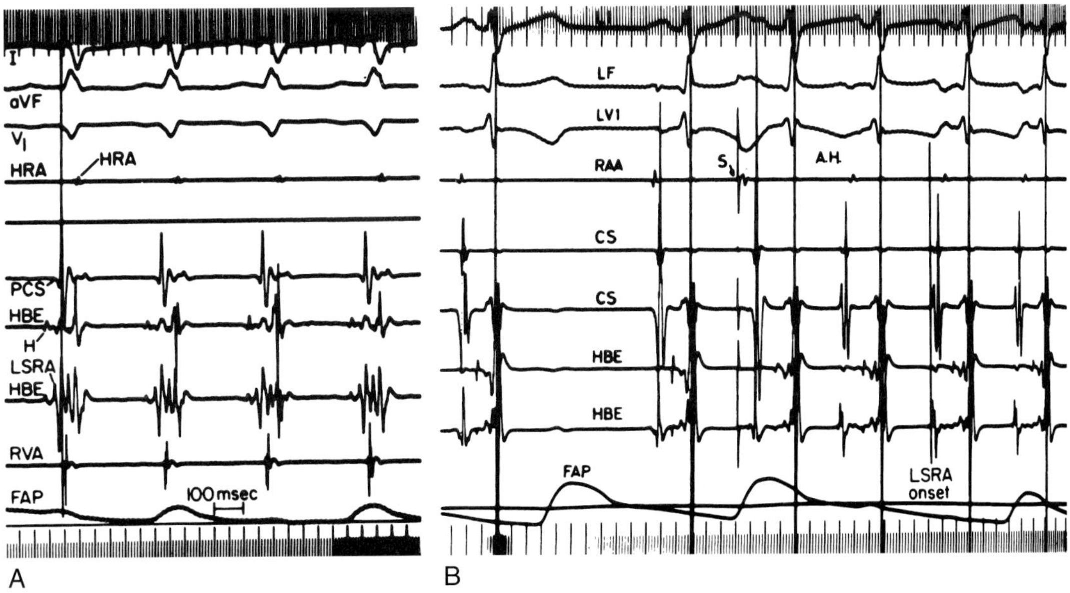

FIGURE 7–11. Intracardiac electrograms and surface electrocardiographic characteristics in two forms of atrioventricular node re-entrant tachycardia (AVNRT). *A,* In the usual form of AVNRT, conduction is down the slow pathway and back up the fast pathway. P waves are superimposed on the QRS complexes, and intracardiac atrial depolarizations document that atrial and ventricular activations are nearly simultaneous. The atrial activation in the His bundle electrogram (HBE) is slightly in advance of the atrial activation in the proximal coronary sinus (PCS). *B,* In the unusual form of AVNRT, conduction is down the fast pathway and back up the slow pathway. P waves are closer to the subsequent QRS complex than the previous, and atrial activation is slightly earlier in the coronary sinus (CS) than the HBE. (HRA, high right atrium; LSRA, low septal right atrium; RVA, right ventricular apex; FAP, femoral artery pressure; LF, lead AVF; LV1, lead V1; RAA, right atrial appendage.)

rograde His-Purkinje conduction and invasion of the tachycardia circuit. A PVC that terminates the tachycardia without advancing the atrium excludes atrial tachycardia. The atrial activation sequence during tachycardia may help differentiate AVNRT from atrial tachycardia. It should be concentric in AVNRT, but should be earliest near the atrial focus in atrial tachycardia.

The differentiation of the unusual form of AVNRT from atrial tachycardia is usually straightforward, by the same principles stated previously for the usual form of AVNRT. Differentiation from PJRT is much more difficult. Dual AV node physiology on the antegrade AV node conduction study should be absent in PJRT. One may be able to rule in PJRT by the demonstration of advancement of an atrial electrogram by a critically timed PVC placed into tachycardia when the His bundle is refractory (see prior discussion), but the failure to demonstrate advancement does not rule out PJRT; in fact, in most patients with PJRT, advancement cannot be demonstrated. The incessant nature of PJRT may help in the differentiation as well.

Acute Treatment

Acute treatment is directed at achieving a brief episode of AV block. Children may respond to vagal maneuvers. If these measures fail, our first choice of medications is intravenous adenosine. Esophageal or intracardiac atrial overdrive pacing is quite effective. Such patients will also respond to DC synchronous cardioversion.

Chronic Treatment

The long-term management is directed at changing conduction through the slow AV nodal pathway. Oral digoxin, beta blocker, or verapamil may be effective. In active children, however, this effect is quite easily overwhelmed by vigorous exercise, particularly with digoxin, and breakthroughs are common. The use of procainamide, flecainide, or sotalol to affect conduction in the retrograde fast pathway is occasionally successful in such patients.

Radiofrequency Ablation

Permanent AV node modification has been described for the elimination of dual AV node physiology with AVNRT. Initial reports of the technique involved the selective ablation of the anterior or "fast" pathway.[53, 54] Fast pathway ablation left the patient with a longer PR interval and an antegrade AV node conduction curve consistent with retention only of the slow pathway with long AH intervals. Although highly effective and simple to perform, this technique was associated with an unacceptably high incidence of postprocedure complete AV block, as high as 15 to 20%. Subsequently, techniques were developed for the selective ablation of the posterior "slow" AV node pathway by the placement of radiofrequency lesions in the posterior septum near the mouth of the coronary sinus[9] or in the midseptal region.[55] Such an AV node modification leaves the patient with evidence only of fast pathway conduction. Often, however, the fast pathway ERP shortens after successful slow pathway ablation, and the patient is left with an AV node ERP not dramatically different from that of a normal patient. The major advantage of slow pathway ablation is that the incidence of complete AV block after the procedure is much lower than for fast pathway ablation, on the order of 1 to 3%, and the technique is similarly efficacious. Slow pathway ablation is currently the preferred technique for AV node modification in older patients with AVNRT.

As with accessory pathway ablation, there is some uncertainty of the place of catheter ablation for treatment of AVNRT in children. Although in the child a substantial proportion of SVT is accounted for by AVNRT, radiofrequency ablation for treatment of AVNRT is not as widely used in the pediatric population. For example, only 11% of procedures reported to the Pediatric Radiofrequency Ablation Registry were AV node modifications for AVNRT.[11] Because the technique for AV node modification of AVNRT is no more challenging than that for ablation of accessory pathways, it is clear that other factors are responsible. The risk of AV block after AV node modification is low in the adult population, but because of the smaller size of the heart in young children, there is a higher risk of AV block in the younger age groups. Any risk of heart block and subsequent lifelong pacemaker dependence must be viewed with concern. Therefore, although elective accessory pathway ablation may be recommended in patients older than 6 years, the age for elective AV node modification for AVNRT should be greater, perhaps 12 years, when the risks of AV block would be expected to be similar to those in adults. Certainly, as more data become available concerning the actual risks in younger children, these recommendations may change. Finally, the technique is clearly indicated for treatment of AVNRT in younger children who prove to be refractory to standard antiarrhythmic agents.

Surgical Ablation

There were initial reports of the use of surgery for selective fast pathway ablation in patients with AVNRT,[56] and these reports served to guide the approach for subsequent development of transcatheter techniques. However, the transcatheter techniques have now completely supplanted the surgical techniques.

JUNCTIONAL ECTOPIC TACHYCARDIA

ANATOMY

The anatomic substrate for automatic JET is essentially unknown, but it may be assumed to be due to a small focus of abnormal automaticity somewhere in the AV node or bundle of His. Some information is available from the study of Bharati et al,[57] in which congenital abnormalities of the conducting system and coronary sinus were detected in three patients who had had JET and who had autopsies. Experience with transcatheter ablation (see later discussion) has suggested that the substrate is supraventricular, adjacent to, or in the compact AV node, because lesions in the atrial septum have been successful in curing this arrhythmia.[58–60]

CLINICAL PRESENTATION AND NATURAL HISTORY

There are three general modes of presentation of JET. The most common occurrence of JET is in the immediate postoperative period in children after cardiac surgery involving cardiopulmonary bypass and especially with surgery of the atrial or ventricular septum. Postoperative JET develops within several hours of discontinuation of bypass and may last several days. The postoperative presentation of JET is associated with a high mortality rate, because the high rate and the AV dissociation (see later discussion) often lead to hemodynamic decompensation. However, the independent contributions of the arrhythmia and the pre-existing hemodynamic state are difficult to separate.

A second common presentation of JET is as a congenital arrhythmia. It was first described by Coumel et al,[61] and is often referred to as "Coumel tachycardia." Congenital JET is sometimes diagnosed in utero by fetal ultrasound examination, when it may be a cause of nonimmune hydrops fetalis, or more often in the neonatal period or infancy as an incessant tachycardia. In most cases, congenital JET is not associated with immediate hemodynamic decompensation. However, the incessant nature of the accelerated rhythm may lead to the development of cardiomyopathy. A large multicenter survey by Villain et al[62] found a mortality rate of 35% in patients with congenital JET, but spontaneous resolutions were also observed. An interesting feature identified in this study is that approximately 50% of patients with JET will have an affected close family member, suggesting a genetic basis for the arrhythmia. Often other family members are not as severely affected as the index case.

A third presentation of JET is in older children, adolescents, and adults, in whom JET presents as a paroxysmal form of narrow QRS tachycardia. This presentation is often referred to as the "adult form" of JET.[60] Such rhythms are difficult to differentiate from the more common forms of SVT, because they are often seen after exertion and are not incessant.[63] The paroxysmal form of JET does not carry the same grim prognosis of either the postoperative or the congenital form of JET.

ELECTROCARDIOGRAPHIC RECOGNITION OF JET

All three presentations of JET have the same electrocardiographic and electrophysiologic features. JET is classically recognized as a narrow QRS tachycardia with AV dissociation and an atrial rate that is slower than the ventricular rate (Fig. 7–12). Presumably, this appearance results from 1:1 conduction of the rapid impulses from the ectopic focus down the His-Purkinje system, so that ventricular activation is normal. Retrograde conduction from the junctional focus back to the atrium is usually absent, however, so that the atrium is activated by the normal sinus impulses at a much slower rate, explaining the AV dissociation. In patients with AV dissociation resulting from junctional tachycardia, one usually observes capture beats. Capture beats result from occasional antegrade conduction of a normal sinus impulse, causing the next QRS complex to occur slightly earlier than expected. Because they use the same His-Purkinje system as the junctional focus, such capture beats will occur with a QRS morphology identical to that seen with the underlying JET.

In some patients, 1:1 conduction from the junctional focus to the atrium is present. In these patients, AV dissociation will be absent. In this

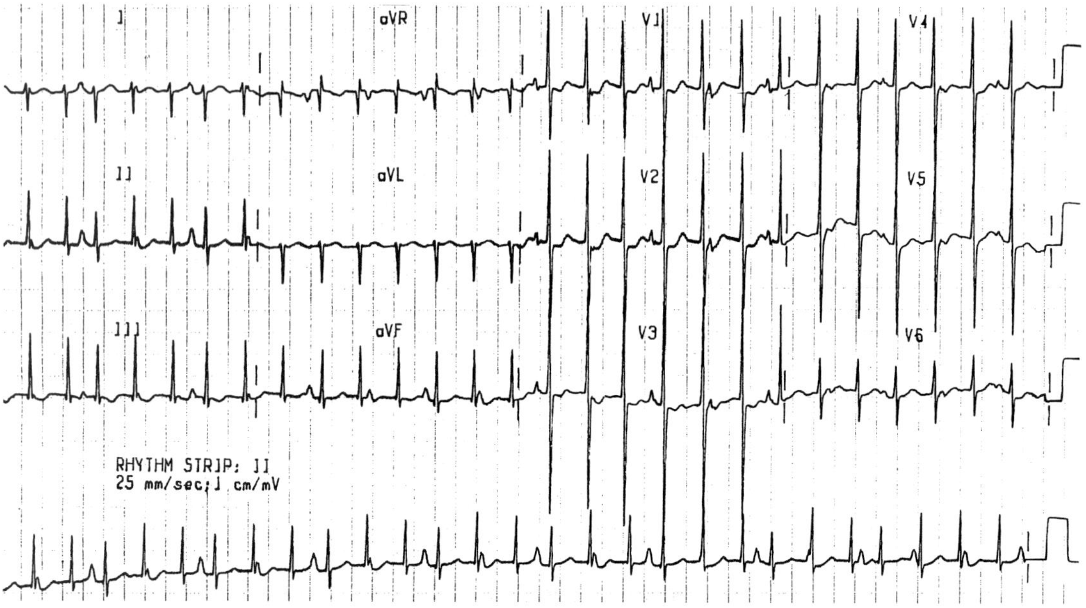

FIGURE 7–12. Twelve-lead electrocardiogram in a patient with congenital junctional ectopic tachycardia (JET). Note that atrioventricular dissociation is easily appreciated, and sudden narrowing of the RR intervals resulting from capture beats is often recorded. From Van Hare GF, Velvis H, Langberg JJ. Successful transcatheter ablation of congenital junctional ectopic tachycardia in a ten-month-old infant using radiofrequency energy. Pacing Clin Electrophysiol 1990;13:730–735. Used with permission.

case, P waves will be superimposed on QRS complexes, just as they are in the usual form of AVNRT. Another exception to the classic electrocardiographic appearance is the occurrence of bundle branch block. This may be rate-dependent aberration, simply because of the rapid rates, or may be fixed and due to surgical damage to the bundle branch. An example of the latter is the patient in whom postoperative JET develops after repair of tetralogy of Fallot, which is often associated with a right bundle branch block.

ELECTROPHYSIOLOGIC STUDY

At electrophysiologic study, the presence of AV dissociation with occasional sinus capture beats is easily confirmed. A His depolarization will be recorded before each QRS complex with a normal HV interval, whereas atrial depolarization will be dissociated from the His bundle electrogram except when a capture beat occurs (Fig. 7–13). In the incessant form of JET, neither atrial nor ventricular stimulation is successful in terminating tachycardia, and entrainment cannot be demonstrated. If AV dissociation is absent (1:1 conduction from junctional focus to atrium), retrograde atrial activation is concentric and earliest near the site of the His bundle electrogram. In the paroxysmal form of JET, tachycardia may be inducible with atrial or ventricular burst pacing. More typically, however, it starts spontaneously with the infusion of isoproterenol.[63]

DIFFERENTIAL DIAGNOSIS

It is usually not difficult to make the diagnosis of JET, because the classic appearance of narrow QRS tachycardia with AV dissociation and capture beats is easily identified (see Table 7–1). However, when a 1:1 AV relationship is present, it must be differentiated from the usual form of AVNRT. One easy way of differentiating these two rhythms is by the intravenous infusion of adenosine.[64] Adenosine may allow tachycardia to continue but elicit AV dissociation by blocking retrograde conduction from the junctional focus. However, it may also terminate tachycardia. At electrophysiologic study, dual AV node pathways should be present in patients with AVNRT, although dual pathways are often absent in patients with documented AVNRT and are often present in normal patients. Initiation by programmed stimulation from the ventricle argues against AVNRT, as does the presence of incessant tachycardia.

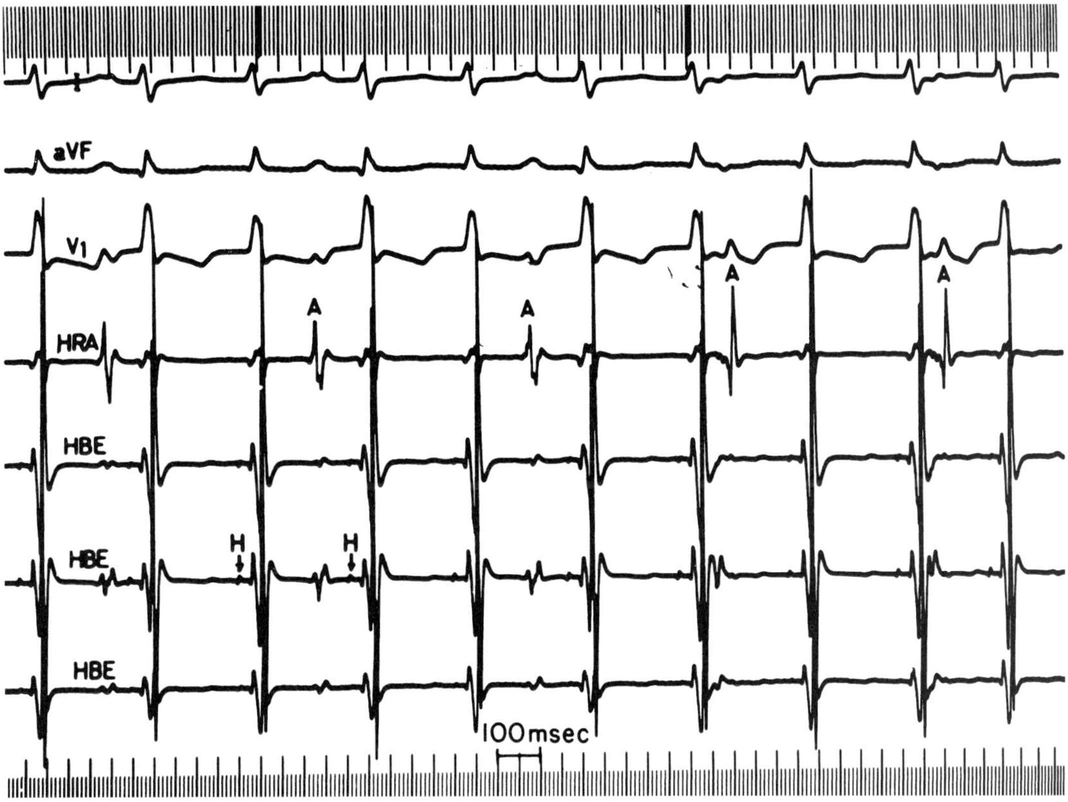

FIGURE 7–13. Intracardiac electrograms in a patient with junctional ectopic tachycardia. Note that the QRS complexes are normal, atrioventricular dissociation is confirmed by the recording of high right atrial (HRA) electrograms, a His bundle electrogram (HBE) precedes each QRS, and the HV interval is normal at 35 ms.

When JET occurs with a wide QRS complex resulting from bundle branch block or aberration, differentiation from ventricular or fascicular tachycardia is necessary. Capture beats are most helpful in this differentiation. Capture beats during ventricular or fascicular tachycardia should narrow or normalize the QRS complex, whereas the QRS should be unchanged or slightly wider during capture beats in JET. This is because, in JET, a wide QRS is caused by abnormal conduction down the His-Purkinje system, and an earlier capture beat will not be expected to encounter improved conduction. In the electrophysiology laboratory, ventricular tachycardia should not be observed with a normal HV interval and His bundle depolarizations preceding each QRS. If there is fascicular tachycardia, one may observe His bundle depolarizations before each QRS, but the HV interval of these should be short, and shorter than on the capture beats.

ACUTE TREATMENT

The treatment of patients with JET who are acutely ill is frequently very difficult. Such tachycardias are generally not amenable to termination by overdrive pacing, and DC cardioversion usually causes the tachycardia to pause only briefly. In the postoperative patient, the tachycardia may be maintained by the infusion of catecholamines, whereas the fast rate and lack of AV synchrony resulting from the JET may make it difficult or impossible to discontinue catecholamine infusion. Several modalities have been shown to be effective in some patients. First, the use of atrial pacing at a rate slightly above the JET rate may capture and overdrive the JET,[65] and the improvement in hemodynamics resulting from restoration of AV synchrony may allow discontinuation of catecholamines or the substitution of a noncatecholamine inotropic agent such as amrinone. Second, surface cooling to a central temperature of 34°C is very effective in lowering tachycardia rates in postoperative JET[66, 67] and may allow the institution of atrial pacing, as previously discussed. Paired ventricular pacing has been used occasionally for short-term management of JET in the postoperative period.[68] In this technique, ventricular pacing with a series of S_1-S_2 ventricular stimuli is timed so that every second ventricular stimulus is successful in capturing ventricular myocardium and suppressing the JET focus, but so early that it does not elicit a mechanical response. Of course, this technique carries with it the hazard of accidental precipitation of ventricular fibrillation.

Intravenous medications have been disappointing in the management of JET. Digoxin, propranolol, and procainamide have been occasionally effective. Intravenous propranolol and procainamide are risky in the immediate postoperative period because of their negative inotropic potential. Propafenone has been used with good success,[69–73] but the intravenous form is not currently available in the United States. Finally, amiodarone, both orally and intravenously, is perhaps the most effective agent for the acute management of JET.[62, 74, 75] The intravenous form is now available in the United States. The use of intravenous amiodarone requires placement of a central venous catheter, but it has not been associated with significant decreases in ventricular function.

Chronic Treatment

The agents available for chronic treatment of JET are similar to those proven effective in the postoperative situation. For patients with the paroxysmal form of JET in which tachycardia is induced by the infusion of isoproterenol, beta blocker therapy is indicated. Patients with incessant JET may respond to sotalol,[76] propafenone,[70] or amiodarone.[62, 65, 77] Of these, amiodarone is probably the most effective.[61]

Radiofrequency Ablation

There is scant experience with radiofrequency ablation for definitive treatment of JET. For the paroxysmal form, there is one report of the successful ablation of the junctional focus with preservation of AV conduction by placement of lesions in the anterior interatrial septum.[60] Such a finding suggests that the substrate for JET does not involve the entire compact AV node. For congenital JET, radiofrequency ablation is effective but clearly carries the high risk of complete AV block with lifelong pacemaker dependence.[58] Clearly, in either form of JET, radiofrequency ablation should be considered as a last resort when antiarrhythmic agents have failed.

Pacemaker Therapy in JET

Some authors suggested that all patients with congenital JET should be considered for placement of a permanent ventricular pacemaker because of the possible occurrence of complete AV block while on antiarrhythmic therapy.[62] This recommendation was prompted by the occurrence of sudden death in several patients who were otherwise well controlled on antiarrhythmic agents[62] as well as the histologically abnormal findings in the AV junction of several patients who died suddenly.[57] However, distal conduction system abnormalities have not been detected at electrophysiologic study in patients with JET, and the observed sudden deaths may well have been explained by a proarrhythmic response to medication. At this time, the place of permanent pacing in the management of congenital JET is unresolved.

EMERGENCY MANAGEMENT OF SUPRAVENTRICULAR TACHYCARDIA

When a child with a previously undiagnosed form of SVT first presents for treatment, planning of therapy must take place without the benefit of knowing the exact mechanism of tachycardia. This may be challenging, but several principles should be observed to allow the therapy to be safe and effective.

Hemodynamic Assessment. When the child with an unknown tachycardia first presents, the hemodynamic state should be rapidly assessed. Is the child entirely asymptomatic except for the sensation of a rapid heart rate? Are there signs or symptoms of hemodynamic compromise, such as tachypnea, pallor, hypotension, hepatomegaly, poor pulses, or altered level of consciousness? If there are such signs, then returning the patient to normal sinus rhythm is more urgent, and more invasive means of achieving sinus rhythm are warranted. For example, in the child who is only mildly symptomatic with no signs of hemodynamic compromise, substantial efforts at vagal maneuvers are reasonable rather than the use of medications or cardioversion. On the other hand, if there are any signs of hemodynamic compromise, such vagal maneuvers should not be used or should be used for only a very brief period of time before progression to medication or cardioversion. Patients with extreme hypotension or altered level of consciousness should have immediate electrical cardioversion.

Vagal Maneuvers. In children, a vagal response with consequent termination of tachycardia may be elicited by a variety of maneuvers. Carotid massage and orbital pressure should not be performed in children. In infants, rectal stimulation (by taking the rectal temperature) is frequently effective. The diving reflex may be elicited by placing a bag filled with ice over the face (and covering the ears) for 15 seconds.[78] Older children may be coached to perform a standard Valsalva maneuver. These maneuvers should be performed with an intravenous catheter in place, and should not be continued for longer than 5 minutes in seriously ill patients before proceeding to other modalities. With all maneuvers, as well as with other interventions such as medications and pacing, it is important to record the ECG continuously. Clues to the mechanism of tachycardia may be evident from the mechanism of termination.

Medications. Adenosine is now considered the drug of choice for the acute pharmacologic conversion of SVT.[79] This agent, when given by rapid intravenous injection, works by inducing a very brief episode of complete AV block, thereby interrupting the re-entrant circuit of SVTs, which involve the AV node as part of the re-entrant circuit, such as AVNRT and AVRT resulting from WPW syndrome. The onset of effect is less than 1 minute, the half-life in blood is less than 10 seconds, and the resulting AV blockade is, therefore, brief and self-limited. It is not usually effective in other forms of tachycardia, although occasional patients with atrial tachycardia or ventricular tachycardia will respond. The successful conversion of SVT with adenosine provides some evidence against other forms of tachycardia, such as atrial tachycardia, that do not involve the AV node as part of the re-entrant circuit.

Several precautions are needed in giving adenosine. There are reports of severe bronchospasm after adenosine infusion in several patients with asthma.[80–82] Although this risk is small, it should be used with caution in such patients. Adenosine may cause atrial fibrillation, which is usually brief and terminates spontaneously.[83, 84] However, if a patient also has WPW syndrome, atrial fibrillation may pose a hazard,[85] and the diagnosis of WPW may not be evident until after conversion to sinus rhythm. For this reason, an electrical cardiovertor-defibrillator should be in the room with the monitoring leads connected to the patient before the administration of adenosine.

Verapamil was also available for the acute intravenous treatment of SVT in children older than 12 months[86, 87] but should rarely be used now. Long sinus pauses with junctional or ventricular escape beats are common as the tachycardia terminates. The drug acts within 2 to 3 minutes. There have been numerous reported cases of hypotension and asystolic cardiac arrests in infants younger than 6 months, and so the drug should not be given in this age group.[88, 89] In any patient given verapamil, the physician must be prepared to manage hypotension with calcium chloride (10 mg/kg), volume infusion, or vasopressor drugs such as dopamine. There is no evidence that verapamil is effective when adenosine is not.

In some patients with AVRT or AVNRT, procainamide may be effective. It probably works by blocking conduction in the accessory pathway or in the retrograde fast limb of AV node reentry. Hypotension is frequent during the loading infusion.

Digoxin is an effective agent for the treatment of most pediatric supraventricular arrhythmias. A disadvantage is the long time period necessary to digitalize a patient safely. One approach to intravenous digitalization is to give 10 μg/kg as a first intravenous dose, followed by a second dose 2 hours later and a third dose at 6 to 12 hours. It should not be given to patients with hypokalemia if there is a suspicion of digoxin toxicity or if WPW syndrome is diagnosed or suspected.

Patients with JET may not respond to any of these measures, and may not be amenable to electrical cardioversion. In these patients, one can only hope to slow the tachycardia rate. For the purpose of slowing the automatic focus, medications such as the beta blockers, class I medications such as procainamide and flecainide, and class III medications such as sotalol and amiodarone may be effective.

Esophageal pacing systems are commercially available. Special pulse generators, which generate long pulse widths (>10 milliseconds) are necessary because the outputs required for capture at conventional pulse widths (< 2 milliseconds) may be very uncomfortable.[90] The esophageal lead is positioned behind the left atrium for pacing. One method of lead positioning is to connect the standard limb leads of an ECG machine to the patient's right and left legs and the right and left arm leads to the two esophageal poles. Lead I will then display a bipolar esophageal electrogram. Positioning to achieve a maximum P-wave amplitude will allow atrial pacing. Use of this lead with a programmable stimulator will allow termination of tachycardias relatively noninvasively by atrial overdrive pacing or atrial extrastimulation. As with adenosine, there is a small risk of causing atrial fibrillation with rapid atrial pacing, and so an electrical cardiovertor-defibrillator should be in the room with the monitoring leads connected to the patient before institution of esophageal pace termination of SVT.

Pacing therapy is the logical choice for nonpharmacologic conversion of atrial flutter, in which adenosine infusion is generally not effective and in which vagal maneuvers often fail.

Electrical Cardioversion. The device used for direct current cardioversion-defibrillation should provide both oscilloscopic display and paper records, come with adult- and infant-sized paddles, allow a choice of several ECG leads from three chest electrodes, function in either asynchronous or synchronous mode, and allow precise outputs for infants (i.e., < 5 J). The correct initial dose for cardioversion or defibrillation is 0.5 to 2.0 J/kg. Narrow QRS tachycardias should always be converted in synchronous mode. In general, no special precautions are necessary in children who are taking normal therapeutic doses of digoxin. If there is a concern of high digoxin levels or digoxin toxicity, an initial bolus of 1 mg/kg of intravenous lidocaine may be given before cardioversion. Adequate sedation or general anesthesia is necessary before cardioversion, unless the patient is critically ill and the delay inherent in administering general anesthesia would be unreasonable.

REFERENCES

1. Keith JD, Rowe RD, Vlad P: Heart Disease in Infancy and Childhood. New York, Macmillan, 1967, pp 1056.
2. Ludomirsky A, Garson A: Supraventricular tachycardia. In Gillette PC, Garson A (eds): Pediatric Arrhythmias: Electrophysiology and Pacing. Philadelphia, WB Saunders, 1990, pp 380–426.
3. Chung KY, Walsh TJ, Massie E: Wolff-Parkinson-White syndrome. Am Heart J 69:1, 1965.
4. Sano S, Komori S, Naitoh A, et al: Incidence of WPW syndrome in school children. Circulation 92(Suppl 1):I-707, 1995.
5. Ko JK, Deal BJ, Strasburger JF, et al: Supraventricular tachycardia mechanisms and their age distribution in pediatric patients. Am J Cardiol 69:1028–1032, 1992.
6. Van Hare GF, Lesh MD, Scheinman M, et al: Percutaneous radiofrequency catheter ablation for supraventricular arrhythmias in children. J Am Coll Cardiol 17:1613–1620, 1991.
7. Dick MD, O'Connor BK, Serwer GA, et al: Use of radiofrequency current to ablate accessory connections in children. Circulation 84:2318–2324, 1991.
8. Jackman WM, Wang XZ, Friday KJ, et al: Catheter ablation of accessory atrioventricular pathways (Wolff-Parkinson-White syndrome) by radiofrequency current. N Engl J Med 324:1605–1611, 1991.
9. Jackman WM, Beckman KJ, McClelland JH, et al: Treatment of supraventricular tachycardia due to atrioventricular nodal reentry, by radiofrequency catheter ablation of slow-pathway conduction. N Engl J Med 327:313–318, 1992.
10. Lesh MD, Van Hare GF, Schamp DJ, et al: Curative percutaneous catheter ablation using radiofrequency energy for accessory pathways in all locations: Results in 100 consecutive patients. J Am Coll Cardiol 19:1303–1309, 1992.
11. Kugler JD, Danford DA, Deal BJ, et al: Radiofrequency catheter ablation for tachyarrhythmias in children and adolescents. The Pediatric Electrophysiology Society. N Engl J Med 330:1481–1487, 1994.
12. Lev M, Givson S, Miller RA: Ebstein's disease with Wolff-Parkinson-White syndrome. Am Heart J 49:724–741, 1955.
13. Smith WM, Gallagher JJ, Kerr CR, et al: The electrophysiologic basis and management of symptomatic recurrent tachycardia in patients with Ebstein's anomaly of the tricuspid valve. Am J Cardiol 49:1223–1234, 1982.
14. Smith RT, Gillette PC, Massumi A, et al: Transcatheter ablative techniques for treatment of the permanent form of junctional reciprocating tachycardia in young patients. J Am Coll Cardiol 8:385–390, 1986.
15. Ticho BS, Walsh EP, Saul JP: Ablation of permanent junctional reciprocating tachycardia. In Huang SKS (ed): Radiofrequency Catheter Ablation of Cardiac Arrhythmias: Basic Concepts and Clinical Applications. Armonk, NY: Futura, 1994, pp 397–409.
16. Gillette PC, Garson A, Cooley DA, et al: Prolonged and decremental antegrade conduction properties in right anterior accessory connections: Wide QRS antidromic tachycardia of left bundle branch block pattern without Wolff-Parkinson-White configuration in sinus rhythm. Am Heart J 103:66–74, 1982.
17. Grogin HR, Lee RJ, Kwasman M, et al: Radiofrequency catheter ablation of atriofascicular and nodoventricular Mahaim tracts. Circulation 90:272–281, 1994.
18. Klein GJ, Guiraudon G, Guiraudon C, et al: The nodoventricular Mahaim pathway: An endangered concept? Circulation 90:636–638, 1994.
19. Gallagher JJ, Smith WM, Kasell JH, et al: Role of Mahaim fibers in cardiac arrhythmias in man. Circulation 64:176–189, 1981.
20. Benditt DG, Pritchett LC, Smith WM, et al: Characteristics of atrioventricular conduction and the spectrum of arrhythmias in Lown-Ganong-Levine syndrome. Circulation 57:454–465, 1978.
21. Perry JC, Garson A: Supraventricular tachycardia due to Wolff-Parkinson-White syndrome in children: Early disappearance and late recurrence. J Am Coll Cardiol 16:1215–1220, 1990.
22. Wu MH, Chang YC, Lin JL, et al: Probability of supraventricular tachycardia recurrence in pediatric patients. Cardiology 85:284–289, 1994.
23. Munger TM, Packer DL, Hammill SC, et al: A population study of the natural history of Wolff-Parkinson-White syndrome in Olmsted County, Minnesota, 1953–1989. Circulation 87:866–873, 1993.
24. Sharma AD, Yee R, Guiraudon G, et al: Sensitivity and specificity of invasive and noninvasive testing for risk of sudden death in Wolff-Parkinson-White syndrome. J Am Coll Cardiol 10:373–381, 1987.
25. Klein GJ, Prystowsky EN, Yee R, et al: Asymptomatic Wolff-Parkinson-White: Should we intervene? Circulation 80:1902–1905, 1989.
26. Deal BJ, Keane JF, Gillette PC, et al: Wolff-Parkinson-White syndrome and supraventricular tachycardia during infancy: Management and follow-up. J Am Coll Cardiol 5:130–135, 1985.
27. Gallagher JJ, Gilbert M, Svenson RH, et al: Wolff-Parkinson-White syndrome: The problem, evaluation and surgical correction. Circulation 51:767–785, 1975.
28. Reddy GV, Schamroth L: The localization of bypass tracts in the Wolff-Parkinson-White syndrome from the surface electrocardiogram. Am Heart J 113:984–993, 1987.

29. Fitzpatrick A, Lesh M: A new statistical appraisal of baseline ECG features for localization of accessory pathways. J Electrocardiol 26(Suppl I):220–226, 1993.
30. Weiss J, Brugada P, Roy D, et al: Localization of the accessory pathway in the Wolff-Parkinson-White syndrome from the ventriculo-atrial conduction time of right ventricular apical extrasystoles. Pacing Clin Electrophysiol 6:260–267, 1983.
31. Sellers TD Jr, Gallagher JJ, Cope GD, et al: Retrograde atrial preexcitation following premature ventricular beats during reciprocating tachycardia in the Wolff-Parkinson-White syndrome. Eur J Cardiol 4:283–294, 1976.
32. Jackman WM, Friday KJ, Scherlag BJ, et al: Direct endocardial recording from an accessory atrioventricular pathway: Localization of the site of block, effect of antiarrhythmic drugs, and attempt at nonsurgical ablation. Circulation 68:906–916, 1983.
33. Jackman WM, Friday KJ, Yeung-Lai-Wah JA, et al: New catheter technique for recording left free-wall accessory atrioventricular pathway activation. Identification of pathway fiber orientation. Circulation 78:598–611, 1988.
34. McClelland JH, Wang X, Beckman KJ, et al: Radiofrequency catheter ablation of right atriofascicular (Mahaim) accessory pathways guided by accessory pathway activation potentials. Circulation 89:2655–2666, 1994.
35. Sellers TD, Bashore T, Gallagher JJ: Digitalis in the preexcitation syndrome: Analysis during atrial fibrillation. Circulation 56:260–267, 1977.
36. Jedeikin R, Gillette PC, Garson A, et al: Effect of ouabain on the antegrade effective refractory period of accessory atrioventricular connections in children. J Am Coll Cardiol 1:869–872, 1983.
37. Perry J, McQuinn R, Smith R, et al: Flecainide acetate for resistant arrhythmias in the young: Efficacy and pharmacokinetics. J Am Coll Cardiol 14:185–191, 1989.
38. Case CL, Gillette PC, Oslizlok PC, et al: Radiofrequency catheter ablation of incessant, medically resistant supraventricular tachycardia in infants and small children. J Am Coll Cardiol 20:1405–1410, 1992.
39. Erickson CC, Walsh EP, Triedman JK, et al: Efficacy and safety of radiofrequency ablation in infants and young children < 18 months of age. Am J Cardiol 74:944–947, 1994.
40. Kugler JD: Radiofrequency catheter ablation for supraventricular tachycardia. Should it be used in infants and small children? [editorial, comment]. Circulation 90:639–641, 1994.
41. Ott DA, Cooley DA, Moak J, et al: Computer-guided surgery for tachyarrhythmias in children: Current results and expectations. J Am Coll Cardiol 21:1205–1210, 1993.
42. Sung RJ, Waxman HL, Saksena S, et al: Sequence of retrograde atrial activation in patients with dual atrioventricular nodal pathways. Circulation 64:1059–1067, 1981.
43. Miller JM, Rosenthal ME, Vassallo JA, et al: Atrioventricular nodal reentrant tachycardia: Studies on upper and lower "common pathways." Circulation 75:930–940, 1987.
44. Josephson ME, Miller JM: Atrioventricular nodal reentry: Evidence supporting an intranodal location [review]. Pacing Clin Electrophysiol 16:599–614, 1993.
45. Sung RJ, Lauer MR, Chun H: Atrioventricular node reentry: Current concepts and new perspectives [review]. Pacing Clin Electrophysiol 17:1413–1430, 1994.
46. Levy AM, Bonazinga BJ: Sudden sinus slowing with junctional escape: A common mode of initiation of juvenile supraventricular tachycardia. Circulation 67:84–87, 1983.
47. Wolff GS, Sung RJ, Pickoff A, et al: The fast-slow form of atrioventricular nodal reentrant tachycardia in children. Am J Cardiol 43:1181–1188, 1979.
48. Sung RJ, Styperek JL, Myerburg RJ, et al: Initiation of two distinct forms of atrioventricular nodal reentrant tachycardia during programmed ventricular stimulation in man. Am J Cardiol 42:404–415, 1978.
49. Brugada P, Vanagt EJ, Dassen WR, et al: Atrioventricular nodal tachycardia with and without discontinuous anterograde and retrograde atrioventricular nodal conduction curves: A reappraisal of the dual pathway concept. Eur Heart J 1:399–407, 1980.
50. Casta A, Wolff GS, Mehta AV, et al: Dual atrioventricular nodal pathways: A benign finding in arrhythmia-free children with heart disease. Am J Cardiol 46:1013–1018, 1980.
51. Silka MJ, Kron J, Halperin BD, et al: Mechanisms of AV node reentrant tachycardia in young patients with and without dual AV node physiology. Pacing Clin Electrophysiol 17:2129–2133, 1994.
52. Wellens HJ, Wesdorp JC, Duren DR, et al: Second degree block during reciprocal atrioventricular nodal tachycardia. Circulation 53:595–599, 1976.
53. Lee MA, Morady F, Kadish A, et al: Catheter modification of the atrioventricular junction with radiofrequency energy for control of atrioventricular nodal reentry tachycardia. Circulation 83:827–835, 1991.
54. Calkins H, Sousa J, El-Atassi R, et al: Diagnosis and cure of the Wolff-Parkinson-White syndrome or paroxysmal supraventricular tachycardias during a single electrophysiologic test. N Engl J Med 324:1612–1618, 1991.
55. Epstein LM, Lesh MD, Griffin JC, et al: A direct midseptal approach to slow atrioventricular nodal pathway ablation. Pacing Clin Electrophysiol 18:57–64, 1995.
56. Ross DL, Johnson DC, Denniss AR, et al: Curative surgery for atrioventricular junctional ("AV nodal") reentrant tachycardia. J Am Coll Cardiol 6:1383–1392, 1985.
57. Bharati S, Moskowitz WB, Scheinman M, et al: Junctional tachycardias: Anatomic substrate and its significance in ablative procedures. J Am Coll Cardiol 18:179–186, 1991.
58. Van Hare GF, Velvis H, Langberg JJ: Successful transcatheter ablation of congenital junctional ectopic tachycardia in a ten-month-old infant using radiofrequency energy. Pacing Clin Electrophysiol 13:730–735, 1990.
59. Young ML, Mehta MB, Martinez RM, et al: Combined alpha-adrenergic blockade and radiofrequency ablation to treat junctional ectopic tachycardia successfully without atrioventricular block. Am J Cardiol 71:883–885, 1993.
60. Scheinman MM, Gonzalez RP, Cooper MW, et al: Clinical and electrophysiologic features and role of catheter ablation techniques in adult patients with automatic atrioventricular junctional tachycardia. Am J Cardiol 74:565–572, 1994.
61. Coumel P, Fidelle JE, Attuel P, et al: Tachycardies focales hissiennes congenitales. Etude cooperative de sept cas. Arch Mal Coeur 69:899–909, 1975.
62. Villain E, Vetter V, Garcia JM, et al: Evolving concepts in the management of congenital junctional ectopic tachycardia. A multicenter study. Circulation 81:1544–1549, 1990.
63. Ruder MA, Davis JC, Eldar M, et al: Clinical and electrophysiologic characterization of automative junctional tachycardia in adults. Circulation 73:930–937, 1986.
64. Rossi AF, Kipel G, Golinko RJ, et al: Use of adenosine in postoperative junctional ectopic tachycardia with 1:1 retrograde atrial conduction. Am Heart J 121:1237–1239, 1991.
65. Case CL, Gillette PC: Automatic atrial and junctional tachycardias in the pediatric patient: Strategies for diagnosis and management. Pacing Clin Electrophysiol 16:1323–1335, 1993.

66. Bash SE, Shah JJ, Albers WH, et al: Hypothermia for the treatment of postsurgical greatly accelerated junctional ectopic tachycardia. J Am Coll Cardiol 10:1095–1099, 1987.
67. Pfammatter JP, Paul T, Ziemer G, et al: Successful management of junctional tachycardia by hypothermia after cardiac operations in infants. Ann Thorac Surg 60:556–560, 1995.
68. Waldo AL, Krongrad E, Kupersmith J, et al: Ventricular paired pacing to control rapid ventricular heart rate following open heart surgery. Observations on ectopic automaticity. Report of a case in a four-month-old patient. Circulation 53:176–181, 1976.
69. Reimer A, Paul T, Kallfelz HC: Efficacy and safety of intravenous and oral propafenone in pediatric cardiac dysrhythmias. Am J Cardiol 68:741–744, 1991.
70. Paul T, Reimer A, Janousek J, et al: Efficacy and safety of propafenone in congenital junctional ectopic tachycardia. J Am Coll Cardiol 20:911–914, 1992.
71. Bryson HM, Palmer KJ, Langtry HD, et al: Propafenone. A reappraisal of its pharmacology, pharmacokinetics and therapeutic use in cardiac arrhythmias [review]. Drugs 45:85–130, 1993. Erratum. Drugs 45:736, 1993.
72. Paul T, Janousek J: New antiarrhythmic drugs in pediatric use: Propafenone [review]. Pediatr Cardiol 15:190–197, 1994.
73. Heusch A, Kramer HH, Krogmann ON, et al: Clinical experience with propafenone for cardiac arrhythmias in the young. Eur Heart J 15:1050–1056, 1994.
74. Perry JC, Knilans TK, Marlow D, et al: Intravenous amiodarone for life-threatening tachyarrhythmias in children and young adults. J Am Coll Cardiol 22:95–98, 1993.
75. Raja P, Hawker RE, Chaikitpinyo A, et al: Amiodarone management of junctional ectopic tachycardia after cardiac surgery in children. Br Heart J 72:261–265, 1994.
76. Maragnes P, Fournier A, Davignon A: Usefulness of oral sotalol for the treatment of junctional ectopic tachycardia. Int J Cardiol 35:165–167, 1992.
77. Fenrich AL Jr, Perry JC, Friedman RA: Flecainide and amiodarone: combined therapy for refractory tachyarrhythmias in infancy. J Am Coll Cardiol 25:1195–1198, 1995.
78. Bisset GS, Gaum W, Kaplan S: The ice bag: A new technique for interruption of supraventricular tachycardia. J Pediatr 97:593–595, 1980.
79. Overholt ED, Rheuban KS, Gutgesell HP, et al: Usefulness of adenosine for arrhythmias in infants and children. Am J Cardiol 61:336–340, 1988.
80. DeGroff CG, Silka MJ: Bronchospasm after intravenous administration of adenosine in a patient with asthma. J Pediatr 125:822–823, 1994.
81. Bennett-Guerrero E, Young CC: Bronchospasm after intravenous adenosine administration [review]. Anesth Analg 79:386–388, 1994.
82. Burkhart KK: Respiratory failure following adenosine administration. Am J Emerg Med 11:249–250, 1993.
83. Crosson JE, Etheridge SP, Milstein S, et al: Therapeutic and diagnostic utility of adenosine during tachycardia evaluation in children. Am J Cardiol 74:155–160, 1994.
84. Cowell RP, Paul VE, Ilsley CD: Haemodynamic deterioration after treatment with adenosine [see comments]. Br Heart J 71:569–571, 1994.
85. Tebbenjohanns J, Pfeiffer D, Schumacher B, et al: Intravenous adenosine during atrioventricular reentrant tachycardia: Induction of atrial fibrillation with rapid conduction over an accessory pathway. Pacing Clin Electrophysiol 18:743–746, 1995.
86. Porter CJ, Garson A Jr, Gillette PC: Verapamil: An effective calcium blocking agent for pediatric patients [review]. Pediatrics 71:748–755, 1983.
87. Porter CJ, Gillette PC, Garson A Jr, et al: Effects of verapamil on supraventricular tachycardia in children. Am J Cardiol 48:487–491, 1981.
88. Epstein ML, Kiel EA, Victorica BE: Cardiac decompensation following verapamil therapy in infants with supraventricular tachycardia. Pediatrics 75:737–740, 1985.
89. Garson A: Medicolegal problems in the management of cardiac arrhythmias in children. Pediatrics 79:84–88, 1987.
90. Benson DW, Dunnigan A, Benditt DG, et al: Transesophageal cardiac pacing: History, application, technique. Clin Prog Pacing Electrophysiol 2:360–372, 1984.

CHAPTER 8

VENTRICULAR ARRHYTHMIAS

Michael J. Silka and Arthur Garson, Jr.

During the past 15 years, a substantial volume of literature has been published regarding ventricular arrhythmias in children; however, many aspects regarding both the evaluation and treatment of these arrhythmias remain controversial. These uncertainties reflect the evolving nature of our understanding of the mechanisms, prognosis, and treatment options for children with ventricular arrhythmias.[1, 2]

Ventricular arrhythmias may be defined as disturbances of cardiac rhythm that originate distal to the bifurcation of the common bundle of His.[3] The clinical significance of these arrhythmias extends in spectrum from benign to lethal, based on the specific type of arrhythmia and associated cardiovascular disease. In this chapter, we discuss current clinical, electrophysiologic, and therapeutic considerations for the various ventricular arrhythmias that may occur during childhood and adolescence.

CLINICAL PRESENTATIONS OF VENTRICULAR ARRHYTHMIAS

Ventricular arrhythmias may be detected as an irregularity of pulse on routine physical examination, during ambulatory monitoring of the patient with cardiovascular disease, and during the evaluation of syncope or unexplained sudden cardiac arrest. Patients with ventricular arrhythmias may be asymptomatic or may have symptoms ranging from chest pain or palpitations, similar to supraventricular tachycardia, to potentially lethal compromised cardiac output.[4] Furthermore, responses to interventions such as atrial pacing or the administration of adenosine or verapamil may result in termination of certain ventricular as well as supraventricular arrhythmias in children. Given the diverse presentations and responses to empiric treatment, initial considerations in the evaluation of ventricular arrhythmias in young patients are careful analysis of the electrocardiogram (ECG) and assessment for the presence of any associated cardiovascular disease.

ELECTROCARDIOGRAPHIC CHARACTERISTICS OF VENTRICULAR ARRHYTHMIAS

Premature ventricular contractions (PVCs) are one of the most common causes for an irregular pulse in a young patient. PVCs have been evident on routine ECGs in 0.8 to 2.2% of children with no known heart disease[5, 6] and in 18% of newborns and up to 50% of adolescents during 24-hour ambulatory ECG monitoring.[7, 8] In comparison, PVCs are present on 8% of routine ECGs and 46% of 24-hour ambulatory recordings in patients who have undergone surgical treatment for tetralogy of Fallot.[1]

PVCs are defined by five electrocardiographic criteria (Fig. 8–1):

1. The QRS is premature. Although a definition of "premature" is based on the underlying rhythm, a QRS occurring 80 milliseconds or more earlier than anticipated during a regular rhythm has been suggested as premature.[9]
2. The morphology of the QRS complex is different than that of the regular QRS complex. PVCs in children are not always "wide" but do have a different QRS from sinus rhythm. Evaluation of multiple simultaneous ECG channels is required because the morphology of a PVC may be similar to the QRS in sinus rhythm in one channel.
3. The QRS complex is usually, but not always, prolonged in duration (> 0.08 second in infants and > 0.09 second in children older than 3 years).
4. There are abnormalities of the ST segment and T wave; the vector of the T wave is usually discordant to that of the QRS complex.
5. The premature QRS complex is not preceded by a premature atrial depolarization.

PVCs may demonstrate fusion, thus confirming their ventricular origin. A fusion complex is defined as one in which the QRS is intermediate in morphology between two other distinct QRS morphologies (Fig. 8–2). For fusion to occur, the ventricle must be activated simultaneously from

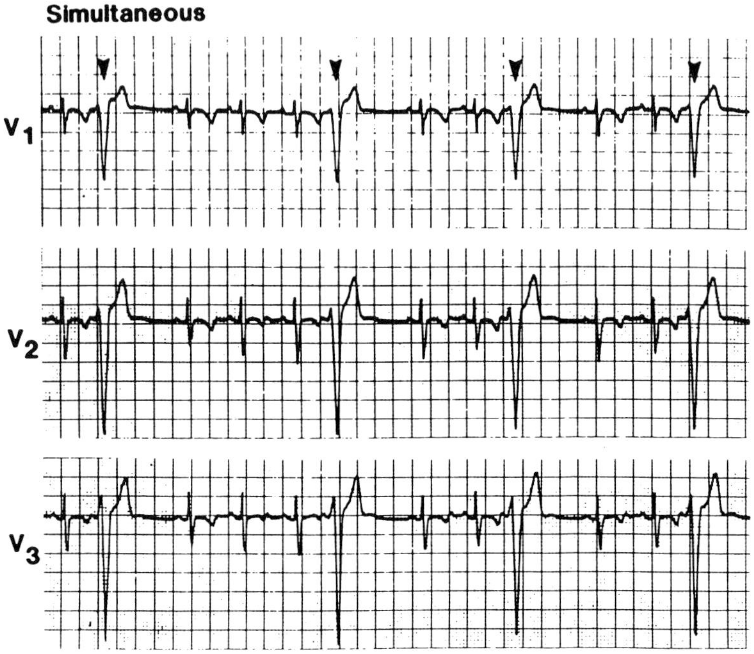

FIGURE 8–1. Electrocardiographic features of premature ventricular contractions (QRS complexes with *arrows*). Premature ventricular depolarizations are premature, occurring 0.38 s before the next anticipated sinus QRS; the morphology of the premature QRS is different and wider than the sinus QRS; there is QRS–T-wave discordance; and the premature QRS complexes are not preceded by a sinus P wave.

two different directions. Most commonly, this occurs as fusion between a conducted sinus beat and a PVC originating in the ventricular myocardium.

In the differential diagnosis of PVCs in children, there are three common arrhythmias: (1) premature atrial depolarizations with aberrant ventricular conduction; (2) premature junctional depolarizations with aberrant conduction; and (3) intermittent antegrade conduction over an accessory atrioventricular connection.

PREMATURE ATRIAL CONTRACTIONS WITH ABERRANT VENTRICULAR CONDUCTION

In children, nearly 50% of premature atrial contractions (PACs) are conducted aberrantly. QRS duration or morphology may not differentiate PACs with aberrancy from PVCs. Premature atrial depolarizations may be identified either by an early P wave or by distortion of the T wave preceding the premature QRS complex. If a premature QRS complex of different morphology from sinus rhythm is not preceded by an identifiable P wave, then the diagnosis is a PVC. Both PACs with aberrancy and PVCs may be interpolated in children. The basic underlying rhythm is not disturbed by the premature beat. When interpolation occurs, the sinus node is not reset by the premature beat, and conduction of the next sinus impulse is not blocked.

If the underlying rhythm is a primary atrial tachycardia (atrial flutter/fibrillation or ectopic atrial tachycardia), it is possible to have either aberrant conduction of the atrial rhythm or PVCs. This differentiation is important, because primary atrial tachycardias commonly occur in postoperative congenital heart disease patients. Schamroth proposed four rules that indicate probable aberrant conduction of atrial impulses rather than PVCs[10]:

1. A relatively fast average ventricular rate. PVCs tend to occur more often with slower intrinsic ventricular rates.
2. QRS morphology variation. Rapid atrial impulses may be conducted to the ventricle at various phases of recovery of the distal conduction system, resulting in QRS morphology variation. Conversely, PVCs tend to have a fixed morphology.
3. Variation of the coupling interval. PVCs usually have fixed coupling intervals.
4. No attempt at a compensatory pause. PVCs may be followed by a pause.

In practice, it may be difficult to distinguish between PVCs and aberrant conduction on ECG during supraventricular tachycardia. With intracardiac electrophysiologic study, aberrantly conducted atrial depolarizations are identified by the presence of a His bundle electrogram preceding

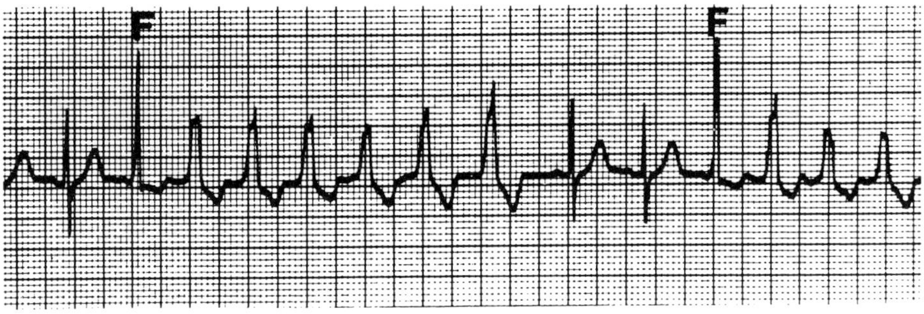

FIGURE 8–2. Fusion (F) beats. The 2nd and 11th QRS complexes are of intermediate morphology between the sinus beats (1st, 9th, and 10th beats) and ventricular tachycardia (other QRS complexes in this rhythm strip). The fusion beats are preceded by P waves, immediately before onset of the fusion QRS complex.

each QRS with a normal or prolonged HV interval, whereas PVCs are usually not preceded by a His bundle electrogram or may be preceded by a shorter than normal HV interval.

PREMATURE JUNCTIONAL DEPOLARIZATIONS WITH ABERRANT CONDUCTION

If a QRS complex with a different morphology from the regular QRS is premature and has no preceding premature P wave, it could be either a premature junctional depolarization with aberrancy or a PVC. The distinction is possible only with the use of intracardiac recordings: in a premature junctional depolarization, the HV interval is either normal or prolonged; in a PVC, either a His potential does not precede the QRS complex or the HV interval is shorter than normal.

If only the surface ECG is available, such complexes are considered PVCs. The only exception may be in the patient with premature junctional beats (i.e., premature QRS complexes of normal morphology not preceded by a premature atrial depolarization).

INTERMITTENT ANTEGRADE CONDUCTION OVER AN ACCESSORY CONNECTION

The distinction between a PVC occurring in late diastole and intermittent conduction of a sinus beat over an accessory connection may be difficult. The transition to conduction over an accessory pathway may occur gradually over several beats, with gradual pre-excitation of the QRS complex. The change to accessory pathway conduction usually accompanies a change in heart rate, either an increase or decrease. Conversely, PVCs tend to occur singly or in pairs, and a rate change may not accompany the appearance of PVCs.

PVC MORPHOLOGIES: MONOMORPHIC AND POLYMORPHIC

PVCs with a consistent QRS morphology in several ECG leads are termed *uniform* or *monomorphic*, whereas those with varying QRS morphologies are *multiform* or *polymorphic*. Fusion complexes should not be mistaken for multiform PVCs. If the wide QRS complex is not preceded by a premature P wave, fusion cannot have occurred between a normally conducted QRS and a PVC.

The terms *unifocal* and *multifocal* have been used to describe PVCs with the assumption that PVCs of a single morphology originate from a single focus in the ventricle, whereas PVCs of differing morphologies originate from multiple sites. However, intracardiac electrophysiology studies have demonstrated that PVCs of the same morphology may originate from different sites,[1, 2] PVCs with different morphologies may originate from the same site with different exit pathways, and QRS morphology is an unreliable guide to PVC origin, particularly in septal sites of ventricular ectopy.[3]

COUPLING INTERVALS AND VENTRICULAR PARASYSTOLE

The coupling interval of a PVC is defined as the time between the onset of the preceding

QRS complex and the onset of the PVC. For each morphology of a PVC, the coupling interval may be fixed or variable (Fig. 8–3). Variable coupling is defined as a change in the coupling interval of 0.08 second or greater. With multiform PVCs, each morphology may have an intrinsic coupling interval in relation to the preceding QRS.

Most PVCs in children demonstrate a fixed coupling interval. If there is variable coupling with the same QRS morphology, the interectopic intervals (time between each PVC) should be measured. If the interectopic intervals are a multiple of a basic single interval, then ventricular parasystole is diagnosed.

The shorter the coupling interval, the closer the PVC is to the apex of the preceding T wave. The period of 10 to 50 milliseconds after the apex of the T wave has been termed the *ventricular vulnerable period*, because ventricular extrastimuli applied during this period (R on T) have been reported to result in ventricular tachycardia (VT) or fibrillation. However, Holter monitor recordings of sudden cardiac arrest frequently demonstrate that a PVC with a long coupling interval initiates VT or fibrillation.[11] The R on T phenomenon is important during attempted cardioversion or defibrillation because a shock delivered at the apex of the T wave may result in ventricular fibrillation in children as well as in adults (see Chapter 12 on antitachycardia devices).

ELECTROCARDIOGRAPHIC PATTERNS OF PVCs: BIGEMINY, TRIGEMINY, AND COUPLETS

Ventricular bigeminy is a regular rhythm, in which a PVC alternates with an underlying sinus QRS. Bigeminy frequently is a stable and self-sustaining rhythm. The reason for this is provided by the rule of bigeminy, which is based on the observation that PVCs are common with slow heart rates (long cycle lengths).[12] If a PVC is followed by a compensatory pause (longer cycle length than the sinus beat), the long cycle length of the compensatory pause will favor another PVC (Fig. 8–4). This PVC generates another compensatory pause, and the rhythm continues as bigeminy. Ventricular trigeminy is a regular alternation of a PVC with two normal QRS complexes. A couplet is defined as two PVCs in a row without an intervening normal QRS complex.

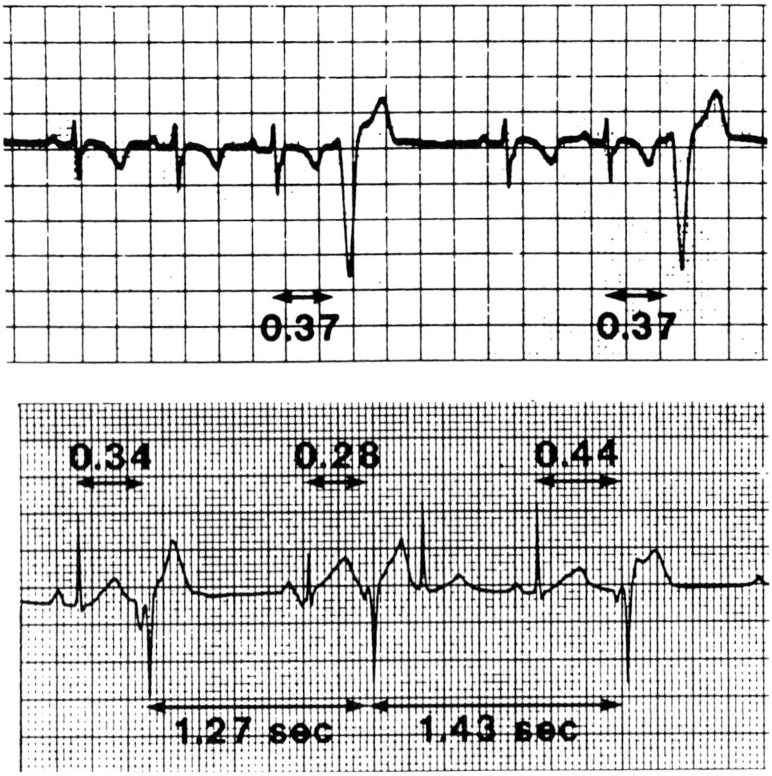

FIGURE 8–3. Coupling intervals. The upper rhythm strip demonstrates a fixed or constant interval of 0.37 s between the sinus beats and premature ventricular depolarizations. In contrast, the lower panel demonstrates variable sinus to PVC intervals, consistent with variable coupling. Because the interectopic interval is not constant, this suggests a non-parasystolic focus (see text for details).

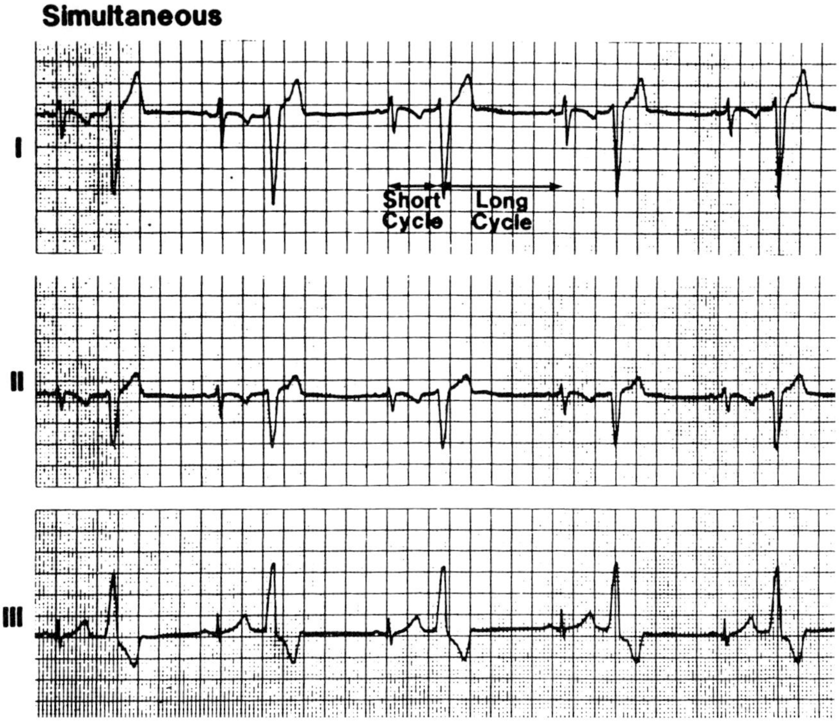

FIGURE 8–4. Ventricular bigeminy. Each sinus QRS is followed by a premature ventricular depolarization. The long cycle length preceding the sinus beat predisposes to a premature ventricular contraction in the subsequent ventricular depolarization.

VENTRICULAR TACHYCARDIA: ELECTROCARDIOGRAPHIC CHARACTERISTICS

VT is a series of three or more consecutive depolarizations that originate from the ventricle at a rate greater than 120 bpm. On the surface ECG, each QRS is different from the sinus morphology. This is a most important consideration because the QRS may not be wide for age.

ECG criteria that favor the diagnosis of VT include

1. Atrioventricular (AV) dissociation, which is reported to be present in the majority of children with VT. If AV dissociation with a wide or different QRS is present, the diagnosis is VT with very rare exception (Fig. 8–5). However, the absence of AV dissociation is not helpful, because VT may occur with 1:1 retrograde VA conduction.
2. Intermittent fusion or sinus capture beats.
3. Morphology of VT similar to single PVCs. If the patient had a prior ECG with PVCs, the VT should be compared to the PVCs. However, if the morphologies of the PVCs and VT are not similar, the diagnosis may still be VT.
4. Rate. In children, it is unusual for sustained VT to have a rate greater than 250/minute. However, this criterion is not helpful in infants, in whom VT rates between 167 and 500 have been reported.[13]

In infants, the most common QRS morphology during VT is right bundle branch block with left axis deviation with a QRS duration from 0.06 to 0.11 second (Fig. 8–6). With increasing age, the QRS duration is often prolonged during VT (> 0.09 second), with a left bundle branch QRS morphology more commonly observed.[14]

VT must be differentiated from supraventricular tachycardia with a "different QRS." (The term *wide QRS* is not used because the QRS frequently is not wide.) Persistent aberrancy of the QRS during supraventricular tachycardia has been reported in 8 to 26% of pediatric series reports.[15] When aberrancy of supraventricular tachycardia occurs, it most frequently is of a right bundle branch morphology; in contrast, VT in children most commonly demonstrates left bundle branch aberrancy.

CATEGORIES OF VENTRICULAR TACHYCARDIA

The definition of VT as three or more consecutive abnormal QRS complexes not initiated by

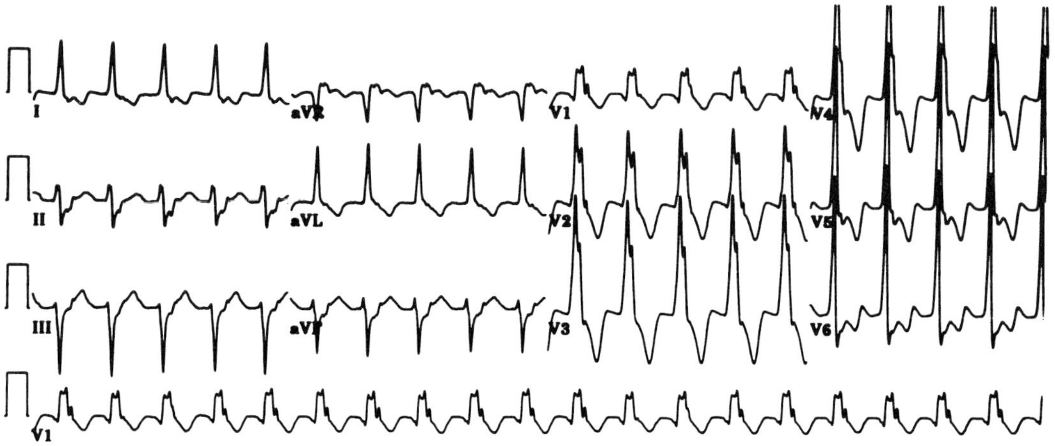

FIGURE 8–5. Ventricular tachycardia. This 12-lead electrocardiogram and rhythm strip demonstrates an inconsistent atrioventricular (AV) relationship, best demonstrated in lead V_1. The persistence of tachycardia, with an intermittent AV dissociation, confirms the ventricular origin of this tachycardia.

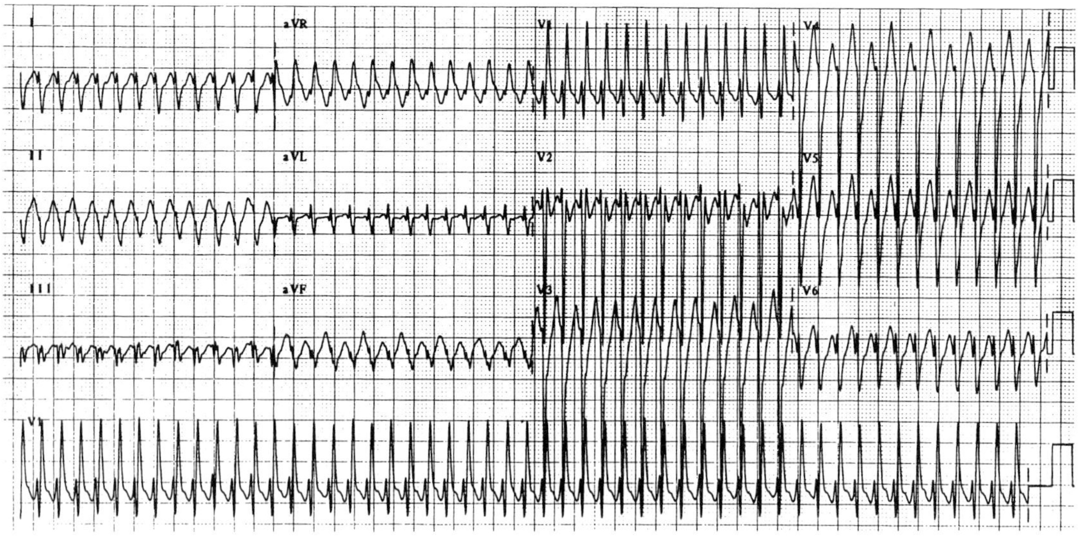

FIGURE 8–6. Ventricular tachycardia in a newborn infant. The electrocardiogram demonstrates a rate of 300 beats/minute with right bundle branch pattern. The differential diagnosis of this tachycardia includes ventricular tachycardia, atrial flutter, and supraventricular tachycardia with aberrancy. Atrioventricular dissociation during tachycardia (with the ventricular rate faster than the atrial rate) was demonstrated during electrophysiology testing, confirming the diagnosis of ventricular tachycardia.

atrial depolarization is nonspecific. Hence, the following definitions of VT have been proposed:[16]

1. *Nonsustained VT:* three beats to 10 seconds of spontaneous VT
2. *Sustained VT:* spontaneous VT lasting 10 seconds or longer
3. *Inducible nonsustained VT:* 10 beats to 30 seconds of VT in response to programmed electrical stimulation
4. *Inducible sustained VT:* 30 seconds or longer VT or an episode requiring termination as a result of hemodynamic compromise in response to programmed stimulation
5. *Accelerated ventricular rhythm:* a rhythm with the ECG characteristics of VT, with a rate approximately the same as the prevailing sinus rate (usually < 120/minute) (Fig. 8–7)

As with PVCs, VT may be classified as monomorphic or polymorphic. This classification is based on the evaluation of the QRS morphologies in multiple simultaneous ECG leads.

VENTRICULAR FIBRILLATION

Ventricular fibrillation (VF) is a state of uncoordinated ventricular depolarizations resulting in no effective cardiac output. On the surface ECG, VF is a series of low-amplitude, irregular deflections without identifiable QRS complexes. This ECG morphology is similar to that observed when an ECG electrode has lost contact with the patient. Therefore, when VF is suspected, the electrodes should be rapidly checked for contact and the absence of a pulse in the patient confirmed.

VF is considered rare in children. In a study of the terminal electrical activity in 100 chronically ill patients younger than 18 years, VF was the terminal rhythm in only 6 (6%).[17] However, with improvements in emergency response systems, VF has been identified as the initial cardiac rhythm during attempted resuscitation in nearly 20% of patients younger than 18 years.[18] A primary determinant of the initial rhythm at attempted resuscitation was time to first response; VF was more common when resuscitative efforts were initiated within 4 minutes of cardiovascular collapse.

CLINICAL SIGNIFICANCE OF VENTRICULAR ARRHYTHMIAS IN CHILDREN

The clinical significance of a ventricular arrhythmia is based on the potential for trouble-

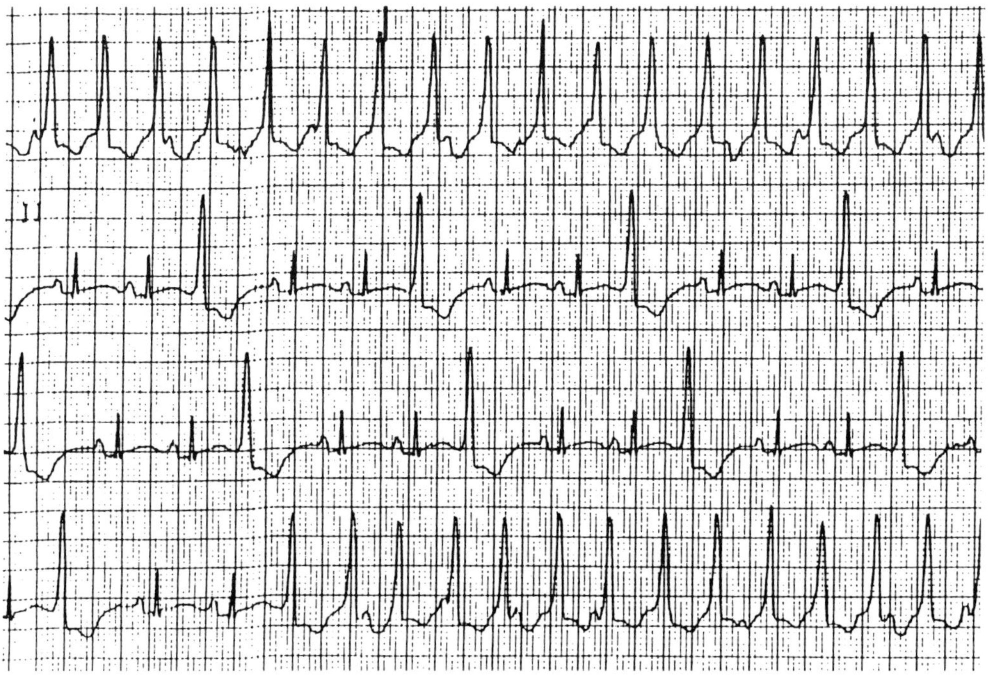

FIGURE 8–7. Accelerated idioventricular rhythm. This electrocardiogram from a newborn demonstrates a wide QRS complex rhythm with atrioventricular dissociation. The rate of the ventricular rhythm is 140 to 150/min compared with a sinus rate of 120/min.

some symptoms (palpitations, syncope) and the risk of sudden cardiac arrest. Evaluation of the clinical significance of a ventricular arrhythmia requires comprehensive evaluation of both the arrhythmia and the cause and severity of any associated cardiovascular disease. Prognostic implications are based on the characteristics of the arrhythmia and the forms and severity of associated cardiovascular disease.

Benign Ventricular Arrhythmias. A large percentage of ventricular arrhythmias in children are nonsustained, produce no hemodynamically significant effects, and are not associated with identifiable heart disease. These arrhythmias do not appear to be associated with an increased risk of sudden death and may been termed "benign." In general, treatment is not warranted for this class of arrhythmias.[9]

Potentially Malignant Ventricular Arrhythmias. A substantial percentage of ventricular arrhythmias in children are nonsustained but are associated with structural heart disease. These arrhythmias are considered as potentially malignant. Similarly, sustained ventricular arrhythmias in the absence of identifiable heart disease may also be of prognostic significance. This class is heterogeneous and associated with variable risk of sudden cardiovascular collapse. These ventricular arrhythmias need to be considered in the specific context of the associated form of cardiovascular disease, which is discussed in detail in the next section.

Malignant Ventricular Arrhythmias. A small percentage of ventricular arrhythmias in young patients are malignant or life threatening. These include hemodynamically significant sustained VT, torsades de pointes, and ventricular fibrillation. Arrhythmias in this category are associated with symptoms of hypotension, syncope, or cardiac arrest and require comprehensive evaluation and definitive treatment.

CARDIOVASCULAR DISEASES ASSOCIATED WITH VENTRICULAR ARRHYTHMIAS

Ventricular arrhythmias are associated with a number of diverse cardiovascular diseases in young patients. To a significant extent, the type of cardiac disease in the young patient with a ventricular arrhythmia will determine the evaluation required, the end points of treatment, and prognostic significance of the arrhythmia. Thus, definition of the presence and type of cardiovascular disease allows a rational approach to the evaluation of the young patient with a ventricular arrhythmia.

Acute Causes of Ventricular Arrhythmias. Sudden-onset complex ventricular ectopy or tachycardia in children may be due to metabolic or electrolyte abnormalities. These include hypoxia, acidosis, and hyperkalemia or hypokalemia. Thus, metabolic considerations are of particular importance in the critically ill or postoperative patient.[19] A second category of agents resulting in ventricular arrhythmias is pharmacologic. This includes sympathomimetic agents, inhalational anesthetics (halothane), and antiarrhythmic drugs. Additionally, several "street" drugs such as amphetamines, hallucinogens, and marijuana may inhibit norepinephrine uptake at synaptic terminals, resulting in ventricular arrhythmias. Myocardial injury may also cause ventricular arrhythmias. This includes myocardial contusion, myocardial injury resulting from myocarditis or pericarditis, and myocardial irritation caused by intravascular catheter placement.[20]

The primary evaluation of the patient with an acute ventricular arrhythmia is directed toward defining the cause and evaluation of the hemodynamic status. Single PVCs are generally well tolerated by children irrespective of the clinical situation. However, unexplained multiform PVCs, couplets, and nonsustained VT may indicate electrical instability of the ventricle and the potential to degenerate into a malignant ventricular arrhythmia. In this setting, acute medical therapy such as intravenous lidocaine may be indicated until the causative factor has been identified and corrected.

VENTRICULAR ARRHYTHMIAS ASSOCIATED WITH CONGENITAL HEART DISEASE

Sudden death and ventricular arrhythmias have been reported in several forms of congenital heart disease, both before and after surgical intervention.[1, 21] It has been hypothesized that most cases of sudden death in these patients were due to a malignant ventricular arrhythmia. Multiple causes for ventricular arrhythmias in patients with congenital heart disease have been proposed and include chronic volume or pressure overload, incomplete myocardial preservation at the time of surgery, residual postoperative defects, and fibrosis at the site of ventriculotomy.[22, 23]

Postoperative Tetralogy of Fallot. Ventricular arrhythmias have been studied extensively in patients who are postoperative for tetralogy of Fallot, and form the basis for most recommendations regarding patients with diverse forms of congenital heart disease. A review of 39 studies on this topic defined the following features (Table 8–1):[1]

1. PVCs were frequent, occurring on an average of 8% (range, 1–33%) of routine ECGs. PVCs were also noted on an average of 18% (range, 13–45%) of exercise tests and 46% (range, 2–77%) of Holter monitors.
2. VT (both sustained and nonsustained) was reported in 17% (range, 14–34%) of electrophysiology studies.
3. Sudden death occurred in 57 patients (1.8%) during a mean follow-up of 8.7 years. The mean age at surgery was 7.3 years; the average age at follow-up was 16.7 years.

The following factors were associated with ventricular arrhythmias after repair of tetralogy of Fallot: (1) greater length of follow-up after surgery, (2) an older age at repair, and (3) abnormal hemodynamics (elevated right ventricular systolic or diastolic pressures or left ventricular dysfunction). Symptoms (sustained palpitations, syncope) before sudden death were reported in only 11 of the 57 patients (19%). However, both ventricular arrhythmias on the Holter monitor and abnormal hemodynamics were present in 80% of patients who died suddenly compared with 8% of the surviving patients.

The significance of PVCs and nonsustained VT in patients with congenital heart disease remains controversial. Initial reports suggested that there is a significant correlation between PVCs on the routine ECG and sudden death in patients with tetralogy of Fallot and that this risk could be reduced with antiarrhythmic treatment.[24, 25] Class 1B antiarrhythmic agents (phenytoin [Dilantin], mexiletine) were most effective in PVC suppression, with minimal effect on ventricular function. However, acceptance of PVC treatment as an end point of therapy has been tempered by the observations that (1) suppression of PVCs does not correlate with suppression of inducible VT at electrophysiology testing[26] and (2) treatment of asymptomatic ventricular arrhythmias with certain antiarrhythmic drugs (class 1C) may be associated with an increased risk of sudden death.[27]

Controversy also exists regarding programmed electrical stimulation in postoperative tetralogy of Fallot patients to identify those with inducible sustained VT. In a multicenter series,[26] VT was inducible in 60 of 359 patients (17%). No patient with VT died suddenly during follow-up. In comparison, sudden death occurred in 5 patients in whom tachycardia was noninducible. The main conclusion of this study was that noninducibility at electrophysiology testing in tetralogy of Fallot patients does not necessarily confer a good prognosis, particularly in the presence of abnormal hemodynamics.

Electrophysiology study has provided some insight into VT in patients with tetralogy of Fallot. Re-entry is the probable mechanism, because the arrhythmia may be reproducibly initiated and terminated with programmed stimulation.[28] The tachycardia also demonstrates entrainment, suggesting a zone of slow conduction as a critical link in the re-entrant arrhythmia circuit.[29] Conversely, some experimental data also support a triggered mechanism of tachycardia.[30] Catheter and operative mapping of tachycardia have localized the arrhythmia circuit to the right ventricular outflow tract at the site of the ventriculotomy. Debate continues whether the tachycardia circuit is a macro–re-entrant circuit around the ventriculotomy[31] or a micro–re-entrant circuit, related to areas of local fibrosis.[32] Third, pharmacologic testing has suggested catecholamine dependency for the induction of tachycardia in some patients as well as noninducibility of tachycardia with beta-adrenergic blockade.[33, 34]

The age of onset of VT after surgery for tetralogy of Fallot or other forms of congenital heart disease is an important consideration. Walsh et al[35] suggested that repair of tetralogy of Fallot during the first 18 months of life may result in a lower incidence of late ventricular arrhythmias. The time of follow-up in this study was 5 years. In the report by Altman on VT after surgery for diverse forms of congenital heart disease, the mean age at onset of VT was 15.2 years.[4] Several studies have also been published reporting the

Table 8–1. Postoperative Tetralogy of Fallot: Prevalence of ECG-EPS Abnormalities (N = 4627)

ABNORMALITY	TEST	AVERAGE FREQUENCY (%)	RANGE (%)
PVC	ECG	8	1–33
PVC	Exercise	18	13–45
PVC	Holter	46	2–77
VT	EPS	17	14–34
Sudden death		1.8	0.5–5

PVC, premature ventricular contraction; VT, ventricular tachycardia; ECG, electrocardiogram; EPS, electrophysiology study.

Modified from Garson A, Jr: Ventricular arrhythmias after repair of congenital heart disease: who needs treatment? Cardiol Young 1:177, 1991.

onset of clinically apparent ventricular arrhythmias in early adulthood after surgery for congenital heart disease during childhood.[24, 36] The substrate for ventricular arrhythmias may evolve as a function of age, possibly related to ongoing fibrosis at the site of the ventriculotomy, ventricular distention caused by chronic valvar insufficiency, or late effects of ischemia on the abnormal myocardium.

The optimal methods of evaluation and treatment for patients with ventricular arrhythmias after repair of tetralogy of Fallot continue to be a matter of debate. In the absence of symptoms, Holter monitoring may be used for arrhythmia screening. Exercise testing before participation in vigorous physical activities or sports should be performed. These noninvasive tests need to be interpreted in conjunction with an echo-Doppler evaluation of hemodynamics. The indications for and interpretation of programmed electrical stimulation in these patients remain in dispute. The presence of abnormal hemodynamics and frequent PVCs (> 30/hr), couplets or VT, or unexplained syncope are proposed as indications for electrophysiologic testing. Indications for catheter evaluation may evolve with increasing experience in radiofrequency catheter ablation for VT in these patients.[37, 38]

VENTRICULAR ARRHYTHMIAS IN OTHER FORMS OF CONGENITAL HEART DISEASE

Ventricular arrhythmias and sudden death have been reported in several forms of congenital heart disease other than tetralogy of Fallot.[39, 40] Most observations that have been made regarding the prevalence and significance of ventricular arrhythmias after surgery for tetralogy of Fallot appear valid for other forms of congenital heart disease. In general, the following factors appear associated with higher incidence of prognostically significant ventricular arrhythmias: (1) hemodynamic abnormalities; (2) complex surgical procedures (e.g., Fontan); and (3) longer duration of follow-up.

A 1995 analysis of patients with congenital heart disease who underwent surgery in the current era identified the following defects as most commonly associated with VT: tetralogy of Fallot; transposition of the great arteries; functional single ventricle requiring Fontan procedure and aortic stenosis.[4] Ten of 76 patients with VT (13%) experienced cardiac arrest, which occurred primarily in patients with poor or fair clinical status.

Syncope is a concerning symptom in the patient with ventricular arrhythmias after surgery for congenital heart disease, and has been associated with inducible or spontaneous ventricular arrhythmias.[41] Unexplained syncope remains one indication for formal electrophysiologic testing in the patient with congenital heart disease.

Formal evaluation and Holter or electrophysiologically guided therapy are required for patients with congenital heart disease and sustained or symptomatic VT. However, the overall incidence of sudden death remains low in these patients compared with the prevalence of asymptomatic, nonsustained ventricular arrhythmias. The utility of routine programmed stimulation or absolute PVC suppression in these patients remains controversial. On the basis of retrospective data analysis, pharmacologic treatment appears warranted in those patients with frequent (> 30/hr) or complex PVCs and abnormal postoperative hemodynamics.[1] Hemodynamic status should also be evaluated because correction of residual abnormalities may prevent arrhythmias.[42]

VENTRICULAR ARRHYTHMIAS ASSOCIATED WITH CARDIOMYOPATHIES

Concern has increased regarding the association between ventricular arrhythmias and sudden cardiac deaths in patients with primary disorders of the ventricular myocardium. Although the prevalence of primary myocardial diseases is much less than that of congenital heart defects among children and adolescents, ventricular arrhythmias in this context appear to be of greater prognostic significance. Thus, a high index of suspicion for subtle forms of these diseases is warranted in young patients with unexplained ventricular arrhythmias.

Hypertrophic Cardiomyopathy. Several studies have reported a significant risk of sudden death (2–6%/yr) in young patients with hypertrophic cardiomyopathy.[43–45] This has resulted in evaluation of both hemodynamic factors and cardiac arrhythmias as predictors of an increased risk of sudden death in such patients. A collaborative study of the Pediatric Electrophysiology Society evaluated these factors in 135 patients with a mean age of 8.8 years.[43] On Holter monitoring, 31% of patients had isolated PVCs, 14% had multiform PVCs or couplets, and 7% had VT. During a mean follow-up of 7 years, the incidence of sudden death was 13%. However, the presence of neither an arrhythmia nor hemodynamic variables was predictive of sudden death. The primary factor predictive of sudden death was a family history of hypertrophic cardiomyopathy, particularly if associated with sudden death.

McKenna et al[44] reported a series of 53 young patients with hypertrophic cardiomyopathy. Fifteen patients were classified as "high risk" on the basis of the presence of VT, syncope, or a family history of sudden death; these patients were treated with amiodarone (1.5–3 mg/kg/day) and experienced no subsequent adverse events. Conversely, of 37 "low-risk" patients, 5 died suddenly and 2 were resuscitated from ventricular fibrillation. None of these 7 patients had ventricular or sustained supraventricular arrhythmias recorded during a median of 3 days of Holter monitoring. This study differs from those of adults with hypertrophic cardiomyopathy, in which VT on a Holter monitor is a sensitive (69%) and specific (80%) marker for sudden cardiac death.

Later data have suggested that myocardial ischemia, rather than VT, may be the primary cause of sudden cardiac arrest in young patients with hypertrophic cardiomyopathy.[45] This may account for the apparent lack of correlation between ambient ventricular arrhythmias and sudden death in these patients. The long-term efficacy with anti-ischemic treatment in these patients has yet to be demonstrated. Further advances in understanding and stratifying the risk of sudden death in these patients may be provided by genetic linkage analysis.[46]

Dilated Cardiomyopathy. Several reports have evaluated the clinical course and prognostic factors for young patients with idiopathic dilated cardiomyopathies.[47–49] VT has been observed during Holter monitoring in 10 to 30% of these patients. However, a causal relationship between ventricular arrhythmias and sudden death has not been established. Congestive heart failure or pulmonary embolism has been reported as causes of death.[50] Additionally, the terminal cardiac rhythm may be bradycardia progressing to asystole rather than VT or fibrillation.[51]

Ventricular arrhythmias in patients with dilated cardiomyopathies appear to be a manifestation of advanced ventricular dysfunction and correlate with total rather than sudden cardiac mortality.[52] Responses to electrophysiologic testing in these patients have been nonspecific, with polymorphic nonsustained VT or VF the primary responses. Age greater than 2 years at presentation and persistent systolic dysfunction appear to be unfavorable prognostic factors.[48] Young patients with moderate (but not complete) improvement in systolic function in response to therapy have been reported to remain at risk for subsequent cardiac arrest.[49]

Arrhythmogenic Right Ventricular Dysplasia. Arrhythmogenic right ventricular dysplasia (ARVD) is a diagnosis to be considered when VT occurs in a previously healthy young patient. This entity is characterized by regional or diffuse contraction abnormalities of the right ventricle and a left bundle branch QRS morphology during tachycardia. ARVD may be the cause of VT in up to 33% of young patients with an ostensibly normal heart, including a normal echocardiogram. Furthermore, ARVD is one cause of unexplained sudden death during exertion.[53]

ARVD is characterized by VT originating in one of three areas of the right ventricle, in what has been termed the *triangle of dysplasia*.[54] The extent of myocardial involvement, in which the myocardium is replaced by fibrofatty tissue, is variable and may evolve over time. These localized abnormalities result in areas of right ventricular dyskinesis or aneurysm. Given the focal nature of the disease, angiography or magnetic resonance imaging is required to establish the diagnosis.[55]

Several ECG features have been reported as characteristic of ARVD. These include T-wave inversion in the anterior precordial leads during sinus rhythm, which may be normal in a pediatric patient, and postexcitation waves at the ST segment. Because tachycardia may originate from several areas of the right ventricle, multiple left bundle branch QRS morphologies may be present during tachycardia (Fig. 8–8).

Exercise-induced tachycardia in ARVD may be difficult to differentiate from "idiopathic right ventricular outflow tract tachycardia." Multiple morphologies of tachycardia, ECG changes during sinus rhythm, and right ventricular enlargement favor the diagnosis of ARVD.[54] Efforts at a correct diagnosis are essential because the prognosis of ARVD is more ominous than that of idiopathic right ventricular outflow tract tachycardia.

A variable long-term prognosis has been reported for patients with ARVD. Initial therapy is pharmacologic with some form of beta blockade, although sotalol may be superior to other pharmacologic modalities.[56] The prognosis may be favorable for patients with tachycardia suppression on medical therapy. Catheter ablation, surgical isolation of the right ventricular free wall, and

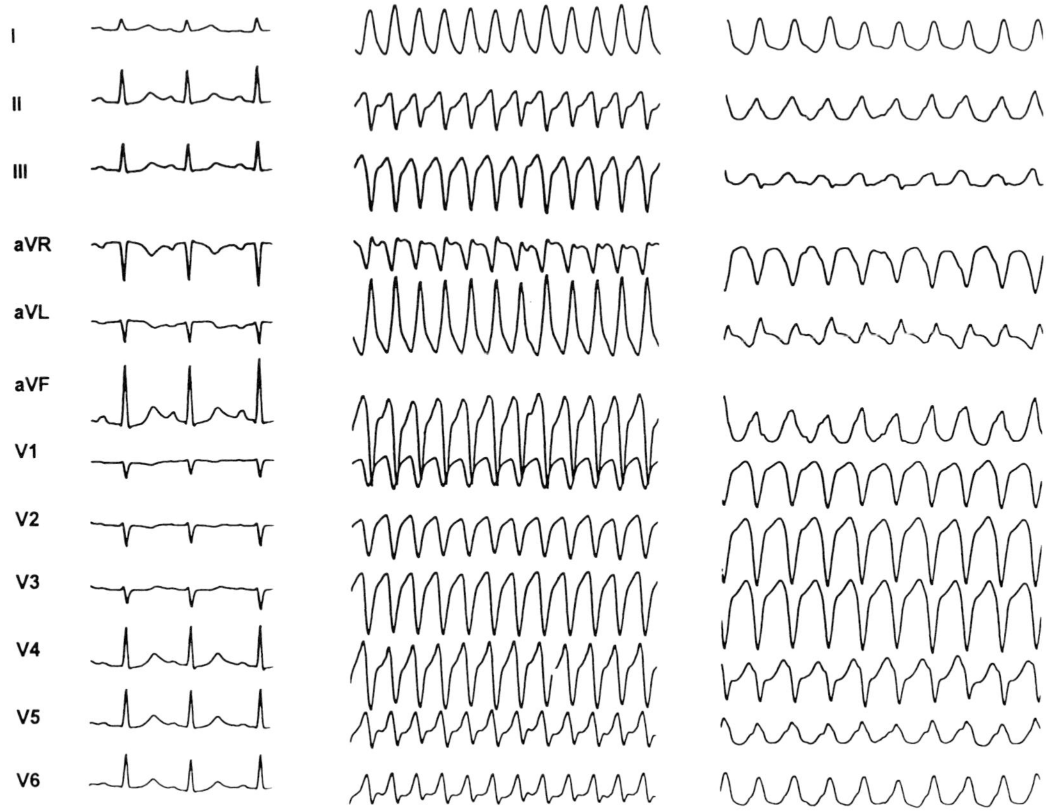

FIGURE 8–8. Multiple QRS morphologies during ventricular tachycardia. The electrocardiograms were recorded from a patient with arrhythmogenic right ventricular dysplasia. The left panel demonstrates three sinus beats for reference. In the middle panel, ventricular tachycardia with a left bundle branch pattern and superior-directed QRS axis with a cycle length of 230 ms is demonstrated. The right panel also demonstrates ventricular tachycardia with a left bundle branch pattern, but with an inferior directed QRS axis and cycle length of 270 ms.

implantable cardioverter defibrillators have been used in a small number of patients with drug refractory or intolerant states.[57, 58]

Ventricular Tachycardia Associated With Myocardial Tumors. Cardiac tumors are an important cause of VT, particularly in infants. The histology of the tumor appears to be the primary determinant of the prognosis and treatment course.

VT may be the initial presentation of rhabdomyomas in 5 to 10% of infants with tuberous sclerosis. In general, VT is well tolerated in these infants and resolves within the first week of life.[59] The primary risk of VT occurs when a large rhabdomyoma obstructs an AV valve orifice. This may result in profound hemodynamic compromise during tachycardia.

Myocardial hamartomas are an important cause of incessant (present > 10% of the time) VT in infants. Hamartomas are usually epicardial and thus not amenable to diagnosis by echocardiography or angiography. It is imperative that the diagnosis of VT be established in these infants, because therapy with digoxin for presumed supraventricular tachycardia may result in ventricular fibrillation. The cycle length of tachycardia may be very short and should not be used as a criterion for a diagnosis of supraventricular tachycardia. In 1984, Garson and Gillette reported surgical treatment of VT in these infants.[60] When discrete and epicardial, these hamartomas are amenable to surgical removal without cardiopulmonary bypass (Fig. 8–9). However, these tumors may also be endocardial and multifocal, presenting a significant surgical risk. Pharmacologic therapy has also been reported as an effective form of treatment for this type of VT during the first year of life.[61] It appears that some hamartomas may undergo involution, similar to rhabdomyomas.

Histiocytic or oncocytic tumors represent a diffuse, infiltrative cardiomyopathy associated with VT. This rare syndrome presents between 6

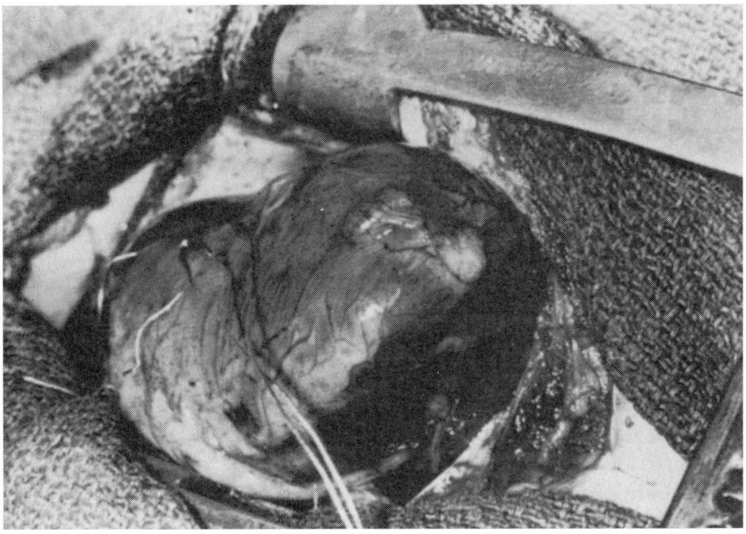

FIGURE 8–9. Epicardial ventricular tumor in a newborn with ventricular tachycardia. The pale area near the cardiac apex was the site of earliest ventricular activation during tachycardia. Resection of this 8-mm tumor resulted in cure of tachycardia. Histology of this tumor identified a Purkinje cell hamartoma.

and 24 months of age and is another cause of incessant VT in infants.[62] Pathologically, this disease is characterized by myocyte degeneration into large, foamy cells resembling histiocytes. This degenerative process may also affect the conduction system. Sudden cardiac arrest may be the initial presentation of this disease process.

VENTRICULAR ARRHYTHMIAS IN THE ABSENCE OF STRUCTURAL CARDIOVASCULAR DISEASE

There has been increased recognition of the occurrence of ventricular arrhythmias in the absence of identifiable heart disease. Both the causes of and optimal treatment for these arrhythmias remain a concern because of the unpredictable clinical course and potentially poor prognosis. With exception of the long QT syndrome, this is a diagnosis of exclusion established only after thorough investigation has failed to identify any anatomic or functional evidence of cardiovascular disease.

Congenital Prolonged QT Syndromes. The prolonged QT syndromes are an established cause of ventricular arrhythmias, exercise- or stress-related syncope, and sudden cardiac arrest in young patients. Thus, evaluation of the corrected QT interval (QTc) is an important consideration in the evaluation of the young patient with a ventricular arrhythmia or syncope. The relationship between QT interval and heart rate was described in 1920 by Bazett[63] as

Corrected QT = measured QT/square root of the preceding RR interval

Although this concept is simple, precise measurement of the QT may be difficult for a number of reasons: (1) prominent U waves are common in children; (2) QT interval is not the same in all leads; and (3) sinus arrhythmia may result in variable QTc measurements in the same patient. In general, calculation of the QTc is determined from lead II, with inclusion of the U wave if it is greater than 50% of the T wave amplitude. The prolonged QT syndrome may be suspect in any child with a QTc greater than 0.44 second; however, this needs to be evaluated in context of additional criteria.

Torsades de pointes ("twisting of the peaks") refers to the polymorphic VT characteristic of the long QT syndromes. Described by Desertenne in 1966, the QRS morphology during tachycardia gradually changes from one morphology to another.[64] The onset of tachycardia characteristically occurs with a PVC in late diastole; although most episodes of torsades de pointes terminate spontaneously, degeneration to VF may occur.

Hereditary syndromes of QT prolongation associated with polymorphic ventricular arrhythmias and sudden death were described by Jervell and Lange-Nielsen (associated with congenital deafness) in 1957 and by Romano and Ward (autosomal dominant without deafness) in 1963 and 1964 in separate reports. Genetic linkage analysis has identified several potential subtypes of this syndrome, possibly associated with different defects in ion channels, with heterogeneous ECG features as an expression of the different basic defects.[65]

Criteria for the diagnosis of prolonged QT syndrome were updated in 1993, as the diverse clinical features of this syndrome became apparent (Table 8–2).[66] ECG findings were graded on the basis of the degree of corrected QT prolongation, the presence of torsades de pointes, T-wave alternans, and a low heart rate for age (Fig. 8–10). Clinical criteria included unexplained syncope with or without stress, a family history of the long QT syndrome, and unexplained sudden death at an age younger than 30 years in the immediate family.

The significant prognostic factors, clinical course, and treatment strategies for young patients with the long QT syndrome were the subject of a 1993 collaborative study of the Pediatric Electrophysiology Society.[67] Several differences between children and adults with prolonged QT syndromes were identified:

1. In 9% of 287 children, cardiac arrest was the presenting symptom; this is in contrast to adults, in whom recurrent syncope usually precedes sudden cardiac arrest.
2. Twenty percent of patients had bradycardia; 2:1 AV block was observed in 5% (only 2 patients had complete AV block); sinus bradycardia was present in 15%.
3. The risk of sudden death was related to QTc prolongation, with the highest risk in patients with QTc greater than 0.55 second.

Table 8–2. Updated Criteria for Diagnosis of Prolonged QT Syndromes

VARIABLE	POINTS
ECG Findings	
QTc	
> 480 ms	3.0
460–470 ms	2.0
450 ms (males)	1.0
Torsades de pointes	2.0
T-wave alternans	1.0
Notched T wave in three leads	1.0
Low heart rate for age	0.5
Clinical History	
Syncope	
with stress	2.0
without stress	1.0
Congenital deafness	0.5
Family History	
Family members with definite long QT	1.0
Unexplained sudden cardiac death at age < 30 years among immediate family members	0.5

Scoring: ≤ 1 point, low probability of long QTS; 2–3 points, intermediate probability of long QTS; ≥ 4 points, high probability of long QT.

Modified from Schwartz PJ, et al: Diagnostic criteria for the long QT syndrome: An update. Circulation 88:782, 1993.

Treatments with propranolol compared with other forms of beta blockade were equally effective, with elimination of symptoms in 76% and ventricular arrhythmias in 60% of patients. One uncontrolled study suggested that a cardioselective beta blocker was less effective than propranolol. Pacemaker therapy, left cervicothoracic sympathectomy, and implantable cardioverter-defibrillators have been reported to be effective in small numbers of pediatric patients in whom beta-blockade therapy was not effective.[68, 69]

Two hypotheses have been proposed regarding the mechanism of QT prolongation and torsades de pointes in these patients: sympathetic imbalance, resulting in regional dispersion of refractoriness of the ventricular myocardium as advocated by Schwartz,[70] and an intrinsic abnormality in sodium or potassium ion channel function that predisposes to repolarization abnormalities, early afterdepolarizations, and triggered activity, as advocated by others.[65] It appears that many molecular or genetic defects will be demonstrated to account for the various forms of the long QT syndrome. As advances in molecular biology provide further insight into the fundamental defects, specific therapies may be defined for variant forms of the long QT syndrome.

An acquired prolonged QT syndrome, secondary either to medication or metabolic disturbance, must be also be considered in the patient with torsades de pointes. This syndrome was initially recognized in patients with recurrent syncope after initiation of treatment with quinidine,[71] but has now been extended to include multiple antiarrhythmic drugs such as procainamide and amiodarone. Drug-induced QT prolongation has been further extended to include tricyclic antidepressants, phenothiazine, terfenadine, and erythromycin.[72] Other factors that have been associated with QT prolongation include central nervous system trauma, hypokalemia, and myocardial ischemia. Although experience is limited, the primary treatment for these arrhythmias is correction of the underlying disorder and either overdrive pacing or an isoproterenol infusion; both measures reduce the dispersion of myocardial refractoriness. Prophylactic long-term therapy after the QT has returned to normal does not appear to be required.

POLYMORPHIC VT OR VF IN THE ABSENCE OF QT PROLONGATION OR STRUCTURAL HEART DISEASE

In approximately 5 to 10% of patients resuscitated from sudden cardiac arrest, a specific cause will not be defined despite an extensive evalua-

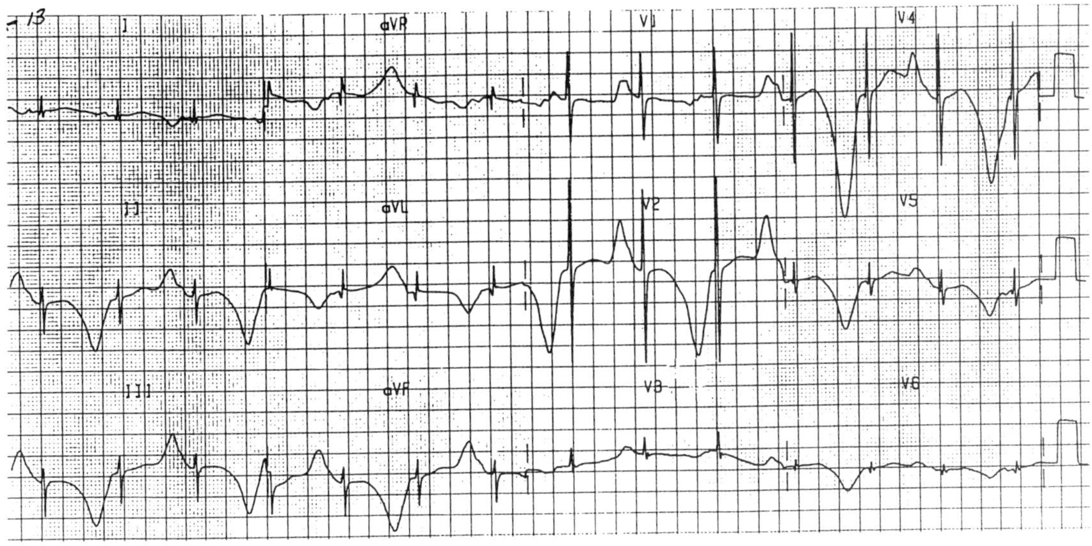

FIGURE 8–10. Electrocardiographic features of the long QT syndrome. The corrected QT interval in this 12-lead electrocardiogram is 0.76 s. Secondary features of the long QT are also present, including sinus bradycardia and T-wave alternans. This 2-year-old infant had repeated episodes of torsades de pointes during febrile illnesses.

tion. These patients have been identified as having idiopathic or primary VF.[73] Because the capability to fibrillate is inherent to the ventricular myocardium, some investigators have argued that idiopathic VF may represent an "electrical accident" occurring in a normal heart.[74] This accidental stimulus may be either a physical stimulus (commotio cordis) or a critically timed PVC.[75] Conversely, others have proposed that abnormalities such as catecholamine hypersensitivity and occult focal myocarditis may be causes of VF in the absence of overt heart disease. In the absence of a defined cause of VF, empiric therapies have ranged from beta blockade to implantable cardioverter-defibrillators. Preliminary reports from the European Unexplained Cardiac Arrest (EUCARE) Registry have suggested an annual recurrence risk of 5%/year.[76]

A syndrome of polymorphic VT in the absence of QTc prolongation or identifiable myocardial ischemia has also been reported in young patients.[77] It is debated whether these patients should be considered as having a variant form of the prolonged QT syndrome. A report of 21 patients (9.9 ± 4 years of age) has detailed the clinical aspects of catecholaminergic polymorphic VT in children. In general, these patients were recognized after referral for exercise- or emotion-related syncope and found to have either polymorphic or bidirectional VT induced by various forms of adrenergic stimulation. A family history of syncope or sudden death was identified in 30% of the patients. Therapy with beta blockade appeared to be effective in preventing further episodes; however, 2 patients died suddenly and 3 experienced recurrent syncope attributed to noncompliance with medical therapy.

REPETITIVE MONOMORPHIC VT IN THE NORMAL HEART

Although most sustained ventricular arrhythmias in young patients are a manifestation of cardiovascular disease, two distinct forms of monomorphic VT have been recognized to occur in the absence of identifiable heart disease. Both of these arrhythmias may terminate with either adenosine or verapamil, which may suggest an incorrect diagnosis of supraventricular tachycardia with aberrancy.[78]

The most common form of VT in the normal heart originates from the right ventricular outflow tract and demonstrates left bundle branch aberrancy with an inferior QRS axis (Fig. 8–11). Episodes of tachycardia may be nonsustained and repetitive and have a constant QRS morphology. In general, this tachycardia has a relatively long cycle length and is tolerated hemodynamically. In contrast to other forms of VT, idiopathic right ventricular outflow tract tachycardia is usually not inducible with programmed extrastimulation; however, exercise or adrenergic stimulation are common clinical and laboratory methods for tachycardia initiation.

In most cases, this arrhythmia has a benign

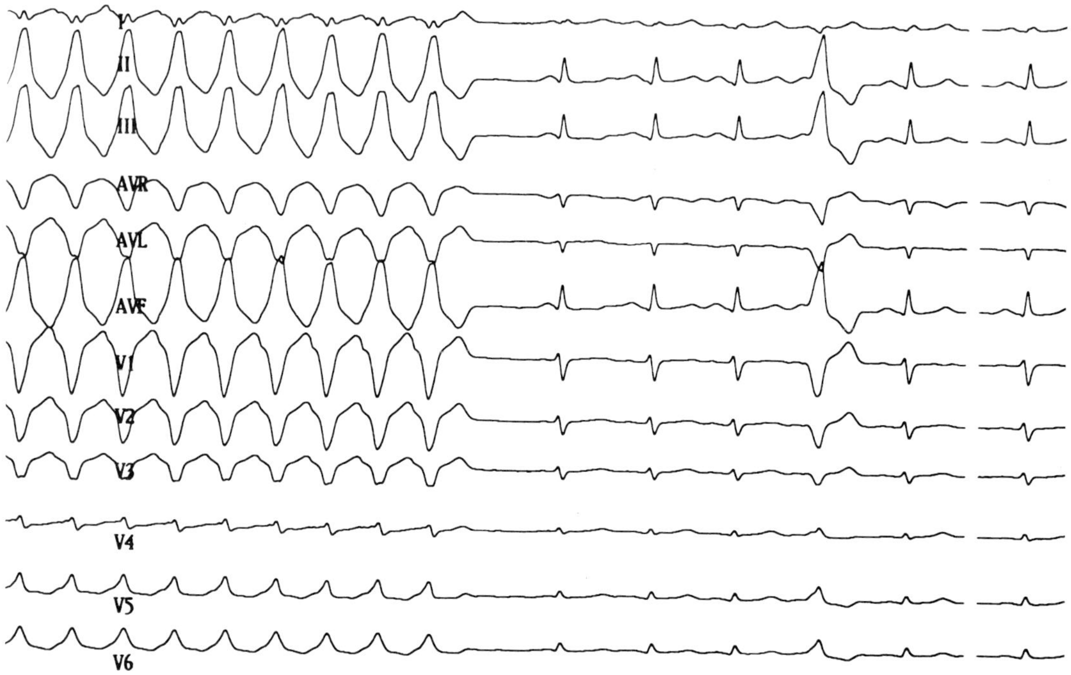

FIGURE 8–11. Idiopathic right ventricular outflow tract tachycardia. The electrocardiographic characteristics of this arrhythmia include an inferior-directed QRS axis, left bundle branch QRS morphology, and recurrent spontaneous onset and termination of tachycardia. Intracardiac mapping identified the earliest activation at the anterolateral aspect of the right ventricular outflow tract immediately beneath the pulmonary valve annulus.

prognosis in the young patient.[79] Differentiation from subtle forms of arrhythmogenic right ventricular dysplasia may be difficult and thus requires caution in evaluation. Although the cycle length of tachycardia is relatively long in most cases, it may shorten with marked exertion, resulting in secondary compromise of cardiac output.

Although the precise anatomic and histologic bases for right ventricular outflow tract tachycardia have not been defined, it appears to arise from a discrete focus in the infundibulum. Because this arrhythmia appears to be adrenergically mediated or dependent, treatment with beta blockade may be effective in reducing, if not completely suppressing, episodes of tachycardia. Conversely, given the focal anatomic basis, this arrhythmia may be treated with radiofrequency catheter ablation, with short-term follow-up suggesting treatment efficacy.[80] Whether this is a benign treatment without late or long-term sequelae in the young patient remains to be determined.[81]

A second form of recurrent sustained monomorphic VT in young patients without heart disease demonstrates a right bundle branch morphology and left axis deviation (Fig. 8–12). This arrhythmia has been termed Belhassen tachycardia and frequently is misdiagnosed as supraventricular tachycardia with aberrancy.[82] Catheter evaluation of this arrhythmia may identify a discrete mid-diastolic potential at the midseptal aspect of the left ventricle.[83] The application of radiofrequency energy at this site may result in an effective cure for this arrhythmia.

NONINVASIVE EVALUATION OF VENTRICULAR ARRHYTHMIAS

The prognostic significance of most ventricular arrhythmias in young patients is determined by the presence of associated cardiovascular disease. Thus, identification of any abnormality that may be implicated as an acute or chronic cause of the ventricular arrhythmia is essential. The history should be reviewed for use of sympathomimetic agents, previous cardiac symptoms, or possible basis for an electrolyte disorder. A history of palpitations should be reviewed, although this finding is nonspecific. Any prior near-syncopal or syncopal events should be reviewed in detail. Family history is equally important. The physical exam may demonstrate subtle features of unrec-

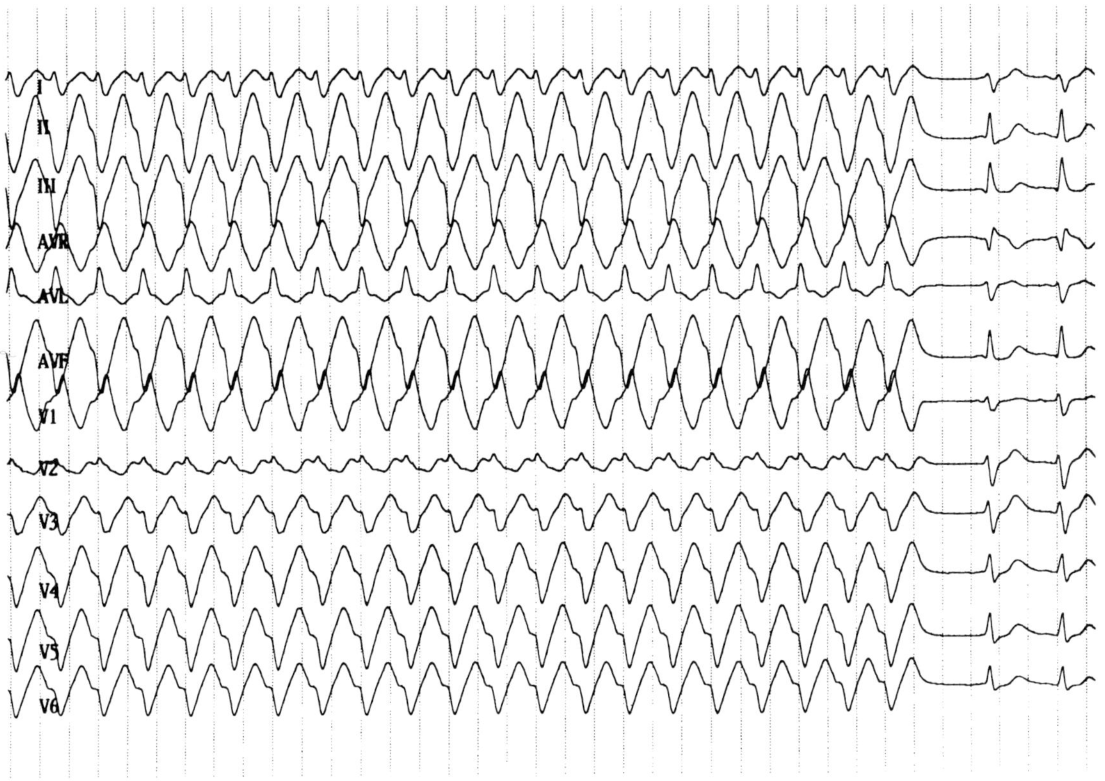

FIGURE 8–12. Left ventricular septal, or "fascicular," tachycardia. This electrocardiogram of this tachycardia demonstrates right bundle branch block and left axis deviation. Termination of the arrhythmia in response to adenosine resulted in a presumptive diagnosis of supraventricular tachycardia with aberrancy. However, there was atrioventricular dissociation during tachycardia at electrophysiology testing and tachycardia was inducible only with left ventricular stimulation.

ognized cardiac disease, such as mitral valve prolapse or an early systolic murmur of hypertrophic cardiomyopathy.

The two-dimensional echocardiogram is essential, for both identification of unrecognized structural cardiovascular disease as well as evaluation of ventricular function. It is also important to recognize the limitations of echocardiography in the identification of cardiovascular diseases associated with ventricular arrhythmias such as right ventricular dysplasia, focal epicardial tumors in infants, and myocarditis.

As previously discussed, precise measurement of the QT interval on the electrocardiogram is an important consideration in the evaluation of any child with ventricular arrhythmias. The ECG should also be evaluated for any form of conduction system disease, which may be a manifestation of organic heart disease, and ST-repolarization abnormalities suggestive of ischemia.[84]

Exercise or treadmill testing may provide further insights beyond the resting ECG. In most children with a normal heart, PVCs are suppressed by sinus tachycardia during exercise and recur in the immediate postexercise period. The purpose of the exercise test is to demonstrate that VT does not develop during exercise, as may occur in arrhythmogenic right ventricular dysplasia or idiopathic right ventricular outflow tract tachycardia. In children with known structural heart disease, there is no characteristic response to exercise: the arrhythmia may not change, worsen, or improve in response to exertion. Sudden death has been reported in patients with prior repair of tetralogy of Fallot who demonstrated complete PVC suppression during exercise.[85] Thus, in patients with an abnormal heart, the exercise test is used to screen for the provocation of PVCs and tachycardia.

The exercise test may also be used in evaluation of the patient with borderline prolongation of the QT syndrome and symptoms or a positive family history. The normal response is for the QT interval to shorten proportionally with increased heart rate. Patients with a borderline prolonged QTc may demonstrate unequivocal QTc prolongation with increased heart rates (Fig. 8–13).[86] Because of the difficulty in exact measurement

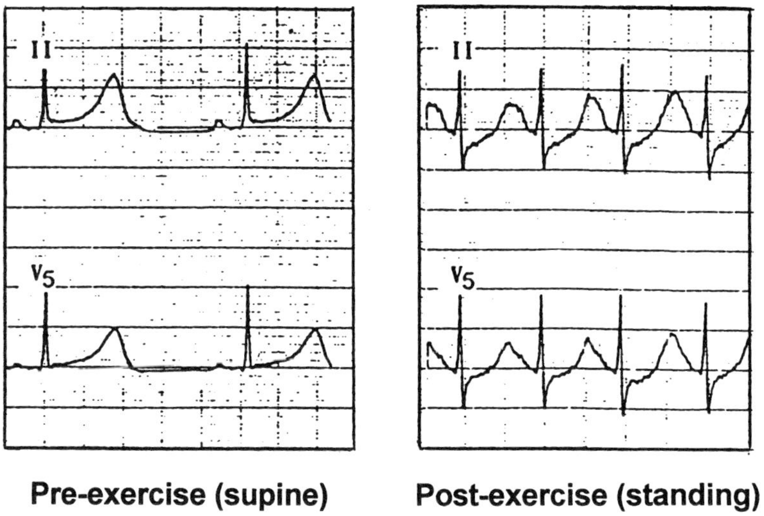

FIGURE 8–13. Exercise testing to establish the diagnosis of prolonged QT. The left panel demonstrates resting rhythm with a corrected QT of 0.45 s. However, the right panel, recorded immediately after exercise, demonstrates a corrected QT of 0.56 s.

of the QT interval during exercise as a result of motion, Schwartz recommended measurement of the QTc at 1 minute after exercise.

Twenty-four-hour continuous ambulatory ECG (Holter) monitoring is an essential aspect of the evaluation of the child with ventricular ectopy. Quantitative assessment of PVC frequency is most commonly described with the Lown criteria, which were developed initially to assess the significance of PVCs after myocardial infarction (Table 8–3).[87] Because the Lown criteria were based on adult patients, they require modification for younger patients with higher heart rates. Because the heart rate of a young child is approximately twice that of an adult, it may be reasonable that 60 PVCs per hour (or 1 per minute) may be frequent in children. Also the high Lown grades for ventricular couplets or bigeminy in the absence of organic heart disease do not appear consistent with the relatively good prognosis that has been established in young patients.[88]

Table 8–3. Lown Criteria for Classification of Premature Ventricular Contractions (PVCs)

GRADE	COMPLEXITY OF PVCs
0	No PVCs
1	< 30 PVCs/hr
1A	< 1 PVC/min
1B	> 1 PVC/min
2	> 1 PVC/min and > 30 PVCs/hr
3	Multiform PVCs
4	Repetitive PVCs
4A	Couplets
4B	Salvos or ventricular tachycardia
5	Early PVCs (R on T phenomenon)

Another use of Holter monitoring is to assess the efficacy of antiarrhythmic drug therapy, based on a comparison of ventricular ectopy before and after treatment. Because of considerable day-to-day variability in the amount of ventricular ectopy, two consecutive 24-hour recordings may be required for an accurate estimation of the basal state before initiation of antiarrhythmic therapy.

INTRACARDIAC EVALUATION OF VENTRICULAR ARRHYTHMIAS

Catheter-based evaluation for young patients with ventricular arrhythmias is generally reserved for those with a sustained tachyarrhythmia or a symptom such as syncope in the context of a probable ventricular arrhythmia. Although primarily used for electrophysiologic evaluation, invasive evaluation may also include endomyocardial biopsy to rule out myocarditis and angiography to evaluate ventricular anatomy. The role of electrophysiology testing in evaluation of the young patient with a ventricular arrhythmia continues to be refined as new insights into arrhythmia mechanisms and treatment modalities become available. The principal goals of electrophysiology study in the evaluation of VT are (1) confirm the diagnosis; (2) evaluate the mechanism of the arrhythmia; (3) map the location of the origin of tachycardia; and (4) select and evaluate the therapy: drug, device, or catheter ablation.

The techniques of programmed ventricular stimulation were developed for the evaluation of VT in adults with chronic ischemic heart disease.[89] Many of these patients had prior infarction or aneurysm formation, which provides an anatomic substrate for recurrent sustained monomorphic VT. This finding differs from young patients with VT or sudden cardiac arrest, who are a heterogeneous group with a spectrum of cardiovascular diseases discussed earlier in this chapter. Sustained monomorphic VT in this group may be evaluated by electrophysiology testing. The role and results of programmed stimulation in patients with polymorphic or nonsustained VT or VF remain controversial.[89, 90]

Electrophysiologic Diagnosis of VT. The intracardiac definition of VT is a tachycardia in which a His bundle electrogram does not precede the onset of ventricular depolarization. The His bundle electrogram is dissociated from or may follow the ventricular electrogram, similar to ECG criteria for the diagnosis of VT based on dissociation of P waves from the QRS complexes (Fig. 8–14). This approach assumes that a stable His bundle electrogram was present before the onset of tachycardia and reappears with the return of sinus rhythm. One exception to this rule may occur in "fascicular tachycardia," which originates from a proximal bundle branch and activates the His bundle before or coincident with the QRS.

VT may be differentiated from a wide QRS tachycardia because of antegrade conduction over an accessory AV connection by the following:

1. If AV dissociation is present, the diagnosis is VT.

2. If the tachycardia morphology can be reproduced with atrial pacing with gradual loss of the His bundle at shorter atrial cycle lengths, the diagnosis is pre-excitation.

Electrophysiologic Mechanisms of VT. Laboratory studies have demonstrated that electrophysiologic mechanisms for VT in children include re-entry, abnormal automaticity, and triggered activity. *Abnormal automaticity,* perhaps the most common mechanism of idiopathic right ventricular outflow tachycardia, may be inferred from two criteria.[91] First is the phenomenon of "warm-up," which is spontaneous initiation of the tachycardia with progressive shortening of the cycle lengths. Second is the inability to initiate or terminate the rhythm with programmed stimulation. One limitation of this criterion is that if tachycardia cannot be initiated or terminated by programmed stimulation, it could be due to any mechanism.

Triggered activity has received increased attention as a potential mechanism for arrhythmias in patients with prolonged QT syndromes and possibly for postoperative tetralogy of Fallot patients.[30, 92] Although debate continues regarding the clinical significance of these arrhythmias, the following criteria have been proposed:

1. Tachycardia is inducible with pacing over a narrow range of cycle lengths, with the cycle length of tachycardia similar to that of the paced interval.

2. The interval from the last paced to the first spontaneous interval is shorter at more rapid cycle lengths.

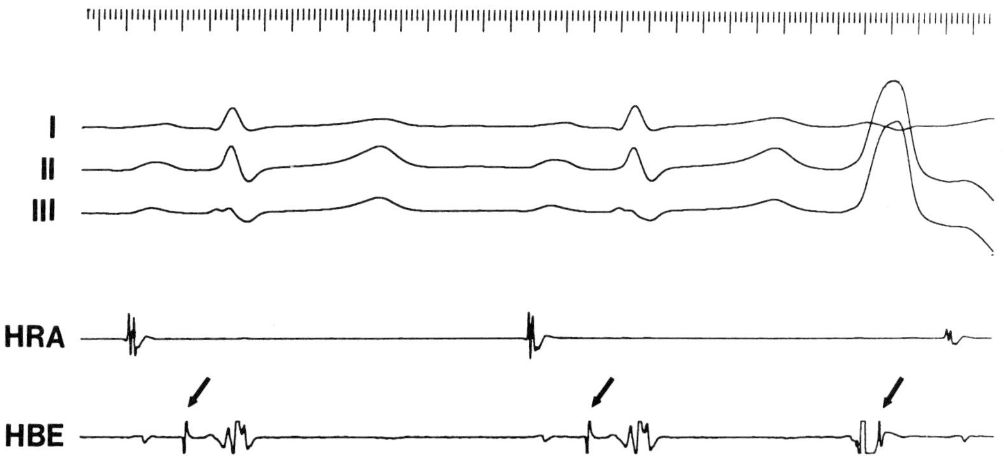

FIGURE 8–14. Electrophysiologic criteria for a premature ventricular depolarization. The first two beats are sinus, with a normal atrial-His-ventricle (A-H-V) sequence of activation. The third beat is premature, with the ventricular electrogram preceding the His, confirming the ventricular origin of this beat. (HRA, high right atrium; HBE, His bundle electrogram.)

3. There are decreasing cycle lengths (warm-up) at the onset of tachycardia.

Re-entry appears to be the mechanism of monomorphic VT in most patients with structural or congenital heart disease, ischemic heart disease, or arrhythmogenic right ventricular dysplasia. The fundamental criterion for re-entry is the reproducible initiation and termination of sustained tachycardia with programmed stimulation (Fig. 8–15). The re-entrant circuit may be due to an anatomic obstacle, such as a scar at a ventriculotomy incision, or may be functional as a result of anisotropic conduction in diseased segments of the ventricular myocardium. The use of pacing at cycle lengths slightly shorter than the tachycardia to demonstrate entrainment also supports re-entry.[29]

Insight into the mechanism of tachycardia may be defined by interventions for termination of the arrhythmia. If tachycardia terminates in response to rapid pacing, it is likely the result of re-entry or triggered activity. In most circumstances, the ventricle is paced at rates 10 to 20 beats faster than the rate of tachycardia, with shortening of the cycle length until tachycardia stops or inconsistent capture occurs. Synchronized DC cardioversion (0.5–2.0 J/kg) may be used both diagnostically and therapeutically. Cardioversion should be performed if the patient becomes symptomatic or tachycardia is not terminated by other methods. The response to cardioversion may not be diagnostic, because both re-entry and triggered activity may respond. If not successful, VT may still be caused by re-entry or triggered activity with "concealed perpetuation" (i.e., tachycardia continues even though the majority of the heart is depolarized).

Mapping the Sequence of Ventricular Activation. After initiation of tachycardia, the catheters may be positioned at multiple sites within the right and left ventricles. The purpose is to identify the earliest local ventricular activation in relation to the QRS complex, which correlates with the endocardial breakthrough point of the tachycardia.[32] Catheter mapping may also identify an area of continuous electrical activity, which may represent slow conduction and corre-

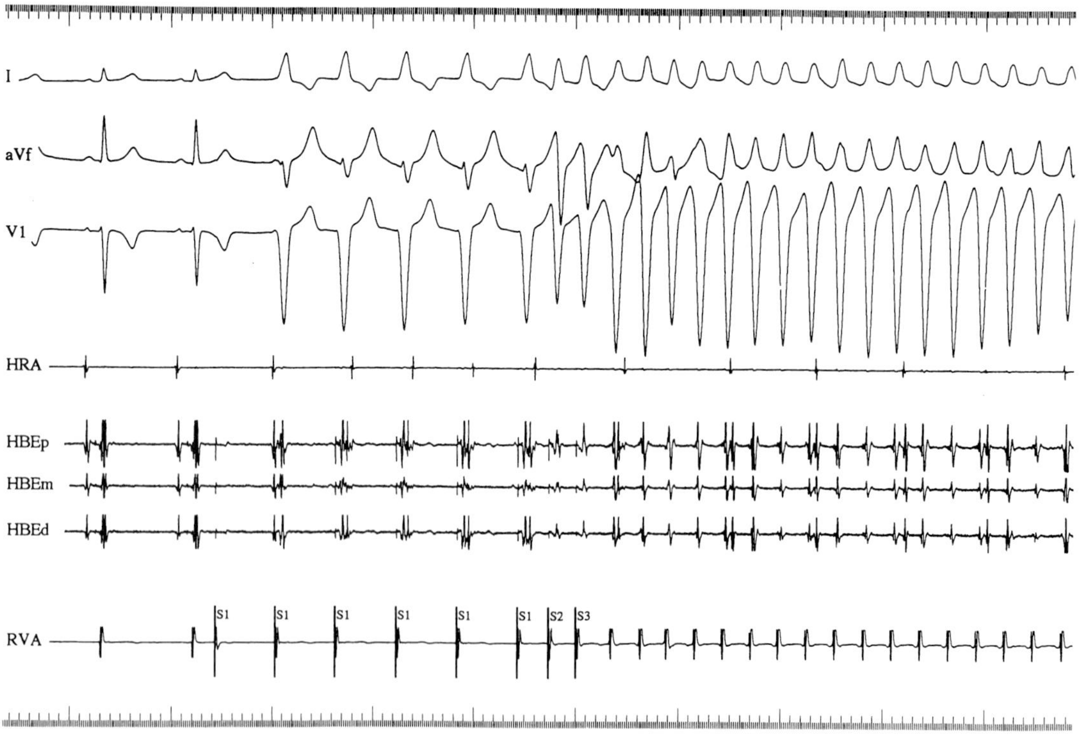

FIGURE 8–15. Induction of sustained ventricular tachycardia. A series of six ventricular stimuli at a cycle length of 600 ms (S_1) are followed by two premature stimuli at coupling intervals of 300 (S_2) and 280 (S_3) ms. Sustained monomorphic ventricular tachycardia at a cycle length of 290 ms was induced. The diagnosis of ventricular tachycardia is confirmed by atrioventricular dissociation, based on comparison of the QRS complexes and atrial electrograms on the high right atrial (HRA) and His bundle (HBE) recordings. (RVA = right ventricular apex.)

late with the site of onset of VT. The significance of slow conduction as related to the origin of VT requires confirmation by either catheter or surgical ablation.[93] With the development of radiofrequency catheter ablation, endocardial mapping has assumed greater importance in evaluation of the patient with sustained monomorphic VT. Catheter mapping may be guided by the surface ECG, which may suggest an apical or basal focus of tachycardia as well as either a right or left ventricular focus. Septal sites of VT may be ambiguous as regards the ventricle of origin.

Electrophysiology Testing in Selection of Therapy for VT. Programmed electrical stimulation is primarily indicated for patients with either sustained tachycardia or symptoms suggestive of circulatory collapse. In these patients, it is imperative to select the therapy most likely to prevent or terminate future recurrences of the arrhythmia. In general, these therapies are pharmacologic, ablative (either surgical or catheter), or device activated (implantable cardioverter-defibrillator).

For the patient with sustained monomorphic VT, the objective is to prevent recurrences of tachycardia. Electrophysiology testing may be used to assess the inducibility of tachycardia before and after drug infusion and to determine whether an antiarrhythmic drug renders tachycardia noninducible.[94] Conversely, ambulatory monitoring may be used to assess frequency of complex ventricular ectopy before and after antiarrhythmic treatment. Both techniques have limitations, which need to be considered in the patient with a potentially lethal condition.

Surgical or catheter ablation may offer a definitive cure for select patients with a discrete focus of VT, such as infantile Purkinje cell hamartomas or VT in the older child with a structurally normal heart. One other role of surgery may be an improvement in hemodynamic condition as a means to prevent recurrent tachycardia, as in patients with severe right ventricular enlargement caused by pulmonary insufficiency after repair of tetralogy of Fallot.[42] Hemodynamic improvement may not equate with arrhythmia-free status.

There appears to be a minimal role for electrophysiology testing in patients with polymorphic VTs, such as associated with the prolonged QT syndromes.[95, 96] Similar caution in use and interpretation of programmed electrical stimulation is also required in patients with unexplained ventricular fibrillation.[89, 90]

LIMITATIONS, TECHNIQUES, AND SENSITIVITY AND SPECIFICITY OF ELECTROPHYSIOLOGY TESTING

Sustained and nonsustained monomorphic VTs are evaluated by programmed ventricular stimulation to confirm the diagnosis, to provide information regarding the mechanism of the arrhythmia, and to assess responses to therapies. A number of protocols for programmed stimulation have been devised, with various degrees of sensitivity and specificity. In general, more aggressive protocols (three or four extrastimuli) have a higher yield of tachycardia induction[89, 90] and are indicated in patients with documented sustained tachycardia. Such protocols also have a high incidence of false-positive or nonspecific responses, such as nonsustained polymorphic VT or VF in the patient with documented monomorphic tachycardia. Thus, selection of the stimulation protocol needs to be based on the clinical arrhythmia.

The use of programmed ventricular stimulation for patients without clinically documented monomorphic VT is controversial and the cause of considerable confusion regarding patient care. Several studies have evaluated inducibilty of VT in patients with tetralogy of Fallot who were without symptoms or clinically documented arrhythmias.[1, 26] Ewing et al[97] reported that, after undergoing repair for tetralogy of Fallot, 8% of patients have inducible ventricular arrhythmias.

Programmed electrical stimulation for patients with polymorphic VT has not been demonstrated to be of clinical utility or validity. This is due to both the lack of specificity of this response as well as the low sensitivity of this testing for induction of this arrhythmia. In general, the more disorganized the arrhythmia induced (e.g., polymorphic VT or VF) and the more aggressive the stimulation protocol (e.g., four extrastimuli), the less specific is the response. In the patient resuscitated from VF, the purpose of electrophysiology testing is to exclude the presence of a treatable arrhythmia or other reversible organic heart disease.

Programmed ventricular stimulation may be indicated in the evaluation of patients with syncope and organic heart disease. The evaluation should include both sinus and AV node function as well as consideration of supraventricular arrhythmias. Benson et al[41] reported a high incidence of inducible sustained ventricular arrhythmias in young patients with syncope and complex ventricular ectopy on Holter monitoring.

VENTRICULAR ARRHYTHMIAS IN YOUNG PATIENTS: TREATMENT SELECTION AND END POINTS

The objectives and treatment methods for ventricular arrhythmias in young patients continue to evolve on the basis of both ongoing clinical trials and progress in medical technology. Specific aspects of these therapies are considered in detail in several chapters in this book. In general, the primary goals in treating ventricular arrhythmias are to prevent or reduce the risk of sudden cardiac death and eliminate symptoms associated with cardiovascular compromise. Treatment objectives and end points need to graded on the basis of clinical presentation in the context of several different categories of risk, as discussed earlier in this chapter.

Most ominous is the patient resuscitated from a malignant ventricular arrhythmia. Several clinical studies of implantable cardioverter-defibrillators in young patients have reported a 35 to 50% recurrence rate of the malignant arrhythmia during a mean follow-up of 2 years.[98, 99] Given this high risk, these patients require "definitive" therapy. This may include hemodynamic improvement with surgery, pharmacologic therapy, implantable device, or some combination thereof. A primary objective of electrophysiologic evaluation in the next decade is the prospective identification of patients at highest risk for sudden death before their index event.

A second category of risk stratification is represented by patients with either cardiovascular disease and nonsustained tachycardia or VT in the absence of identifiable heart disease. Treatment end points are primarily suppression of ambient or inducible complex ectopy and definitive treatment of the arrhythmia if reasonable. Selection of therapy is an important issue in these patients because treatment may have an inherent risk, such as proarrhythmia or depression of ventricular function associated with antiarrhythmic drug use.[100] The decision and method of treatment are based on an estimation of the potential risk of a life-threatening arrhythmia.

Young patients with hypertrophic cardiomyopathy or long QT syndrome are at a clearly defined high risk of sudden arrhythmic death. Prophylactic antiarrhythmic treatment with the possible addition of permanent cardiac pacing are reasonable "preventive" and potentially beneficial measures in this setting. Conversely, patients who have undergone surgery for congenital heart disease are an extremely heterogeneous group and, overall, appear to have a lower individual risk of sudden death. Selection criteria for patients' treatment and method, and end point of treatment continue to be studied and redefined. Current evidence supports prophylactic antiarrhythmic drug treatment in patients with postoperative ventricular dysfunction and complex or inducible ventricular ectopy. Antiarrhythmic drugs with a low potential for depression of ventricular function such as phenytoin (Dilantin) or mexiletine generally have been recommended as initial therapies. Alternatively, surgical therapy for residual volume or pressure overload may correct the ventricular distention or remodeling, which may be a cause of the arrhythmia.

The treatment of sustained or nonsustained VT in the absence of associated cardiovascular disease has been revised with the development of radiofrequency catheter ablation. Because most of these arrhythmias appear to be due to discrete foci of cells, catheter ablation may provide a means for definitive cure. Alternatively, pharmacologic therapy with beta blockade may provide effective arrhythmia prophylaxis for these arrhythmias.

The decision regarding treatment or observation for patients with "benign" ventricular arrhythmias requires caution, but is defensible after a careful evaluation. In general, patients with isolated PVCs, bigeminy, and couplets may be followed up by sequential ambulatory monitoring in the absence of associated cardiovascular disease and clinical symptoms. In the future, newer methods of risk stratification may allow further insight into which young patients with ventricular arrhythmias require definitive, prophylactic, or no treatment.

REFERENCES

1. Garson Jr A: Ventricular arrhythmias after repair of congenital heart disease: Who needs treatment? Cardiol Young 1:177, 1991.
2. Silka MJ, Kron J: Radiofrequency catheter ablation for idiopathic right ventricular tachycardia. First, last or only therapy—Who decides? J Am Coll Cardiol 27:869–874, 1996.
3. Josephson M, Horowitz LN, Farshidi A, et al: Recurrent sustained ventricular tachycardia. 1. Mechanisms. Circulation 57:431, 1978.
4. Altman CA, Vick GW III, Perry JC, et al: Ventricular tachycardia after repair of congenital heart disease. Prog Pediatr Cardiol 4:229, 1995.
5. Jacobsen JR, Garson A, Gillette PC, et al: Premature ventricular contractions in normal children. J Pediatr 92:36, 1978.
6. Nagashima M, Tsushima M, Ogawa A, et al: Cardiac arrhythmias in healthy children revealed by 24-hour ambulatory monitoring. Pediatr Cardiol 8:103, 1987.
7. Southall DP, Richards J, Mitchell P: Study of cardiac rhythm in healthy newborn infants. Br Heart J 43:14, 1980.

8. Brodsky M, Wu D, Denes P, et al: Arrhythmias detected by 24-hour continuous ambulatory monitoring in 50 male medical students without apparent heart disease. Am J Cardiol 39:390, 1977.
9. Yabek SM: Ventricular arrhythmias in children with an apparently normal heart. J Pediatr 119:1, 1991.
10. Schamroth L: The Disorders of Cardiac Rhythm. Oxford, England, Blackwell, 1970, pp 85–94.
11. Han J: Ventricular vulnerability to fibrillation. In Dreifus LS, Likoff W (eds): Cardiac Arrhythmias. New York, Grune & Stratton, 1973, pp 87–95.
12. Langendorf R, Pick A, Winternitz M: Mechanisms of intermittent ventricular bigeminy. 1. Appearance of ectopic beats dependent upon length of the ventricular cycle, the "rule of bigeminy." Circulation 11:422, 1955.
13. Davis AM, Gow RM, McCrindle BW, et al: Clinical spectrum, therapeutic management and follow-up of ventricular tachycardia in infants and young children. Am Heart J 131:186, 1996.
14. Pederson DH, Zipes DP, Foster PR, et al: Ventricular tachycardia and ventricular fibrillation in a young population. Circulation 60:988, 1979.
15. Garson A Jr, Gillette PC, McNamara DG: Supraventricular tachycardia in children: Clinical features, response to treatment and long-term follow-up in 217 patients. J Pediatr 98:875, 1981.
16. Buxton AE, Waxman HL, Marchlinski FE, et al: Electrophysiologic studies in nonsustained ventricular tachycardia: Relation to underlying heart disease. Am J Cardiol 52:985, 1983.
17. Walsh C, Krongrad E: Terminal cardiac electrical activity in pediatric patients. Am J Cardiol 43:421, 1979.
18. Mogayzei C, Quan L, Graves JR, et al: Out of hospital ventricular fibrillation in children and adolescents. Ann Emerg Med 25:484, 1995.
19. Wiles HB, Gillette PC, Harley RA: Cardiomyopathy and myocarditis in children with ventricular ectopic rhythm. J Am Coll Cardiol 20:359, 1992.
20. Dyckner T, Wester PO: Potassium/magnesium depletion in patients with cardiovascular disease. Am J Med 82:11, 1987.
21. Garson A Jr, McNamara DG: Sudden death in a pediatric cardiology population: Relation to prior arrhythmias. J Am Coll Cardiol 5:134B, 1985.
22. Sullivan JD, Presbitero P, Gooch VM, et al: Is ventricular arrhythmia in repaired tetralogy of Fallot an effect of operation or a consequence of the course of the disease? Br Heart J 58:40, 1987.
23. Deanfield JE, Anderson RH, Hallidie-Smith KA: Late sudden-death after repair of tetralogy of Fallot. A clinicopathologic study. Circulation 67:626, 1983.
24. Garson A Jr, Nihill MR, McNamara DG, et al: Status of the adult and adolescent following repair of tetralogy of Fallot. Circulation 59:1232, 1979.
25. Garson A Jr, Randall DC, Gillette PC, et al: Prevention of sudden death after repair of tetralogy of Fallot: Treatment of ventricular arrhythmias. J Am Coll Cardiol 6:221, 1985.
26. Chandar JS, Wolff GS, Garson A Jr, et al: Ventricular arrhythmias in postoperative tetralogy of Fallot. Am J Cardiol 65:655, 1990.
27. Echt DS, Liebson PR, Mitchell LB, et al: Mortality and morbidity in patients receiving encainide, flecainide or placebo: The cardiac arrhythmia suppression trial. N Engl J Med 324:781, 1991.
28. Horowitz LN, Vetter VL, Harken AH, et al: Electrophysiologic characteristics of sustained ventricular tachycardia occurring after repair of tetralogy of Fallot. Am J Cardiol 46:446, 1980.
29. Kremers MS, Wells PJ, Black WH, et al: Entrainment of ventricular tachycardia in postoperative tetralogy of Fallot. Pacing Clin Electrophysiol 11:1310, 1988.
30. Garson A Jr: Ventricular arrhythmias after congenital heart surgery: A canine model. Pediatr Res 18:1112, 1980.
31. Harken AH, Horowitz LN, Josephson ME: Surgical correction of recurrent sustained ventricular tachycardia following complete repair of tetralogy of Fallot. J Thorac Cardiovasc Surg 80:779, 1980.
32. Downar E, Harris L, Kimber S, et al: Ventricular tachycardia following surgical repair of tetralogy of Fallot: Results of intraoperative mapping. J Am Coll Cardiol 20:648, 1992.
33. Silka MJ, Cutler JE, Kron J: Catecholamine dependent ventricular tachycardia induction following repair of tetralogy of Fallot. Am Heart J 122:568, 1991.
34. Kugler JD, Pinsky WW, Fleming WW: Sustained ventricular tachycardia after repair of tetralogy of Fallot: New electrophysiologic findings. Am J Cardiol 51:1137, 1983.
35. Walsh EP, Keana JF, Hougen TJ: Late results in patients with tetralogy of Fallot repaired during infancy. Circulation 77:1062, 1988.
36. Waien SA, Liu PP, Ross BL, et al: Serial follow-up of adults with repaired tetralogy of Fallot. J Am Coll Cardiol 20:295, 1992.
37. Burton ME, Leon AR: Radiofrequency catheter ablation of right ventricular outflow tract tachycardia late after complete repair of tetralogy of Fallot using the pace mapping technique. Pacing Clin Electrophysiol 16:2319, 1993.
38. Biblo LA, Carlson MD: Transcatheter radiofrequency ablation of ventricular tachycardia following surgical correction of tetralogy of Fallot. Pacing Clin Electrophysiol 17:1556, 1994.
39. Shen WK, Holmes DR, Poter CJ, et al: Sudden death after repair of double-outlet right ventricle. Circulation 81:128, 1990.
40. Oh J, Holmes D, Hayes D, et al: Cardiac arrhythmias in patients with surgical repair of Ebstein's anomaly. J Am Coll Cardiol 6:1351, 1985.
41. Seliem MA, Benson DW Jr, Strasburger HF, et al: Complex ventricular ectopic activity in patients less than 20 years of age with or without syncope, and the role of ventricular extrastimulus testing. Am J Cardiol 68:745, 1991.
42. Zahka KG, Horneffer PJ, Rowe SA, et al: Long-term valvular function after total repair of tetralogy of Fallot. Relation to ventricular arrhythmias. Circulation 78:III-14, 1988.
43. Hordof A, Keuhl K, Vetter V, et al: Risk factors for sudden death in patients with hypertrophic obstructive cardiomyopathy. Circulation 78:II-595, 1988.
44. McKenna W, Harris L, Rowland E, et al: Amiodarone for long-term management of patients with hypertrophic cardiomyopathy. Am J Cardiol 53:1614, 1984.
45. Fananapazir L, Epstein SE: Hemodynamic and electrophysiologic evaluation of patients with hypertrophic cardiomyopathy surviving cardiac arrest. Am J Cardiol 67:280, 1991.
46. Watkins H, McKenna WJ, Thierfelder L, et al: Mutations in the genes for cardiac troponin T and tropomyosin in hypertrophic cardiomyopathy. N Engl J Med 332:1058, 1995.
47. Friedman RA, Moak JP, Garson A Jr: Clinical course of idiopathic dilated cardiomyopathy in children. J Am Coll Cardiol 18:152, 1991.
48. Chen C, Naori S, Balfour J, et al: Clinical profile of congestive cardiomyopathy in children. J Am Coll Cardiol 15:189, 1990.

49. Burch M, Sidden SA, Cleremajer DS, et al: Dilated cardiomyopathy in children: determinants of outcome. Br Heart J 72:246, 1994.
50. Hsu DT, Addonizio LJ, Hordof AJ, et al: Acute pulmonary embolism in pediatric patients awaiting heart transplantation. J Am Coll Cardiol 18:1835, 1991.
51. Luu ML, Stevenson WG, Stevenson LW, et al: Diverse mechanisms of unexpected cardiac arrest in advanced heart failure. Circulation 80:1675, 1989.
52. Packer M: Sudden unexpected death in patients with congestive heart failure: A second frontier. Circulation 72:681, 1985.
53. Thiene G, Nava A, Corrado D, et al: Right ventricular cardiomyopathy and sudden death in young people. N Engl J Med 318:129, 1988.
54. Marcus FI, Fontaine GH, Guiraudon G, et al: Right ventricular dysplasia. A report of 24 cases. Circulation 65:382, 1982.
55. Auffeman W, Wichter T, Breithardt G, et al: Arrhythmogenic right ventricular disease: MR imaging versus angiography. Am J Roentgenol 161:549, 1993.
56. Wichter T, Borgreffe M, Haverkamp W, et al: Efficacy of antiarrhythmic drugs in patients with arrhythmogenic right ventricular disease: Results in patients with inducible and noninducible ventricular tachycardia. Circulation 86:29, 1992.
57. Fontaine G, Frank R, Rougier I, et al: Electrode catheter ablation of resistant ventricular tachycardia in arrhythmogenic right ventricular dysplasia. Heart Vessels 5:172, 1990.
58. Cox JL, Bardy GH, Damiano RJ Jr, et al: Right ventricular isolation procedures for nonischemic ventricular tachycardia. J Thorac Cardiovasc Surg 90:212, 1985.
59. Holley DG, Martin GR, Brenner JI, et al: Diagnosis and management of fetal cardiac tumors: A multicenter experience and review of published reports. J Am Coll Cardiol 26:516, 1995.
60. Garson A Jr, Gillette PC, Titus JL, et al: Surgical treatment of ventricular tachycardia in infants. N Engl J Med 310:1443, 1984.
61. Zeigler VL, Gillette PC, Crawford FA, et al: New approaches to treatment of incessant ventricular tachycardia in the very young. J Am Coll Cardiol 16:681, 1990.
62. Malhotra V, Ferrans VJ, Virmani R: Infantile histiocytoid cardiomyopathy: Three cases and literature review. Am Heart J 128:1009, 1994.
63. Bazett HC: Analysis of the time relations of electrocardiograms. Heart 7:353, 1920.
64. Desertene F: La tachcardie ventriculaire a deux foyers opposes variables. Arch Mal Coeur 59:263, 1966.
65. Moss AJ, Zareba W, Benhorin J, et al: ECG T-wave patterns in genetically distinct forms of the hereditary long QT syndrome. Circulation 92:2929, 1995.
66. Schwartz PJ, Moss AJ, Vincent GM, et al: Diagnostic criteria for the long QT syndrome: An update. Circulation 88:782, 1993.
67. Garson A Jr, Dick M II, Fournier A, et al: The long QT syndrome in children. An international study of 287 patients. Circulation 87:1866–1872, 1993.
68. Eldar M, Griffin JC, Abbott JA, et al: Permanent cardiac pacing in patients with long QT syndrome. J Am Coll Cardiol 10:600, 1987.
69. Schwartz PJ, Locati EH, Moss AJ, et al: Left cardiac sympathetic denervation in the therapy of the congenital long QT syndrome: A worldwide report. Circulation 84:503, 1991.
70. Schwartz PJ: The long QT syndrome: Progress and questions. Am Heart J 109:399, 1985.
71. Webb CL, Dick M II, Rocchini AP, et al: Quinidine syncope in children. J Am Coll Cardiol 9:1031, 1987.
72. Martyn R, Somberg JC, Kerin NZ: Proarrhythmia of nonantiarrhythmic drugs. Am Heart J 126:201, 1993.
73. Wever EFD, Hauer RNW, Oomen A, et al: Unfavorable outcome in patients with primary electrical disease who survived an episode of ventricular fibrillation. Circulation 88:1021, 1993.
74. Zipes DP: Electrophysiological mechanisms involved in ventricular fibrillation. Circulation 51:III-120, 1975.
75. Maron BJ, Poliac LC, Kaplan JA, et al: Blunt impact to the chest leading to sudden death from cardiac arrest during sports. N Engl J Med 333:380, 1995.
76. Priori S, Borgreffe M, Camm AJ, et al: Role of the implantable cardioverter defibrillator in patients with idiopathic ventricular fibrillation. Pacing Clin Electrophysiol 18:799, 1995.
77. Leenhardt A, Lucet V, Denjoy I, et al: Catecholaminergic polymorphic ventricular tachycardia in children: A 7 year follow-up of 21 patients. Circulation 91:1512, 1995.
78. Lerman B, Belardinelli L, DiMarco J: Adenosine sensitive ventricular tachycardia: Evidence suggesting cyclic AMP mediated triggered activity. J Am Coll Cardiol 7:155, 1986.
79. Fulton DR, Chung KJ, Tabakin BS, et al: Ventricular tachycardia in children without heart disease. Am J Cardiol 55:1328, 1985.
80. O'Connor BK, Case CL, Sokolowski M, et al: Radiofrequency catheter ablation of right ventricular tachycardia in children. J Am Coll Cardiol 27:869, 1996.
81. Saul JP, Hulse JE, Papagiannis J, et al: Late enlargement of radiofrequency lesions in infant lambs: Implications for ablation procedures in small children. Circulation 90:492, 1994.
82. Lin FC, Finley D, Rahimtoola SH, et al: Idiopathic paroxysmal ventricular tachycardia with a QRS pattern of right bundle branch block and left axis deviation: A unique clinical entity with specific properties. Am J Cardiol 52:95, 1983.
83. Nakagawa H, Beekman KJ, McClelland JH, et al: Radiofrequency catheter ablation of idiopathic left ventricular tachycardia guided by a Purkinje potential. Circulation 88:2607, 1993.
84. Brugada P, Brugada J: Right bundle branch block, persistent ST segment elevation and sudden cardiac death: A distinct clinical and electrocardiographic syndrome. J Am Coll Cardiol 20:1391, 1992.
85. Garson A Jr, Gillette PC, Gutgessell HP, et al: Stress-induced ventricular arrhythmia after repair of tetralogy of Fallot. Am J Cardiol 46:1006, 1980.
86. Martin AB, Perry JC, Robinson JL, et al: Calculation of QTc duration and variability in the presence of sinus arrhythmia. Am J Cardiol 75:950, 1995.
87. Lown B, Calvert AF, Armington R, et al: Monitoring for serious arrhythmias and high risk of sudden death. Circulation 52:III-89, 1975.
88. Paul T, Marchall C, Garson A Jr: Ventricular couplets in the young: Prognosis related to underlying substrate. Am Heart J 119:577, 1990.
89. Wellens HJ, Schuilenburg RM, Durrer D: Electrical stimulation of the heart in patients with ventricular tachycardia. Circulation 46:216, 1972.
90. Silka MJ, Kron J, Cutler JC, et al: Analysis of programmed stimulation methods in the evaluation of ventricular arrhythmias in patients 20 years old and younger. Am J Cardiol 66:826, 1990.
91. Calkins H, Kalbfleisch SJ, El-Attassi R, et al: Relation between efficacy of radiofrequency catheter ablation and site of origin of idiopathic ventricular tachycardia. Am J Cardiol 71:827, 1993.
92. Antzelevitch C, Sicouri S: Clinical relevance of cardiac

arrhythmias generated by afterdepolarizations. J Am Coll Cardiol 23:259, 1994.
93. Misaki T, Tsubota M, Watanabe G, et al: Surgical treatment of ventricular tachycardia after surgical treatment of tetralogy of Fallot. Circulation 90:264, 1994.
94. Brugada P, Green M, Abdollah H, et al: Significance of ventricular arrhythmias initiated by programmed ventricular stimulation: Importance of the type of ventricular arrhythmia induced and the number of premature stimuli required. Circulation 69:87, 1984.
95. Bhandari AK, Shapiro WA, Morady F, et al: Electrophysiologic testing in patients with long QT syndrome. Circulation 71:63, 1985.
96. Case C, Gillette PC: Treatment of ventricular arrhythmias in children without structural heart disease with class IC agents as guided by invasive electrophysiology. Am J Cardiol 66:1265, 1990.
97. Ewing L, Gillette PC: Only 8% of postoperative tetralogy patients have inducible dysrhythmias. J Am Coll Cardiol 9:36A, 1987.
98. Silka MJ, Kron J, Dunnigan A, et al: Sudden cardiac death and the use of implantable cardioverter defibrillators in pediatric patients. Circulation 87:800, 1993.
99. Hamilton RM, Dorian P, Gow RM, et al: Five-year experience with implantable defibrillators in children. Am J Cardiol 77:524, 1996.
100. Fish F, Gillette PC, Benson DW Jr: Proarrhythmia, cardiac arrest and death in young patients receiving encainide and flecainide. J Am Coll Cardiol 18:365, 1991.

SECTION III

Treatment

CHAPTER 9

ACUTE TREATMENT OF ARRHYTHMIAS

Amy T. Winslow, John Papagiannis, and Ronald J. Kanter

Advances in nonpharmacologic techniques and availability of newer pharmacologic agents to convert cardiac arrhythmias to a normal or safe rhythm now permit control of nearly any tachy- or bradyarrhythmia in children. The newer available modalities and agents include transthoracic external pacing, esophageal pacing, intravenous adenosine, and intravenous amiodarone. In this chapter, we consider the therapies available by arrhythmia category and suggested treatment algorithms by specific arrhythmia type.

BRADYCARDIAS

PHARMACOLOGIC MANAGEMENT

Sinus bradycardia, sinus node arrest with a delayed junctional or ventricular escape rhythm, and varying degrees of atrioventricular (AV) block are the most common lethal pediatric arrhythmias[1] and usually are secondary to profound systemic disease. Positive chronotropic agents are of value in such cases, but are only temporizing if the underlying disorder cannot be corrected.

Epinephrine, an alpha- and beta-adrenergic receptor agonist, is the first-line medication when treating secondary symptomatic bradycardia from a nonvagal entity. The recommended dose of epinephrine via the intravenous or intraosseous route is 0.01 mg/kg of the 1:10,000 solution and can be repeated every 3 to 5 minutes.[2]

There is a limited role for the use of drugs to augment heart rate in instances of primary acute AV block or severe sinus bradycardia. Special circumstances merit further comment.

Cardiac manifestations of digitalis toxicity may include profound sinus bradycardia or sinoatrial exit block or second- or third-degree AV block.[3] These bradycardias may be treated with digoxin-specific sheep Fab fragments. The decision to use this treatment should be based on multiple factors. In any patient receiving digoxin in whom there is an arrhythmia known to be caused by digoxin toxicity, and if there is cardiovascular compromise, this agent should be used. The commercially available product, Digibind, comes as 40-mg vials. The total dose administered is based on the estimated total body load of digoxin and the plasma concentration:

$$\text{Total load (mg)} = \frac{\text{plasma concentration (ng/ml)} \times 5.6 \times \text{weight (kg)}}{1000}$$

or

$$\text{Total load (mg)} = \text{ingested digoxin (mg)} \times 0.8$$

The Digibind dose is then calculated using the following formula:

$$\text{Digibind dose (mg)} = \text{total load (of digoxin from above)} \times 66.7$$

Digibind is administered intravenously over 15 to 30 minutes through a 0.22-micron filter. The response to this drug is nearly immediate, but the arrhythmia may recur as tissue-bound digoxin is released into the plasma, requiring repeat dosing. Every effort should also be made to eliminate factors that predispose patients to toxicity, including myocardial hypoxia, hypokalemia, hypercalcemia, hypomagnesemia, alkalosis, sympathomimetic drugs, and some anesthetic agents. Transthoracic or transvenous temporary ventricular pacing may be necessary until Digibind is available for unacceptable bradycardia.

Atropine sulfate, the drug of choice in the treatment of vagally induced bradycardia, is a parasympatholytic agent that enhances sinus node or atrial pacemakers and AV conduction.[2] The recommended dose is 0.02 mg/kg with a minimum dosage of 0.1 mg and a maximum initial dose of 0.5 mg for a child and 1 mg for an adolescent. This dose can be repeated after 5 minutes to a maximum cumulative dose of 1.0 mg for a child and 2.0 mg for an adolescent.[2] Paradoxic bradycardia can occur if a vagolytic dosage of atropine sulfate is not administered.[4] This drug may also be used to treat permanent bradyarrhythmias while the patient is being prepared for temporary pacing. It has been given as a continuous infusion at a dosage of 0.01 mg/kg/

hr in rare instances of postoperative Bezold-Jarisch reflex-mediated asystole in infants.[5]

Isoproterenol, a beta-adrenergic receptor agonist, may be used for symptomatic bradycardia as a result of third-degree AV block unresponsive to atropine. The American Heart Association recommends noninvasive temporary pacing before isoproterenol administration when treating symptomatic bradycardia or asystole.[2] Isoproterenol is administered via continuous intravenous infusion starting at 0.02 to 0.05 μg/kg/min.[2] This drug has a large side effect profile, including hypotension and life-threatening ventricular arrhythmias resulting from an increase in oxygen consumption and direct effects on myocyte excitability.

NONPHARMACOLOGIC THERAPY

The technique of transthoracic external pacing for severe bradycardia was first described by Zoll in 1952.[6] The original energy delivery method was very painful, but refinements in technique have made this a widely accepted short-term means of chronotropic support. Beland et al first described the effectiveness and safety of external pacing in 21 children.[7, 8] It is most frequently administered as a temporizing pacing method for any patient with acute bradycardia before temporary transvenous pacing wire placement. Such clinical circumstances might include late AV block after congenital heart surgery, severe sinus bradycardia or AV block secondary to myocarditis or drug ingestion, or sudden pacemaker failure in a patient who is pacemaker dependent.

Transcutaneous pacing involves the application of two large patch electrodes to the skin in an anteroposterior or base-apex configuration, an external pulse generator, and a pacing cable. The pacing threshold should be tested in advance whenever possible and is usually 40 to 75 mA at a pulse width of 40 milliseconds. This relatively high current is necessary because bone and muscle lie between the electrodes and the heart. Large skin electrodes are preferred even in the pediatric patient. They lower the pacing threshold and minimize the discomfort for the nonsedated patient; however, pacing thresholds are highly individualized. Taylor suggested that the adult-size electrodes should be used for patients down to 5 kg.[9] Younger children typically require sedation with intravenous infusion of benzodiazepines, sometimes with a narcotic. Taylor did not recommend transcutaneous pacing for more than 1 hour when other pacing modalities exist.[9] Younger pediatric patients have the potential of impairment of skin integrity at electrode sites.

Advantages of transcutaneous pacing include the relatively noninvasive nature of the technique, the briefer set-up period compared with the transvenous approach, and the fact that physician assistants, registered nurses, and other trained personnel can utilize this device in an acute clinical situation. Disadvantages of transcutaneous pacing include discomfort, potential for skin burns, and the time required for sedation and possible secondary endotracheal intubation in younger patients before external pacing.

Temporary transvenous pacing is a reliable means of chronotropic support for children having any of the conditions just described. It may be used reliably for days until the underlying condition has been corrected or a permanent pacemaker is implanted. The technique requires vascular access, usually to a ventricle. An internal jugular vein, subclavian vein (contralateral to where the permanent pacing lead would be placed), axillary vein, or, less desirably, a femoral vein may be used. After a Fontan-type operation or placement of a prosthetic tricuspid valve, arterial access to a ventricle is necessary. Balloon-directed bipolar electrode catheters as small as 4 French are available. In the presence of a structurally normal heart, right ventricular access may be accomplished from an upper body vein using such a catheter without fluoroscopic guidance, although we always prefer such help. At the time of placement, the catheter should be directed through a long accordion-like sterile cover, which is secured to the sheath, to later permit repositioning of the catheter if the pacing threshold should rise. Once the electrode catheter is in position, the pacing and, if there is an intrinsic rhythm, sensing thresholds should be measured and the pacing output and sensing amplitude values on the temporary pacemaker set to be three times these thresholds. The most important complications of this pacing technique include cellulitis, bacteremia, cardiac perforation with tamponade, catheter-induced tachyarrhythmias, and thrombus formation with pulmonary or systemic embolization. The addition of heparin should be considered in patients known to be prone to thrombus formation, in the presence of low cardiac output, or if there are systemic-to-pulmonary circulation connections.

At the conclusion of a congenital heart operation, two epicardial pacing wires are routinely sewn onto the atrial epicardium and two onto the ventricular epicardium. The safety and efficacy of this practice were demonstrated by Waldo and MacLean in more than 9000 adult patients[10] and by Yabek et al in more than 100 pediatric patients.[11] The stainless steel wires are coated with polyethylene and are primarily used to maintain AV synchrony or to provide rate support appropriate for the patient's metabolic needs. Their use for postoperative tachyarrhythmias is discussed later. They are employed as a bradycardia back-up pacemaker in children after atrial surgery having transient sinus bradycardia, in those with severe right ventricular dysfunction with atrial stretch and sinus bradycardia, and in those with potentially reversible postoperative AV block. Pacing and sensing thresholds in both bipolar configurations should be measured for each lead pair at the conclusion of the case once the patient is normothermic. It should be remembered that pacing thresholds will be altered by high catecholamine states, hypothermia, alkalosis, hypoxia, and hypokalemia. The thresholds should be remeasured daily. The stability of the thresholds is highly individualized; thresholds may be stable for weeks or may deteriorate within days. At the conclusion of their usefulness, and in the presence of normal clotting status, they may be percutaneously removed. The major complication of their use is pericardial tamponade after they are removed. Infection is very uncommon.

TACHYCARDIAS

PHARMACOLOGIC TREATMENT

In the United States, the antiarrhythmic drugs that are helpful to acutely terminate pathologic tachycardias and to prevent their recurrences and that are conveniently delivered intravenously include procainamide, lidocaine, phenytoin, esmolol, propranolol (and several other beta-adrenergic blocking drugs), bretylium, amiodarone, digoxin, adenosine, phenylephrine, and edrophonium. These drugs, their classification, arrhythmia types for which they are efficacious, dosing technique, acute side effects, and other considerations pertinent to acute use are listed in Table 9–1. The cellular and clinical electrophysiologic properties, considerations for long-term therapy, and chronic side effects are discussed in detail in Chapter 13. Adenosine is only provided for acute termination of tachyarrhythmias, and intravenous amiodarone has just been released in the United States. They are discussed next.

Adenosine

Adenosine is an endogenous nucleoside formed by either dephosphorylation of adenosine monophosphate or metabolism of *S*-adenosyl homocysteine. It binds to the A_1 receptors on atrial myocytes and sinoatrial nodal and AV nodal cells. Using a guanine nucleotide-binding protein (G_1) as a transduction molecule, it directly activates an outward potassium current (Ik_{AChAdo}),[12] resulting in shortening of the action potential and hyperpolarization of these cells.[13, 14] The clinical electrophysiologic effects of this drug in pharmacologic doses include reduction in impulse formation in the sinus and AV nodes (N region especially) and in atrial myocytes and reduction in sinoatrial and AV nodal conduction velocity, resulting in sinus bradycardia and arrest and any degree of AV nodal block. The elimination half-life is 0.5 to 5.0 seconds,[15, 16] making this an exceedingly short-acting drug. It is rendered ineffective by therapeutic blood levels of theophylline but not by caffeine after usual caffeinated beverage intake. Dipyridamole delays adenosine clearance, making dose selection difficult.

Adenosine at doses of 37.5 to 300 μg/kg as rapid intravenous bolus terminated paroxysmal supraventricular tachycardia in 86 to 100% of 59 patients in four pediatric series.[17–20] As predicted from its electrophysiologic effects, adenosine terminates orthodromic reciprocating tachycardia in the antegrade (or slow) AV node, following the atrial electrogram (Fig. 9–1). In patients having decrementally conducting accessory pathways, block within the pathway may occur, with termination after the ventricular electrogram.

Adenosine does not terminate atrial flutter, atrial re-entry tachycardia, or atrial fibrillation,[21] but will cause a brief period of reduced AV conduction, better revealing the underlying persisting atrial rhythm (Fig. 9–2). It thus serves as a good diagnostic tool if discrimination between a primary atrial tachycardia and paroxysmal supraventricular tachycardia (PSVT) is necessary. In our experience, adenosine will transiently terminate some mostly right-sided foci of atrial ectopic tachycardia. Some patients having ventricular tachycardia emanating from the right ventricular outflow tract, and thus having an inferior axis left bundle branch block morphology, experience tachycardia termination with adenosine.[22] This type of ventricular tachycardia generally also responds to verapamil and likely has a triggered mechanism.

Adenosine delivery should be as central in the circulation as possible. Nonrhythm side effects lasting less than 1 minute occur in 40 to 60% of patients and include flushing, dyspnea, bronchospasm, and chest pressure. Brief periods of sinus bradycardia, AV block, and ventricular ectopic beats after PSVT termination are ubiquitous and benign,[23] but atrial fibrillation and torsades de pointes[24] have also been observed. This drug should probably not be given to a patient known to have a long QT interval, and should be given

Table 9–1. Intravenous Use of Antiarrhythmic Drugs for Acute Termination of Tachyarrhythmias

DRUG	CLASS	USES	DOSING	ACUTE SIDE EFFECTS	OTHER CONSIDERATIONS
Procainamide	Ia	AFl, PSVT, VT, JET	10–15 mg/kg over 15–60 min (load); 20–60 μg/kg/min (infusion)	Hypotension; more rapid ventricular response during AFl	Additional AV node blockade for AFl
Lidocaine	Ib	VT, VF	1 mg/kg q 5 min × 3 (load); 20–50 μg/kg/min (infusion)	Tinnitus; perioral paresthesias; altered sensorium; seizure; rarely decreases CO	Lower dose with heart or liver failure
Phenytoin	Ib	VT from digoxin intoxication; occasionally other VTs	15 mg/kg over 60 min (q 5 min pushes)	Hypotension	Increases verapamil effect
Propranolol	II	Rapidly recurrent TDP in known LQTS	0.05–0.15 mg/kg	Bronchospasm; sinus arrest; AV block; hypotension, shock	Should not be used with verapamil or severe CHF
Esmolol	II	Same as propranolol	500 μg/kg bolus; then 50 μg/kg/min; repeat load every 4 min, and increase infusion by 50 μg/kg/min up to 400 μg/kg/min, as needed	Same as propranolol	May require very large doses in young children
Bretylium	III	VF (especially with digoxin toxicity), VT	5 mg/kg over 1 min; may be doubled	Hypotension	Quinidine antagonizes effect
Amiodarone	III	VT, JET, resistant recurrent PSVT, AFl, very rapid AET	5 mg/kg/30 min up to 20 mg/kg as load; 10–15 mg/kg/24 hr as continuous infusion	Hypotension; sinus bradycardia or AV block if intrinsic disease	Increases level of digoxin, procainamide, quinidine
Diltiazem	IV	PSVT; ventricular rate control for AFib/Fl	0.25 mg/kg up to 20 mg bolus over 2 min; repeat at 0.35 mg/kg up to 25 mg 15 min later, if necessary; 0.1–0.3 mg/kg/hr up to 15 mg/hr as infusion	Hypotension; sinus bradycardia; AV block	Use with caution if oral digoxin or beta blocker in use
Adenosine	Purinergic	PSVT; diagnostically to diagnose primary atrial re-entry, some JET, causes of WCT	100 μg/kg rapid bolus; increase by 50 μg/kg up to 250 μg/kg max	Sinus arrest; AV block; PVCs; AFib (all transient)	Not useful if therapeutic theophylline; low dose in presence of dipyridamole
Digoxin	Digitalis glycoside	PSVT; AFl or AFib for ventricular rate control; postoperative JET; AET	*Total po load* (½/¼/¼ q 8 hr): premature, 20 μg/kg; term–6 mo, 30 μg/kg; >6 mos, 40 μg/kg; maximum, 1.0 mg *Total IV load:* (as above, but ¾ po doses)	Sinus bradycardia; AV block; atrial tachy; accelerated junctional; PACs; PVCs; nausea; lethargy; visual changes	Quinidine, amiodarone, verapamil ↑ digoxin level; toxicity more likely if low K^+ or high Ca^{+2}

Table 9–1. Intravenous Use of Antiarrhythmic Drugs for Acute Termination of Tachyarrhythmias *Continued*

DRUG	CLASS	USES	DOSING	ACUTE SIDE EFFECTS	OTHER CONSIDERATIONS
Phenylephrine	Alpha-agonist	PSVT	0.01 mg/kg; double q 5 min until SBP twice baseline or PSVT termination	Sinus bradycardia; AV block; hypertension	Atropine for excessive vagal response; less effective in infants
Edrophonium	Cholinesterase inhibitor	PSVT	0.04 mg/kg test for bronchospasm; then 0.16 mg/kg over 2 min	Sinus bradycardia; AV block; bronchospasm; abdominal pain	Atropine for excessive vagal response; less effective in infants

AET, atrial ectopic tachycardia; AFib, atrial fibrillation; AFl, atrial flutter; AV, atrioventricular; CHF, congestive heart failure; CO, cardiac output; JET, junctional ectopic tachycardia; LQTS, long QT syndrome; PAC, premature atrial contraction; PSVT, paroxysmal supraventricular tachycardia; PVC, premature ventricular contraction; SBP, systolic blood pressure; TDP, torsades de pointes; VT, ventricular tachycardia; VF, ventricular fibrillation; WCT, wide-complex tachycardia.

only if electrical countershock is available and if Wolff-Parkinson-White syndrome is believed to be present, because a rapid ventricular response from atrial fibrillation after tachycardia termination could occur. Adenosine at low dose (50 μg/kg) should always be used initially in children also receiving dipyridamole.

Amiodarone

Amiodarone is a potent antiarrhythmic agent because of its potassium channel and lesser sodium channel, beta-adrenergic, and calcium channel blocking effects. Oral amiodarone is highly efficacious in preventing recurrences of most tachyarrhythmias in children,[25, 26] but it requires a 5- to 10-day oral loading period. Although this drug has many long-term noncardiac side effects, it does not have negative inotropic properties and is an attractive agent in children with poor ventricular function. Figa[27] and Perry[28] and their colleagues reported excellent effectiveness and safety of intravenous amiodarone for acute treatment of otherwise drug-resistant arrhythmias. In Figa's series, 94% of children with supraventricular and ventricular tachyarrhythmias benefited from amiodarone, including partial responses in 45% and complete responses in 55% of those having chaotic atrial, atrial ectopic, and junctional ectopic tachycardias.[27] Perry et al reported an 80% response of postoperative ventricular tachycardia to amiodarone.[28] Junctional ectopic tachycardia that is difficult to manage appears to be especially responsive to this drug. A suggested dosing regimen is 5 mg/kg over 30 to 60 minutes, with continuous blood

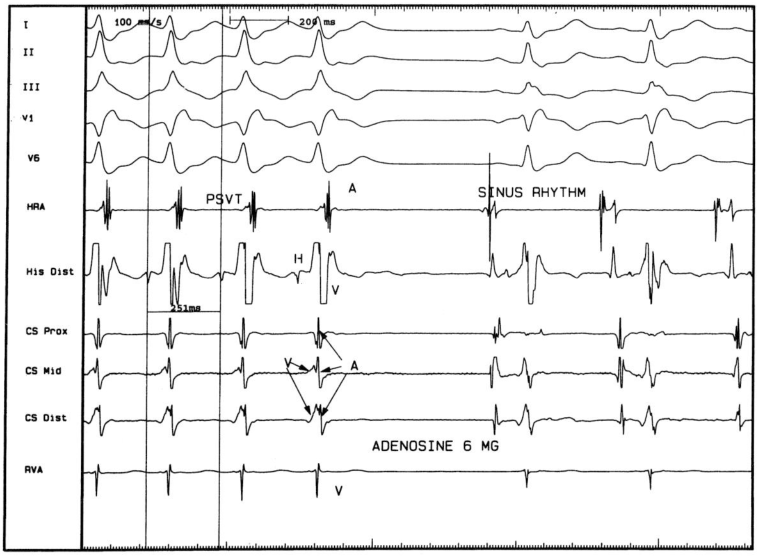

FIGURE 9–1. Surface and intracardiac electrograms from an 11-year-old with the typical variety of atrioventricular (AV) node re-entry tachycardia, illustrating the effect of adenosine. Tachycardia terminates after the atrial electrogram and, thus, in the AV node. (A, atrial electrogram; H, His bundle electrogram; PSVT, paroxysmal supraventricular tachycardia; V, ventricular electrogram.)

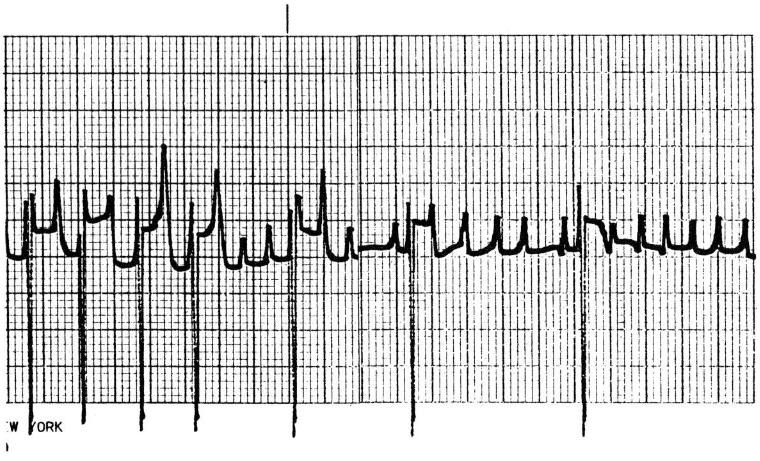

FIGURE 9–2. A rhythm strip from a 2-day-old with congenital atrial tachycardia. The P wave and QRS relationship are not obvious during the first second of this strip, but the effects of adenosine, 0.6 mg, then demonstrate a slightly irregular atrial rate at about 340 bpm with higher grade atrioventricular block.

pressure monitoring. This may be repeated as necessary up to a total of 20 mg/kg. This should be followed by maintenance dosing of 10 to 15 mg/kg/24 hr as a continuous infusion, until conversion to oral medication or definitive therapy is possible. The only side effects during loading included severe sinus bradycardia requiring temporary postoperative pacing[27] and transient hypotension responsive to volume or calcium chloride infusions.[28]

NONPHARMACOLOGIC THERAPY

Arrhythmia Diagnosis: Techniques for Recording Atrial Activity

The identification of atrial electrograms and their relationship to the QRS complex during tachyarrhythmias is often impossible from surface ECGs because of QRS and T-wave interference and the small size of the atrial signals. Knowledge of these electrogram relationships is critical for tachycardia diagnosis and proper treatment selection. Techniques available to provide this information include transesophageal catheter placement, temporary epicardial pacing wire placement (postoperatively), and signal-averaged ECGs.

Transesophageal electrode catheter placement may be performed relatively painlessly after providing local anesthesia to the nasopharynx and by using a soft silicone rubber–coated electrode catheter (Electro-Catheter Corporation, Rahway, NJ) or, in older children, a "pill" electrode (Arzco Medical Electronics, Chicago, IL). The electrode pair should be advanced to a position behind the atrial mass. This depth may be estimated in advance by measuring the distance from the nares to the xyphoid and confirmed by fluoroscopy. The catheter is advanced similarly to a nasogastric tube. Once in position, the electrode catheter poles should be connected to a preamplifier in a bipolar configuration, filtered at 30 to 500 Hz, and displayed along with at least one surface channel. Alternately, a standard ECG machine may be used wherein the electrode catheter poles are connected to the V_1 and V_2 inputs using alligator clips, and the limb and V_3 inputs are normally attached. Continuous display of the V_1, V_2, and V_3 montage will provide two esophageal (V_1 and V_2) and one surface (V_3) recording. The catheter is then advanced or pulled back until the largest atrial signal is identified. Additional information may be learned by recording signals during attempted tachycardia termination using vagal maneuvers or intravenous adenosine or procainamide (Fig. 9–3). This technique is valuable in diagnosing atrial tachyarrhythmias in the presence of low- amplitude P waves, such as after the atrial switch operation for transposition[29] or after the Fontan operation, and for discriminating typical variety AV nodal re-entry tachycardia from AV reciprocating tachycardia.[30] Continuous 24-hour ambulatory esophageal recordings may provide useful information in up to 76% of cooperative patients,[31, 32] particularly in those having wide-complex nonsustained tachycardias.

Temporary atrial epicardial pacing wires, when placed intraoperatively, may also provide diagnostic information during tachycardias critical to therapy selection. These wires may be attached to a standard ECG machine as just described for esophageal recordings. We have found this technique valuable in discriminating sinus tachycardia or PSVT from junctional ectopic tachycardia, PSVT with bundle branch aberrancy from ventricular tachycardia, and atrial tachyarrhythmias with varying AV block from sinus rhythm with junctional or atrial premature beats (Table 9–2).

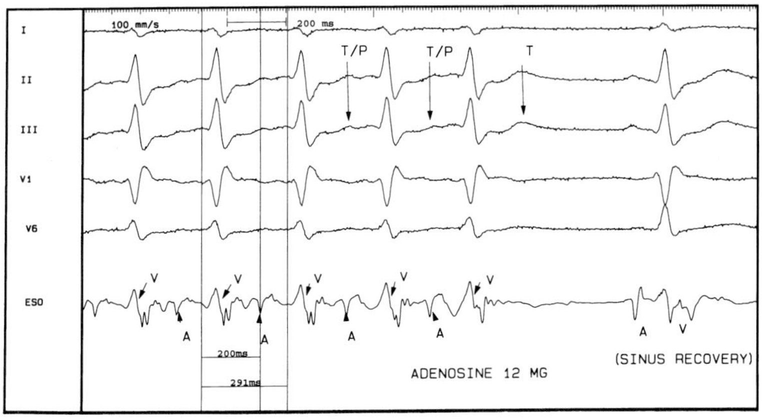

FIGURE 9–3. Surface leads and esophageal electrograms from a 16-year-old boy with exercise-induced palpitations. Under the influence of isoproterenol and atropine, this long RP tachycardia was induced. A rapid intravenous bolus of adenosine, 12 mg, terminated tachycardia after the ventricular electrogram. This helped limit the differential diagnosis to the atypical variety of atrioventricular (AV) node re-entry tachycardia, an unusual form of AV reciprocating tachycardia using an adenosine-sensitive accessory pathway, or an unusual type of atrial re-entry tachycardia. At invasive electrophysiologic study, the patient was demonstrated to have the atypical variety of AV node re-entry. The surface P waves were difficult to interpret because they were buried in the T wave. (A, atrial electrogram; V, ventricular electrogram.)

Valsalva and Vagal Maneuvers

Sudden enhanced parasympathetic influences may acutely terminate paroxysmal tachycardias that use the AV node or sinoatrial node as part of their circuit. Firm massage of the carotid sinus for 10 seconds may occasionally provide the vagal response necessary in older children. This is best performed in a supine position.[33] The right carotid sinus should be massaged first, followed by the left. Simultaneous massage of both carotid sinuses should never be performed. Bisset et al[34] described the technique of placing an ice bag over the face for 5 to 10 seconds to promote a

Table 9–2. Use of Temporary Epicardial Pacing Wires for Discrimination of Postoperative Arrhythmias

VARIABLE	ELECTROGRAM RELATIONSHIPS	EFFECTS OF ADENOSINE
1. Junctional ectopic tachycardia	Dissociated or short V-A	V-V unaffected; V-A block
vs.		
Sinus tachycardia	1 : 1 with V-A > A-V	A-V block; asystole
2. Paroxysmal supraventricular tachycardia with bundle branch aberrancy	1 : 1 with V-A < A-V	Termination after A
vs.		
Atrial re-entry with bundle branch aberrancy	1 : 1 A-V or more As than Vs	A-A unaffected; fewer Vs
vs.		
Ventricular tachycardia	Dissociated sometimes	V-V unaffected; V-A block
3. Atrial flutter with 2 : 1 A-V conduction	2 : 1 A-V	A-A unaffected; fewer Vs
vs.		
Sinus rhythm	1 : 1 with V-A > A-V	A-V block; asystole
vs.		
Paroxysmal supraventricular tachycardia	1 : 1 with V-A < A-V	Termination after A
4. Atrial flutter with variable A-V conduction	Regular A-A; variable A-V	A-A unaffected; fewer Vs
vs.		
Sinus rhythm with PACs/PJCs	Early atrial electrograms after sinus As	A premature; A unaffected; A-V block; asystole
5. Sinus bradycardia	1 : 1 with V-A > A-V	
vs.		
Nonconducted atrial bigeminy	Early atrial electrogram without QRS	
6. Junctional rhythm	1 : 1 V-A with short V-A	
vs.		
Atrial flutter with 4 : 1 A-V conduction and low-amplitude P waves	4 : 1 A-V	

A, atrial electrogram; V, ventricular electrogram or QRS; PACs, premature atrial contractions; PJCs, premature junctional contractions.

diving reflex with resulting hypervagotonia. This may be performed in infants, but precautions should be taken to prevent prolonged bradycardia or aspiration. The ophthalmic division of the trigeminal nerve seems to be most sensitive to this stimulation. Other vagal maneuvers that have been reported to be helpful include coughing, gag reflex stimulation by a tongue blade, squatting, and Trendelenburg position. Eyeball pressure is strongly discouraged, because retinal detachment has been reported to occur. It is preferable to perform vagal maneuvers in the hospital setting with continuous ECG monitoring and availability of atropine. This is not practical for children who have been taught methods to self-terminate PSVT, but should always be considered for infants subjected to the diving reflex.

The older child or adolescent can be taught to perform a rather complete Valsalva maneuver (attempted forced expiration against a closed glottis). Younger children may be instructed to take a deep breath and hold it as long as they can, to strain as if having a bowel movement, or to blow against their thumb. These maneuvers enhance vagal tone after the release phase (phase 4) and have additional mechanical influences on right-side heart filling during phases 2 and 4. Such changes in right atrial dimensions may account for the occasional patient who can terminate bona fide atrial flutter with these maneuvers.

Antitachycardia Pacing

The technique of rapid pacing will terminate most cases of re-entry tachyarrhythmia, including atrial flutter, atrial re-entry tachycardia, sinoatrial node re-entry tachycardia, AV node re-entry tachycardia, AV reciprocating tachycardia, and re-entry forms of ventricular tachycardia. The basic premise of this method is that by pacing the heart at a constant rate faster than the tachycardia rate (overdrive pacing) or by placing a sequence of premature beats into tachycardia (programmed stimulation), the first paced wave front will collide in an antidromic direction with the last tachycardia wave front and, with subsequent beats, will eventually be premature enough to encounter an area of refractoriness in the orthodromic direction (Fig. 9–4), thus terminating tachycardia. Thus, "entrainment with termination" will have been accomplished. For PSVT and atrial flutter, this requires a paced cycle length 65 to 85% of the tachycardia cycle length and is greatly influenced by the distance between the pacing electrode and the circuit; the more distant it is from the circuit, the shorter the cycle length that is required. Termination generally requires bursts of 10 to 20 seconds (average, 11 seconds).[35] Rapid pacing of the atrium is more effective (93% of episodes) than programmed stimulation (73% of episodes) for PSVT,[36] although atrial fibrillation may result in about 25% of cases.[36–38] This may be prevented by pretreatment with procainamide.[39] Overdrive pacing using the transesophageal method has been reported to terminate 47 to 94% of atrial flutter episodes,[29, 37, 40] including patients who had undergone the Mustard operation.[29] Another burst-pacing technique involves progressively faster pacing beginning at a cycle length only 10

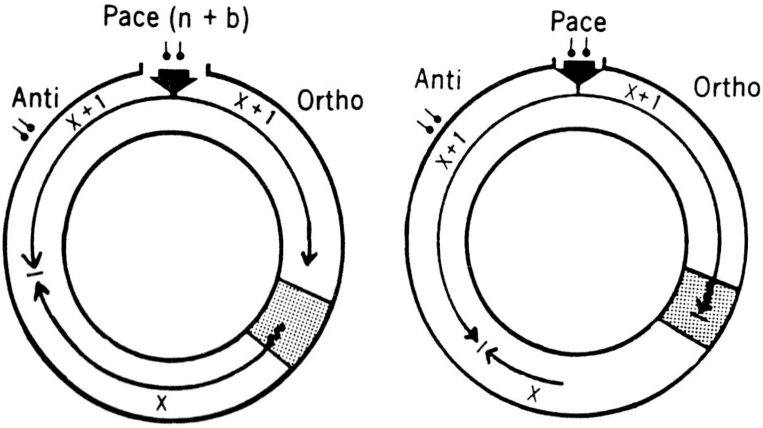

FIGURE 9–4. Concept of overdrive termination of a re-entry tachycardia. On the left, a paced wavefront (X + 1) collides with the previous tachycardia wavefront (X) in the antidromic direction, but continues tachycardia in the orthodromic direction. Transient entrainment with tachycardia perpetuation is said to have occurred. On the right, pacing at a faster rate results in a wavefront (X + 1) that collides with the previous wavefront (X) in the antidromic direction earlier in the cycle and, in addition, is early enough to encounter a portion of the circuit still refractory in the orthodromic direction. It is then said that entrainment with termination has occurred.

to 20 milliseconds shorter than the tachycardia cycle length. "Ramp pacing" continues until a P-wave morphology change is noted, representing entrainment, and pacing is abruptly discontinued. If atrial flutter does not convert, this maneuver is repeated with further decrement in pacing cycle length.

Transesophageal stimulation may be performed using any programmable stimulator capable of delivering a constant current square wave pulse of 10-millisecond duration. The pacing threshold is influenced by the pulse width delivered and the optimal catheter depth, but not by the interelectrode distance.[41] The technique for catheter placement has been discussed. Once in position, atrial pacing is begun at a pulse width of 10 milliseconds and a current of 10 mA. The current strength is increased until capture occurs or the patient experiences chest pain (usually 15–18 mA). Failure to capture at greater than 20 mA requires catheter repositioning. Complications of transesophageal pacing are uncommon but include esophageal erythema, atrial fibrillation, and ventricular, diaphragm, or brachial plexus pacing.[42] Other indications for transesophageal pacing are listed in Table 9–3.

Overdrive pacing using a transvenous approach requires fluoroscopic guidance, more time to achieve vascular access, and higher degree of skill. However, it permits greater opportunity to pace nearer to the tachycardia circuit and is probably more efficacious than transesophageal pacing for converting atrial flutter.[37] It is also a safer technique if there is risk of AV block during rapid atrial pacing and, of course, is the only means to overdrive terminate sustained ventricular tachycardia.

Almost any ventricular or supraventricular tachyarrhythmia using a re-entry mechanism can be converted to sinus rhythm by the passage of high-energy direct current across the chest. When the discharge is synchronized with the R wave, the risk of accidental discharge during the ventricular vulnerable period is avoided, and the risk of converting the tachyarrhythmia to ventricular fibrillation is reduced. If the patient is already in ventricular fibrillation, the R-wave amplitude is too low, and synchronization is not possible, then defibrillation must be performed. The specific tachyarrhythmias that may be cardioverted include atrial fibrillation, atrial flutter, atrial re-entry tachycardia, sinoatrial node re-entry tachycardia, AV node re-entry tachycardia, AV reciprocating tachycardia, and re-entrant forms of ventricular tachycardia. Defibrillation is mandatory for ventricular fibrillation, and cardioversion is the treatment of choice for any of these tachyarrhythmias in a patient who is in extremis.

Direct current countershock may result in transient myocardial damage, as suggested by ST-segment changes, elevation of plasma cardiac enzymes,[43, 44] depression of left ventricular dp/dt, and increase in left ventricular diastolic pressure.[45] Although these changes are usually reversible, transient hypotension often occurs. The combination of underlying myocardial ischemia and multiple high-energy shocks may result in more significant myocardial damage.

Direct current countershock may predispose the patient to additional arrhythmias, including atrial fibrillation, ventricular tachycardia, ventricular fibrillation, sinus bradycardia, AV block, and bundle branch block. Bradycardias may occur in patients on certain antiarrhythmic drugs or who have underlying conduction system disease. Fortunately, many newer models of cardioverter-defibrillators permit postcardioversion transthoracic external pacing. Malignant ventricular arrhythmias after cardioversion are a particular concern in the presence of digitalis toxicity[46] and hypokalemia. If the digoxin level is in the therapeutic range, this risk is not significantly increased.[47] The defibrillation threshold may be increased in the presence of other antiarrhythmic agents, especially amiodarone, quinidine, phenytoin, and flecainide.[48–50] Bretylium and probably lidocaine do not increase this threshold.

Special considerations exist for patients with permanent pacemakers who require cardioversion or defibrillation. The electrode paddles or patches should be placed as far from the pulse generator as possible, and the energy selected should be the lowest appropriate for the specific arrhythmia. The pacemaker should be noninvasively evaluated after countershock to ensure that

Table 9–3. Indications for Transesophageal Pacing

1. Termination of re-entry supraventricular tachyarrhythmias (atrial flutter, atrial re-entry, sinoatrial re-entry, AV node re-entry, AV reciprocating)
2. Assessment of antiarrhythmic drug efficacy
3. Inducibility of AV reciprocating tachycardia in infants younger than 1 year after neonatal PSVT and no clinical recurrences
4. Minimally invasive determination of accessory pathway properties in Wolff-Parkinson-White syndrome (ERP, shortest pre-excited and average intervals in atrial fibrillation)
5. Emergency atrial pacing for sinus bradycardia
6. Evaluation of PSVT type
7. Moderate term improvement of hemodynamics by creation of 2 : 1 block

AV, atrioventricular; PSVT, paroxysmal supraventricular tachycardia; ERP, effective refractory period.

no changes in pacing mode have occurred. Altamura et al[51] described a significant rise in ventricular pacing threshold, including transient loss of capture in 50% of such patients. In addition, worsening of sensing function was present in a large minority of cases, and two pulse generators required replacement.

Electrical countershock, when possible, should be performed in the postprandial state, and no sooner than 4 hours after the last dose of digoxin. Elective cardioversion should be performed in the intensive care unit or cardiac catheterization laboratory, with an intravenous catheter in place and continuous blood pressure monitoring. Sedation should include anesthetic or hypnotic agents, and someone should be on hand to manage the airway. We prefer the use of methohexital, in 10-mg doses every 30 seconds, until the patient does not respond to his or her name. The incidence of apnea is very low in our experience. The patient is connected to an ECG monitor capable of R-wave synchronization. Before anesthesia, the patient is attached to the electrode patches. The cardioversion threshold is reduced with larger electrodes, and the pediatric-sized electrodes should be restricted to children weighing less than 15 kg. Once R-wave synchronization is ensured, the patient undergoes cardioversion at the first selected dose. If unsuccessful, additional shocks are applied at approximately double the energy until cardioversion has succeeded. Whenever possible, each shock should be separated by at least 2 minutes to reduce myocardial injury. The patient's rhythm should be monitored after successful cardioversion for 2 hours before the patient's return to his or her ward room.

Atrial flutter is the most common arrhythmia requiring elective cardioversion in the pediatric age group. The association of this arrhythmia with sick sinus syndrome requires that back-up pacing be available after cardioversion. Atrial overdrive pacing is our preferred means of conversion of this tachyarrhythmia, but direct current cardioversion is occasionally necessary. An energy level of 0.5 J/kg is usually sufficient to convert atrial flutter, but occasionally this must be increased to as much as 4 J/kg.

If medical therapy fails, atrial fibrillation can only be converted using direct current cardioversion. Sustained atrial fibrillation is almost exclusively a postoperative arrhythmia in the pediatric age range. If it has been present for more than 48 hours or if its duration is unknown, a transesophageal echocardiogram is performed to evaluate the patient for intra-atrial thrombi. If present, and if the patient's clinical status is stable, the patient is placed on warfarin for 3 weeks before cardioversion. This is based on adult experience in which there is a 0.7% risk of thromboembolism after atrial defibrillation.[52] If additional ventricular rate reduction is necessary, diltiazem is generally preferred because it has minimal negative inotropic effects.[53] Children and teenagers who have atrial thrombi probably require maintenance of anticoagulation for several weeks after return of sinus rhythm[54] because of continued atrial stunning. The energy dose required to convert atrial fibrillation begins at 1.0 J/kg, but may not even be successful at 360 J. We have reported efficacy of intracardiac cardioversion for resistant atrial fibrillation in two young adults with complex congenital heart disease by using two decapolar electrode catheters placed along opposite sides of the atrial mass. Cardioversion was accomplished with 5 to 10 J using a biphasic waveform.[55]

AV node re-entry and AV reciprocating tachycardias seldom require countershock, except for the occasional neonate who presents in shock after a long period of undiagnosed PSVT. Even in these patients, adenosine is presently the treatment of choice. Cardioversion using an energy level of 0.25 to 0.5 J/kg is nearly always successful, but doses of up to 1.0 J/kg may be required. In a multicenter investigation of Wolff-Parkinson-White syndrome and PSVT in infants younger than 4 months, cardioversion was successful in 73% of 59 patients.

Ventricular tachycardia in a patient with hemodynamic compromise who is unresponsive to intravenous lidocaine can be successfully terminated with synchronized direct current cardioversion beginning at 0.5 to 1.0 J/kg.

Ventricular fibrillation is very uncommon in children. Among 100 children 18 years of age and younger who suffered sudden death, only 6% had as their terminal rhythm ventricular fibrillation.[1] In all others, the terminal rhythm was a bradycardia. When defibrillation is required, we begin with an energy level of 2.0 J/kg without synchronization. If unsuccessful, urgent consideration of such issues as hypoxia, acidosis, and hypoglycemia must be given. The energy dose is doubled, and the treatment algorithm as defined by pediatric advanced life support is followed.[2]

Treatment Algorithms for Specific Arrhythmias

Figures 9–5 to 9–10 represent suggested algorithms for acute conversion of atrial flutter–atrial re-entry tachycardia, atrial fibrillation, PSVT, junctional ectopic tachycardia, ventricular tachy-

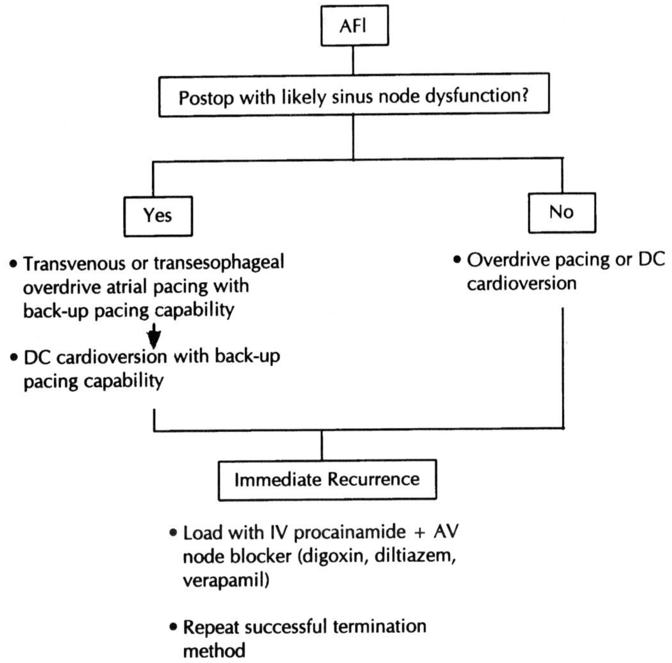

FIGURE 9–5. Suggested algorithm for acute therapy for atrial flutter (AFl). In this and subsequent figures, arrows indicate failure of previous step. Multiple actions, when suggested, are demarcated by dots. (AV, atrioventricular.)

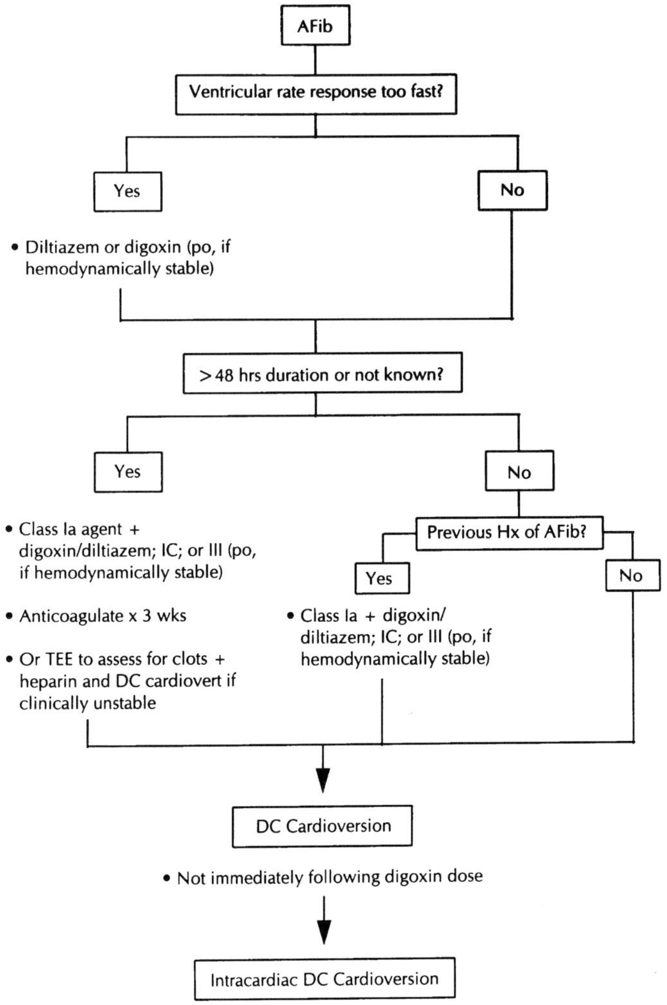

FIGURE 9–6. Suggested treatment algorithm for atrial fibrillation (Afib). (TEE, transesophageal echocardiogram.)

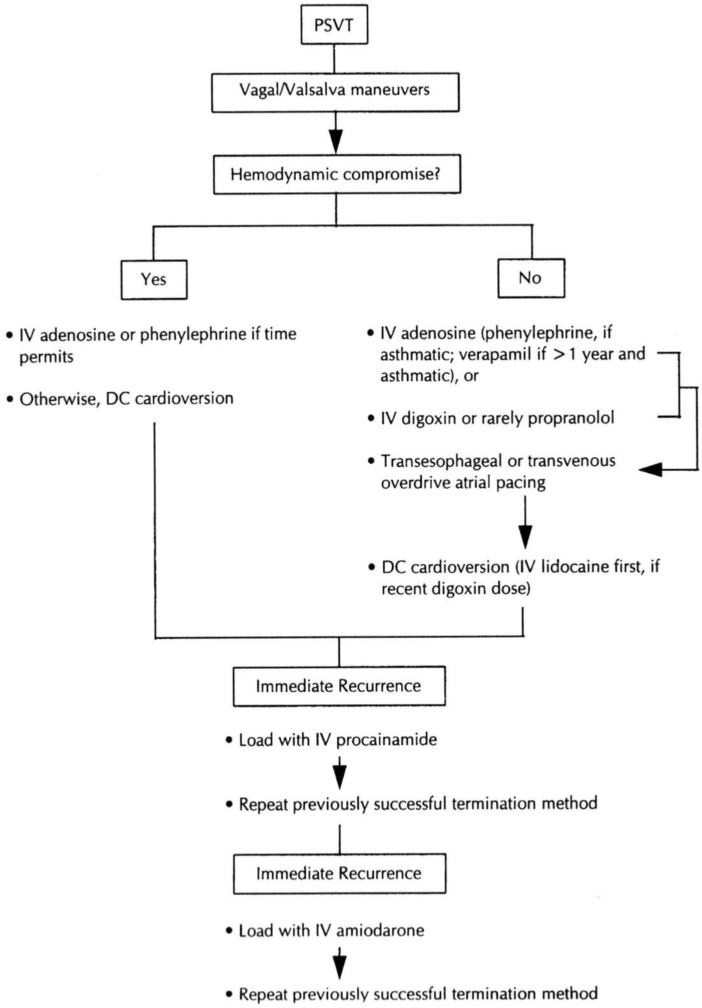

FIGURE 9–7. Suggested algorithm for acute termination of atrioventricular (AV) node requiring forms of paroxysmal supraventricular tachycardia (PSVT), including AV node re-entry tachycardia and AV reciprocating tachycardia.

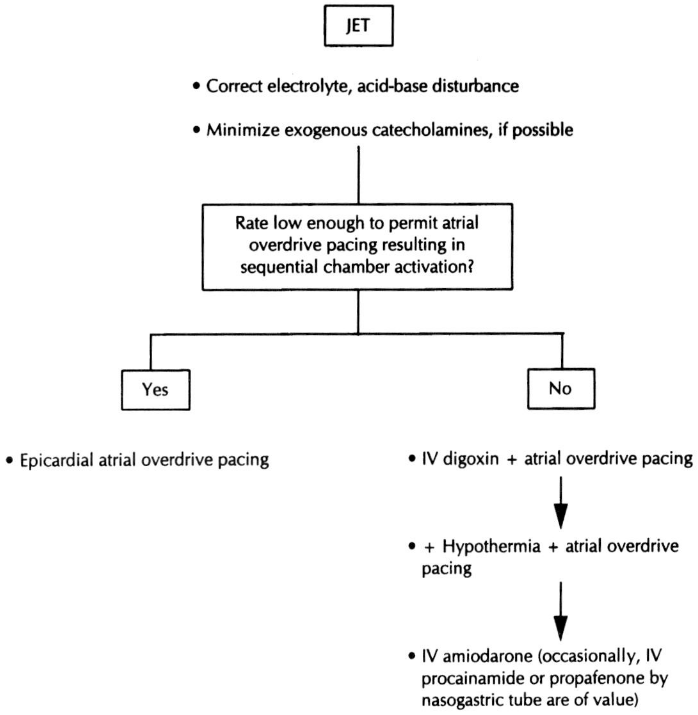

FIGURE 9–8. Suggested algorithm for acute treatment for junctional ectopic tachycardia (JET).

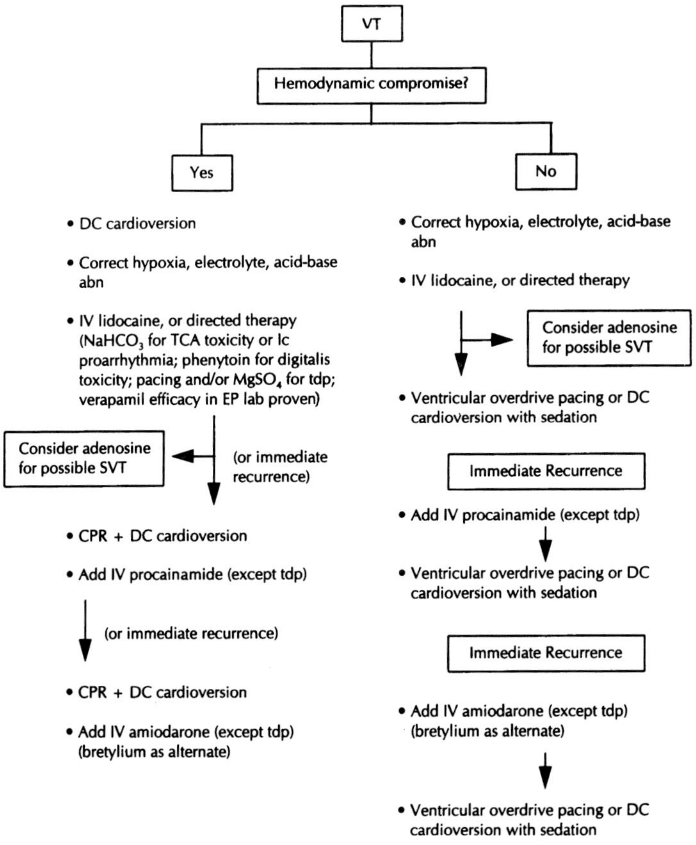

FIGURE 9–9. Suggested algorithm for acute termination of ventricular tachycardia (VT). (TCA, tricyclic antidepressant; tdp, torsades de pointes; abn, abnormalities; EP, electrophysiology; SVT, supraventricular tachycardia; CPR, cardiopulmonary resuscitation.)

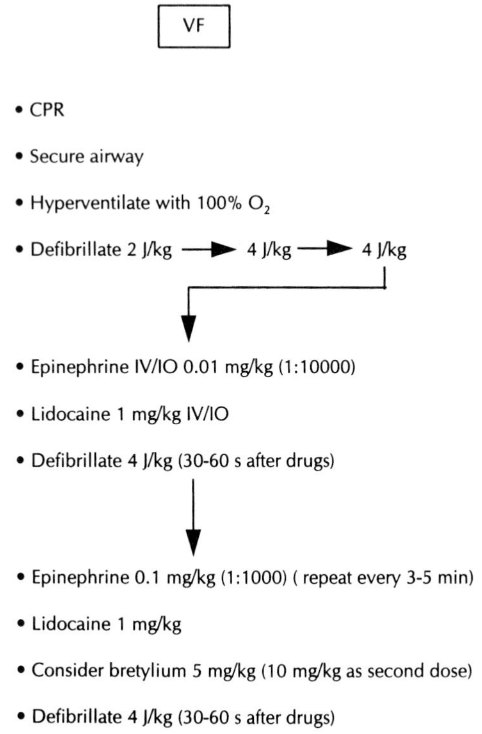

FIGURE 9–10. Suggested algorithm for treatment of ventricular fibrillation (VF) based upon the recommendations of the American Heart Association. (CPR, cardiopulmonary resuscitation; O_2, oxygen.)

cardia, and ventricular fibrillation. In each algorithm, arrows (↓) indicate failure of the previous step to convert the arrhythmia, and some steps require multiple actions, each prefixed by a solid bullet (•). Immediate recurrences of the arrhythmia sometimes occur after successful conversion, and this is also included in some of the algorithms.

REFERENCES

1. Walsh CK, Krongrad E: Terminal cardiac electrical activity in pediatric patients. Am J Cardiol 51:557–561, 1983.
2. American Heart Association: Cardiac rhythm disturbances. In Chameides L, Hazinski, MF (eds): Textbook of Pediatric Advanced Life Support 1994, 7-1–7-12.
3. Marcus FI: Use and toxicity of digitalis. Heart Disease and Stroke 1:27–31, 1992.
4. Dauchot P, Gravenstein JS: Effects of atropine on the electrocardiogram in different age groups. Clin Pharmacol Ther 12:274–280, 1971.
5. Fullerton DA, St. Cyr JA, Clarke DR, et al: Bezold-Jarisch reflex in postoperative pediatric cardiac surgical patients. Ann Thorac Surg 52:534–536, 1991.
6. Zoll PM: Resuscitation of the heart in ventricular standstill by external electrical stimulation. N Engl J Med 248:768–771, 1952.
7. Beland MJ, Hesslein PS, Finlay CD, et al: Noninvasive transcutaneous cardiac pacing in children. Pacing Clin Electrophysiol 10:1262–1270, 1987.
8. Quan L, Graves JR, Dinder DR, et al: Transcutaneous cardiac pacing in the treatment of out-of-hospital pediatric cardiac arrests. Ann Emerg Med 21:905–909, 1992.
9. Taylor S: Temporary pacing in children. In Gillette PC, Zeigler VL (eds): Pediatric Cardiac Pacing, Armonk, NY, Futura, 1995, p 118.
10. Waldo AL: Diagnosis and Treatment of Cardiac Arrhythmias Following Open Heart Surgery. Mount Kisco, NY, Futura, 1980.
11. Yabek SM, Bechara FA, Berman W, et al: Use of atrial epicardial electrodes to diagnose and treat postoperative arrhythmias in children. Am J Cardiol 46:285–289, 1980.
12. Belardinelli L, Isenberg G: Isolated atrial myocytes: Adenosine and acetylcholine increase potassium conductance. Am J Physiol 244(Heart Circ Physiol 13):H734–H737, 1983.
13. West GA, Belardinelli L: Correlation of sinus slowing and hyperpolarization caused by adenosine in sinus node. Pflugers Arch 403:75–81, 1985.
14. Song Y, Thecford S, Lerman BB, Belardinelli L: Adenosine-sensitive afterpolarizations and triggered activity in guinea pig ventricular myocytes. Circ Res 70:743–753, 1992.
15. Shryock JC, Boykin MT, Hill JA, Belardinelli L: A new method of sampling blood for measurement of plasma adenosine. Am J Physiol 258(4, Pt 2):H1232–H1239, 1990.
16. Moser GH, Schrader J, Deussen A: Turnover of adenosine in plasma of human and dog blood. Am J Physiol 256:C799–C806, 1989.
17. Overholt ED, Rheuban KS, Gutgesell HP, et al: Usefulness of adenosine for arrhythmias in infants and children. Am J Cardiol 61:336–340, 1988.
18. Clarke B, Till J, Rowland E, et al: Rapid and safe termination of supraventricular tachycardia in children by adenosine. Lancet 1:299–301, 1987.
19. Till J, Shinebourne EA, Rigby ML, et al: Efficacy and safety of adenosine in the treatment of supraventricular tachycardia in infants and children. Br Heart J 62:204–211, 1989.
20. Rossi AF, Steinberg LG, Kipel G, et al: Use of adenosine in the management of perioperative arrhythmias in the pediatric cardiac intensive care unit. Crit Care Med 20:1107–1111, 1992.
21. Sellers TN, Kirchhoffer JB, Modesto TA: Adenosine: A clinical experience and comparison with verapamil for the termination of supraventricular tachycardias. In Pelleg A, Michelson EL, Dreifus LS (eds): Cardiac Electrophysiology and Pharmacology of Adenosine and ATP: Basic and Clinical Aspects. New York: Alan R. Liss, 1987, pp 283–299.
22. Lerman BB, Belardinelli L, West GA, et al: Adenosine-sensitive ventricular tachycardia: Evidence suggesting cyclic AMP-mediated triggered activity. Circulation 74:270–280, 1986.
23. DiMarco JP, Miles W, Akhtar M, et al: Adenosine for paroxysmal supraventricular tachycardia: Dose ranging and comparison with verapamil in placebo-controlled, multicenter trials. Ann Intern Med 113:104–110, 1990.
24. Wesley RC Jr, Turnquest P: Torsades de pointes after intravenous adenosine in the presence of prolonged QT syndrome. Am Heart J 123:794–796, 1992.
25. Coumel P, Fidelle J: Amiodarone in the treatment of cardiac arrhythmias in children: One hundred thirty-five cases. Am Heart J 100:1063–1069, 1980.
26. Garson A Jr, Gillette PC, McVey P, et al: Amiodarone

treatment of critical arrhythmias in children and young adults. J Am Coll Cardiol 4:749–755, 1984.
27. Figa FH, Gow RM, Hamilton RM, Freedom RM: Clinical efficacy and safety of intravenous amiodarone in infants and children. Am J Cardiol 74:573–577, 1994.
28. Perry JC, Knilans TK, Marlow D, et al: Intravenous amiodarone for life-threatening tachyarrhythmias in children and young adults. J Am Coll Cardiol 22:95–98, 1993.
29. Butto F, Dunnigan A, Overholt ED, et al: Transesophageal study of recurrent atrial tachycardia after atrial baffle procedures for complete transposition of the great arteries. Am J Cardiol 57:1356–1362, 1986.
30. Gallagher JJ, Smith WM, Kasell J, et al: Use of the esophageal lead in the diagnosis of mechanisms of reciprocating supraventricular tachycardia. Pacing Clin Electrophysiol 3:440–451, 1980.
31. Schuchard GH, Tristani FE: A new use of the esophageal lead: Continuous telemetry monitoring. Am Heart J 111:1007–1009, 1986.
32. Schnittger I, Rodriquez I, Winkle RA: Esophageal electrocardiography: A new technology revives and old technique. Am J Cardiol 57:604–607, 1986.
33. Kienzle MG: Parasympathetic influence in cardiac electrophysiology. In Podrid PJ, Kowey PR (eds): Cardiac Arrhythmia: Mechanisms, Diagnosis and Management. Baltimore, Williams & Wilkins, 1995, pp 168–181.
34. Bisset GS, Gaum WE, Kaplan S: The ice bag: A new technique for interruption of supraventricular tachycardia. J Pediatr 97:593–595, 1980.
35. Waldo AL, McLean WAH, Karp RB, et al: Entrainment and interruption of atrial flutter with atrial pacing: Studies in man following open heart surgery. Circulation 56:737–745, 1977.
36. German LD, Strauss HC: Electrical termination of tachyarrhythmias by discrete pulses. Pacing Clin Electrophysiol 7:514–521, 1984.
37. Campbell R, Dick M, Jenkins J, et al: Atrial overdrive pacing for conversion of atrial flutter in children. Pediatrics 75:730–736, 1985.
38. Ward DE, Camm AJ, Spurrell RAJ: The response of regular re-entrant supraventricular tachycardia to right heart stimulation. Pacing Clin Electrophysiol 2:586–595, 1979.
39. Olshansky B, Okumura K, Hess PG, et al: Use of procainamide with rapid atrial pacing for successful conversion of atrial flutter to sinus rhythm. J Am Coll Cardiol 11:359–364, 1988.
40. Dunnigan A, Benson DW, Benditt DG: Atrial flutter in infancy: Diagnosis, clinical features, and treatment. Pediatrics 75:725–729, 1985.
41. Benson DW, Sanford M, Dunnigan A, et al: Transesophageal atrial pacing threshold: Role of inter-electrode spacing, pulse width and catheter insertion depth. Am J Cardiol 53:63–76, 1984.
42. Porter CJ: Premature atrial contractions and atrial tachyarrhythmias. In Gillette PC, Garson A Jr (eds): Pediatric Cardiac Arrhythmias: Electrophysiology and Pacing. Philadelphia, WB Saunders 1990, pp 328–359.
43. Eysmann SB, Marchlinski FE, Buxton AE, et al: Electrocardiographic changes after cardioversion of ventricular arrhythmias. Circulation 73:73–81, 1986.
44. Pauletto P, Scannapieco G, Compostella L, et al: Myocardial damage after d.c. countershock: Myoglobin and ck-mb radioimmunoassay evaluation. Acta Cardiol 39:115–120, 1984.
45. Geddes LA, Niebauer MJ, Babbs CF: Fundamental criteria underlying the efficacy and safety of defibrillating current waveforms. Med Biol Eng Comput 23:122–130, 1985.
46. Lown B, Kleiger R, Williams BJ: Cardioversion and digitalis drugs: Changed threshold to electric shock in digitalized animals. Circ Res 17:519–531, 1965.
47. Mann DL, Maisel AS, Atwood E, et al: Absence of cardioversion-induced ventricular arrhythmias in patients with therapeutic digoxin levels. J Am Coll Cardiol 5:882–890, 1985.
48. Babbs CF, Yim GKW, Whistler SJ, et al: Elevation of ventricular defibrillation thresholds in dogs by antiarrhythmic drugs. Am Heart J 98:345–350, 1979.
49. Tacker WA Jr, Niebauer MJ, Babbs CF, et al: The effect of new antiarrhythmic drugs on defibrillation threshold. Crit Care Med 8:177–180, 1980.
50. Van Gelder IC, Crijns HJGM, Van Gilst WH, et al: Effects of flecainide on the atrial defibrillation threshold. Am J Cardiol 63:112–114, 1989.
51. Altamura G, Bianconi L, Lo Bianco F, et al: Transthoracic DC shock may represent a serious hazard in pacemaker dependent patients. Pacing Clin Electrophysiol 18:194–198, 1995.
52. Kinch JW, Davidoff R: Prevention of embolic events after cardioversion of atrial fibrillation. Current and evolving strategies (review). Arch Intern Med 155:1353–1360, 1995.
53. Salerno DM, Dias VC, Kleiger RE, et al: Efficacy and safety of intravenous diltiazem for treatment of atrial fibrillation and atrial flutter. The diltiazem atrial fibrillation/flutter study group. Am J Cardiol 63:1046–1051, 1989.
54. Missault L, Jordaens L, Gheeraert P, et al: Embolic stroke after unanticoagulated cardioversion despite prior exclusion of atrial thrombi by transesophageal echocardiography. Eur Heart J 15:1279–1280, 1994.
55. Cooper RAS, Johnson EE, Kanter RJ, et al: Internal cardioversion in two patients with atrial fibrillation refractory to external cardioversion. Pacing Clin Electrophysiol 19:872–875, 1996.
56. Walsh CK, Krongrad E: Terminal cardiac electrical activity in pediatric patients. Am J Cardiol 51:557–561, 1983.
57. Yabek SM, Bechara FA, Berman W, et al: Use of atrial epicardial electrodes to diagnose and treat postoperative arrhythmias in children. Am J Cardiol 46:285–289, 1980.

CHAPTER 10

CATHETER AND SURGICAL ABLATION THERAPIES

Christopher L. Case, Ronald J. Kanter, Fred A. Crawford, Jr, and Paul C. Gillette

THE ABLATION REVOLUTION

In less than one decade, there has been a revolution in the treatment of arrhythmias in both adults and children. This revolution in arrhythmia therapeutics has been facilitated largely by refinement of catheter ablation techniques, which allows arrhythmias to be diagnosed and "cured" in one session in the catheterization laboratory. This movement toward more definitive ablation therapies has also been spurred by studies that have emphasized the rare yet real potential of proarrhythmia caused by the use of certain antiarrhythmic agents in specific disease processes.[1, 2] Thus, drug therapy of arrhythmias, previously the mainstay of treatment options, has in many circumstances become a second-line therapeutic alternative. The 1990s started with surgical ablation of pediatric arrhythmias being performed for only the most recalcitrant of cases; however, catheter ablation of pediatric rhythm disturbances will become a very common procedure in many pediatric catheterization laboratories.

The purpose of this chapter is to discuss the role of catheter ablation techniques in the treatment of specific pediatric arrhythmias. Data concerning the performance and outcomes of this new procedure are presented to help the practitioner properly place this therapy in management strategies for pediatric arrhythmias. Finally, surgical ablation techniques that are still important for controlling certain pediatric rhythm disturbances are reviewed.

CATHETER ABLATION: WHAT DOES IT INVOLVE?

In its most simple form, catheter ablation is a procedure during which a patient's cardiac conduction system is tested for its ability to sustain an arrhythmia. Once the arrhythmia is diagnosed, its substrate is electrically identified and anatomically localized. Subsequently, a critical component of the arrhythmia's substrate is destroyed using energy delivered through the tip of a catheter. Currently, the energy most commonly used is radiofrequency energy. This energy source has been used for years in the operating room in the form of electrocautery. The catheter ablation procedure is usually performed in conjunction with an invasive electrophysiology study (see Chapter 3). The electrophysiology study identifies and localizes the arrhythmogenic substrate of a pathologic tachycardia. This substrate may be an accessory connection responsible for atrioventricular (AV) reciprocating supraventricular tachycardia (SVT) or Wolff-Parkinson-White (WPW) syndrome; an irritable focus in the atrium or ventricle responsible for an atrial ectopic tachycardia (AET) or ventricular tachycardia (VT); a scar in the atrium or ventricle forming a component of a re-entrant tachycardia circuit (atrial flutter or VT); or an area of slow AV node conduction that is critical for the perpetuation of AV node re-entry tachycardia.

Once the substrate responsible for the child's clinical arrhythmia is identified and localized, the ablation catheter is positioned in very close proximity to the targeted area. This catheter is connected to a radiofrequency generator, which delivers energy. Close contact of the catheter tip to the endocardium is critical as the underlying tissue (substrate) is heated to 50 to 60°C. At this temperature, irreversible cell death and tissue injury ensue. If the catheter is properly placed on the arrhythmogenic substrate and proper contact is maintained during the delivery of energy, the arrhythmogenic substrate will be destroyed.

The catheter ablation procedure usually involves an overnight hospital stay. Catheter ablation is most often performed in children under deep sedation or general anesthesia. The procedure sometimes may be lengthy (average procedure time, between 4 and 6 hours), and adequate anesthesia is a necessity. A type and cross-match for one unit of blood is sometimes performed in complicated cases, but rarely is it necessary to give blood during the catheter ablation procedure. The equipment needed to perform a catheter ablation procedure is similar to that used during an invasive electrophysiology study (see Chapter 3).

In addition, a radiofrequency energy generator is a necessity to perform the ablation procedure. Several radiofrequency units are commercially available. Most generators are capable of monitoring the temperature at the catheter tip during the delivery of energy. To monitor temperature, one must use a catheter that has a temperature-sensing device (thermistor or thermocouple) incorporated into the distal ablation electrode. Monitoring catheter temperature during energy applications can yield valuable information about the stability of the electrode–tissue interface. With good stability, temperatures in the 50 to 60°C range will be recorded. The ability to monitor the temperature of the ablation catheter tip is also important to avoid coagulum formation during the application of energy. Excessive catheter tip temperatures during energy application can result in coagulum production with the possibility of subsequent embolization. Temperature monitoring during energy application with feedback inhibition of excessive energy delivery can mitigate coagulum formation and its associated morbidity.[3]

Many pediatric ablation procedures require obtaining access to the left atrium. This is most often accomplished by performing a transseptal puncture (see Chapter 3). To perform a transseptal puncture safely, biplane fluoroscopy is needed. Biplane fluoroscopy is also an invaluable aid in positioning catheters during complex ablation procedures in patients with congenital heart disease. During many catheter ablation procedures, especially those involving left-sided substrates, the patient is fully anticoagulated using heparin. This anticoagulation is important to mitigate clot formation on catheters introduced into the left side of the heart. Coagulum formation secondary to excessive radiofrequency energy is thought to be decreased with proper anticoagulation. Many laboratories monitor the activated clotting times (ACTs) during the heparinized course of the catheter ablation procedures. The ACT is usually maintained in the range of 300 seconds.

In summary, catheter ablation of most pediatric arrhythmias can be safely performed during a 3- to 4-hour procedure in the context of a 23-hour admission to the hospital. In an experienced, properly equipped pediatric electrophysiology laboratory, the efficacy and simplicity of a catheter ablation procedure make it an attractive alternative to chronic medical therapy in the treatment of many pediatric arrhythmias.

PEDIATRIC ARRHYTHMIAS AMENABLE TO ABLATION

Almost all common pediatric arrhythmias can be treated with catheter ablation. Each common pediatric arrhythmia substrate is individually discussed next. Perhaps the best information source concerning ablation of specific pediatric arrhythmias is provided by the data base from the pediatric ablation registry. This registry was started in January 1991 by the Pediatric Electrophysiology Society, and it compiles data on ablation procedures performed on children from 47 centers. Data from the registry have been published in journal and abstract form, and it is updated every 6 months and presented to registry members.[4–7] All in all, pooled data from the registry allow the pediatric practitioner to track the average changing trends and outcome expectations of this new therapy.

ACCESSORY ATRIOVENTRICULAR CONNECTIONS

The most common sustained SVT in children is secondary to accessory AV connections (ACs). This substrate for SVT can be manifest on the surface electrocardiogram (ECG) and be responsible for WPW syndrome. These pathways can also be "concealed" (not apparent during normal sinus rhythm) and yet still be responsible for AV reciprocating tachycardia. It is safe to say that ACs are the most common substrate for pediatric catheter ablation procedures. During the initial 6 years of the registry, 4135 children underwent catheter ablation procedures for AV reciprocating SVT; 3110 children had accessory pathways and 920 children had AV node re-entry tachycardia. The total registry population during that time period was approximately 5000 children.[7]

The overall acute success rate for accessory connection ablation in the registry is 90%. This success rate is highest for left-sided ACs (95%) followed by septal ACs (87%) and right free wall ACs (86%). Long-term follow-up shows a 3-year freedom of recurrence of 77%. The freedom of recurrence from left-sided ACs was statistically greater when compared with that for septal and right-sided ACs.

The registry data show that the average pediatric procedure time is approximately 4 hours. The time for successful procedures is less than that for unsuccessful procedures. Procedure time is greatly influenced by the "wait time" after the pathway has been ablated. Some laboratories wait up to 1 hour after the "successful" ablation lesion is placed before terminating the procedure. Mitigating fluoroscopy time is also a concern during the pediatric ablation procedure. Over the years of registry data collection, the average fluoroscopy time of the successful ablation procedure has decreased from 60 minutes to 47 minutes. Average fluoroscopy time of unsuccessful registry ablation is unchanged over 6 years (approximately 85 minutes).[7]

ACs are destroyed at the point that they cross the AV groove. In the past, the cornerstone of successful surgical ablation therapies involved interruption of the accessory connection at the AV groove by incision or cryoablation techniques. In the catheterization laboratory, the initial step in the ablation procedure involves mapping the AC's location. To accomplish this, the ablation catheter is placed along the AV groove and electrograms are displayed. The atrial end of the AC can be localized by finding the earliest atrial activation or shortest ventriculoatrial (VA) interval during reciprocating tachycardia (Fig. 10–1A and B). Alternatively, one can pace the ventricle and map retrograde conduction in the same manner (recording earliest atrial activation or shortest VA intervals); however, when using ventricular pacing to map AC location, care must be taken to avoid fusion through the AV node and the pathway, which can confound mapping accuracy. Alternatively, if the pathway has manifest pre-excitation, the ventricular end of the pathway can be mapped in sinus rhythm or with atrial pacing to maximize pre-excitation. When mapping the ventricular end of the pathway, the earliest ventricular signal or shortest AV interval localizes the pathway location (Fig. 10–2A and B). Other electrogram characteristics that may help in localizing AC position include electrogram complexity and the presence of pathway potentials. Sometimes these factors are more important than measured intervals in the exact localization of AC position.

Catheter manipulation techniques for AC mapping and energy delivery may vary. For right-sided ACs, the AV groove is approached via a catheter introduced up the inferior vena cava and inserted on the atrial side of the tricuspid annulus (see Fig. 10–2B). Some physicians use a long sheath with a variable curve to stabilize the catheter. Occasionally, the catheter is introduced into the right ventricle, and the tip is turned upward under the tricuspid annulus. Anterior septal and midseptal ACs are usually approached from the atrial side of the annulus. Posterior septal ACs sometimes involve delivering energy in the mouth of the coronary sinus (Fig. 10–3). The posterior septum is a very complex structure, and pathways in this area may also necessitate a right or left ventricular approach.

The most meaningful variation in pediatric catheter ablation techniques involves the approach to left-sided accessory connections. In general, the left AV groove can be approached via the atrium or retrograde via the ventricle. Access to the atrial side of the left annulus usually involves placing the catheter across a patent foramen ovale or performing a transseptal puncture (see Fig. 10–1B). Alternatively, access to the left AV annulus via the left ventricle involves coursing a retrograde transarterial catheter up the femoral artery and across the aortic valve, and looping the catheter in the left ventricular cavity to place the catheter tip under the mitral apparatus (Fig. 10–4).

There are theoretical advantages for each approach to pediatric left-sided ACs. According to the registry, 60% of left-sided ACs in children are approached via the atrium. This is due to size limitation, wherein the pediatric arterial system, aortic valve, mitral valve, and left ventricle may be more susceptible to injury from retrograde catheter manipulation. In contrast, the pediatric atrium, even in the smallest of patients, can accommodate most catheter sizes and curves to address all left-sided ACs.

The disadvantage of the left-sided atrial approach is that catheter stability may be more problematic. AC insertion on the atrial side of the annulus may be more diffuse than on the ventricular side of the mitral annulus. Energy applications on the atrial side may have to be more extensive. Some laboratories believe that the transseptal procedure is a drawback to using a transatrial approach. In reality, in a normal heart with biplane fluoroscopy, the transseptal procedure is very safe if performed by an experienced operator. Most pediatric laboratories are well versed in the transseptal approach; however, adult laboratories are more apt to favor a retrograde approach.

The question of the arrhythmogenicity of radiofrequency lesions may favor an atrial approach to left-sided ACs. Although well-positioned annular lesions delivered via the atrium or ventricle will injure tissues on both sides of the annulus, some

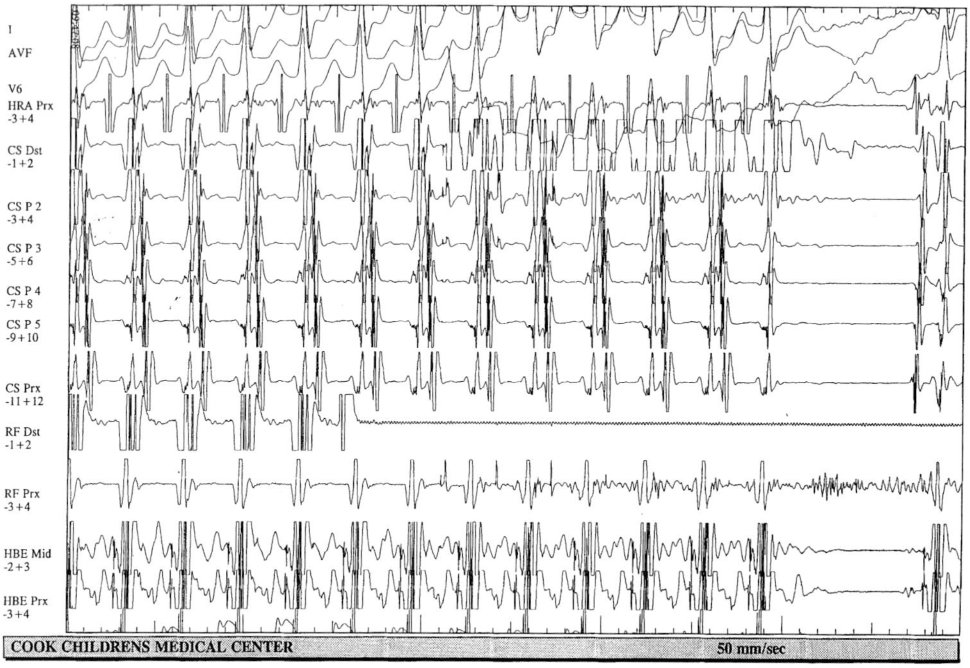

A

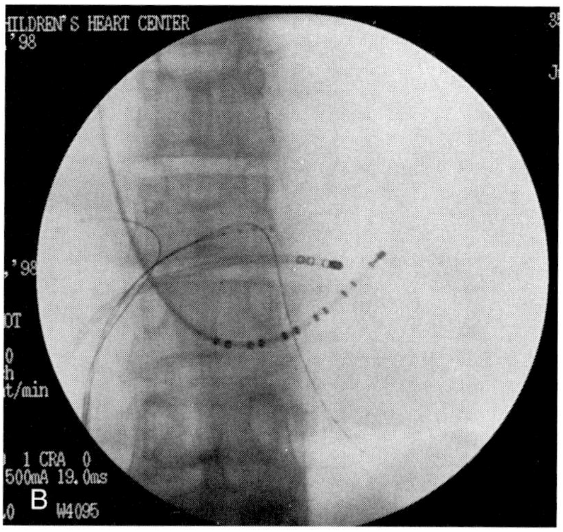

B

FIGURE 10–1. *A*, Orthodromic supraventricular tachycardia successfully terminated with radiofrequency energy. From top to bottom: Surface electrocardiogram leads I, aVF, and V_6 with electrograms from the following: high right atrium, coronary sinus (CS; distal through proximal), radiofrequency catheter (distal and proximal), and His bundle (HBE; mid and proximal). Note the short ventriculoatrial interval as demonstrated on the electrogram from the distal radiofrequency (RF) electrode. Also the tachycardia is terminated very quickly in the retrograde limb. *B*, Catheter positions corresponding to the electrograms displayed in *A*. The RF catheter is positioned along the left AV groove via transseptal puncture.

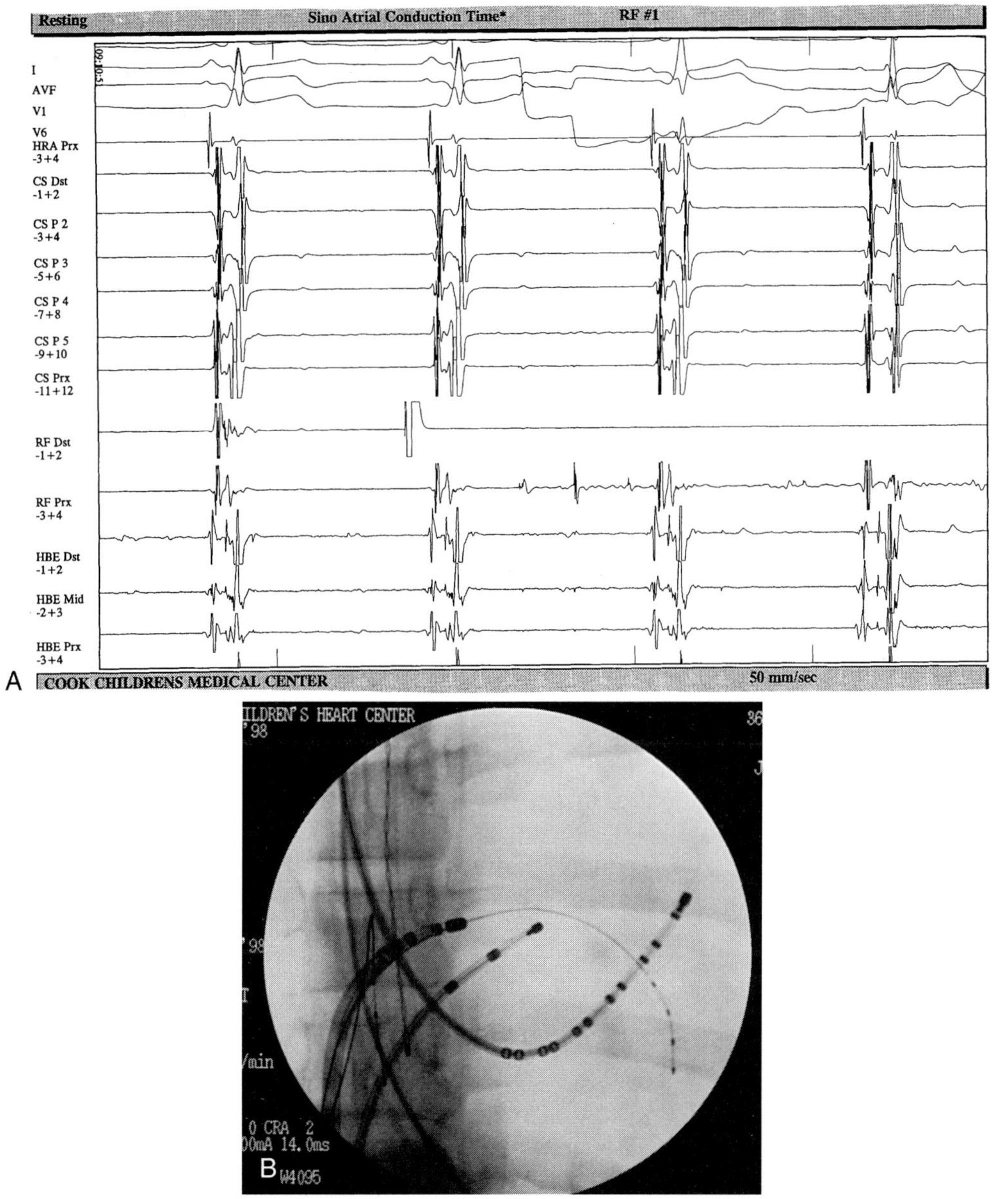

FIGURE 10–2. *A*, Successful ablation of Wolff-Parkinson-White syndrome. From top to bottom: Surface electrocardiogram (ECG) leads I, aVF, V_1 and V_6 and electrograms from the following: high right atrium, coronary sinus (CS; distal through proximal), radiofrequency (RF) catheter (distal and proximal electrodes), and His bundle (HBE; distal, mid, proximal). The electrogram recorded from the distal RF electrode during the first beat exhibits a short atrioventricular interval with a possible pathway potential. Note that the surface ECG changes two beats after RF energy application with disappearance of the delta wave. *B*, Catheter positions corresponding to the electrograms displayed in *A*. Note that the RF catheter is placed on the atrial side of the tricuspid valve via the inferior vena cava.

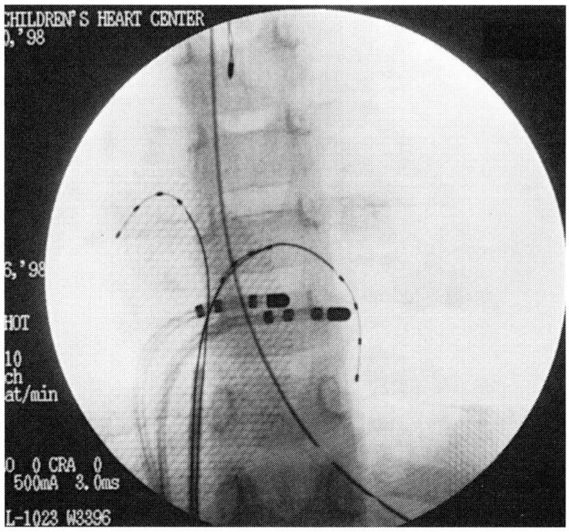

FIGURE 10–3. Catheter position exhibiting radiofrequency (RF) energy delivery in the mouth of the coronary sinus.

radiofrequency lesions do "miss the mark." In view of the concern of the arrhythmogenicity of these lesions, theoretically, it seems better to minimize direct ventricular damage, which may result in more associated morbidity. To optimize success for left-sided AC ablation, it is best to be proficient in multiple approaches. Although the transatrial approach is probably the best and most frequently used technique for ablating left-sided pediatric ACs, certain pathways are best

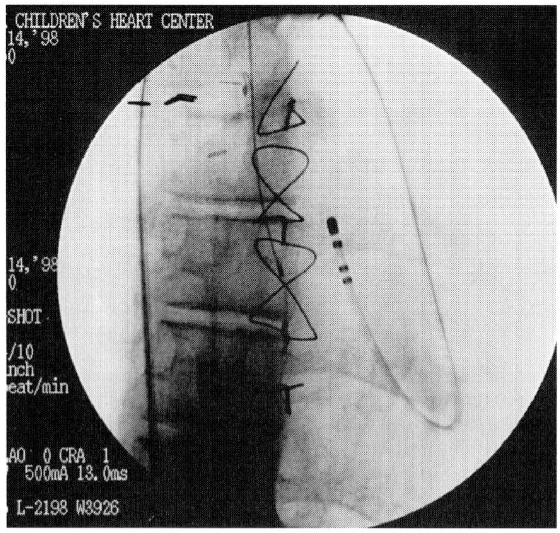

FIGURE 10–4. Demonstration of the retrograde approach to ablation of a left-sided accessory connection. The catheter is introduced via the aortic valve and turned upward in the ventricle with the tip positioned on the ventricular side of the mitral annulus.

approached by a very specific technique. Crossing over from one approach (atrial, via the coronary sinus, or retrograde) to another approach can maximize success rate.[8]

The complication rate from catheter ablation techniques in children is 7.8%, as compiled by the registry; 3.1% of these complications are major, including second- or third-degree AV block (45/5782 cases), perforation (40/5782 cases), emboli (13/5782 cases), and pneumothorax (10/5782 cases). There have been six procedure-related deaths, giving approximately a 0.1% mortality rate.

The issue of operator experience is very important when deciding when, how, and who to ablate an accessory connection in a pediatric patient. For virtually every ablation outcome measurement (i.e., ablation success rate, fluoroscopy time, procedure length, and complication rate), operator experience is important. This fact has been highlighted by registry data[5] as well as by a study at a single institution with only two operators.[9] The latter study showed that a plateau for success rate was achieved only after 70 cases. There are some patients with accessory connections who do seem to present a greater challenge to ensure success and avoid complication. Patients with congenital heart disease and AC-mediated SVT can be especially challenging. In the registry data, the patients with concomitant congenital heart disease constitute about 10% of the ablation population. Tachycardias in these patients may be particularly difficult to ablate because of anatomic variations, limited vascular access, and hemodynamic instability during tachycardia. In the registry data, many of these patients have Ebstein's anomaly or ventricular inversion.

Children who are small also pose problems for accessory pathway ablation, especially in terms of complication rate. Catheter ablation is more problematic in small children and infants; however, there are infants and small children in whom AC-mediated tachycardia can occasionally cause significant morbidity and even mortality. Therefore, catheter ablation in this population is sometimes a necessity. Some centers do have extensive experience in catheter ablation of small children, and referral to one of these centers may be indicated.[10]

ATRIOVENTRICULAR NODE RE-ENTRY TACHYCARDIA

AV nodal re-entry tachycardia (AVNRT) is an important cause of SVT in children of school age and older, and rarely may occur in children younger than 2 years. It is nearly as prevalent as AV reciprocating tachycardia in older teenagers[11] and is the most common cause of SVT in adults. Since Moe et al demonstrated in dogs[12] and Wit et al demonstrated in humans[13] the existence of functional duality of AV nodal conduction, the possibility of an anatomic separation of inputs to the compact AV node has been entertained. We now know that the occurrence of AVNRT depends on different conduction and refractoriness characteristics among two or more such anatomic inputs (and outputs). Our understanding of anatomic and functional correlates of the AV node has been greatly enhanced by radiofrequency ablation techniques for AVNRT, atrial fibrillation, atrial flutter, septal accessory pathways, and foci of AET.

Anatomy

On the basis of histologic examinations, atrial myocardium is separated from ventricular tissue by a transitional cell zone between atrial myocardium and the compact AV node (containing so-called AN cells), the compact AV node itself (containing N cells), and the bundle of His. These tissues are contained within the triangle of Koch, an anatomic region that has as its anterosuperior apex the central fibrous body; the anterior-to-anteroinferior side, the tricuspid annulus; the posterior-to-posteroinferior side, the tendon of Todaro; and the posteroinferior base, a perpendicular line from the tricuspid annulus to the coronary sinus (Fig. 10–5). In an adult, the distance from the central fibrous body to the nearest edge of the coronary sinus ostium is 17 ± 3 mm, and from the tricuspid valve to the nearest edge of the coronary sinus ostium measures 13 ± 3 mm.[14] The compact node lies inferoposterior to the central fibrous body just off of the tricuspid annulus and within the septum itself; it measures 6 mm in length and 3.5 mm in width in an adult. These dimensions are all roughly one half as large in a 5-year-old child.

Cellular electrophysiologic techniques have shown distinctive characteristics of the AN cell and N cell with gradual transition from one cell zone to another in the mammalian species studied. There are at least two functionally distinct regions of the AN zone in humans: the rapidly conducting "fast pathway" (also referred to as the β zone) and the "slow pathway" (α zone). Sung et al[15] demonstrated that the fast and slow AV node pathways have distinct anatomic atrial insertions during retrograde conduction in humans with dual AV nodal pathways. The fast AV node pathway is located just posterior to the His bundle recording site, and the slow AV node pathway is located posterior and inferior to the compact node, between the coronary sinus ostium and the tricuspid annulus. Jazayeri et al[16] popularized the artificial division of the tricuspid annulus into six regions—posterior (P_1, P_2), midseptal (M_1, M_2), and anterior (A_1, A_2)—to standardize the approach to radiofrequency ablation of AVNRT (Fig. 10–6). In this scheme, most slow inputs to the compact node are in zones P_1, P_2, and M_1. Retrograde and antegrade fast pathway inputs to the atrium are in zones A_1 or A_2 in 75% of cases, although they may be located in the middle and even the posterior thirds of this region in an important minority.

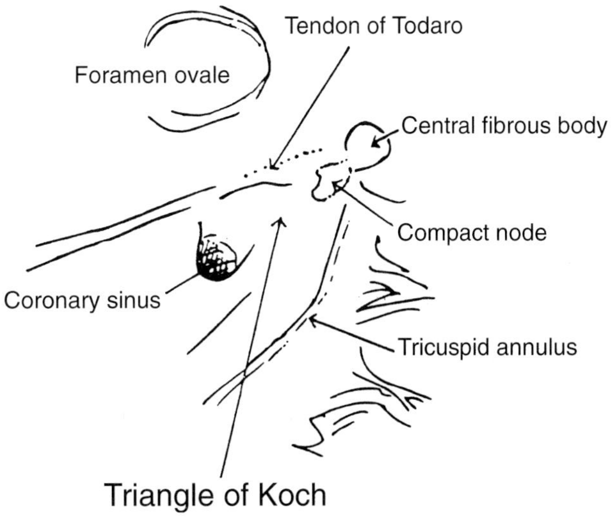

FIGURE 10–5. Schematic of the triangle of Koch, illustrating its borders and the location of the compact node. The right side is anatomically anterior, and the top is anatomically superior. From Sung RJ, Lauer MR, Chun H: Atrioventricular node reentry: Current concepts and new perspectives. Pacing Clin Electrophysiol 17:1414, 1994. Used with permission.

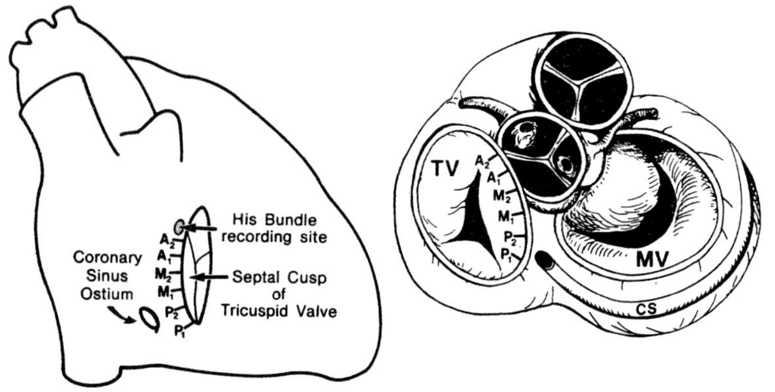

FIGURE 10–6. The anatomic region of the interatrial septum at the level of the tricuspid annulus, which is important for radiofrequency modification of atrioventricular nodal re-entrant tachycardia from the right anterior oblique projection (left) and the base of the heart (right). (MV, mitral valve; TV, tricuspid valve; CS, coronary sinus.) From Akhtar M, Jazayeri MR, Sra J, et al: Atrioventricular nodal reentry: Clinical, electrophysiological, and therapeutic considerations. Circulation 88:292, 1993. Used with permission.

Clinical Electrophysiology

There are two major clinical types of AVNRT: the common type (slow-fast) and the uncommon type (fast-slow). In the common form, antegrade inputs to the compact node are via the slow pathway, and the retrograde limb of the circuit is through the fast pathway (Fig. 10–7). Conversely, in the uncommon form, antegrade conduction is by the fast pathway, and the retrograde limb, which results in atrial activation, is by the slow pathway (Fig. 10–8).

The common form of AVNRT is most readily induced in the electrophysiology laboratory with atrial extrastimuli. According to traditional teaching, the common variety of AVNRT occurs when a critically timed atrial extrastimulus results in antegrade block in the fast pathway and continued conduction down the slow pathway. Specifically, when this atrial extrastimulus (A_1-A_2 interval) is placed 10 ms earlier than the previous A_1-A_2 interval, resulting in an A_2-H_2 interval 50 ms or more than the previous A_2-H_2 interval, dual AV nodal conducting curves are said to be present. If that "jump" in the A_2-H_2 interval is associated with an extra atrial electrogram occurring nearly simultaneous with the H_2 or V_2 electrogram and if that electrogram appears first at the His bundle catheter (or occasionally on time between the His bundle catheter and the coronary sinus ostium pole of that catheter), it is said that a typical AV nodal echo beat has occurred. This represents conduction up a recovered fast pathway, and if it perpetuates in another H-V sequence after the long AH interval, the common variety of AVNRT is the diagnosis; however, in children, the finding of dual AV nodal conduction curves is neither specific for AVNRT nor a necessary observation in children having AVNRT.[17]

The relationship between ventricular and atrial electrograms during the common variety of AVNRT is dependent on the location of the fast pathway and its retrograde conduction time compared with antegrade conduction time through that part of the lower compact AV node and His bundle distal to the fast pathway turnaround point (see Fig. 10–7). By definition, the VA interval (usually from the His bundle catheter) is less than or equal to 60 ms. To measure this, very premature ventricular beats must be introduced during tachycardia from the right ventricular apex to "pull the ventricular electrogram off of the atria."

Pertinent to this discussion and to catheter ablation, intranodal versus partially extranodal origin of the re-entry circuit is an unsettled issue. The concept of a lower common pathway within the AV node bridging antegrade penetration from the previous slow input and retrograde conduction up the next fast output is supported by (1) the occasional observation of block in the His bundle without affecting the tachycardia cycle length; (2) the finding that the HA interval during tachycardia is less than that occurring during ventricular pacing at the AVNRT cycle length; and (3) the observation that a critically placed premature ventricular beat alters the timing of the next His bundle electrogram without affecting the tachycardia (atrial) cycle length.

More difficult to demonstrate is the presence of an upper common pathway bridging the previous retrograde impulse of the fast pathway with the next antegrade impulse down the slow pathway. In Figure 10–9, proof of such an intranodal connection appears in the form of continuation of AVNRT during HA block. Successful treatment of this tachycardia using slow pathway modification in the P_1 and P_2 zones ruled out intra-His bundle re-entry as an alternative explanation in this patient. However, Keim et al were unable to demonstrate an upper common path-

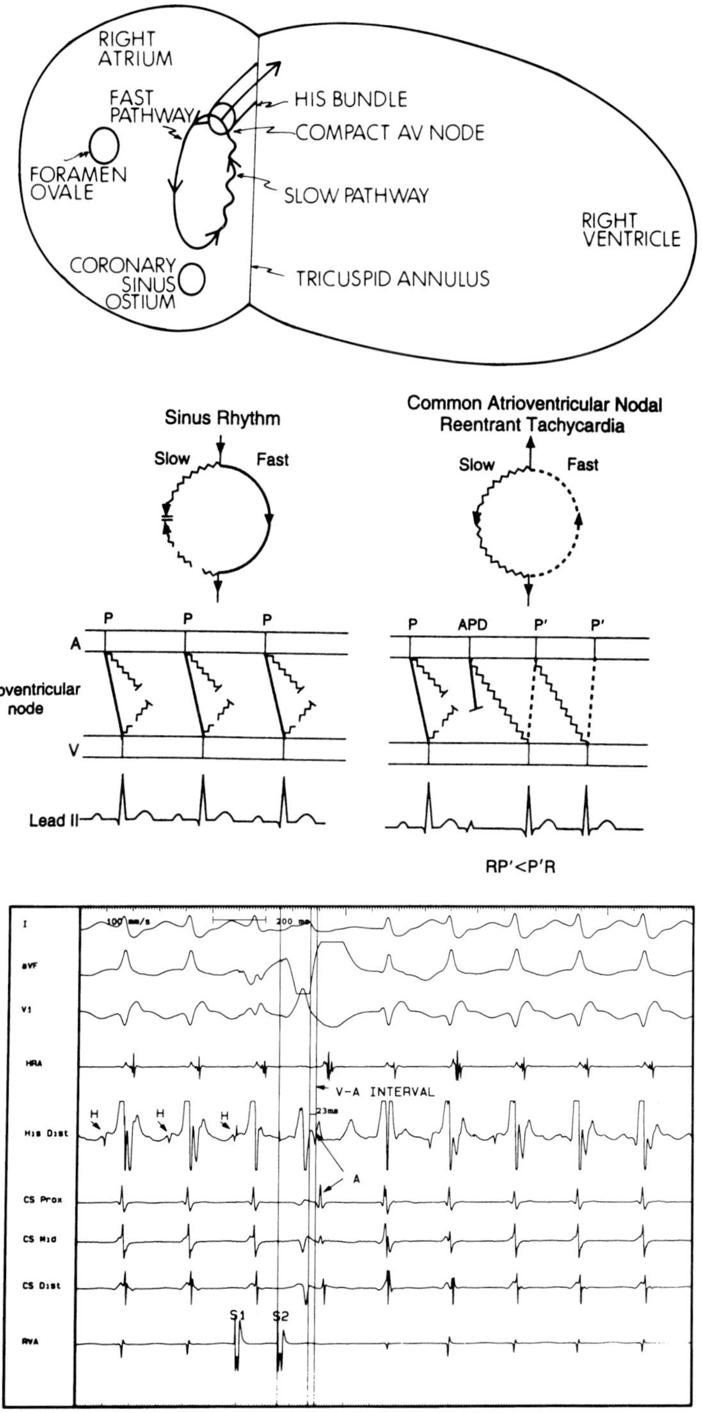

FIGURE 10–7. Common form of atrioventricular nodal re-entrant tachycardia (AVNRT) illustrating a schematic of the proposed anatomic circuit (top) and ladder diagram of sinus rhythm and AVNRT mechanism initiated by an atrial premature depolarization (APD; middle). Bottom panel, The atrial activation sequence during the common type of AVNRT is revealed by the placement of two ventricular premature beats (S_1 and S_2), which "pull the ventricular electrogram off the atrial" from the His bundle catheter channel (His dist) without disturbing the tachycardia (atrial) cycle length. The ventriculoatrial (VA) interval is measured from the expected onset of unaltered ventricular activation to the local atrial electrogram from the His dist channel. (HRA, high right atrium; CS, coronary sinus.) Middle panel from Ganz LI, Friedman PL: Supraventricular tachycardia. N Engl J Med 332:163, 1995. Used with permission.

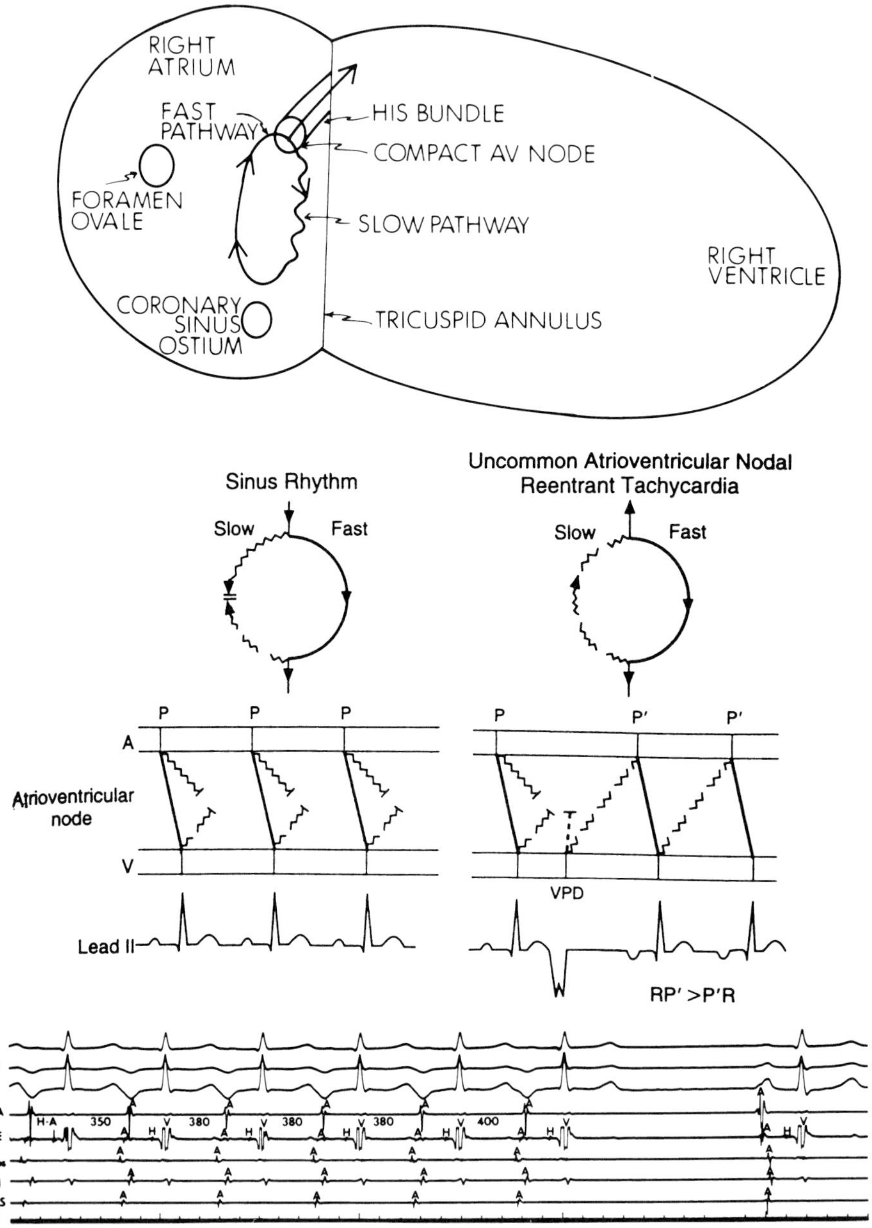

FIGURE 10–8. Uncommon form of atrioventricular nodal re-entrant tachycardia (AVNRT), illustrating a schematic of the proposed anatomic circuit (top) and ladder diagram of sinus rhythm and AVNRT mechanism initiated by a ventricular premature depolarization (VPD; middle). Bottom panel, The uncommon form of AVNRT terminates (during carotid sinus massage) in the retrograde slow pathway after a ventricular (V) electrogram and after a sequence of prolongation of His-to-atrial (HA) intervals. Middle panel from Ganz LI, Friedman PL: Supraventricular tachycardia. N Engl J Med 332:163, 1995. Used with permission. Lower panel from Josephson M (ed): Clinical cardiac electrophysiology: Techniques and interpretations. Philadelphia, Lea & Febiger, 1993. p 224. Used with permission.

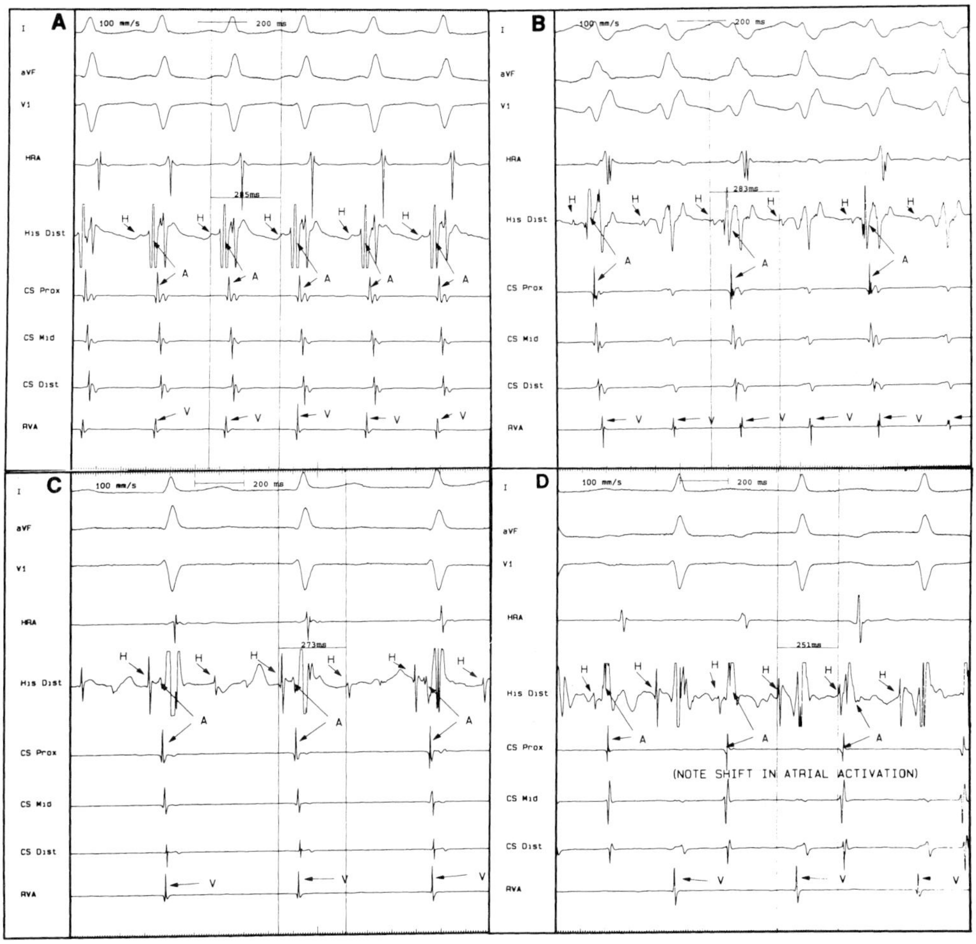

FIGURE 10–9. Four episodes of the common form of atrioventricular nodal re-entrant tachycardia (AVNRT) in an 18-year-old man before radiofrequency ablation. In Panel A, there is 1:1 relationship among atrial (A), His (H), and ventricular (V) electrograms; the earliest atrial electrogram is from the His bundle catheter, and there is a very short ventriculoatrial interval. In Panel B, there are two His bundle and two ventricular electrograms for every atrial electrogram, with the same HV interval as in Panel A and the same atrial activation sequence. In Panel C, there is slight shortening of the HH interval with two His electrograms for each atrial and ventricular electrogram. In Panel D, the HH interval is even shorter, with alternating atrial and ventricular electrograms for every His electrogram. There is also a shift in retrograde atrial activation from the His distal to CS proximal. Tachycardia was rendered noninducible after ablation in the P_1 and P_2 zones. Panels B, C, and D suggest the occurrence of block in an upper common pathway, and Panels C and D suggest the occurrence of block in a lower common pathway. The retrograde atrial exit point is capable of shifting to a more posterior location, as evidenced in Panels C and D. The successful treatment of AVNRT by a slow pathway approach proves that the alternative possibility, His bundle re-entry, was not the mechanism.

way during reversible cooling of portions of the atrial septum between areas of demonstrated fast and slow conduction during surgical ablation of AVNRT.[18]

Before the ablation portion of the procedure, complete data should be obtained, including AVNRT types and functional characteristics of antegrade and retrograde fast and slow pathways. When children are studied under general anesthesia, in particular, induction of AVNRT may not be possible because of sympathetic or parasympathomimetic dependence of antegrade conduction in the slow pathway; hence, isoproterenol and sometimes atropine are required to sustain tachycardia. In older teenagers not studied using general anesthesia, the natural differences between the fast and slow pathways may be problematic. For example, the effective refractory period of the fast pathway is usually more responsive to autonomic influences than the slow pathway. If slow pathway function predominates at rest, isoproterenol may be necessary to preferentially shorten the retrograde refractory period of the fast pathway, and if the fast pathway function predominates, esmolol may preferentially lengthen the antegrade effective refractory period of the fast pathway. AV nodal re-entry tachycardia may only then be inducible. These examples not withstanding, the usual observations include a shorter effective refractory period in the antegrade slow versus fast pathway, allowing "dual AV nodal conduction curves"; a shorter effective refractory period in the retrograde fast versus slow pathway; and an antegrade AV nodal Wenckebach cycle length longer than the AVNRT cycle length.

In summary, the diagnosis of the common variety of AVNRT depends on the induction of re-entry SVT having a VA interval less than 60 ms and with concentric atrial activation. The diagnosis is supported by the observation that induction follows an "A_2-H_2 jump" of greater than or equal to 50 ms, that inductions are dependent on a critical H_1-H_2 interval but not A_1-A_2 interval, and that an adenosine bolus terminates tachycardia after an atrial electrocardiogram, and after a sequence of AH interval increments and VA interval constancy. The differential diagnosis includes atrial re-entry tachycardia emanating from the low anterior or midseptum and having a coincidental short VA interval relationship. In this case, a late premature atrial beat will advance the subsequent His and ventricular electrograms, but in the case of AVNRT, a late premature atrial beat would not be expected to penetrate the tachycardia circuit. AV nodal independence of atrial tachycardia may also be demonstrated pharmacologically.

In most cases of the uncommon (fast-slow) form of AVNRT (see Fig. 10–8), the tachycardia circuit is thought to include antegrade conduction to the compact node and His bundle using the fast pathway and retrograde conduction from the distal turnaround point to atrial breakthrough using the slow pathway. The earliest atrial activation site is usually in the P_1, P_2, or M_1 regions along the tricuspid annulus, but it may exist anywhere in the atrial septum, the posteromedial tricuspid annulus, or for a short distance within the coronary sinus.[19] A 1995 report in adults comparing the fast and slow pathway responses to intravenous adenosine in patients having uncommon versus common forms of AVNRT showed disparate responses inconsistent with the notion that these tachycardias are simple mirror images of one another.[20] During extrastimulus testing, the effective refractory period of the slow pathway in the retrograde direction is typically shorter than that of the fast pathway, and retrograde dual AV nodal function curves may be present. This type of AVNRT is most easily inducible using ventricular extrastimuli. In the antegrade direction, dual AV nodal physiology may not be demonstrated, because antegrade conduction down the fast pathway will persist until refractoriness is reached. Silka suggested that the physiology of AVNRT may evolve as a function of age; the uncommon form is relatively more common in younger children.[17] Both forms may coexist in the same patient.

The uncommon form of AVNRT is one of the long RP interval types of SVT and, before ablation, must be discriminated from the permanent form of junctional reciprocating tachycardia (PJRT), using a decrementally conducting posteroseptal accessory pathway; septal atrial re-entry tachycardia; and low AET. In the case of the PJRT, a relatively late premature ventricular extrastimulus introduced when the His bundle is refractory (50 ms or less before the next expected tachycardia ventricular electrogram) will pre- or postexcite the next atrial electrogram. However, only a very early premature ventricular extrastimulus (at least 100 ms premature) will perturb the next atrial electrogram of the uncommon form of AVNRT. Uncommon AVNRT is favored over septal atrial re-entry tachycardia if retrograde dual AV nodal refractory curves can be demonstrated or if initiation is related to specific H_1-A_2 intervals instead of A_1-A_2 intervals. Termination by vagal maneuvers after the ventricular electrogram is also more likely in the case of uncommon AVNRT (see Fig. 10–8). Atrial automatic tachycardia cannot be terminated by pacing or cardioversion. Single premature extrastimuli given into AET may manifest a reset curve.

Methodology

Once the diagnosis of common variety AVNRT is made, radiofrequency ablation is usually performed during sinus rhythm or during atrial pacing. The favored approach is presently slow pathway modification or ablation rather than fast pathway ablation, although the latter is also described. Ablation should be performed with catheters positioned in the right ventricle (should unintended AV block occur), in the His bundle region, and in the coronary sinus. Atrial pacing during radiofrequency energy delivery is often desirable to ensure that AV conduction persists and that the AH interval is stable once accelerated junctional rhythm is induced by energy application. Such pacing is usually provided from a right atrial catheter. The ablation catheter used has a 4-mm distal electrode and is tip deflectable. Among children undergoing ablation using general anesthesia, ventilation is held during energy delivery to maximize ablation catheter stability. Occasionally, the coronary sinus ostium is directed more anteriorly than usual, such that the coronary sinus catheter interferes with stable placement of the ablation catheter along the posteroseptal tricuspid annulus; thus, in such cases, it should be removed.

The proper catheter location to effect fast pathway ablation appears in Figure 10–10. The catheter is first placed in the His position and withdrawn to a more proximal (actually posterior) and superior location. The atrial electrogram should be at least twice the amplitude of the ventricular electrogram, and the His bundle electrogram should be < 0.1 mV. With clockwise torque, power is applied until first-degree AV block or junctional tachycardia occurs. End points for successful ablation include prevention of AVNRT inducibility and at least prolongation of the retrograde AV nodal effective refractory period. The antegrade AV nodal effective refrac-

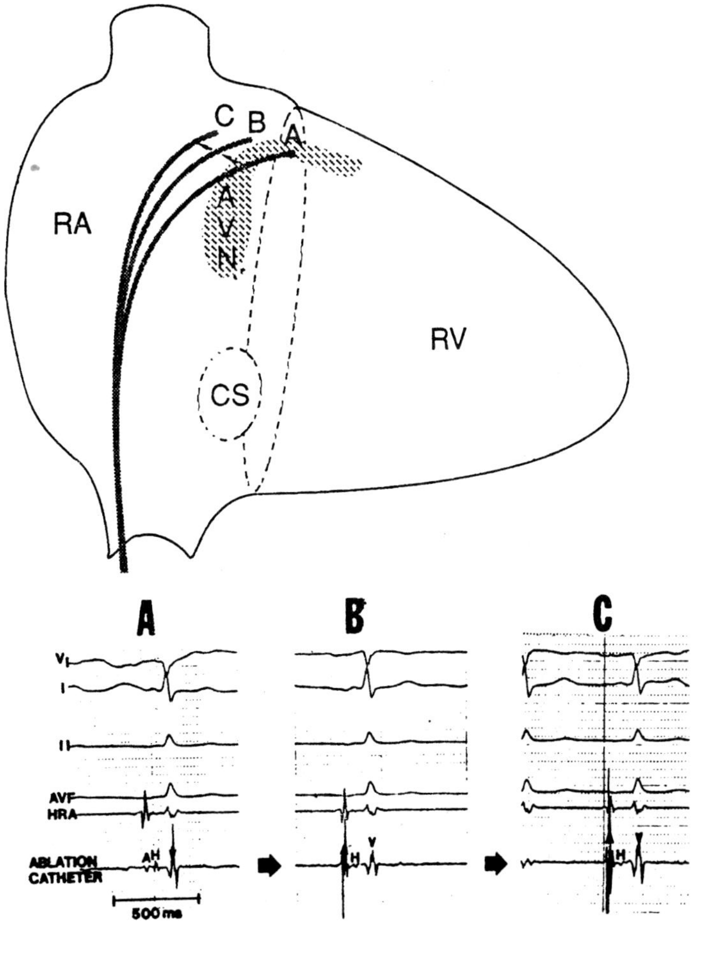

FIGURE 10–10. Schematic of catheter manipulation to perform fast pathway ablation and the electrogram associated with each catheter location. In the diagram of the right anterior oblique projection, the ablation catheter tip is placed at the site of maximal His bundle electrogram (A). At this location, the atrial electrogram is small. As the catheter is positioned more posteriorly and superiorly (B to C), the atrial electrogram increases, and the His bundle and ventricular electrograms diminish in size. At the target site (C), the atrial electrogram is more than twice the amplitude of the ventricular electrogram, and the His bundle electrogram is barely visible. (RA, right atrium, RV, right ventricle; CS, coronary sinus; AVN, atrioventricular node.) From Langberg JL, Harvey M, Calkins H, et al: Titration of power output during radiofrequency catheter ablation of atrioventricular nodal reentrant tachycardia. Pacing Clin Electrophysiol 16:467, 1993. Used with permission.

tory period and Wenckebach cycle length are unaffected. Langberg et al[21] showed that gradual increases in power application resulted in a lower incidence of third-degree AV block than fixed power delivery. Nevertheless, in adults, the incidence of third-degree AV block using this approach is 8 to 23%.[21–23] There are no published data regarding this risk in children, but considering the expected size of the lesions, radiofrequency ablation at this site is considered at least as likely to cause high-grade AV block as it is in adults. Langberg et al[24] also described the occurrence of inducible uncommon AVNRT after incomplete fast pathway ablation in 9 of 88 patients. The clinical significance of this laboratory finding was uncertain.

After successful fast pathway ablation, patients (including children) with multiple slow inputs to the compact node and at least one with retrograde conduction properties are still at risk for the "slow-slow" type of AVNRT. Rigorous provocative pacing maneuvers may be necessary to demonstrate this. Additional ablation of the slow inputs may increase the likelihood of third-degree AV block. The presence of more than one functional slow input to the compact AV node should be suspected in a child who has a long RP, long PR re-entry tachycardia, and concentric atrial activation *or* in a patient with common AVNRT and at least two distinct populations of AH intervals during tachycardia.

Slow pathway ablation and modification are the techniques of choice to treat common variety AVNRT. Slow pathway ablation is said to have been accomplished when (1) the antegrade AV node effective refractory period has been prolonged,[16] (2) dual AV nodal conduction curves, once present, are now absent,[25] and (3) AVNRT of any type that uses the slow pathway is rendered noninducible. Typical AV nodal echo beats are also absent. Retrograde AV nodal conduction properties are usually unaffected. Modification of the slow inputs to the AV node results in noninducibility of common variety AVNRT but with preservation of slow pathway physiology during testing of antegrade conduction properties. Single typical AV nodal echo beats are usually still inducible. This method has been found to be adequate in preventing tachycardia recurrences at a mean follow-up of 17 months (Table 10–1).

This technique may be performed using either anatomic or electrophysiologic guidelines; however, in practice, both approaches are usually used. The ablation catheter is either placed in the His bundle region and flexed posteroinferiorly along the tricuspid annulus or advanced into the posterobasilar right ventricle and pulled back to the tricuspid annulus. In either instance, the target sites are along the tricuspid annulus at the P_2, M_1, or P_1 zones (Fig. 10–11). It is here that a complex atrial electrogram or a low-frequency, low-amplitude atrial electrogram followed by a high-frequency component (the so-called slow pathway potential) may be found (Fig. 10–12).

Data by Hummel et al[26] suggest that the morphology of the slow pathway electrogram is dependent on the direction of atrial activation and does not represent a discrete "pathway." The slow pathway potential serves only as a catheter target, because this potential is present in most individuals and persists after successful slow pathway ablation. The anatomic approach requires catheter manipulation as described previously, but using the uppermost portion of the coronary sinus ostium as the superoinferior level of the tricuspid annulus at which to begin energy delivery. This is roughly equivalent to the P_2 zone, and the ventricular electrogram amplitude is usually at least twice as large as the atrial. Constant clockwise torque on the catheter is necessary to maintain septal contact. A sensitive but relatively nonspecific indication of successful ablation is the occurrence of accelerated junctional rhythm during energy delivery,[27] usually at a rate only slightly faster than the prevailing sinus rate (see Fig. 10–12). A more accelerated junctional rhythm and the occurrence of VA block are useful indicators for pending third-degree AV block

Table 10–1. Atrioventricular (AV) Nodal Function in 31 Children Immediately Before and After Radiofrequency Modification of the Slow Inputs to the AV Node

VARIABLE	SCL	aAVNERP	rAVNERP	aAVNWBCL
Preablation	833 ± 147	298 ± 83	303 ± 93	375 ± 102
Postablation	577 ± 109	288 ± 72	258 ± 34	344 ± 93
Value of P	< 0.001	NS	NS	NS

SCL, sinus cycle length; aAVNERP, antegrade AV nodal effective refractory period; aAVNWBCL, antegrade AV nodal Wenckebach cycle length; rAVNERP, retrograde AV nodal effective refractory period.

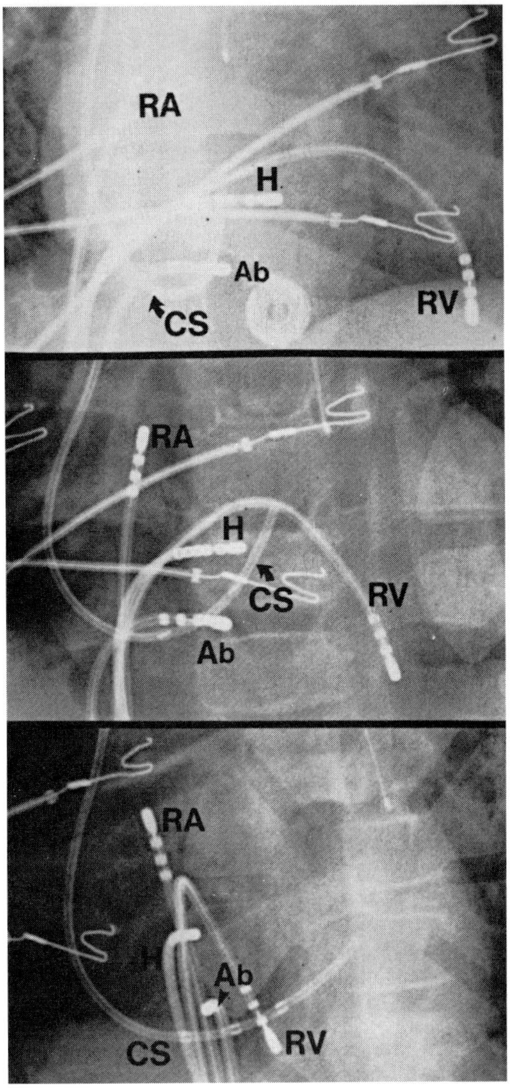

FIGURE 10–11. Right anterior oblique 30° (top), anteroposterior (middle), and left anterior oblique 30° (bottom) projections from a patient having the common type of atrioventricular nodal re-entrant tachycardia, illustrating ablation (Ab) catheter location at the P_2 zone before successful modification of the slow inputs to the atrioventricular node. (RA, right atrium; H, His bundle; RV, right ventricle; CS, coronary sinus.)

and require immediate discontinuation of energy delivery.[28]

Many operators will intermittently pace the atrium during accelerated junctional rhythm to be certain that the AH interval is stable. Some advocates of the anatomic approach have described a "drag technique," whereby the ablation catheter is withdrawn during energy delivery from its tricuspid annular position atrialwise toward the upper rim of the coronary sinus ostium, in effect, transecting the slow AV nodal inputs.[29] During this procedure, nonsustained atrial tachycardia can be expected. Moulton et al were successful in all of their 30 adult clients using this technique, requiring only one to three energy applications.[30] When the two approaches are compared, the slow potential electrogram and anatomic approaches are of equal efficacy.[29]

Our approach relies on slow pathway potential identification and ablation in the P_2 zone, followed by ablation attempts in the P_1, M_1, and then M_2 zones until an energy application occurs, during which there is accelerated junctional rhythm. A total of 30 to 60 seconds of energy delivery is then provided. If still unsuccessful, the coronary sinus is mapped for slow pathway potentials, followed finally by ablation attempts on the atrial side of the tricuspid annulus, anterior to the roof of the coronary sinus ostium. Catheter stabilization in the P_1 and P_2 zones without "falling into" the coronary sinus ostium is difficult to achieve in some patients. This is probably due to the relatively large ostium that the patient with AVNRT tends to have.[31] After each energy application, during which there is an acceptable episode of accelerated junctional rhythm, tachycardia induction is attempted using whatever method was required during the diagnostic portion of the procedure. The persistence of single typical (slow-fast) AV nodal echo beats and dual AV nodal conduction curves are accepted.

Once the diagnosis of the uncommon type of AVNRT is made, slow pathway modification is again the technique of choice. This is usually performed in sinus or atrial paced rhythm, but, unlike common AVNRT, atrial mapping during tachycardia may more precisely identify the earliest atrial breakthrough of retrograde conduction; therefore, analogous to radiofrequency ablation of primary atrial tachycardia, energy may be delivered during tachycardia. Catheter movement toward the compact node and the risk of third-degree AV block when tachycardia abruptly terminates is a hazard of this approach. During the uncommon form of AVNRT, the proper catheter location for ablation may reveal a slow pathway potential preceding the earliest, low-frequency, low-amplitude atrial electrogram.

Results and Follow-Up

The early success rate of radiofrequency ablation for AVNRT among children enrolled by contributing members of the Pediatric Electrophysiology Society was 83% of 76 patients, including 11 of 12 fast pathways and 52 of 64 slow path-

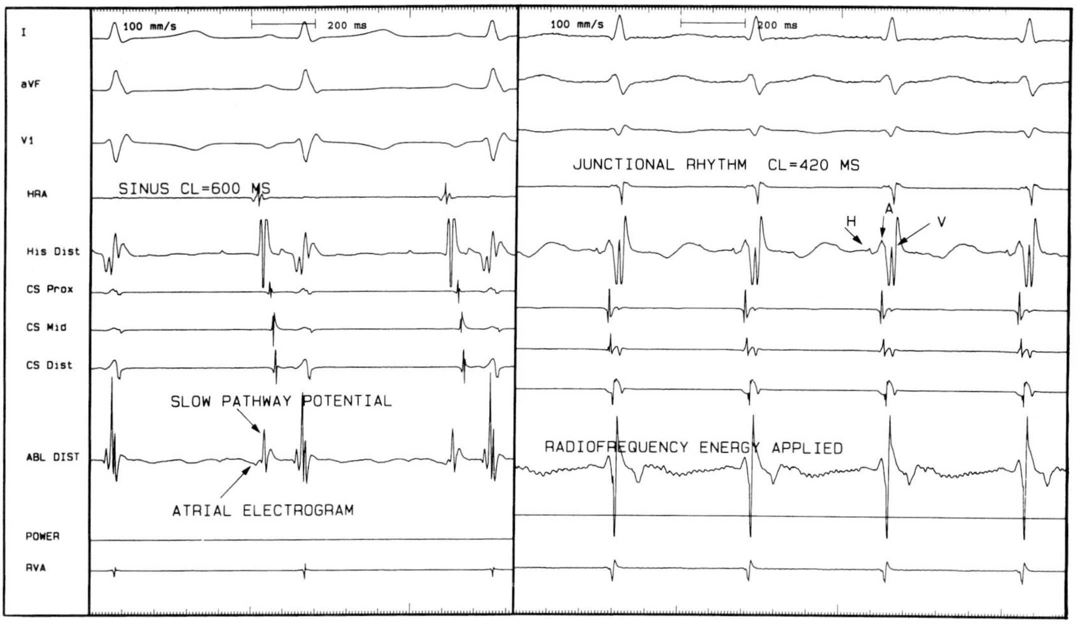

FIGURE 10–12. Electrograms from the same patient as in Figure 10–11, illustrating a so-called slow pathway electrogram at the site of successful energy delivery from the ablation catheter (abl dist, left panel). During energy delivery (right panel), an accelerated junctional rhythm developed with intact retrograde conduction to the atrium. (HRA, high right atrium; CS, coronary sinus.)

ways.[32] In a separate report, Teixiera et al[33] reported the initial experience at the Medical University of South Carolina of radiofrequency ablation of AVNRT in 18 consecutive children (mean age, 13.6 years; range, 8.2–17.9 years), 14 of whom underwent slow pathway modification-ablation. Sixteen patients were successfully treated, 4 of whom had transient second- or third-degree AV block. The average energy used for these procedures was 33 watts (range, 24–50 watts), and the average fluoroscopy time was 29.9 minutes (range, 7–73 minutes). Two patients had late recurrences, both of whom underwent a successful second procedure.

The Duke University experience with children having common variety AVNRT includes 32 consecutive patients (mean age, 12.5 years; range, 4–20 years); only the first underwent fast pathway ablation, and the remainder underwent slow pathway modification. The procedural end points for successful modification included attainment of accelerated junctional rhythm during energy delivery followed by the inability to induce greater than a single AV nodal echo beat during retesting. The immediate pre- and postablation AV nodal conduction characteristics appear in Table 10–1. Antegrade refractoriness properties were unaffected, and there was a trend toward shortening of the retrograde (fast pathway) effective refractory period. There are conflicting reports regarding the postulate that transient vagal denervation to the AV node occurs in adults during this procedure,[34–37] which would be one plausible explanation for this observation. The observed relative sinus tachycardia after the procedure generally persisted for the remainder of the hospitalization (12–18 hours) but was not present at 1 month follow-up.

In Ehlert et al's[37] report of several adults having long-term inappropriate sinus tachycardia after radiofrequency ablation of AVNRT, only the anterior (fast pathway) approach had been used. Only 16 of our patients (50%) had dual AV nodal conduction curves demonstrated by atrial extrastimulus testing: in 11 it was absent during restudy, in 4 it was still present, and in 1 it was only noted during restudy. At procedure conclusion, a 6-year-old child had permanent first-degree AV block and a teenager had transient second-degree AV block. At a mean of 17.5 months (range, 2–44 months) follow-up, there was one recurrence in the third patient studied, which occurred 6 weeks after the procedure. She was also the youngest (4 years old), and during a second ablation attempt, she suffered permanent third-degree AV block requiring pacemaker implantation. The balance between achieving a low recurrence rate and avoiding permanent AV block may be more difficult to achieve in children younger than about 8 years than in adults. Baker et al demonstrated a 7.4% recurrence rate at 20 months follow-up among adults undergoing slow pathway ablation.[38] In that report, dual antegrade AV nodal conduction properties and single AV nodal echo beats had been present at the conclusion of the study in a disproportionately large number of individuals who later had recurrences than in those who had not. The reported incidence of symptomatic second- or third-degree AV block after slow pathway ablation or modification in adults ranges from 0 to 3%.[29, 30, 39, 40]

In a report by Silka et al,[41] immediately after slow pathway modification of common AVNRT, 9 of 18 young patients (mean age, 12.9 years) had inducible AVNRT with 2:1 block, atypical (fast-slow) AVNRT, or sustained accelerated junctional rhythm. This compared with only 2 of 59 adults having unusual forms of AVNRT after ablation in the same laboratory ($p = .01$). Additional applications of radiofrequency energy rendered all pediatric patients noninducible, but common variety AVNRT recurred in 1 and uncommon variety AVNRT occurred in 2 patients at an average of 9.8 months follow-up. The authors concluded that the different response to modification of antegrade conduction of slow pathway fibers in children, compared with adults, suggests differences in anatomic or electrophysiologic substrates that may evolve as a function of age.

ATRIAL ECTOPIC TACHYCARDIA

The importance of ablation therapy for AETs in the pediatric population was first established in the 1970s and 1980s with the surgical experience.[42] These tachycardias are characterized by their resistance to pharmacologic therapy, so surgical ablation was often needed for effective control. Spurred on by the successful application of catheter ablation techniques to cure AC-mediated tachycardia, it soon became evident that many AETs also could be mapped and "cured" by catheter ablation therapy, thus avoiding the morbidity of the surgical procedure.[43]

Approximately 6% of the cases in the pediatric registry are AET; 60% originate from the right atrium and 40% from the left. Acute success rates are reported to be 85% for the right AETs and 89% for the left AETs. Recurrence rates, however, are high for AETs, with long-term success rates between 50 and 66%. This high recurrence rate is probably because the substrates for AET, in many cases, may be multifocal. Common areas for AETs in the right atrium include the area in and around the atrial appendage and crista terminalis region. On the left side, AETs are often in the orifices of the pulmonary veins.

There are important technical considerations for ablation of AET in the pediatric patient. The substrates for AET can be very easily suppressed by anesthetic agents. Because most pediatric catheter ablation procedures require deep sedation or general anesthesia, accurate mapping of the ectopic substrate may be compromised. Manipulation of anesthetic agents and the use of light sedation may help efficiency of the procedure by more consistently eliciting the clinical tachycardia. The elusive nature of AETs under anesthesia may account for this tachycardia's high recurrence rate. Mapping techniques for AET involve the recording of early electrograms from the atrial focus during tachycardia. The initial deflection of the surface P wave is used as the reference, and electrograms from the tip of the ablation catheter are compared with the onset of the surface P wave. Signals that are 30 to 50 milliseconds in front of the P wave are indicative of the focus location (Fig. 10–13A and B). Sometimes, electrograms recorded from the focus area are not only early in reference to the P wave but are also fractionated. Energy applications placed in the targeted area occasionally accelerate the focus for a few beats before its complete termination.[44]

Another feature of AETs in children is the propensity for the tachycardia to be incessant resulting in ventricular dysfunction. AETs may cause few acute symptoms and patients thus present with "chronic" ventricular dysfunction. Patients with AET and ventricular dysfunction are poor surgical candidates and are also less than ideal candidates for antiarrhythmic drug therapy. Catheter-based ablation therapy is the treatment of choice for such patients. Even in the catheterization laboratory, patients with AET and depressed cardiac function may exhibit poor hemodynamics when sedated for the ablation procedure. Rapid atrial pacing to produce 2:1 AV block and a slower ventricular rate can occasionally be used to stabilize the hemodynamics in the early stages of the ablation procedure. Despite these technical concerns and the resistance of the ectopic foci to respond to medical therapy, catheter ablation is fast becoming the initial procedure of choice for this arrhythmia in the pediatric age group.

ATRIAL MUSCLE RE-ENTRY TACHYCARDIA

There is no more problematic tachycardia treated by pediatric cardiology practitioners than

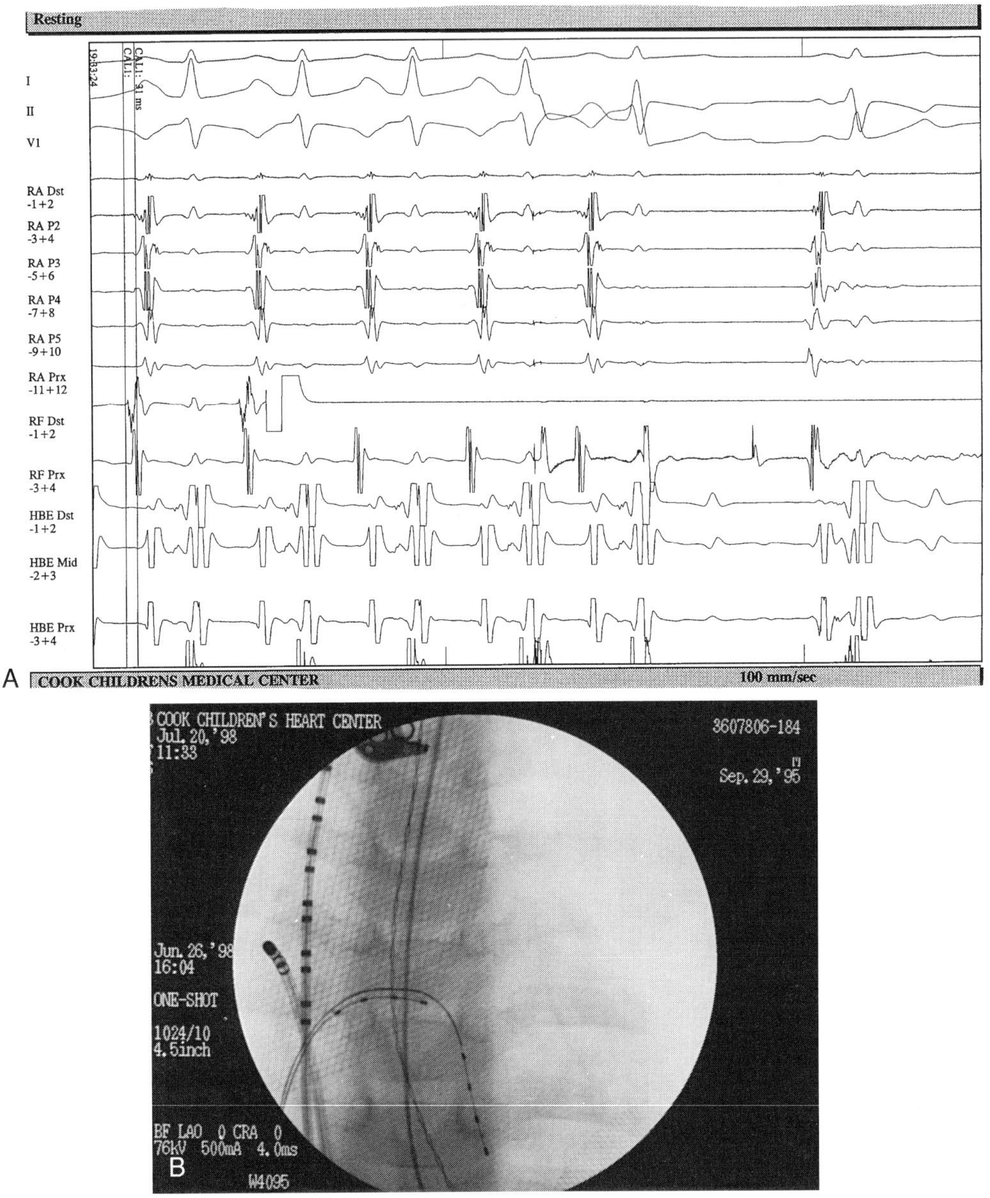

FIGURE 10–13. *A*, Electrograms from a patient with atrial ectopic tachycardia (AET), which is successfully ablated. From top to bottom: surface leads I, II, and V_1 and electrograms from the following: high right atrium (HRA; pairs 1–6), radiofrequency (RF) distal and RF proximal, and His bundle (HBE; distal, mid, and proximal). Note that the electrogram on the distal tip of the RF catheter is 31 ms in front of the P wave. Application of RF energy results in immediate termination of the tachycardia. *B*, Catheter positions corresponding to the electrograms shown in *A*.

atrial muscle re-entry tachycardia (AMRT). Typically, this arrhythmia is encountered in children who have had surgery for congenital heart lesions, specifically those procedures which necessitate extensive atrial incisions and suturing. Patients who have had atrial switch procedures for transposition of the great vessels (Mustard, Senning), those who have had Fontan operations, and those who have had atrial septal defect repairs often are the subgroups in which AMRT is encountered.[45] This arrhythmia is re-entrant in nature and has some similarities to atrial flutter. It is a primary atrial tachycardia with a slower atrial cycle length than that of classic atrial flutter. Like atrial flutter, the mechanism of AMRT is re-entry, and the substrate involves surgical scar tissue, which facilitates re-entry. Animal models of AMRT simulating those encountered in Mustard and Fontan patients have been reported. These models have identified critical areas in the atrium that are important for the perpetuation of AMRT.[45–50]

Uncontrolled AMRT has been associated with significant morbidity and mortality in patients with surgically corrected congenital heart disease.[51] Treatment of AMRT can be quite problematic. Strategies for treatment have been proposed, yet none are absolutely effective.[52] Class I and III antiarrhythmic medications are often effective but may necessitate back-up bradycardia pacing caused by drug-induced exacerbation of preexisting sinus bradycardia. Antitachycardia pacing may help control the arrhythmia especially in Mustard and Senning patients, but antitachycardia pacing in Fontan patients has proved to be more problematic.[53]

Catheter ablation techniques have been applied to AMRT, yet this therapy has not been a panacea for this condition. Approximately 5% of catheter ablations in the pediatric registry involve AMRT. Acute success ranges between 75% and 90%, and yet recurrences are frequent.[54–59] Actual long-term success rates are reported to be in the 30 to 50% range.[60] This high recurrence rate may be attributable to different forms of AMRT that appear over time.

Ablation of AMRT presents specific technical considerations. Concealed entrainment techniques similar to those used in classic atrial flutter ablation procedures are useful to identify areas of slow conduction, which can be targeted for ablation. Knowledge of the previously performed anatomic repair, specifically atriotomy sites and baffle suture lines, is imperative. These scars and baffle lines form areas of conduction block, which are needed for circuit formation. Corridors of tissue (isthmi), which are critical components of the AMRT circuit, are usually bounded by surgical scars, natural barriers (tricuspid valve, inferior vena cava), and baffle lines. Knowledge of the surgical anatomy along with concealed entrainment techniques may identify where radiofrequency lesions can be placed to interrupt conduction.[55]

In some cases, a discrete lesion may be enough to stop the tachycardia and ablate the circuit; however, in many cases, large linear lesions are needed to cut off the critical isthmus of conduction. It may be that certain AMRT circuits are more epicardial in location, so radiofrequency lesions may need to achieve some depth to destroy a circuit completely.

Catheter positioning in AMRT may also be challenging because of the vast permutations of surgical anatomy. No "standard" catheter positions are applicable. In such complex hearts, anatomic variation in the position of the AV conduction axis, coronary sinus, caval and pulmonary vein positions, and AV valve location must be kept in mind to maximize efficiency and mitigate complications. Thus, the intricate nature of the AMRT circuits in the context of some unique cardiac anatomic variations makes ablation of some circuits very difficult.

Despite these limitations, catheter ablation of AMRT is an attractive alternative for certain patients. This rhythm abnormality can be quite debilitating in patients with an abnormally structured heart. Because of the relative nonefficacy and potential proarrhythmic potential of antiarrhythmic therapy, nonpharmacologic therapy is a compelling option. The chance to return some of these patients to a normal lifestyle by permanently or even temporarily destroying a recalcitrant AMRT circuit justifies the use of this invasive therapy.

VENTRICULAR TACHYCARDIA

VT is another rare arrhythmia encountered in children that may be amenable to catheter ablation techniques. In the pediatric ablation registry, 3% of catheter ablation procedures involved a VT substrate with an overall acute success rate of 65%.

The most common ventricular tachycardia encountered in children undergoing catheter ablation involves automatic foci in the right ventricle. Commonly, the VT focus resides in the region of the right ventricular outflow tract and is referred to as right ventricular outflow tract (RVOT) VT. The characteristic morphology seen on the surface ECG is a wide QRS with a left bundle branch block pattern and an inferior axis. These automatic foci are sensitive to autonomic tone and may be catecholamine and exercise sensitive. The cardiac structure and function of patients with RVOT VT is normal, although some abnormalities have been described in certain patients using MRI.[61] Medical treatment of these tachycardias is preferred by many practitioners. Beta blockers and verapamil therapy are usually the chosen therapies. Also some children with these tachycardias need no treatment because of the slow, intermittent nature of the VT.

Catheter ablation techniques for RVOT VT have been performed in patients who are "medicine intolerant" (asthmatics) and those who have extreme symptoms with exercise. Some patients with athletic aspirations choose to have their tachycardia cured with an ablation procedure. The technique for catheter ablation is quite similar to that used with any automatic focus tachycardia. Multipolar mapping catheters are placed in the body of the right ventricle and in the outflow tract. An ablation catheter is then moved around in the ventricular cavity to perform "activation mapping" of the VT. The ablation catheter is used to record an early ventricular signal (electrogram), which starts 40 to 60 milliseconds in front of a QRS complex that exhibits the morphology of the clinical tachycardia[62] (Fig. 10–14A and B).

Pace-mapping techniques can also be used to locate the focus. Pace-mapping attempts to create a QRS morphology that is identical to the QRS morphology of the VT focus. The QRS morphologies created by pacing in a certain area are compared on a 12-lead surface ECG to the typical QRS morphologies of the VT. Pace mapping can elucidate the general area in which the VT focus resides. Activation mapping can fine tune the mapping. Radiofrequency energy placed in an area of the VT focus will sometimes accelerate the tachycardia before termination. Similar to other automatic tachycardias, there are some difficulties ablating RVOT VT with the sedation protocols used in the pediatric catheterization laboratory. These tachycardias can be suppressed by anesthesia, making accurate mapping difficult. In some instances, mapping single premature ventricular contractions with a similar morphology to the clinical VT is all that is possible in the laboratory. If one maps single premature ventricular contractions, care must be taken to avoid fusion with sinus beats. Fusion can make accurate ventricular activation mapping difficult. Also, as is the case with AET, RVOT VTs can sometimes emanate from a wide dysplastic area of ventricular myocardium. Such larger foci may be difficult to destroy by catheter techniques. Care must be taken to limit excessive energy application in the areas of the right ventricular myocardium, such as the anterior wall of the RVOT where the perforation potential is high. Also some RVOT tachycardias actually can arise from an area in close proximity to the His bundle, so the potential for AV block can be real. There have been reports of using catheter ablation for RVOT tachycardia with 80 to 90% long-term success rates. Controversy does exist as to the exact place for catheter ablation techniques in the treatment strategies of pediatric RVOT VT.[63]

Patients with normal cardiac structure may also have VT originating from a left ventricular focus. The characteristic appearance of the tachycardia is a wide QRS with a right bundle branch morphology and a superior axis. This is a re-entrant tachycardia with a substrate that involves the Purkinje network of the left posterior fascicle; thus, this tachycardia is sometimes termed *posterior fascicular VT* or *verapamil sensitive* because of its propensity to be terminated with the intravenous form of verapamil. Chronic arrhythmia control can also be achieved with oral verapamil but sometimes stronger antiarrhythmics such as class I drugs are often needed to avoid recurrences. Catheter ablation techniques to control this arrhythmia have described the recording of high-frequency potentials, which occur 15 and 40 milliseconds in front of the QRS complex during the characteristic VT.[64] Application of energy targeted to this potential will terminate the tachycardia. Inducibility of this tachycardia in the catheterization laboratory can be problematic because of the effects of anesthetic agents.

Other types of VT that are ablated in pediatric patients are re-entrant ventricular arrhythmias secondary to the repair of congenital heart disease. These are often encountered in patients who have had ventricular septal defect repair or repaired tetralogy of Fallot.[65, 66] For years, the propensity for such patients to have ventricular arrhythmias with subsequent morbidity and mortality has been described. Medical treatment has been problematic because of nonefficiency and the propensity for proarrhythmia. Similar to congenital heart patients with AMRT, patients with VT secondary to congenital heart disease are intolerant of strong antiarrhythmic medications because of pre-existing sinus node dysfunction. Back-up bradycardia pacing is sometimes necessary in the face of antiarrhythmic therapy; thus, catheter ablation techniques are an important part of the treatment strategy in these patients.

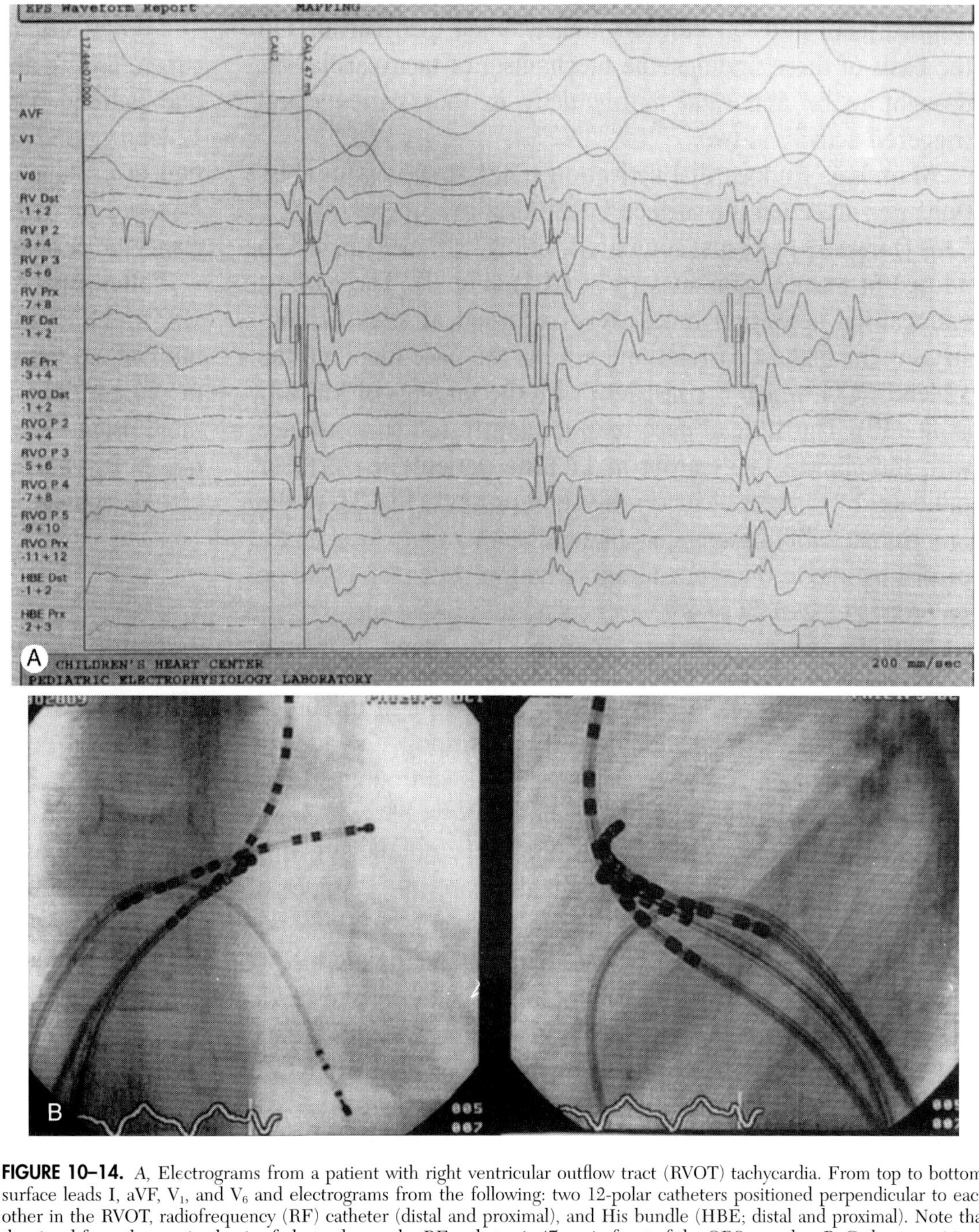

FIGURE 10–14. *A*, Electrograms from a patient with right ventricular outflow tract (RVOT) tachycardia. From top to bottom: surface leads I, aVF, V_1, and V_6 and electrograms from the following: two 12-polar catheters positioned perpendicular to each other in the RVOT, radiofrequency (RF) catheter (distal and proximal), and His bundle (HBE; distal and proximal). Note that the signal from the proximal pair of electrodes on the RF catheter is 47 ms in front of the QRS complex. *B*, Catheter positions, anteroposterior (left) and lateral (right), corresponding to the electrograms in *A*. *A* and *B* from O'Connor B, Case C, Sokoloski M, et al: Radiofrequency catheter ablation of right ventricular outflow tachycardia in children and adolescents. J Am Coll Cardiol 27:871, 1996. Used with permission of the American College of Cardiology.

Techniques to ablate VT in these patients have similarities to those used with AMRT ablation. Because these are re-entrant arrhythmias, concealed entrainment techniques are useful to identify critical components of the re-entrant circuits. Anatomic details of the surgical repair also are important to help localize areas of conduction block. Surgical scars, valves, and patches can form corridors of tissue (isthmi), which are critical to the VT circuit. These corridors may need to be targeted and ablated with a single lesion or a larger linear lesion. Long-term success of ablation procedures in these children is approximately 50%. If the targeted arrhythmia has caused near sudden death symptoms in a patient, care must be taken to prove success of the procedure. As is the case with "acutely successful" ablation procedures in adults with ischemic VT who have had near sudden death events, placement of a back-up defibrillator may be necessary in certain congenital heart patients after "successful " ablation of a VT substrate. The severity of the presenting symptoms and probability of chronic recurrence should guide this decision.

CONGENITAL JUNCTIONAL ECTOPIC TACHYCARDIA

Abnormal automaticity of the His bundle can cause junctional ectopic tachycardia (JET) in the newborn, resulting in significant morbidity and mortality. This arrhythmia is often amenable to amiodarone therapy, but occasionally catheter ablation is necessary if ventricular dysfunction occurs. Certainly, if catheter ablation is considered, there is an inherent possibility of AV block with the need for permanent cardiac pacing; however, there have been multiple reports of successful ablation of JET with preservation of AV conduction.[67]

INDICATIONS FOR CATHETER ABLATION IN CHILDREN

The indications for the use of catheter ablation procedures in children are controversial. Some believe that the long-term effects of this therapy are unknown, and this precludes its use in all except extreme cases. Others believe that it should be offered as a potential curative therapy for most arrhythmias encountered in children. There are unknowns about the long-term effects of radiofrequency lesions on the developing heart. Also many arrhythmia substrates in children change in severity with maturation. These two uncertainties make absolute indications for the use of catheter ablation a controversial subject in the pediatric age group.

It is clear, however, that an absolute indication for ablation is the occurrence of any pathologic tachycardia in any child (regardless of age) who has life-threatening symptoms, provided that the substrate is amenable to ablation. It has been shown that catheter ablation can be safe and effective even in infants. Only 9% of ablation attempts in children are performed for life-threatening events. A common scenario is a near sudden death event in a patient with WPW syndrome. Another compelling indication for catheter ablation is any arrhythmia causing ventricular dysfunction. In this scenario (often seen with incessant tachycardia such as AET and JET), antiarrhythmic therapy can further exacerbate ventricular dysfunction. Catheter ablation therapy is best performed before the development of severe dysfunction, which can increase the likelihood of procedure-related morbidity. Tachycardia-induced dysfunction accounts for only 3% of procedures performed in the pediatric registry.

Other compelling indications for catheter ablation include children who have arrhythmias secondary to corrected congenital heart disease. As previously stated, these arrhythmias include AMRT in patients who have had atrial septal defect repair, the Senning or Mustard procedure, and the Fontan procedure. Also included are children with VT after certain congenital surgeries (i.e., ventricular septal defect (VSD), tetralogy of Fallot repair). The propensity for morbidity and mortality of these arrhythmias, coupled with the nonefficacy and adverse effects of pharmacologic therapy, makes catheter ablation an attractive therapeutic alternative.

The indications for most catheter ablation procedures in children involve an element of patient choice. According to the registry data, patient choice is the largest (and still growing) indication for catheter ablation procedures, comprising 46% of all indications.[7] The second most common indication (34%) is failure of medical therapy. Undoubtedly, the failure of medical therapy indication does involve patient choice issues. In reality, the indications for nearly 90% of catheter ablation procedures involve patient choice factors. The practitioner can help the family make an informed choice by formulating the risk-benefit analysis of catheter ablation in regard to each pediatric arrhythmia. This analysis should include the age of the patient, expertise of the ablation operator, natural history of the arrhythmia, lifestyle consideration for the parents and the child, expected outcome of an ablation, known complications and potential risks of the procedure, known efficacy and potential risks of alternative therapies, and other medical conditions that complicate pharmacologic or alternative arrhythmia treatment. It is clear that, with all these factors outlined, many parents will choose to have catheter ablation procedures, even for the most common sustained pediatric arrhythmias encountered in children.

Another factor to consider in the use of catheter ablation is medical costs. It has been proposed that catheter ablation is a less expensive medical alternative for children older than 7 years with WPW syndrome and tachycardia recurrences on chronic medical therapy. With these thoughts in mind, it can be proposed that catheter ablation should be a therapeutic consideration for any child older than 5 years with re-entrant AV tachycardia who needs combination drug therapy (e.g., digoxin and propranolol) or class I or III antiarrhythmic therapy for tachycardia control. At this age, catheter ablation can be offered as an equal alternative to any medical therapy. In children younger than 5 years, catheter ablation seems to have higher risks, and more stringent indications are reasonable; however, with potentially life-threatening symptoms, catheter ablation is the procedure of choice regardless of patient age.

SURGICAL ABLATION

Although most pediatric arrhythmias requiring ablation can be safely and effectively performed with a catheter, there is still a role for surgical ablation in children.[68] Certain arrhythmias that are multifocal can best be corrected by surgical excision or extensive cryothermia applications. This includes some types of AET and infantile VT caused by hamartomas. Also there are rare ACs that are not accessible with a catheter that may be more safely destroyed in the operating room. ACs in the posterior septum comprise many of these exceptions. Arrhythmias encountered in children with congenital heart disease can also be addressed in the operating room. This is especially indicated when concomitant structural abnormalities need surgical revision. In the operating room, patients with tetralogy of Fallot and residual pulmonary stenosis or insufficiency may have their structural problem corrected and at the same time have cryolesions placed in critical areas that are responsible for ventricular arrhythmogenicity. Similarly, patients who undergo Fontan revision and have recalcitrant atrial muscle re-entry tachycardia can have cryolesions placed in certain anatomic regions to interrupt real or anticipated areas critical to re-entrant circuits. These procedures in children with congenital heart disease usually require a presurgical electrophysiology study to ascertain the location of the arrhythmogenic substrate. Close cooperation between the surgeon and the electrophysiologist in the preoperative, operative, and postoperative phases of treatment is imperative to guarantee efficacy and avoid complications.

FUTURE DIRECTIONS

Future directions in pediatric catheter ablation therapies will most likely be directed by advances in catheter technology and the potential use of alternative energy sources. Technology will most likely lead to the development of smaller catheters, which are more amenable to use in smaller children for the treatment of more common types of pediatric arrhythmias (re-entrant SVTs). Advances in mapping catheter designs will help with more accurate mapping of complex arrhythmias encountered in children with postoperative heart disease (AMRT, VT). Alternative energy sources (which create larger, deeper lesions) may be explored to help increase the long-term efficacy of such recalcitrant arrhythmias such as AMRT. Finally, informed parental acceptance of catheter ablation as a first-line therapy for most pediatric arrhythmias will become common.

REFERENCES

1. The Cardiac Arrhythmia Suppression Trial (CAST) Investigators: Preliminary report: Effect of encainide and flecainide on mortality in a randomized trial of arrhythmia suppression after myocardial infarction. N Engl J Med 321:406–412, 1989.
2. Fish F, Gillette P, Benson DW: Proarrhythmia, cardiac arrest and death in young patients receiving encainide and flecainide. J Am Coll Cardiol 1991:18:356–365, 1991.
3. Calkins H, Prystowsky E, Carlson M, et al: Temperature monitoring during radiofrequency catheter ablation procedures using closed loop control. Circulation 90:1279–1286, 1994.
4. Kugler J, Danford D, Deal B, et al: Radiofrequency catheter ablation for tachyarrhythmias in children and adolescents. N Engl J Med 330:1481–1487, 1994.
5. Danford D, Kugler J, Deal B, et al: The learning curve for radiofrequency ablation of tachyarrhythmias in pediatric patients. Am J Cardiol 75:587–590, 1995.
6. Schaffer M, Silka M, Ross B, et al: Inadvertent atrioventricular block during radiofrequency catheter ablation: Results of the pediatric radiofrequency ablation registry. Circulation 94:3214–3220, 1996.
7. Kugler J, Danford D, Houston K, et al: Radiofrequency catheter ablation for paroxysmal supraventricular tachy-

cardia in children and adolescents without structural heart disease. Am J Cardiol 80:1438–1443, 1997.
8. Vora AM, Jazayeri MR, Dhala A: Ablation of atrial insertion sites of left-sided accessory pathways in children: Efficacy and safety of transseptal versus transaortic approach. Pediatr Cardiol 18:322–338, 1997.
9. Bubolz B, Case C, McKay C, et al: Learning curve for radiofrequency catheter ablation in pediatrics at a single institution. Am Heart J 131:956–960, 1996.
10. Case C, Gillette P, Oslizlok P, et al: Radiofrequency catheter ablation of incessant, medically resistant supraventricular tachycardia in infants and small children. J Am Cardiol 20:1405–1410, 1992.
11. Ko JK, Deal BJ, Strasburger JF, et al: Supraventricular tachycardia mechanisms and their age distribution in pediatric patients. Am J Cardiol 69:1028–1032, 1992.
12. Moe GK, Preston JB, Burlington H: Physiologic evidence for a dual A-V transmission system. Circ Res 4:357–375, 1956.
13. Wit AL, Weiss MB, Berkowitz WD, et al: Patterns of atrioventricular conduction in the human heart. Circ Res 27:345–356, 1970.
14. McGuire MA, Johnson DC, Robotin M, et al: Dimensions of the triangle of Koch in humans. Am J Cardiol 70:829–830, 1992.
15. Sung RJ, Waxman HL, Juma Z, et al: Sequence of retrograde atrial activation in patients with dual atrioventricular nodal pathways. Circulation 64:1053–1067, 1981.
16. Jazayeri MR, Hempe SL, Sra JS, et al: Selective transcatheter ablation of the fast and slow pathways using radiofrequency energy in patients with atrioventricular nodal reentry tachycardia. Circulation 85:1318–1328, 1992.
17. Silka MJ, Kron J, Halperin BD, et al: Mechanisms of AV node reentrant tachycardia in young patients with and without dual AV node physiology. Pacing Clin Electrophysiol 17:2129–2133, 1994.
18. Keim S, Werner P, Jazayeri M, et al: Localization of the fast and slow pathways in atrioventricular nodal reentrant tachycardia by intraoperative ice mapping. Circulation 86:919–924, 1992.
19. Jackman WM, Bechman KJ, McClelland JH, et al: Treatment of supraventricular tachycardia due to atrioventricular nodal reentry by radiofrequency catheter ablation of slow-pathway conduction. N Engl J Med 327:313–318, 1992.
20. Hill JN, Freedberg NA, Zimerman L, et al: Are typical and atypical AV node re-entry "mirror image" tachycardias? Response to adenosine suggests otherwise. Circulation 92(Suppl I):594, 1995 (abstract).
21. Langberg JJ, Harvey M, Calkins H, et al: Titration of power output during radiofrequency catheter ablation of atrioventricular nodal reentrant tachycardia. Pacing Clin Electrophysiol 16:465–470, 1993.
22. Mitrani RD, Klein LS, Hackett FK, et al: Radiofrequency ablation for atrioventricular node reentrant tachycardia: Comparison between fast (anterior) and slow (posterior) pathway ablation. J Am Coll Cardiol 21:432–441, 1993.
23. Lee MA, Morady F, Kadish A, et al: Catheter modification of the atrioventricular junction with radiofrequency energy for control of atrioventricular nodal reentry tachycardia. Circulation 83:827–835, 1991.
24. Langberg JJ, Kim Y-N, Goyal R, et al: Conversion of typical to "atypical" atrioventricular nodal reentrant tachycardia after radiofrequency modification of the atrioventricular junction. Am J Cardiol 69:503–508, 1992.
25. Natale A, Wathen M, Wolfe K, et al: Comparative atrioventricular node properties after radiofrequency ablation and operative therapy of atrioventricular node reentry. Pacing Clin Electrophysiol 16:971–9711, 1993.
26. Hummel J, Strickberger A, Kalbfleisch S, et al: Effect of pacing site on the atrial electrogram at target sites for slow pathway ablation in patients with atrioventricular nodal reentrant tachycardia. Pacing Clin Electrophysiol 17:585–589, 1994.
27. Jentzer JH, Goyal R, Williamson BD, et al: Analysis of junctional ectopy during radiofrequency ablation of the slow pathway in patients with atrioventricular nodal reentrant tachycardia. Circulation 90:2920–2926, 1994.
28. Thakur RK, Klein GJ, Yee R, et al: Junctional tachycardia: A useful marker during radiofrequency ablation for atrioventricular node reentrant tachycardia. J Am Coll Cardiol 22:1706–1710, 1993.
29. Kalbfleisch SJ, Strickberger A, Williamson B, et al: Randomized comparison of anatomic and electrogram mapping approaches to ablation of the slow pathway of atrioventricular node reentrant tachycardia. J Am Coll Cardiol 23:716–723, 1994.
30. Moulton K, Miller B, Scott J, et al: Radiofrequency ablation for AV nodal reentry: A technique for rapid transection of the slow AV nodal pathway. Pacing Clin Electrophysiol 16:760–768, 1993.
31. Hiraoka A, Karakawa S, Muraoka Y, et al: The structural characteristic of coronary sinus in patients with atrioventricular nodal reentrant tachycardia (AVNRT). Circulation 92(Suppl I):594, 1995 (Abstract).
32. Kugler JD, Danford DA, Deal BJ, et al: Radiofrequency catheter ablation for tachyarrhythmias in children and adolescents. N Engl J Med 330:1481–1487, 1994.
33. Teixeira OHP, Balaji S, Case CL, et al: Radiofrequency catheter ablation of atrioventricular nodal reentrant tachycardia in children. Pacing Clin Electrophysiol 17:1621–1626, 1994.
34. Biehl M, Keelan ET, Underwood D, et al: Temporal changes in atrioventricular nodal refractoriness post slow pathway ablation. Circulation 92(Suppl I):213, 1995 (abstract).
35. Garratt CJ, Stafford PJ, Skehan JD: Effect of slow pathway atrioventricular node ablation on chronotropic and dromotropic responses to the Valsalva maneuver. Circulation 92(Suppl I):213, 1995 (abstract).
36. Olsovsky MR, Belz MK, Stambler BS, et al: Does selective slow pathway ablation alter vagal input to the fast pathway of the AV node? Circulation 92(Suppl I):213, 1995 (abstract).
37. Ehlert FA, Goldberger JJ, Brooks R, et al: Persistent inappropriate sinus tachycardia after radiofrequency current catheter modification of the atrioventricular node. Am J Cardiol 69:1092–1095, 1992.
38. Baker JH, Plumb VJ, Epstein AE, et al: Predictors of recurrent atrioventricular nodal reentry after selective slow pathway ablation. Am J Cardiol 73:765–769, 1994.
39. Wu C, Yeh S-J, Wang C-C, et al: A simple technique for selective radiofrequency ablation of the slow pathway in atrioventricular node reentrant tachycardia. J Am Coll Cardiol 21:1612–1621, 1993.
40. Lindsay BD, Chung MK, Gamache C, et al: Therapeutic end points for the treatment of atrioventricular node reentrant tachycardia by catheter-guided radiofrequency current. J Am Coll Cardiol 22:733–740, 1993.
41. Silka MJ, Kron J, Park JK, et al: Atypical forms of supraventricular tachycardia due to atrioventricular node reentry in children after radiofrequency modification of slow pathway conduction. J Am Coll Cardiol 23:1363–1369, 1993.
42. Case C, Gillette P: Automatic atrial and junctional tachycardias in the pediatric patient: Strategies for diagnosis and management. Pacing Clin Electrophysiol 16:1323, 1993.

43. Walsh E, Saul P, Hulse E, et al: Transcatheter ablation of ectopic atrial tachycardia in young patients using radiofrequency current. Circulation 86:1138–1146, 1992.
44. Perry J, Fenrich A, Legras M, et al: Acceleration of atrial ectopic tachycardia as a guide to successful radiofrequency ablation. Pacing Clin Electrophysiol 16:2007, 1993.
45. Kanter R, Garson A Jr: Atrial arrhythmias during chronic follow-up of surgery for complex congenital heart disease. Pacing Clin Electrophysiol 20(Pt II):502–511, 1997.
46. Cronin C, Nitta T, Mitsuno M, et al: Characterization and surgical ablation of acute atrial flutter following the Mustard procedure. Circulation 88(Pt 2):461–471, 1993.
47. Gandhi S, Bromberg B, Schuessler R, et al: Characterization and surgical ablation of atrial flutter after the classic Fontan repair. Ann Thorac Surg 61:1666–1679, 1996.
48. Gandhi S, Bromberg B, Rodefeld M, et al: Lateral tunnel suture line variation reduces atrial flutter after the modified Fontan operation. Ann Thorac Surg 61:1299–1309, 1996.
49. Rodefeld M, Gandhi S, Huddleston C, et al: Anatomically based ablation of atrial flutter in an acute canine model of the modified Fontan operation. J Thorac Cardiovasc Surg 112:898–907, 1996.
50. Rodefeld M, Bromberg B, Schuessler R, et al: Atrial flutter after lateral tunnel construction in the modified Fontan operation: A canine model. J Thorac Cardiovasc Surg 111:514–526, 1996.
51. Garson A, Bink-Boelkens M, Hesslein PS, et al: Atrial flutter in the young: A collaborative study of 380 cases. J Am Coll Cardiol 6:871–878, 1985.
52. Balaji S, Johnson TB, Sade RM, et al: Management of atrial flutter after the Fontan procedure. J Am Coll Cardiol 23:1209–1215, 1994.
53. Case C, Gillette P, Zeigler V, et al: Problems with permanent atrial pacing in the Fontan patient. J Am Coll Cardiol 12(Pt. 1):92–96, 1989.
54. Lesh M, Van Hare G, Epstein L, et al: Radiofrequency catheter ablation of atrial arrhythmias. Circulation 89:1074–1089, 1994.
55. Kalman J, Van Hare G, Olgin J, et al: Ablation of "incisional" reentrant atrial tachycardia complicating surgery for congenital heart disease. Circulation 93:502–512, 1996.
56. Van Hare G, Lesh M, Ross B, et al: Mapping and radiofrequency ablation of intraatrial reentrant tachycardia after the Senning or Mustard procedure for transposition of the great arteries. Am J Cardiol 77:985–991, 1996.
57. Baker B, Lindsay B, Bromberg B, et al: Catheter ablation of clinical intraatrial reentrant tachycardias resulting from previous atrial surgery: Localizing and transecting the critical isthmus. J Am Coll Cardiol 28:411–417, 1996.
58. Triedman J, Jenkins K, Colan S, et al: Intra-atrial reentrant tachycardia after palliation of congenital heart disease: Characterization of multiple macroreentrant circuits using fluoroscopically based three-dimensional endocardial mapping. J Cardiovasc Electrophysiol 8:259–270, 1977.
59. Triedman J, Saul P, Weindling S, et al: Radiofrequency ablation of intra-atrial reentrant tachycardia after surgical palliation of congenital heart disease. Circulation 91:707–714, 1995.
60. Triedman J, Bergau D, Saul P, et al: Efficacy of radiofrequency ablation for control of intraatrial reentrant tachycardia in patients with congenital heart disease. J Am Coll Cardiol 30:1032–1038, 1997.
61. Globits S, Kreiner G, Frank H, et al: Significance of morphological abnormalities detected by MRI in patients undergoing successful ablation of right ventricular outflow tract tachycardia. Circulation 8:2633–2640, 1997.
62. O'Connor B, Case C, Sokoloski M, et al: Radiofrequency catheter ablation of right ventricular outflow tachycardia in children and adolescents. J Am Coll Cardiol 27:869–874, 1996.
63. Silka M, Kron J: Radiofrequency catheter ablation for idiopathic right ventricular tachycardia: First, last or only therapy—Who decides? J Am Coll Cardiol 27:875–876, 1996.
64. Nakagawa H, Beckman K, McClelland J, et al: Radiofrequency catheter ablation of idiopathic left ventricular tachycardia guided by a Purkinje potential. Circulation 88:2607–2617, 1993.
65. Chinushi M, Aizawa Y, Kitazawa H, et al: Successful radiofrequency catheter ablation for macroreentrant ventricular tachycardias in a patient with tetralogy of Fallot after corrective surgery. Pacing & Clinical Electrophysiol 18(Pt. I):1713–1716, 1995.
66. Gonska B, Kejiang C, Raab J, et al: Radiofrequency catheter ablation of right ventricular tachycardia late after repair of congenital heart defects. Circulation 94:1902–1908, 1996.
67. Ehlert F, Goldberger J, Deal B, et al: Successful radiofrequency energy ablation of automatic junctional tachycardia preserving normal atrioventricular nodal conduction. Pacing Clin Electrophysiol 16:54–56, 1993.
68. Crawford FA Jr, Gillette PC: Surgical treatment of cardiac dysrhythmias in infants and children. Ann Thorac Surg 58:1262–1268, 1994.

C H A P T E R 11

CARDIAC PACING

Paul C. Gillette, Jeffrey S. Heinle, and Vicki L. Zeigler

Permanent cardiac pacing was originally used in the pediatric population to keep children alive after attempted repair of congenital heart defects.[1] Indications for cardiac pacemakers in children and young adults have evolved over the past few decades to include a variety of patients, including those with anatomically normal hearts. This broadening of indications is due to an improved understanding of the mechanisms, hemodynamic consequences, and natural history of bradydysrhythmias. The pulse generators and pacing leads have also dramatically improved technologically, and now, in addition to prolonging life, they can improve quality of life as well.[2]

Pediatric patients constitute only a small portion of the overall pacemaker population. Although no pacemakers are made specifically for children, certain programmable parameters allow the customization of most devices to fit the needs of most pediatric patients. The fact that most pacemaker recipients are elderly makes very small pulse generators popular, which indirectly benefits the smallest of pediatric patients.[3–8]

The pediatric pacing team should be led by a physician interested in and trained in pediatric cardiac pacing and arrhythmias and should include a nurse with similar expertise. An extremely organized approach is necessary for optimal outcomes in the pediatric pacemaker recipient and requires not only expertise in caring for children and families but a working knowledge of congenital heart disease as well. This chapter includes an overview of the pacing indications in children, selection of individualized hardware, implant techniques, both endocardial and epicardial, intraoperative testing, postoperative care, pacing system follow-up, and special considerations.

INDICATIONS

The American College of Cardiology/American Heart Association guidelines for implantation of cardiac pacemakers and antiarrhythmia devices were published in 1984 and revised in 1991.[9, 10] The 1991 guidelines were updated in 1998 to reflect the advances in pacemaker technology as well as the publication of newer data that have provided increased knowledge regarding the natural history of bradyarrhythmias and tachyarrhythmias, which may benefit from device therapy.[11]

The specific indications for permanent cardiac pacing in children and adolescents are listed in Table 11–1. The standard format remains the same with regard to classification: Class I conditions include patients in whom there is general agreement that the device will be beneficial, Class II conditions include patients in whom there is ambivalence regarding whether the device will be beneficial or not, and Class III conditions include patients in whom there is agreement that the device will not be useful. An addition to the 1998 guidelines is a level of evidence ranking. Level A is assigned if the literature reports data from multiple, randomized clinical trials involving many patients. Level B is assigned if the literature reports data from a small number of trials with a limited number of patients. Level C is assigned when the indication was derived by expert consensus. The pediatric indications include no assignments of Level A in part because of the small number of pediatric patients.

Although the general indications for pacemaker implantation in children are similar to those for adults, several important issues need to be considered in the pediatric and young adult pacemaker recipient.[12] Generally, the child, adolescent, or young adult requiring a permanent cardiac pacemaker will fit into one of four main categories: (1) symptomatic bradycardia, (2) recurrent bradycardia-tachycardia, (3) congenital atrioventricular (AV) block, or (4) surgical/acquired advanced second- or third-degree AV block[11] (Fig. 11–1).

As a result of advances in the field of cardiac surgery for congenital heart disease, many children are living longer. These same children are often "palliated" rather than "corrected," and

Table 11–1. Indications for Permanent Pacing in Children and Adolescents

CLASS	INDICATIONS
I	1. Advanced second- or third-degree AV block associated with symptomatic bradycardia, congestive heart failure, or low cardiac output (level of evidence: C)
	2. Sinus node dysfunction with correlation of symptoms during age-appropriate bradycardia; definition of bradycardia varies with patient age and expected heart rate (level of evidence: B)
	3. Postoperative advanced second- or third-degree AV block that is not expected to resolve or persists for at least 7 days after cardiac surgery (level of evidence: B, C)
	4. Congenital third-degree AV block with a wide QRS escape rhythm or ventricular dysfunction (level of evidence: B)
	5. Congenital third-degree AV block in the infant with a ventricular rate < 50–55 bpm or with congenital heart disease and ventricular rate < 70 bpm (level of evidence: B, C)
	6. Sustained pause-dependent VT, with or without prolonged QT, in which the efficacy of pacing is thoroughly documented (level of evidence: B)
IIa	1. Bradycardia-tachycardia syndrome with the need for long-term antiarrhythmic treatment other than digitalis (level of evidence: C)
	2. Congenital third-degree AV block beyond the first year of life with an average heart rate < 50 bpm or abrupt pauses in ventricular rate that are two to three times basic cycle length (level of evidence: B)
	3. Long QT syndrome with 2 : 1 AV block or third-degree AV block (level of evidence: B)
	4. Asymptomatic sinus bradycardia in the child with complex congenital heart disease with resting heart rate < 35 bpm or pauses in ventricular rate > 3 seconds (level of evidence: C)
IIb	1. Transient postoperative third-degree AV block that reverts to sinus rhythm with residual bifascicular block (level of evidence: C)
	2. Congenital third-degree AV block in the asymptomatic neonate, child, or adolescent with acceptable rate, narrow QRS complex, and normal ventricular function (level of evidence: B)
	3. Asymptomatic sinus bradycardia in the adolescent with congenital heart disease with resting heart rate < 35 bpm or pauses in ventricular rate > 3 seconds (level of evidence: C)
III	1. Transient postoperative AV block with return of normal AV conduction within 7 days (level of evidence: B)
	2. Asymptomatic postoperative bifascicular block with or without first-degree AV block (level of evidence: B)
	3. Asymptomatic type I second-degree AV block (level of evidence: C)
	4. Asymptomatic sinus bradycardia in the adolescent with longest RR interval < 3 seconds and minimum heart rate > 40 bpm (level of evidence: C)

AV, atrioventricular; VT, ventricular tachycardia.

Adapted from Gregoratos G, Cheitlin MD, Conill A, et al: ACC/AHA guidelines for implantation of cardiac pacemakers and antiarrhythmia devices. J Am Coll Cardiol 31:1175–209, 1998. Used with permission.

may experience symptoms of bradycardia at lesser degrees than their counterparts with structurally normal hearts, thus making their pacemaker indication more dependent on symptomatology rather than absolute heart rate criteria. Because bradycardia may be considered age specific, one heart rate in an adolescent athlete may be considered normal, whereas that same heart rate in a neonate with structural heart disease may be a pacemaker indication.

Certain findings in asymptomatic children have been found to result in better outcomes when treated with a cardiac pacemaker. The neonate with congenital complete AV block with no congenital heart disease and a ventricular rate of 55 beats per minute (bpm) or less should receive a permanent cardiac pacemaker. The same neonate with congenital heart disease or respiratory distress with a ventricular rate of 70 bpm or less should undergo pacemaker implantation.[13, 14] A wide QRS escape rhythm as opposed to the usual narrow QRS escape rhythm is an indication for pacemaker implantation.[15] In older children, a ventricular rate of 40 bpm or less or a wide QRS escape rhythm has been found to lead to syncope or sudden death. A rate of 30 bpm or less during sleep and a pause of more than 4 seconds are also indications for permanent pacing. Complex ventricular arrhythmias associated with congenital AV block also require pacemaker therapy.[16] Premature ventricular contractions (PVCs) in these patients generally subside after dual-chamber pacemaker implantation.

Evidence of exit block from an escape focus, such as RR intervals 2 or 3 times the basic escape interval, has been said to predict syncope and sudden death in patients with congenital complete AV block. Michaelsson and colleagues suggested that patients with congenital complete AV block should be permanently paced before adolescence to prevent syncope, death, and irreversible myocardial dysfunction.[17] These recommendations have been positively received by most physicians who routinely implant pacemakers.

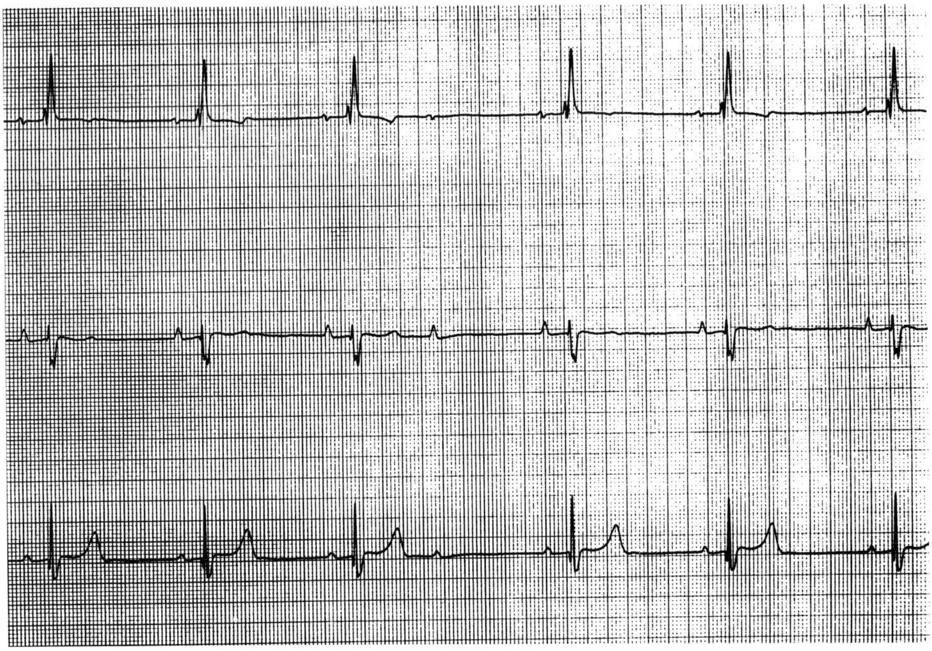

FIGURE 11–1. Simultaneous recording of leads V_1, AVF, and V_6 in a 5-year-old with syncope during exercise. This electrocardiographic tracing exhibits sinus bradycardia, right bundle branch block, left anterior hemiblock, and Mobitz type II second-degree atrioventricular block.

Second-degree AV block may also constitute a pacemaker indication in the pediatric patient. Although rare in children, Mobitz type II second-degree AV block may require permanent pacing. Mobitz type II second-degree AV block is different from fixed 2:1 AV block, which may not require permanent cardiac pacing. Two-to-one block resulting from a markedly prolonged QT interval is a pacemaker indication, whereas block in the AV node may be evaluated on a regular outpatient basis. Progression from 2:1 AV block to third-degree AV block may result in a large rate decrease, so close follow-up is necessary in these patients. Mobitz type I second-degree AV block (or Wenckebach) is not an indication for permanent pacing.

Surgically acquired AV block (i.e., Mobitz type II second-degree, fixed 2:1, or complete AV block) is always an indication for a permanent pacemaker if the block persists for more than 7 to 10 days after surgery. It is not yet known whether transient, complete AV block that alternates with sinus rhythm with or without bifascicular block is likely to recur. Any patient undergoing surgery for correction of a ventricular septal defect is at risk, albeit small, for late AV block. In the postoperative state, "trifascicular block" is usually not associated with late AV block development. Electrophysiology studies in the aforementioned patients showed that the AV node conduction time (AH interval) was found to be prolonged to more than 120 milliseconds. Prolonged HV intervals (from 50 to 75 milliseconds) in postoperative patients with first-degree AV block have not been found to be predictive of late development of AV block.

Nonsurgically acquired AV block is unusual in children. It is usually due to viral or bacterial infections, resulting in cardiac irritability and a severely damaged conduction system; thus, a permanent pacemaker is usually indicated. The exception to this is Lyme disease, which occasionally results in complete AV block and generally resolves with medical therapy (i.e., antibiotics).

Pacemakers can also be used in patients with hypertrophic cardiomyopathy to decrease aortic outflow tract gradients by pre-exciting the right ventricular apex. This indication is very controversial but has worked well in select patients.[18, 19] The availability of implantable defibrillators capable of dual-chamber pacing is an attractive option for older children with hypertrophic cardiomyopathy with associated ventricular arrhythmias or aborted sudden death.

CHOOSING INDIVIDUALIZED HARDWARE

The choice as to the most appropriate pulse generator, pacing mode, and pacing leads for a specific patient and the pacing indication is multifaceted. Determining factors include the specific electrophysiologic indication (i.e., sinus bradycardia or AV block), overall cardiac condition, size of the patient, percentage of time that the device will be required to stimulate (vs. sensing), and need for battery longevity. The goal of the pacing system is to mimic the normal conduction system as much as possible and to improve the patient's overall hemodynamics.

PULSE GENERATOR

The specific pulse generator should match the patient's pacing indication as closely as possible. The chosen device should be capable of pacing in a variety of modes (see the pacemaker code in Table 11–2). In the patient with complete AV block with normal sinus node function, a pacemaker capable of atrial synchronous (DDD) pacing is most appropriate. In the patient with complete AV block and sinus node dysfunction, the addition of a sensor (DDDR) might be required. Also, if there is suspicion that the former patient might be predisposed to sinus node dysfunction at a later time, the implanted device should be capable of rate adaptive pacing, although it may not be programmed that way initially.

In patients with sinus node dysfunction with intact AV nodal conduction, atrial pacing (AAICO) is the preferred mode.[20] If there is chronotropic incompetence, rate adaptation in the single-chamber mode is most appropriate. If there is documented intra-atrial re-entrant tachycardia or the suspicion that it may develop in the future, atrial antitachycardia pacing (AAICP) is the mode of choice.[21–23]

Single-chamber ventricular pacemakers are being used less and less in the pediatric population. The patient requiring infrequent pacing might be best suited for a single-chamber ventricular pacemaker without rate adaptation (VVICO). A postoperative patient with intermittent (i.e., 10–20 min/day) AV block 7 to 10 days after open heart surgery is the most likely candidate for this type of device. The patient with extremely poor venous access may benefit from single-chamber pacing with rate adaptation (VVIRO).

Rate adaptive devices are used when there is a need for a sensor that the cardiac electrical system is no longer capable of providing.[24] These sensors include activity-triggered devices such as those with a piezoelectric crystal or accelerometer or minute ventilation, which uses impedance pneumography. Several devices are capable of providing both types of sensors, either alone or in combination.

The decision as to which device to implant can be quite confusing. Size is an important factor when choosing a pulse generator. In the past, the larger devices were thought to be "too large" for most pediatric patients, but the current "downsizing" has resulted in decreased battery longevity in patients who require a lifetime of pacing. The smaller devices are excellent for infants and small children, but the inability to procure larger devices with the same technology has become quite frustrating.

The availability of certain programming options is very important in the pediatric pacing population. In many patients, an upper tracking limit of 180 ppm is desired, so the device must be capable of providing high upper rate limits. Adaptive AV intervals are important in the pediatric pacemaker recipient, as are short postventricular atrial refractory periods (PVARPs) that allow Wenckebach, rather than 2:1, block at the

Table 11–2. Revised NASPE/BPG Pacemaker Code*

POSITION I, CHAMBERS PACED	POSITION II, CHAMBERS SENSED	POSITION III, RESPONSE TO SENSING	POSITION IV, PROGRAMMABILITY, RATE MODULATION	POSITION V, ANTITACHYARRHYTHMIA FUNCTION
0 = none	0 = none	0 = none	0 = none	0 = none
A = atrium	A = atrium	T = triggered	P = simple programmable	P = pacing (antitachyarrhythmia)
V = ventricle	V = ventricle	I = inhibited	M = multiprogrammable	
D = dual (A + V)	D = dual (A + V)	D = dual (T + I)	C = communicating	S = shock
			R = rate modulation	D = dual (P + S)
	S = single (A or V)†	S = single (A or V)†		

*Positions I through III are used exclusively for antibradyarrhythmia function.
†Manufacturers' designation only.

upper rate limit. Because many postoperative congenital heart disease patients are at risk for atrial tachycardia, a device capable of mode switching or providing the DDI pacing mode is an attractive option.

LEAD SELECTION

When choosing the pacing leads most appropriate for each patient, the first decision is to determine which implant technique—epicardial versus endocardial—will be used.[25–27] Because the epicardial technique is more invasive, often results in higher stimulation thresholds and lead fractures, and results in decreased pacemaker longevity, it is generally reserved for those few patients in whom endocardial pacing is contraindicated.[28–30] Candidates for the epicardial technique include infants weighing less than 5.0 kilograms, patients with intracardiac shunts, patients whose superior vena cava does not connect at the atrial level, and patients whose anatomy does not allow venous access to the chamber requiring lead placement, such as the Fontan patient with complete AV block.

When using the epicardial implant technique, the choice of pacing leads is somewhat limited.[31–34] Although there have been some reports of placing endocardial bipolar pacing leads transatrially,[35] the placement of unipolar, epicardial pacing leads is more common. The three most commonly used unipolar leads include the stab-on (or fishhook lead), the screw-in lead (Fig. 11–2), and the steroid-eluting suture-on electrode (Fig. 11–3). The latter has become the epicardial pacing lead of choice at the authors' institution because of its small contact surface area, low chronic pacing thresholds, excellent sensing characteristics, and applicability to both the atria and ventricles for chronic cardiac pacing.[28, 36–39] One potential contraindication of this type of lead is in a patient with severe epicardial fibrosis, in whom a fishhook or screw-in lead might be more optimal for epicardial penetration (Fig. 11–4).

When using the endocardial or transvenous implant technique, bipolar pacing leads are preferable to unipolar leads.[40] Although they are slightly larger than their unipolar counterparts, they are less likely to sense skeletal muscle and cause stimulation of that muscle because of the close spacing of the bipolar electrodes. The type of lead fixation is variable, as is lead length. For atrial placement in small children as well as those postoperative for congenital heart disease, an actively fixated, screw-in lead is clearly preferred.

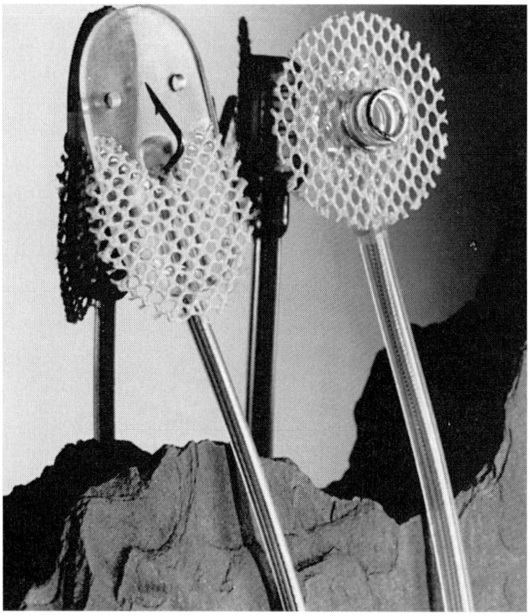

FIGURE 11–2. Actively fixated epicardial pacing leads. The "fishhook" lead on the left can be used for the atrium, whereas the "screw-in" lead on the right is better suited for ventricular placement.

Passively fixated, tined leads can be considered for placement in the ventricle. Overall, silastic insulation has proven to last longer than polyurethane and is favored for pediatric use in which longevity is pivotal.

Steroid-eluting leads, both actively and passively fixated, have proven to result in increased longevity because of lower acute and chronic pacing thresholds.[30, 41] A fixed screw-in, steroid-eluting, Silastic-insulated lead is the bipolar pacing lead of choice at the authors' institution. Chronic pacing leads must be extremely flexible and have a short interelectrode distance for optimal sensing capabilities. Leads with extendable and retractable screws tend to irritate the child's heart because of their inherent stiffness.

The single-pass lead for atrial synchronous pacing in the VDD mode has resulted in some success in children but is not without its problems.[42] The spacing from the ventricular pacing electrode to the atrial sensing electrode is extremely variable during growth and often fails to provide AV synchrony, which was the original intent when this lead was developed. These leads also tend to be somewhat fragile and subject to fracture.

Lead length is also an important consideration. In the smallest of infants, it is not preferable to use very short epicardial pacing leads. If the chronic pacing thresholds are low, the potential

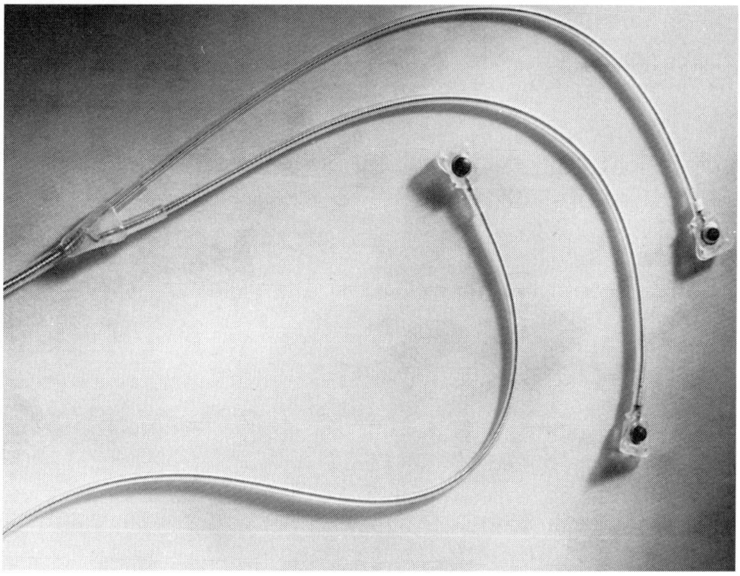

FIGURE 11–3. The epicardial steroid-eluting pacing leads. The active electrode is the black dot. Depicted are both the conventional unipolar type and a bifurcated connection allowing the two unipolar electrodes to function as a bipolar lead.

for the device lasting more than 3 years is very good. With the amount of growth experienced from the newborn to toddler years, a very short lead may become taut enough to fracture. In very young patients requiring epicardial pacing lead placement, a 35-cm lead is preferred. In older patients, a 50-cm lead is used.

For endocardial placement, the size of the child at the time of lead placement is important. The use of an absorbable suture at the site of lead tie-down allows inward migration of the pacing lead as the child grows.[43] Again, a medium length is preferable to a shorter one to get as much use from the original lead as possible. At the authors' institution, in children who have not yet reached adolescence, a 45-cm lead and a 52-cm lead are used for the atrium and ventricle, respectively. In adolescents and young adults, especially those who are very tall or who are expected to become very tall, a 52-cm lead is used in each chamber.

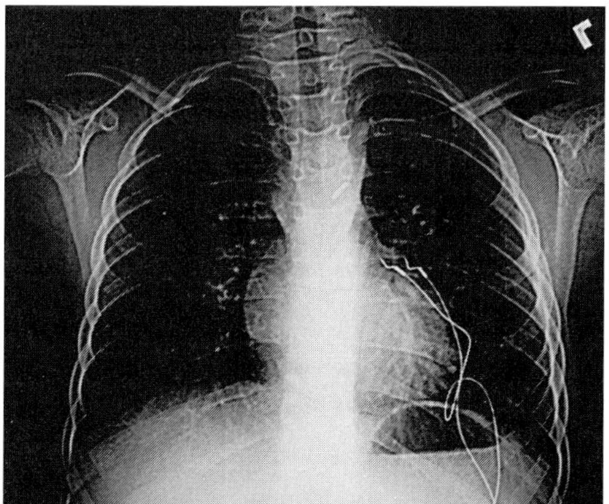

FIGURE 11–4. Chest radiograph of a bipolar atrial antitachycardia pacing system in a postoperative Senning patient. Because of an intracardiac shunt, the epicardial approach was performed. Two epicardial leads were attached to the base of the left atrial appendage and connected to a bipolar pulse generator with the use of an adaptor.

Although it seems somewhat premature at initial implantation, the fact that some of the patient's pacing leads will require removal sometime in the future should be taken into account when determining the type of fixation to use.[44] It is thought that actively fixated leads are generally easier to remove than passively fixated leads.

IMPLANT TECHNIQUE

As previously discussed, the implant technique is determined by the size of the child, the presence of intracardiac shunts, superior vena cava obstruction or lack of a connection at the atrial level, and structural anatomy that precludes endocardial lead placement.[26, 45, 46] All pertinent noninvasive data should be reviewed before system implantation, including electrocardiogram (ECG), 24-hour ambulatory monitoring, exercise stress testing (if applicable), previous operative/catheterization reports, current medications, and, importantly, an echocardiogram. All efforts to determine the presence of intracardiac shunting should be undertaken and, in some cases, may require contrast echocardiography, because the incidence of embolic events is increased in these patients.[47]

ENDOCARDIAL OR TRANSVENOUS TECHNIQUE

The endocardial or transvenous implant technique is best performed by a pediatric cardiologist who is also trained in electrophysiology. The procedure should be undertaken in a pediatric catheterization/electrophysiology laboratory with a team of individuals who routinely care for children. This team should consist of a nurse capable of performing intraoperative testing,[48] an anesthesiologist/nurse anesthetist, nurses who routinely staff the catheterization laboratory, and radiologic and cardiovascular technicians/technologists. The catheterization laboratory itself must meet sterility and air handling/filtration standards consistent with those of the operating room. The implant team must also be trained in sterile technique to a higher degree than usual for the catheterization laboratory. The optimal laboratory is one that implants more than 20 pacemakers per year and is also used for other major interventional procedures.[49]

In consultation with the implanting physician, the pacemaker nurse is responsible for having all necessary pacemakers, leads, programmers, pacing accessories, and pacing system analyzers present for the procedure. Duplicates of each piece of equipment as well as duplicate pacemakers and leads should be made available in case of unexpected problems. A defibrillator with external pacing capabilities, as well as a full range of resuscitation equipment and medications, must be available.

Patient Preparation

Once it has been determined that a pacemaker is required, the patient and family must be prepared.[50, 51] A discussion with the implanting physician and pacemaker nurse will not only prepare them for the procedure but, it is hoped, ease their anxiety as well. This is also a good time to dispel any myths that the patient and family may have about pacemakers and provides an opportunity for visualization of the pacing system. A basic explanation of how the pacemaker works is extremely helpful, because many patients believe that the pacemaker will somehow make them "dependent." Any visual aids about the conduction system, pacemaker, and implant technique can also assist in the patient's and family's understanding. Any written information that can be given to them to take home is also very useful. The implant technique to be used is also discussed, including the site of the pacemaker pocket. Because the left shoulder is preferred, patients who are left-handed must be informed. In rare instances, the right versus the left shoulder can be used for patient preference.

On the day before the procedure, the patient reports to the outpatient department for preoperative testing. A history and physical examination are performed as well as any necessary cardiovascular tests that have not been previously or recently performed. For initial implants, a type and cross-match for one unit of packed red blood cells is performed. Females 12 years or older undergo pregnancy testing, and all patients meet with anesthesia personnel before the procedure to discuss the type of anesthesia to be used. The implanting physician discusses potential complications of the procedure, and the pacemaker nurse provides any further patient education that is necessary. The patient and family are instructed when to withhold food and fluids (i.e., 6–8 hours before the procedure depending on the anesthesia type) and where to report for the procedure.

On the day of the procedure, most patients receive oral premedication with midazolam or diazepam in a holding room just outside of the catheterization laboratory. Once drowsiness occurs, the patient is taken into the catheterization laboratory where the following monitors are placed: ECG, pulse oximetry, end-tidal carbon dioxide, dispersive electrocautery pads, and external pacing/defibrillation pads. Further sedation is given, and an endotracheal tube is placed. A "roll" is placed between the shoulder blades, with the affected arm (usually the left) placed at the patient's side.

The Procedure

Once anesthesia is administered and the patient's groin area is prepared for cardiac catheterization, an arterial puncture is made to place an indwelling arterial catheter (4-French dilator) for invasive blood pressure monitoring and blood gas analysis throughout the procedure. An appropriately sized end-hole catheter is placed via the femoral vein into the right atrium to the superior vena cava, innominate vein, and subclavian and axillary veins. A contrast injection by hand is made at this time to demonstrate venous anatomy. If the subclavian or axillary veins cannot be entered despite the use of flexible guide wires,

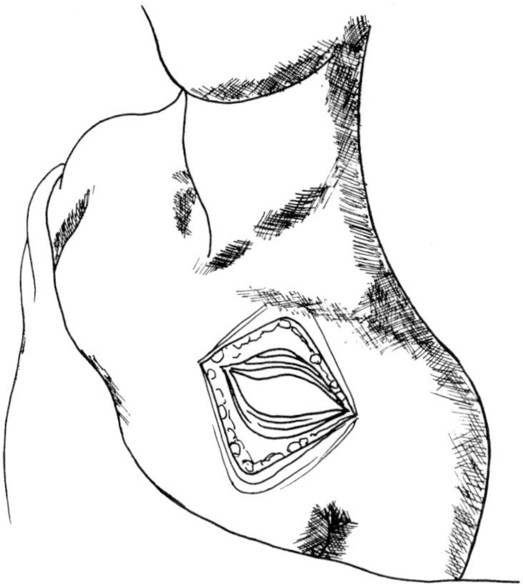

FIGURE 11–5. Line drawing depicting a typical pacemaker pocket incision. Note that the incision is roughly parallel to the clavicle. The pectoralis major muscle is spread, and the lead insertion point is seen under the muscle.

an angiogram is done by injecting the left brachial vein.[52]

If suitable venous access is visualized, the catheter is left in place, and the implanting physician "rescrubs and regowns" before the shoulder area is prepared with alcohol. An Ioban® drape is applied generously to cover the entire shoulder area. The radiopaque sponges are counted, and the electrocautery and suction equipment is attached. Sterile plastic covers are applied to the image intensifier tube as well as to the overhead light. An incision is made to accommodate the pulse generator being implanted and is approximately 125% of the pacemaker's diameter (Fig. 11–5). When the incision is made, the patient is given 12.5 mg/kg of intravenous cefazolin (Ancef) for prophylaxis. If the patient is allergic to cefazolin, vancomycin is used. A second cefazolin dose is given one hour after the initial dose.

The incision starts medially and ends laterally at the deltopectoral groove. It should be 1 to 2 fingerbreadths below the clavicle. Hemostasis is obtained using cautery, which is also used to dissect the layer of subcutaneous fat with the setting of "coagulation" versus "cut." It is not necessary to use the "cut" setting at all during the procedure. When the pectoralis major muscle is visualized, the fibers are spread, rather than cut, with the tips of Metzenbaum or Mayo scissors, with the angle of the muscle fibers being different from that of the pocket incision.[53]

Care must be taken to leave enough muscle superior to the area of muscle separation to allow for later suture closure of the pocket. When the fascia over the pectoralis minor muscle is visualized, blunt dissection between the two muscle layers creates the pocket. Again, the pocket should be made just large enough to accommodate the implanted pacemaker as well as extravascular leads. The pocket should be extended more medially than laterally to avoid the axillary structures.

Once the pocket has been formed and final coagulation with electrocautery is achieved, the axillary/subclavian vein junction is punctured with an 18-gauge needle, the length of which will depend on patient size. The puncture is made below instead of through the pectoralis major muscle, and care must be taken not to direct the needle too deeply or too medially to avoid puncture of the lung or an artery. In patients with deep subcutaneous tissue, the puncture may be made through the pectoralis to help minimize bleeding. The vein is punctured under fluoroscopy by aiming the needle at the previously placed catheter where it crosses the rib cage (Fig. 11–6). This results in an almost 90° angle with the chest wall rather than the usual angle for subclavian vein puncture. Once brisk blood flow is noted, a .038-inch J-tipped guide wire is placed through the needle and passed to the right atrium or inferior vena cava.

Once the guide wire has been advanced, a 10.5-French sheath with a bleed-back valve and side arm is positioned over the wire (Fig. 11–7). At this time, the "aiming" catheter is removed.

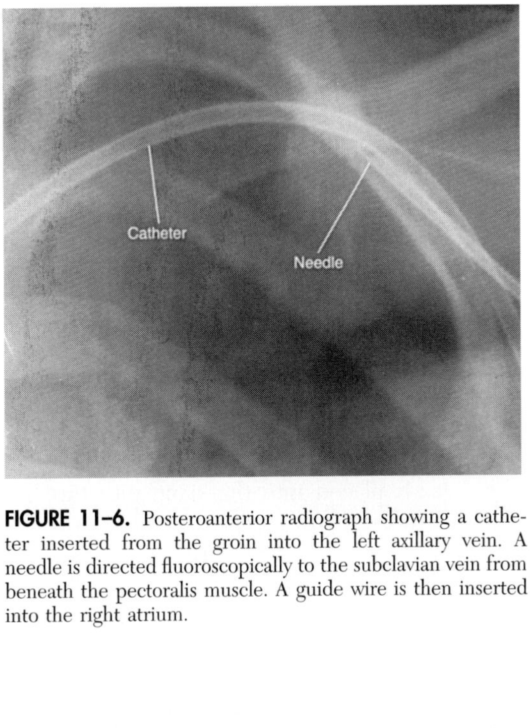

FIGURE 11–6. Posteroanterior radiograph showing a catheter inserted from the groin into the left axillary vein. A needle is directed fluoroscopically to the subclavian vein from beneath the pectoralis muscle. A guide wire is then inserted into the right atrium.

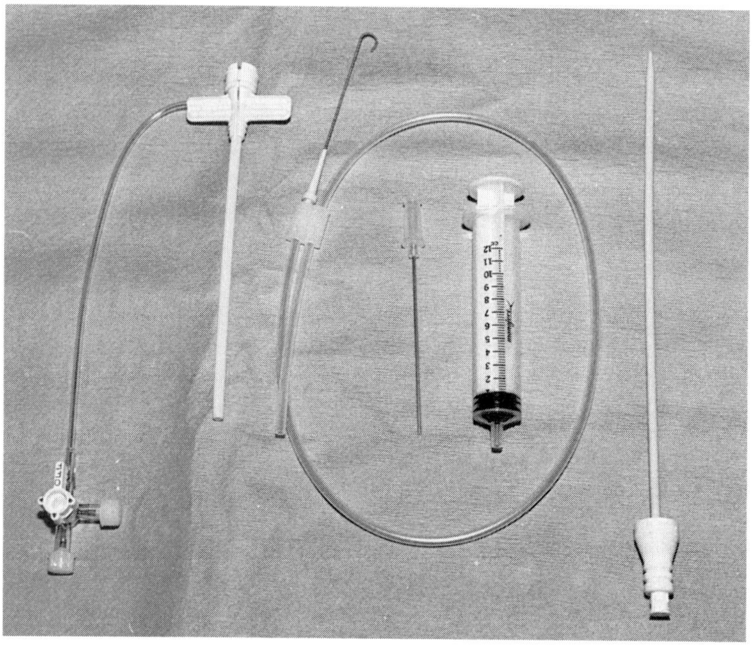

FIGURE 11–7. A typical introducer set for transvenous pacemaker implantation. The sheath can be torn in half after the lead has been positioned. The bleed-back valve and side arm minimize bleeding during lead manipulation.

The tip of the dilator is manipulated fluoroscopically into the right atrium or as far as possible toward the right atrium. The dilator and guide wire are then removed, and the sheath is aspirated and then flushed. The permanent pacing lead is then positioned through the sheath; the first of two leads is advanced into the right ventricle using a curved stylus. The ventricular lead is usually positioned just cephalad to the apex of the right ventricle in the septum to prevent diaphragmatic pacing (Fig. 11–8). In older patients with thicker ventricles, the apex is acceptable (Fig. 11–9). A small, gentle loop may be left in the atrium but should not impinge on the tricuspid valve.

The stylus remains in the lead, with the guide wire reinserted through the same sheath and into the right atrium. The sheath is then torn in half and removed. A second sheath-dilator is then positioned into the right atrium over the guide wire and is left in place; the second lead is positioned in the right atrium, preferably in the right atrial appendage (Fig. 11–10). If placement in the right atrial appendage is not possible, an area high in the right atrium is preferred. In the patient with high central venous pressure, the use of 2 separate punctures is preferable because the 2 leads placed into the same puncture site form a figure-8, allowing more blood loss through the narrow area. The leads are then fixated, and a small amount of extra lead is positioned in the heart. The stylets and sheaths are subsequently removed, and intraoperative testing is performed.

Once adequate pacing and sensing thresholds have been obtained, the leads are secured over the sewing sleeve with absorbable 2-0 Dexon suture. The leads are attached to the pulse generator with visual verification that the connector pins are in the appropriate place. Additionally, a gentle tug on the leads themselves ensures their security. The pocket is then irrigated with a bacitracin-neomycin solution, and any excess lead is placed into the pacemaker pocket under the pulse generator. Before pocket closure, a sponge count is taken; the number should agree with the count at the beginning of the procedure. The pectoral and subcutaneous layers are closed using absorbable 2-0 Dexon; 4-0 Dexon is used to suture the skin. Steri-Strips are placed vertically over the incision to approximate the edges of the skin. A Telfa pad is placed over the Steri-Strips, followed by a gauze dressing secured with paper tape. The venous and arterial catheters are then removed; the usual postcatheterization pressure dressing is placed. The patient generally is admitted to the postanesthesia care unit for 1 to 2 hours before being transferred to a telemetry-monitored hospital bed.

EPICARDIAL TECHNIQUE

Epicardial pacing systems are implanted in the operating room under general anesthesia. Typi-

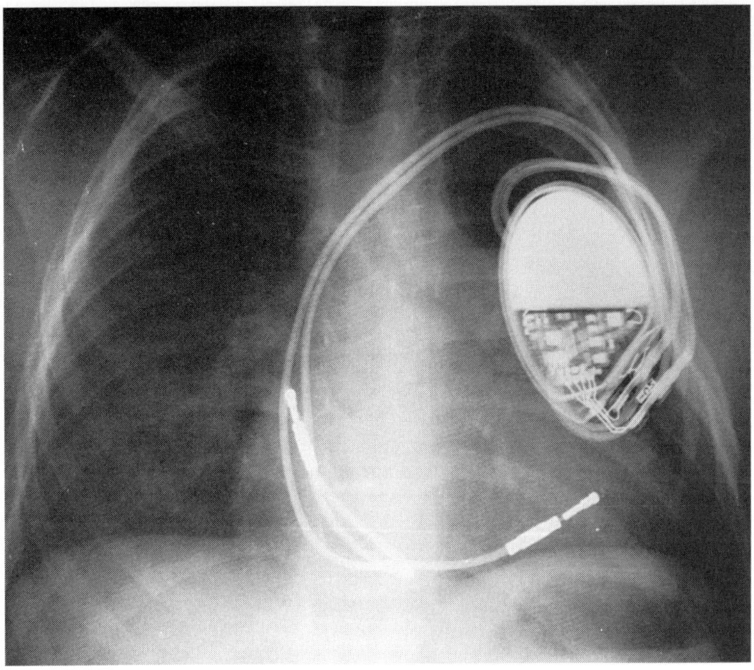

FIGURE 11–8. Common lead positions in an infant with a transvenous dual-chamber pacemaker. The ventricular lead is positioned away from the apex of the right ventricle to prevent diaphragmatic pacing.

cally, the unipolar pacing configuration is used with the body of the pulse generator functioning as the indifferent electrode. The specific approach to pacemaker placement must be individualized for each patient and his or her specific clinical situation. Epicardial pacing electrodes can be placed using the following techniques: median sternotomy, subxiphoid approach, or thoracotomy. The median sternotomy approach is used most often at the authors' institution because of the large number of dual-chamber implants and the excellent results with the steroid-eluting epicardial pacing lead. This approach allows better visualization and pace mapping for the atrial pacing electrode (Fig. 11–11).

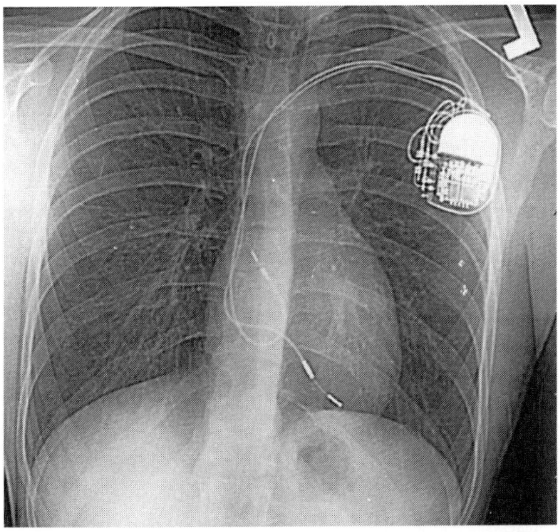

FIGURE 11–9. Typical lead placement in an adolescent with a transvenous dual-chamber pacemaker.

Median Sternotomy

The median sternotomy approach provides excellent access to both the atrial and ventricular surfaces, especially in neonates and small infants. Despite the need for sternal division, this approach results in optimum electrode placement, lower acute and chronic pacing thresholds, excellent sensing of intrinsic deflections, and extended battery longevity.

After adequate general anesthesia has been administered, the chest and abdomen are prepared and draped into the sterile field. A midline incision is performed and may be extended into the upper abdomen if the generator is to be placed through the same incision. Alternately, a separate transverse left upper quadrant abdominal incision can be used to create the pulse generator pocket. Once a median or partial sternotomy is performed, the pocket is created. For a subfascial pocket, the anterior rectus fascia is opened, and electrocautery is used to create the pocket. For a subrectus pocket, the rectus muscle is retracted laterally from the midline, and the dissection is performed by staying anterior to the posterior rectus fascia or by splitting the rectus muscle fibers.

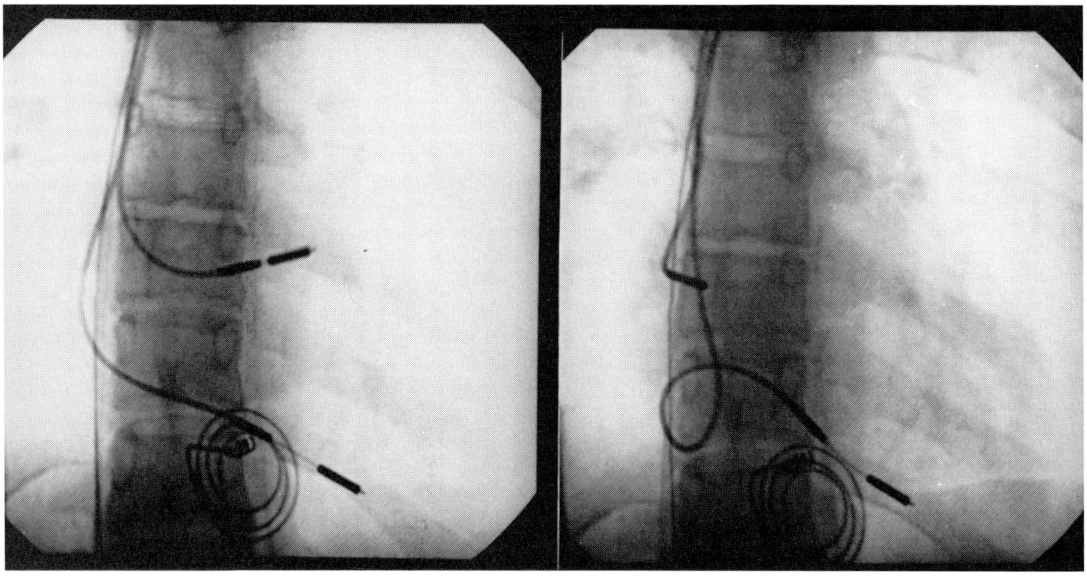

FIGURE 11–10. Demonstration of incorrect (left) and correct (right) positioning of the atrial pacing lead. In the left panel, the upper lead is in the right ventricular outflow tract, as evidenced by the broad low curve. In the right panel, it is in the stump of the right atrial appendage.

The pericardium is then opened to expose the epicardium, and a pericardial well is created with stay sutures. The steroid-eluting leads can then be used to map the atrial and ventricular surfaces by holding the electrode firmly against the epicardial surface. Both intrinsic deflections and pacing thresholds can be measured and performed, respectively. Once a suitable site has been selected, the lead is fixated by securing the surface of the lead with nonabsorbable suture. The fixation is important to prevent motion of the electrode surface against the epicardium, which could potentially lead to chronic irritation, fibrosis, and elevated chronic pacing thresholds. It is also important to avoid ischemia of the underlying myocardium with sutures placed incorrectly or too tightly.[54]

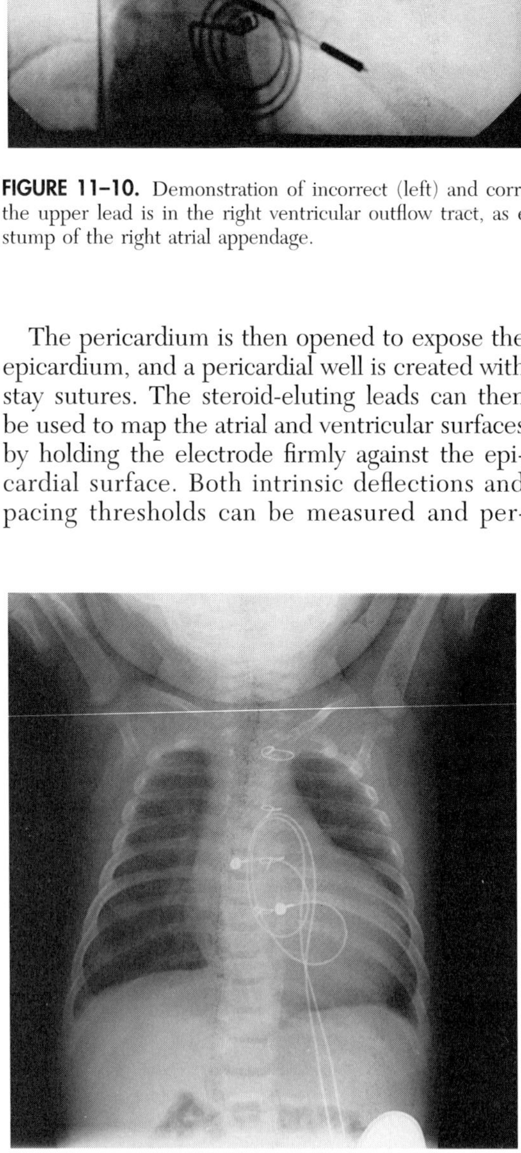

FIGURE 11–11. Epicardial steroid-eluting leads implanted by midline sternotomy in an infant. The pacemaker is seen in the left upper quadrant of the abdomen.

After the leads have been sutured in place, intraoperative testing is performed. If the measurements are acceptable, the leads are tunneled via a subxiphoid route into the pulse generator pocket. To avoid lead fracture, the leads are not tunneled between or over the ribs. Acute bending of the lead at the subcostal border must be avoided to prevent the possibility of lead fracture. A loop of electrode is left within the mediastinum to allow for growth and to prevent stretching of the lead against the rib cage, leading to potential fracture during movement and growth. The leads are connected to the pulse generator and placed into the abdominal pocket with the noninsulated aspect of the generator facing away from the muscle. Redundant lead length is gently looped beneath the pulse generator. Excessive loops are avoided to preclude vascular structure entrapment.[55, 56] The mediastinum is then irrigated with antibiotic saline solution, the pericardial edges are loosely reapproximated, and a temporary drainage catheter is placed within the mediastinum. The sternal edges are reapproximated, and the sternal incision is closed in the usual manner.

Subxiphoid Approach

The subxiphoid approach can also be used for epicardial pacemaker implantation, including the placement of dual-chamber systems.[57, 58] The advantages of this approach include minimal postoperative morbidity and an excellent cosmetic result. Through a single incision, the epicardium can be exposed, electrodes placed, and the pulse generator pocket created.[59] A short upper midline abdominal incision is used, and the rectus fascia is opened to expose the diaphragm and pericardium. With anterior retraction of the sternum, the pericardium is incised and the epicardial surface exposed. Appropriate leads are placed, and intraoperative testing is performed. The leads are then tunneled into the pacemaker pocket, and, as described previously, additional electrode length is left in the mediastinum and the pocket. The edges of the fascia are reapproximated, and the wound is closed in layers.

The subxiphoid approach provides good access to the ventricular epicardium but limited exposure to the atrium, which makes it somewhat difficult when placing the steroid-eluting lead, especially in small infants. This approach may also be problematic in the patient requiring reoperation in whom there is significant epicardial fibrosis.

Thoracotomy

The thoracotomy approach to epicardial pacemaker implantation is being used less frequently than in the past. This approach may be beneficial in patients who have previously undergone cardiac surgery and in very small neonates. Dual-chamber pacing is possible with this approach, although left atrial pacing is required when using a left-sided approach. An anterior thoracotomy through the fourth to sixth intercostal space is used to expose the pericardium. The pericardium itself is opened longitudinally; care is taken to avoid the phrenic nerve. An appropriate site for lead placement is selected, and intraoperative testing is performed. The pulse generator is placed in an abdominal pocket through a separate subcostal incision. The leads are tunneled below the costophrenic angle into the pulse generator pocket. It is important that the leads not be passed above the ribs to avoid lead fracture. Again, a gentle loop of lead is left in the mediastinum, and the redundant lead is looped underneath the pulse generator. Tension on the lead should be avoided as it passes under the costophrenic angle to prevent rubbing of the lead against the rib cage, making it subject to lead fracture. The thoracotomy incision is then closed in the standard fashion.

General Considerations

Epicardial pacing systems are implanted under general anesthesia; prophylactic antibiotics are initiated preoperatively and administered for 24 hours postoperatively. The generator pocket is created first so that the use of electrocautery can be minimized once the electrodes have been placed, reducing the potential for "microburns," scarring at the electrode tip, and potential early lead abandonment.[60, 61] In most cases, the pulse generators are placed on the left side of the abdomen so as not to obscure physical examination of the liver, although generators have been placed on the right side of the abdomen in the presence of a gastrostomy tube.

Subcutaneous abdominal pockets should be avoided in children because of the possibility of migration and erosion of the pulse generator. Additionally, subcutaneous placement generally results in a poorer cosmetic result. The subrectus location provides added protection to the generator, lowers the risk of erosion and wound infection, and is cosmetically superior in small patients.[62]

INTRAOPERATIVE TESTING

PACEMAKER PREPROGRAMMING

The availability of any and all necessary supplies that might be required during pacing system implantation is of paramount importance. If the procedure consists of a generator replacement only, knowledge regarding lead connectors and pulse generator compatibilities is critical in order to have the correct supplies. Although rarely necessary, a duplicate of each lead and pulse generator should be readily available. In addition, the following items are necessary: pacing system analyzer (PSA), test cables, extra lead stylets, indifferent electrode (for unipolar leads), appropriate screwdrivers (for generator replacements), sterile magnet, sterile programming wand, and a pacemaker-specific programmer.[48]

The soon-to-be implanted device is interrogated and preprogrammed still within its sterile packaging before implantation. The lead polarity and pacemaker polarity should be the same, which may or may not require reprogramming. Because most devices are programmed to nominal settings before implantation, certain programmed values will require re-evaluation. Because acute pacing thresholds will rise to a peak value in the first few weeks after implantation,[63] we use a standardized output setting of 5.0 V and 0.5 milliseconds at the time of implantation. The rate of the pulse generator should be programmed to meet the individual needs of the patient (i.e., age, hemodynamic benefit, optimal electrophysiologic benefit). In a dual-chamber system (DDDCO), the lowest acceptable atrial rate for the patient is chosen as the permanently programmed lower rate. In a rate adaptive system, the lower rate chosen should be age appropriate with a higher sensor-driven upper rate. In patients receiving atrial antitachycardia devices (AAICP), a faster than normal bradycardia pacing rate is used in an attempt to decrease ectopy and prevent tachycardia episodes that may be bradycardia induced.

The sensitivity can be programmed before implantation, but may require readjustment on the basis of the intrinsic deflections obtained with lead placement. Although a setting of 1.0 mV is acceptable for atrial sensitivity, we generally use 0.5 mV because the atrial electrogram amplitude decreases with exercise in children.[8] When this setting is used in patients with intra-atrial tachycardia, it often results in R-wave oversensing on the atrial electrogram; however, less sensitive settings may result in undersensing of the atrial tachycardia.[48] The ventricular sensitivity is programmed from 2.8 to 4.0 mV depending on the intrinsic R-wave deflection.

The upper rate limit in a dual-chamber device should be programmed to a value acceptable for the patient's age and hemodynamic status. It may not always be desirable for postoperative patients to sense the atrium to rates of 180 ppm. Also, the "true tracking limit" must be recognized as the total atrial refractory period (i.e., the sum of the AV delay and the PVARP). If the total atrial refractory period is less than the programmed upper rate limit, the device will exhibit 2:1 AV block before Wenckebach block, the latter of which is the preferred upper rate limit behavior in all pediatric patients.

The AV delay is programmed anywhere from 75 to 100 ms in the neonate to 120 to 150 ms in older patients and in those with postoperative congenital heart disease. The availability of rate adaptive AV delays has been of great benefit in pediatric patients, because they mimic the physiologic adaptation to a shorter PR interval with increasing atrial rates.[64]

The ventricular refractory period, used primarily to prevent T-wave oversensing, is generally programmed to 200 ms. Ventricular blanking must be programmed in such a way that premature ventricular events are appropriately sensed while also alleviating the sensing of atrial signals on the ventricular channel. This value can be programmed to the lowest available setting in most pediatric patients without unwanted sequelae.

Rate adaptive parameters are generally programmed to the "nominal settings" until postprocedure testing can be performed to ascertain the most appropriate settings for each individual patient. Specific events in the postoperative period (i.e., chest percussion or ventilatory support) may preclude the programming of rate adaptive parameters at the time of implantation.

Antitachycardia functions can be programmed based on the patient's clinical tachycardia in most cases and should be patient and tachycardia specific. In many patients, a detection algorithm of high rate and sudden onset is sufficient in recognizing most intra-atrial re-entry tachycardias.

ACUTE THRESHOLD TESTING

Once the leads are positioned, the sterile test cables are attached to the leads and the PSA. The pacing mode used for acute lead testing depends on the number of leads that are placed. When placing two leads, we use the DOO mode for testing to obtain a high atrial pacing rate. Once capture is verified in the patient who is minimally paralyzed with muscle relaxants, high output of 10.0 V and 2.0 milliseconds is used to evaluate the presence of diaphragmatic or phrenic nerve stimulation. In some cases, this high-output setting will result in the atrial lead pacing the ventricle; this is of little clinical significance in this setting. If diaphragmatic pacing or phrenic nerve stimulation occurs, the lead is repositioned. This high-output test is not accurate in the patient who is maximally medicinally paralyzed.

Lead resistance (impedance) measurements are obtained at 5.0 V and 0.5 milliseconds and vary according to lead polarity and manufacturer characteristics. An acceptable range for lead resistance in an acute lead is 200 to 1000 Ω. If an extreme measurement is obtained, all connections from the PSA to lead are verified and the measurement is repeated. For chronic lead testing in pulse generator replacements, a difference of 200 Ω from the initial measurement is acceptable.

Pacing thresholds are obtained for one or two leads, depending on the number of leads implanted. The acute pacing threshold is considered to be the lowest output setting (voltage) that captures the chamber being paced 100% of the time. At our institution, a voltage threshold is performed at a constant pulse width, but testing can be performed in the opposite manner also. An acceptable acute pacing threshold range for the atrium is 0.5 to 2.5 V and for the ventricle, 0.5 to 2.0 V. Again, these voltage thresholds are performed at 0.5 millisecond.

Intrinsic deflections should be obtained at implantation whenever possible. These values should be compatible with the available sensitivity settings of the implanted pulse generator. The intrinsic atrial deflection or atrial electrogram should be at least 1.0 mV, with an acceptable range of 1 to 3 mV. Many postoperative patients will have very small atrial signals, which again stresses the importance of available programmable parameters and intrinsic deflection measurement compatibility. The actual intrinsic deflection measurement can be obtained using the PSA or a physiologic recorder (Fig. 11–12). It is preferable to have little or no R wave on the atrial electrogram. The ventricular intrinsic deflection or R-wave electrogram should range from 4 to 7 mV and again be compatible with the available ventricular sensitivity settings within the implanted pulse generator.

Once all acute lead measurements have been obtained and the generator has been attached and placed in the pocket, a telemetry measurement is obtained with the sterile programming wand. This will provide baseline impedance measurements through the programmer and will also verify that there are no connector problems before closing the pocket. A sterile magnet can be used at this time to verify pacing and capture of the implanted device.

In the patient receiving unipolar leads, an indifferent electrode must be used for testing. This electrode provides a ground for the unipolar system. It is placed in the pocket, and the terminal end is attached to the positive clip (vs. the negative clip) on the test cables. The negative clip is attached to the lead's connector pin in order for testing to be accomplished. Additionally, once the unipolar device is attached to the leads, pacemaker function cannot be verified until the device has been placed in the pacemaker pocket.

POSTOPERATIVE CARE

Once the procedure has been completed as just described, the patient is transferred to the postanesthesia care unit or telemetry unit depending on whether general anesthesia or deep

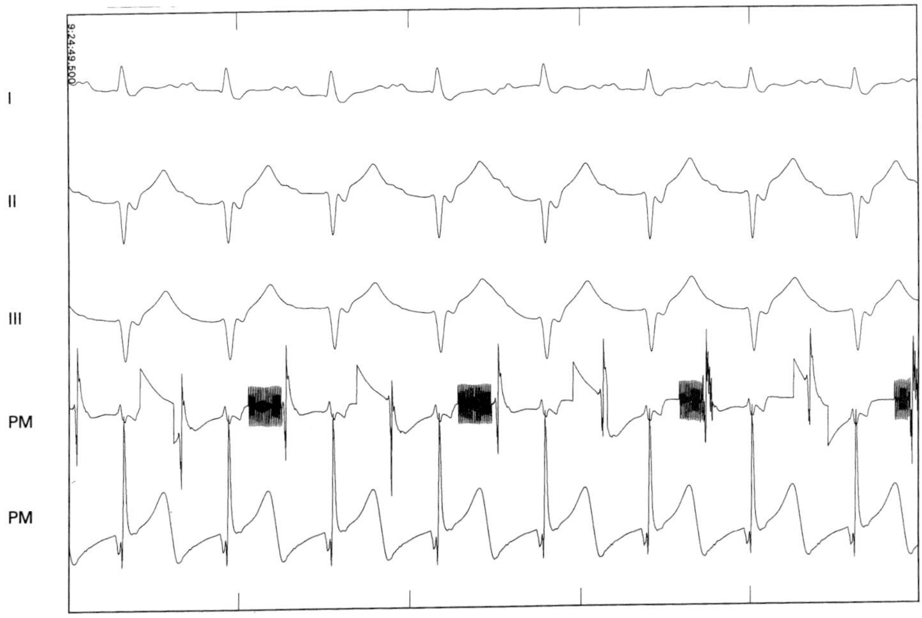

FIGURE 11–12. Atrial (Channel 4) and ventricular (Channel 5) electrograms recorded in the bipolar format through a physiologic recorder. At the time of the recording, a 1-mV calibration was being applied to the atrial signal.

sedation was used, respectively. The postoperative orders include frequent assessment of vital signs, including temperature in the immediate postoperative period. Fluids are allowed only when the patient is fully awake and alert. Ambulation is deferred for overnight but is encouraged the next day. Medications include cefazolin, 12.5 mg/kg every 6 hours for 8 doses, acetaminophen with codeine for pain, acetaminophen for fever or mild pain, dexamethasone (Decadron), 1 to 2 mg every 6 hours for elevated acute pacing threshold, promethazine (Phenergan) for nausea and vomiting, and any medications prescribed before pacemaker implantation. A shoulder immobilizer is used on most patients to decrease the possibility of early lead dislodgment. All patients are monitored on telemetry until discharge by personnel knowledgeable about pacemakers, arrhythmias, and monitor artifacts (Fig. 11–13); the risk of monitor failure to detect cardiac arrest is decreased with the use of an "attended" system.[65]

Before discharge, all patients undergo ECG, chest radiograph, and noninvasive pacemaker testing. The chest radiograph verifies lead position and such complications as pneumothorax and hemothorax. The ECG will depict pacemaker function (i.e., pacing and sensing). The pacemaker testing includes performance of pacing thresholds and sensing thresholds and determination of underlying rhythm. Diagnostic data counters are programmed at this time, as are any other parameters requiring programming or reprogramming.

Before discharge, the dressing is removed from the pacemaker incision. Patients and families are instructed in the use of Polymyxin-bacitracin (Polysporin) powder, which is applied to the wound twice daily. They are instructed not to remove the Steri-Strips and to expect a small amount of serosanguineous drainge with increased ambulation. They are also instructed in the signs and symptoms of wound infection, as well as ways to bathe without getting the incision wet. We require the use of subacute bacterial endocarditis prophylaxis on all transvenous implants even though the American Heart Association and American Dental Association no longer recommend it.

An outpatient follow-up appointment is scheduled for 6 to 8 weeks after implantation. If the wound is thought to be at particular risk, an interim visit is scheduled at 2 to 3 weeks after the procedure. The child's activity level is slowly increased, and strenuous physical activity is moderated according to his or her overall cardiac condition.[66] The pacemaker patient with an anatomically normal heart is allowed to compete at any level of athletics with the exception of varsity football and hockey. The patient with congenital heart disease often has restrictions placed more so because of the structural disorder rather than the conduction system disease.

Last, the patient and family are instructed in the use of a transtelephonic monitor as an adjunct to hands-on outpatient follow-up. The pacemaker nurse provides verbal and written instructions, and each family is required to provide a return demonstration. They are instructed to call weekly for the first six weeks or anytime a problem with the child's rhythm or pacemaker is perceived. This component of pacemaker follow-up has proven to be both valuable and cost effective in the pediatric pacemaker population.[67]

FOLLOW-UP

Pacing system follow-up should ideally begin at the time the decision is made to place a

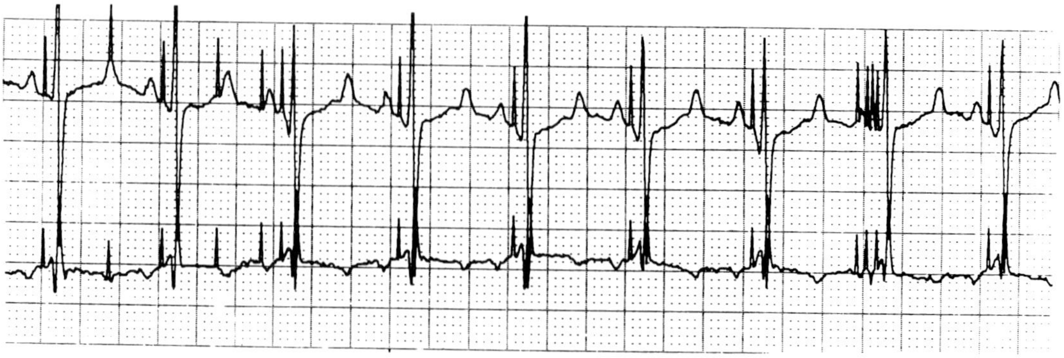

FIGURE 11–13. Artifactual pacemaker spikes generated by the software of a telemetry system with the pacemaker setting "on." This algorithm enhances pacemaker spikes but also detects other rapid rises and falls in the electrocardiogram. The three very rapid spikes on the next to the last beat are impossible.

permanent cardiac pacemaker. This follow-up is equally important to the implant itself and is crucial in maintaining optimal hemodynamics and battery longevity. Additionally, follow-up provides early recognition of inadequate or even inappropriate pacing system performance. Although it is not always feasible, it is desirable to have the implanting physician also be the follow-up physician. It not only is cost efficient but provides continuity in the patient's care. This follow-up care should consist of regular hands-on outpatient clinic visits, with complementary transtelephonic monitoring of pacemaker function in between.

TRANSTELEPHONIC MONITORING

Transtelephonic monitoring can be accomplished by providing an on-site service or by using a centralized service. Although for some pacemaker follow-up centers the use of a centralized service is more cost effective, it is not optimal when caring for children for several reasons.[68] First, the geographic distance between the patient and the service is often very wide with differing time zones, making communication with the service and the follow-up physician more difficult. Second, the service has complete knowledge of the pacing system but does not actually know the patient, which can be problematic in patients with congenital heart disease and a malfunctioning pacemaker. Third, once an abnormal ECG is received by the service, the follow-up physician must be notified to make arrangements for pacemaker adjustment. This procedure is time consuming and could result in occasional unwanted sequelae.

An on-site transtelephonic surveillance system provides a continuum of care unrivaled by an off-site service. Several pieces of equipment as well as personnel knowledgeable about the patient and pacing system are necessary. Many systems are now computerized, obviating the need for much of the equipment used in the early days of pacemaker follow-up. A receiving center capable of providing a single-channel lead is used at our institution (Fig. 11–14). It is attached to an answering machine, which allows the patient and family to transmit at their convenience using a toll-free number for the call. Reminder letters are sent to each patient approximately two weeks before a scheduled transmission. If a transmission is not obtained, pacemaker clinic personnel contact the family to request one.

This system works fairly well, but an adjunct system has been placed for use when problems occur after regular business hours. A second receiving center is located on the inpatient telemetry unit and is attached to an acoustic coupler. If a problem arises, the physician on call simply transfers the call to the nursing unit for a real-time transmission. Once the ECG has been obtained, the physician reviews it, either by facsimile or direct visualization, and proceeds from there. Use of this secondary method is rarely

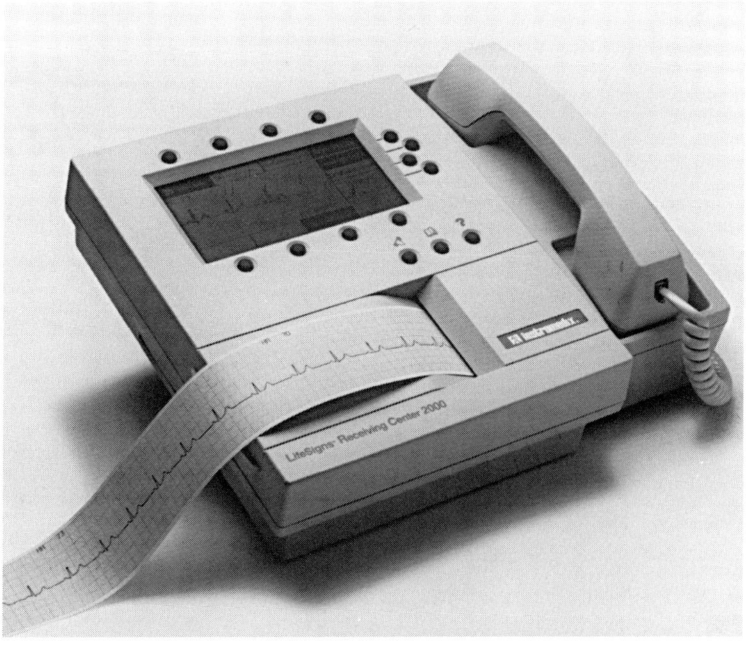

FIGURE 11–14. A transtelephonic system consisting of an answering machine and a receiving center. Transtelephonic electrocardiograms can be either printed directly or stored on computer for complete data management. (Courtesy of Instromedix.)

required, but the few times that it has been used has resulted in prompt identification and treatment of pacemaker-related problems.

It is helpful for the individual receiving the transtelephonic ECG to have some knowledge of the various transmitters used for pacemaker surveillance. At our institution, the nurses who provide patient education regarding transmitter usage also receive the transtelephonic ECGs. On occasion, patients and parents become "flustered" when attempting to send an ECG and may place the telephone backward on the transmitter or in the telephone cradle. Knowledge of the type of transmitter allows the receiver to solve potential problems related to technique in these cases.

The type of transmitter used for transtelephonic follow-up varies from institution to institution (Fig. 11–15). Transmitters with wrist electrodes, finger electrodes, or chest electrodes with leads are not desirable in the pediatric population for several reasons. First, the wrist and finger electrodes, because they are made for adults, are too large for use on small patients. Second, chest electrodes attached to ECG leads are loathed by most children because they "hurt" when being removed. The use of a transmitter with metal "electrodes" on the back or those with a telephone cradle with chest probe are the transmitters of choice for children.[2, 68] The latter allows the operator to hold the chest probe with one hand and soothe the child with the other. Before hospital discharge from the pacemaker implant procedure, the patient and family are instructed in the use of the specific transmitter and are introduced to the transtelephonic service.

Transtelephonic ECGs are received on a routine basis, but the families are told to transmit any time they perceive a problem with the pacing system or the child experiences symptoms (i.e., syncope, dizziness, tachycardia, palpitations). At our institution, transtelephonic ECGs are received weekly for the first 6 to 8 weeks after initial implantation. At this time, a hands-on follow-up visit will determine the frequency of telephone transmissions. If there is a problem, patients may require more intensive telephone follow-up. In most cases, the telephone follow-up proceeds to monthly for the first year and then every three months after the first anniversary of implantation. Once the device is approximately five years of age or shows evidence of battery depletion, transtelephonic surveillance is intensified, as determined by the follow-up physician.

The ECG transmission itself consists of a 30-second ECG without magnet application and a 30-second ECG with magnet application (Fig. 11–16). Knowledge of each device's response to magnet application and elective replacement indicators is important when receiving a transtelephonic recording. Additionally, many manufacturers have included a threshold margin test (TMT) to allow verification that an adequate safety margin has been programmed. In general, the TMT consists of a specific number of beats at a predetermined rate, with a percentage re-

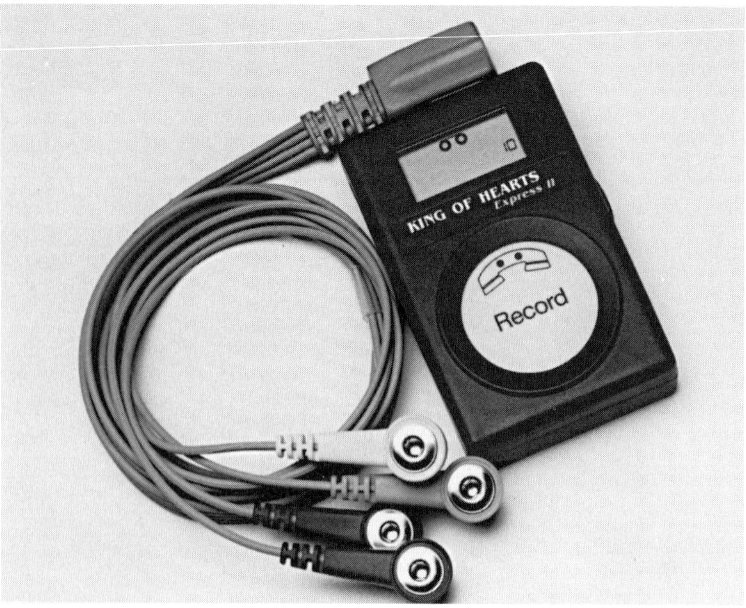

FIGURE 11–15. Transmitter used for transtelephonic pacemaker follow-up. This device has four metal "feet" on the back, which are placed on the patient's chest during transmission. The mouthpiece of the telephone is placed over the front of the transmitter. The arm receptacles on the bottom for wrist, finger, or chest electrodes are not used. (Courtesy of Instromedix.)

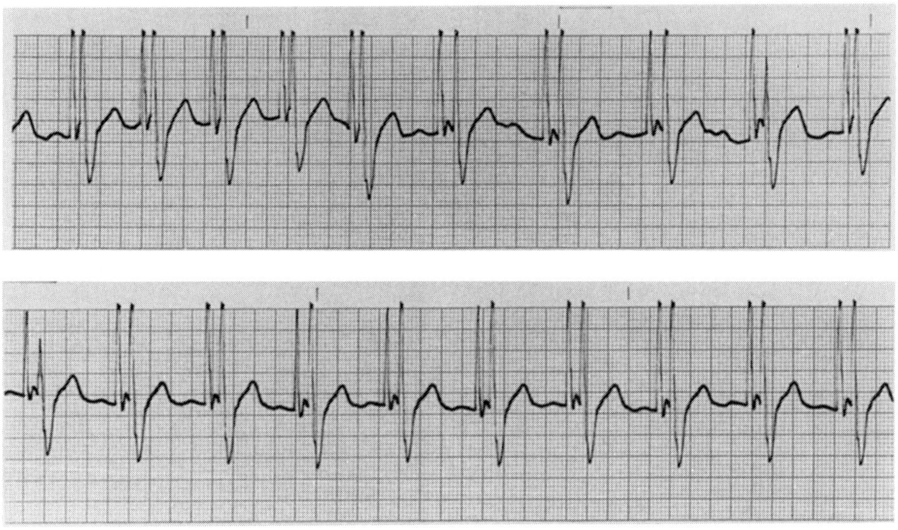

FIGURE 11–16. Single-lead *magnet* and *nonmagnet* transtelephonic tracings in a patient with a DDD pacemaker. The normal pacing rate and atrioventricular (AV) interval are measured on the bottom strip *without magnet*. In the top recording *with magnet*, the rate increases, the AV interval decreases, and the mode is asynchronous.

duction in output on the specified beat. Often the pulse width is temporarily reduced by 25 to 50%, depending on the device manufacturer.

HANDS-ON FOLLOW-UP

Outpatient, hands-on follow-up is scheduled on an individual basis, depending on underlying rhythm, concomitant structural heart disease, patient and device age, and previous pacemaker history (e.g., elevated thresholds, lead fracture). In general, patients younger than 2 years, patients with epicardial pacing leads, patients who are considered pacemaker dependent, patients with complex congenital heart disease, and patients with previous threshold problems are seen every six months. All others are seen annually. Once impending battery depletion is noted, the hands-on as well as transtelephonic follow-up schedule is intensified, as prescribed by the follow-up physician.

The hands-on follow-up visit may include a multitude of tests, depending on each patient's specific needs. All patients should undergo a complete history and physical examination as well as a complete pacemaker evaluation. The value of obtaining a history cannot be overstated because it often reveals problems that might otherwise go unidentified. Symptoms such as dizziness, new-onset exercise intolerance, syncope, and "loss of energy" may be indicative of pacemaker malfunction.[2] The physical examination allows the physician to evaluate the patient's overall physical status, and also provides an opportunity to detect problems that may be directly

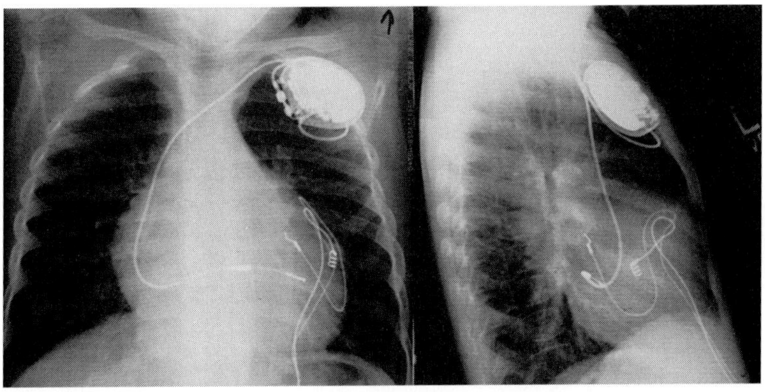

FIGURE 11–17. Posteroanterior (PA) (left) and lateral (right) chest radiographs in a patient who experienced epicardial lead exit block. A transvenous lead was inadvertently positioned in the left ventricle through a patent foramen ovale. The lead position appears satisfactory on the PA view but is clearly posterior in the lateral view.

related to the pacing system, such as irregular heart rhythms, pacemaker pocket infections, changes in valve function, and so on.

Other tests that are important in the follow-up of the pediatric pacemaker patient include chest roentgenogram, exercise stress testing, echocardiography, routine 12- or 15-lead ECG, and twenty-four-hour ambulatory monitoring. Chest roentgenography should be performed at least annually in the growing child (i.e., < 17 years) to assess lead length and position as well as lead migration and interference with cardiac function (Figs. 11–17 and 11–18). Echocardiography is generally performed in those patients with concomitant congenital heart disease and at the discretion of the follow-up physician (Fig. 11–19).

Exercise stress testing is an invaluable tool in the pediatric pacemaker patient.[69] A multitude of information can be obtained regarding the pacemaker's performance that may not be evident during pacemaker testing.[70] The problems identified during exercise stress testing can relate to undesirable upper rate limit behavior, inadequate heart rate increase with exercise, variation of pacing thresholds with exercise, and atrial undersensing as a result of changes in atrial electrogram voltage during exercise.[7, 8, 71–73] Many of these problems are easily corrected by parameter reprogramming.

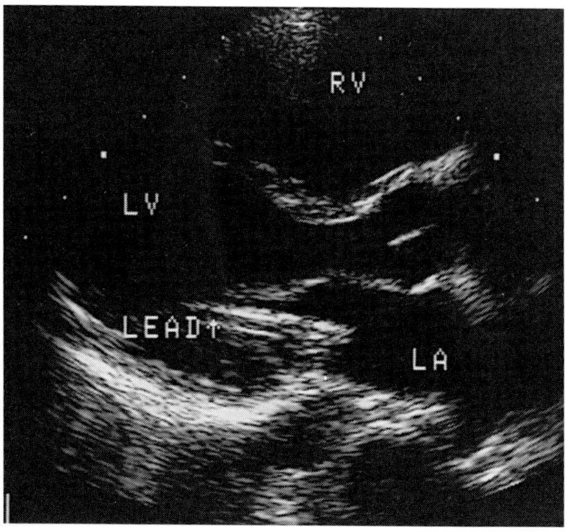

FIGURE 11–19. Long-axis two-dimensional echocardiogram of the left atrium (LA) and left ventricle (LV) showing a pacemaker lead in the left ventricle that had inadvertently been placed there through a patent foramen ovale.

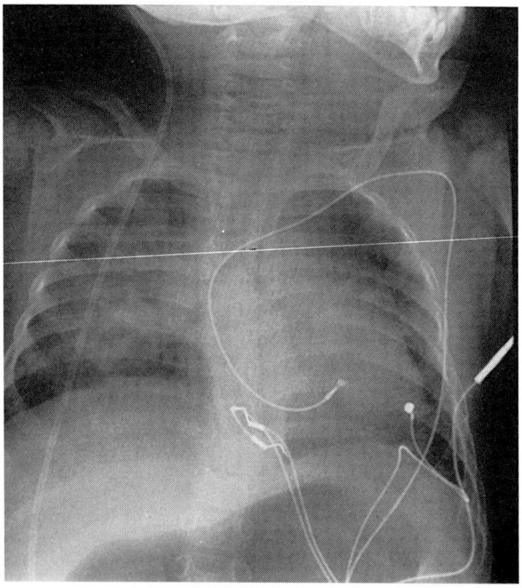

FIGURE 11–18. Posteroanterior chest radiograph in a patient with congenital complete atrioventricular (AV) block. At birth, two epicardial fishhook leads were placed, one atrial and one ventricular, at 1290 g of body weight. The atrial lead functioned well for 6 years, but exit block developed in the ventricular lead, necessitating placement of an epicardial steroid-eluting lead. Exit block developed in this lead also, and a transvenous steroid-eluting lead was placed and tunneled to an abdominal pocket.

Twenty-four-hour ambulatory monitoring is another valuable tool in the follow-up of the pediatric pacemaker patient.[74, 75] It is especially helpful in younger patients who are unable to perform exercise stress testing (Figs. 11–20 to 11–22). Intermittent problems, such as under- or oversensing and noncapture, can be detected by twenty-four-hour ambulatory monitoring (Fig. 11–23). Additionally, competition between the patient's paced and intrinsic rhythm can be identified. Last, any symptomatology that the patient may be experiencing related to the pacing system may be verified in this manner (Fig. 11–24).

Noninvasive pacemaker evaluation in the child should be performed by qualified personnel adept at dealing with children and their families. A calm child is cooperative, allowing complete pacemaker evaluation. Limb leads are attached to the patient for a baseline ECG recording of leads I, II, and III. If available, an ECG cable that hooks into the specific pacemaker programmer is also attached. The pacemaker is then interrogated for programmed settings, measured data, and diagnostic data. Measured data includes performance data such as battery voltage, lead impedance, measured pulse width and amplitude, current flow, and energy delivered.

The programmed values should be evaluated and compared with values from the last visit to ensure that no reprogramming has occurred. Some generators will revert to noise reversion

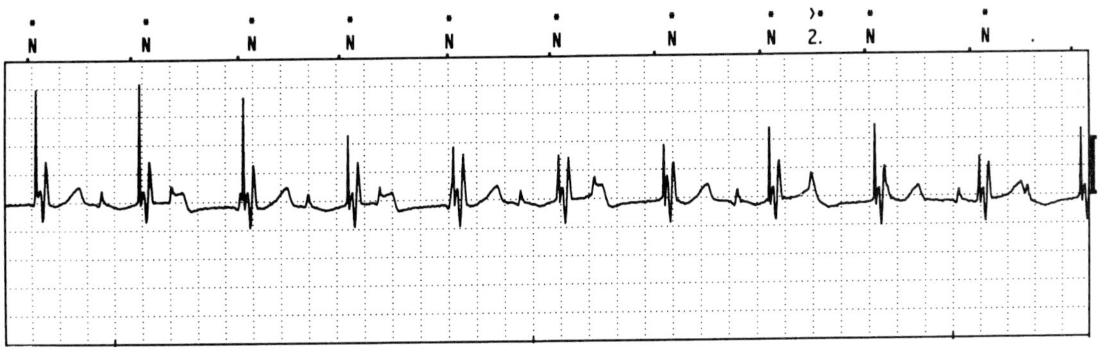

FIGURE 11–20. Ventricular demand rate adaptive pacing in a patient with complete atrioventricular (AV) block. Complete atrial dissociation is seen in the presence of paced ventricular activity.

modes or elective replacement when exposed to electromechanical interference. Although this information is frequently discussed with the patient and parents, exposure to such hazards occasionally occurs.

The measured data are very valuable to the practitioner. The pacemaker's battery voltage and cell impedance should be assessed and compared with the previous values to estimate battery longevity and determine frequency of follow up. In most lithium batteries, the cell impedance will increase as the battery voltage decreases. This does not occur logarithmically and is very hard to predict in devices with very small batteries. Lead impedance is critical because it is a very good indicator of how the lead is functioning. Normal lead impedance measurements vary according to lead polarity and can range from 200 to 1000 Ω,[76] although some leads with very high impedances (i.e., >1200 Ω) are currently being manufactured. The measurements should be compared with previous values to determine any abrupt or subtle changes. A change in either direction of 200 Ω or greater should arouse suspicion, in these cases, repeat measurements should be taken at the same pulse width and pulse amplitude for consistency.[68] In general, an abrupt decrease in the lead impedance is indicative of insulation problems, whereas an increase is indicative of lead wire fracture, pacemaker header problems, electrode tip erosion, or impending exit block.

The pacemaker's diagnostic data are very helpful but vary among device manufacturers. Pacemaker usage as well as heart rate ranges can be assessed using the diagnostic counters (Fig. 11–25). Other useful information that can be obtained includes the incidence of premature beats and runs of tachycardia and the number of tachycardia episodes and subsequent modes of termination; the latter are found in atrial antitachycardia devices (Fig. 11–26).

Intracardiac electrograms and annotation markers are available in most commercially avail-

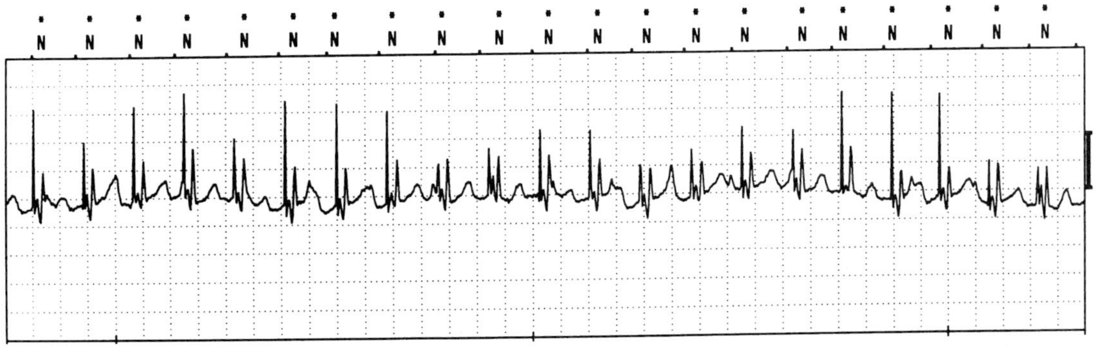

FIGURE 11–21. Pacing in the same patient as in Figure 11–20. The ventricular pacing rate has now accelerated as a result of an increase in the patient's activity.

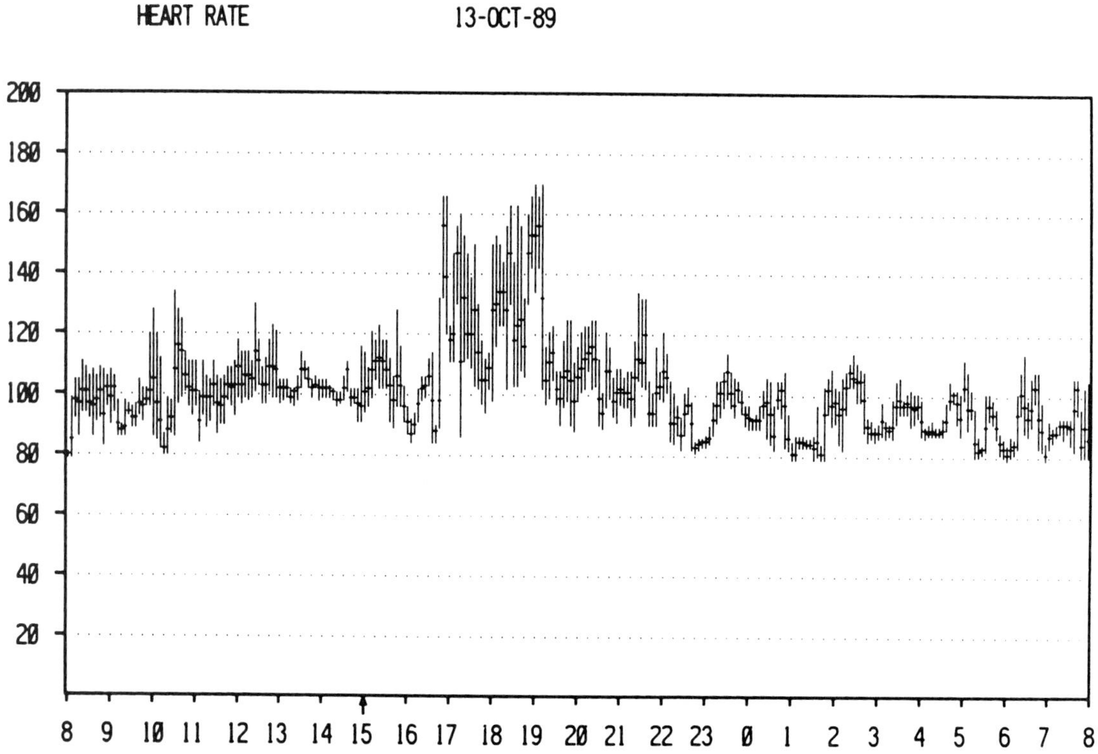

FIGURE 11–22. Heart rate depiction plotted against time in a child with a ventricular rate adaptive device.

able devices (Fig. 11–27). These features can be extremely useful in identifying the source of sensing problems and other unclear problems. A frequently encountered problem in patients with atrial antitachycardia pacemakers with postoperative intra-atrial re-entry tachycardia is the presence of R-wave oversensing on the atrial electrogram. On the surface ECG, it appears that the device is malfunctioning because the paced rate is less than the programmed rate. In evaluating the atrial electrogram, a ventricular intrinsic deflection is present, causing the device to appropriately inhibit. If one were to measure from the atrial pacemaker artifact on the surface ECG to

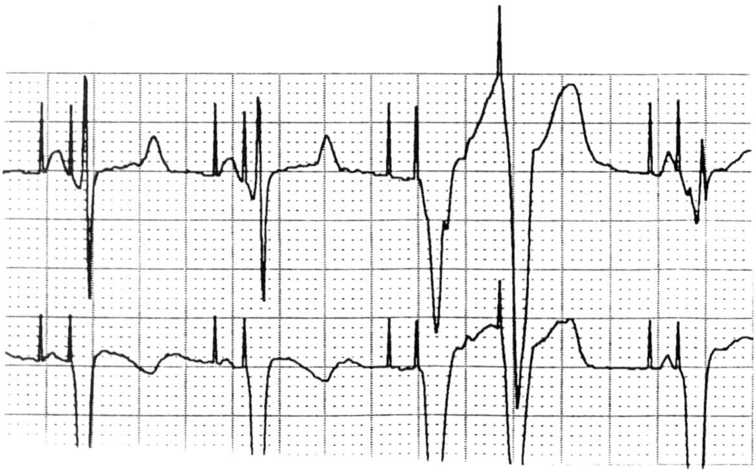

FIGURE 11–23. Loss of atrial capture resulting in a prematurely paced QRS in a patient with a DDD pacemaker. The dual-chamber system begins pacing and capturing in both chambers. On the third beat, atrial noncapture occurs with a sinus escape in the next ST segment, triggering a paced ventricular response on the T wave.

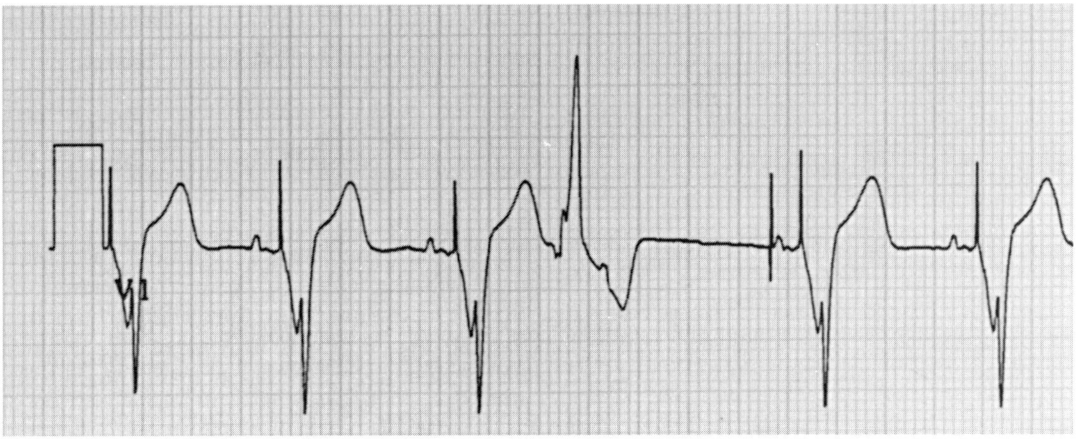

FIGURE 11–24. Atrial synchronous pacing. The first 2 beats are atrial sensing with ventricular pacing. A premature ventricular contraction is appropriately sensed and a stimulus inhibited. The next sinus P wave in the ST segment is also appropriately sensed and a stimulus inhibited. The device next stimulates in an atrioventricular sequential fashion and then resumes atrial sensing followed by ventricular pacing.

the previous QRS complex, the measured interval should correlate to the programmed pacing rate. Intracardiac electrograms are also helpful in identifying obscure atrial arrhythmias that are difficult to ascertain on the surface ECG.

The actual provocative testing of the device includes pacing thresholds, sensing thresholds, and underlying rhythm. The pacing thresholds are performed in the chambers being paced. Pulse width thresholds are performed at various pulse amplitudes. The threshold is considered to be the lowest pulse width value that produces a depolarization 100% of the time. For leads that are older than 6 weeks, the programmed output is permanently programmed as follows: for the atrium, the threshold pulse width value is doubled; for the ventricle, the threshold pulse width value is tripled. Sensing thresholds are also important to evaluate and should correlate with the intracardiac electrogram when using bipolar leads.[77] Because the atrial electrogram voltage decreases with exercise,[8] the atrial sensitivity is left at the maximal setting (i.e., 0.5 mV in most devices). In the case of unipolar leads, the atrial sensitivity is programmed to a slightly less sensitive setting because of the propensity to sense

MEDTRONIC 9760 PROGRAMMER 9858A001 9/29/94 12:36
Copyright (c) Medtronic, Inc. 1992
---------------- HISTOGRAM TABLE REPORT --------------- Page 1 of 1

Pacemaker Model: Legend 8416 Serial Number: XT2138890
Source: Heart Rate Collected: 9/29/94 12:34
Term: Long

Histogram Values:

Rate Bin	Number of Events	% Total Events	% Paced
<= 60			
61 - 70	956160	5	75-100
71 - 80	5361920	27	75-100
81 - 90	5028096	25	75-100
91 - 100	4017408	20	75-100
101 - 110	3196672	16	75-100
111 - 120	1147392	6	75-100
> 120			
	19707648		

MEDTRONIC 9760 PROGRAMMER 9858A001 9/29/94 12:35
Copyright (c) Medtronic, Inc. 1992
-------------- HISTOGRAM GRAPHICS REPORT -------------- Page 1 of 1

Pacemaker Model: Legend 8416 Serial Number: XT2138890

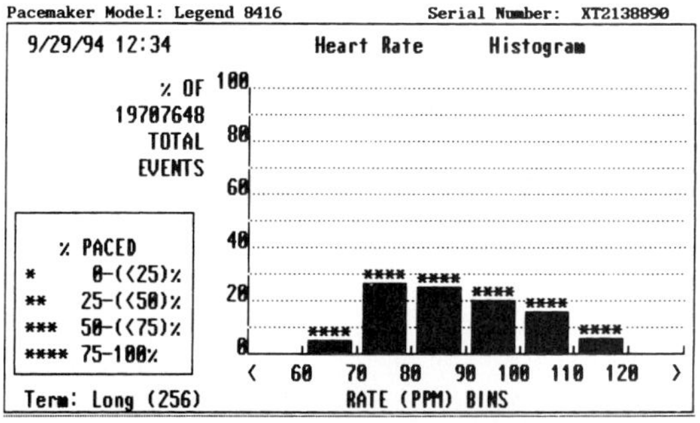

FIGURE 11–25. Heart rate chart and histogram demonstrating pacing rate for more than nearly 2 million beats. A fair response of rate variability is seen. Reprogramming the rate response should result in an improvement of heart rate variability and allow faster heart rates during exercise. (Copyright © Medtronic, Inc., 1992.)

```
262-16-001601                    FEB  2 '94   7:26 AM
              DIAGNOSTIC DATA

MOST RECENT PRIMARY MODALITY:
MEASURED TACHYCARDIA INTERVAL......   215    MSEC
BURST CYCLE LENGTH.................   200    MSEC
DELAY (TS1)........................   172    MSEC

        CONTINUE DISPLAY DIAGNOSTIC DATA
PRINT     CLEAR EVENT COUNTERS          RETURN
```

```
262-16-001601                    FEB  2 '94   7:27 AM
          DIAGNOSTIC DATA CONTINUED

TOTAL TACHYCARDIAS DETECTED........   255
HIGH RATE CRITERION MET............   255  TIMES
SUDDEN ONSET CRITERION MET.........   255  TIMES

PRIMARY MODALITY SUCCESSFUL........   255  TIMES
SECONDARY MODALITY SUCCESSFUL......   108  TIMES

EVENT COUNTERS LAST CLEARED...FEB  3, 10:10 AM

PRINT     CLEAR EVENT COUNTERS          RETURN
```

INTERMEDICS INC.

FIGURE 11–26. Event monitoring log of an antitachycardia pacemaker indicating more than 255 episodes of tachycardia in a one-year period. The cycle length of the most recent tachycardia is also displayed.

skeletal muscle.[78] The ventricular sensitivity is generally programmed to at least two settings more sensitive than the point at which sensing was lost. Again, judgment must be used when programming the sensitivity in a unipolar device.

Determination of the patient's underlying rhythm is important for several reasons. First, it answers the question of pacemaker dependency, which is critical in caring for pacemaker patients of any age. The majority of pediatric pacemaker patients are not pacemaker dependent. Second, it shows the patient and family that merely having a pacemaker does not make one dependent on it. Third, it reassures the cardiovascular caregivers and the patient and family that, in the case of pacemaker or lead malfunction, the child's heart will more often than not revert back to the rhythm that required the pacemaker initially. The optimal way to determine underlying rhythm is not to inhibit the pacemaker suddenly. This results in a brief (sometimes prolonged) period of asystole and is generally despised by the patient. By slowly decreasing (in 10-ppm increments) the programmed pacing rate, the child's underlying rhythm will gradually emerge. In the patient with a DDDCO pacemaker that is atrial tracking or in the patient with rate adaptation, it will first be necessary to program the mode to VVICO. Once this has been accomplished, one can proceed with lowering the rate. Of course, all of the information obtained during pacemaker evaluation should be documented in the patient's record, including all changes made in the programmed settings.

The programmed pacing rate in the pediatric patient requires periodic adjustment with increasing age. Once the child reaches 16 years of age, the lower rate can be programmed as low as 40 ppm in both rate adaptive and atrial synchronous modes. In the child with postoperative bradycardia-tachycardia syndrome, a lower rate

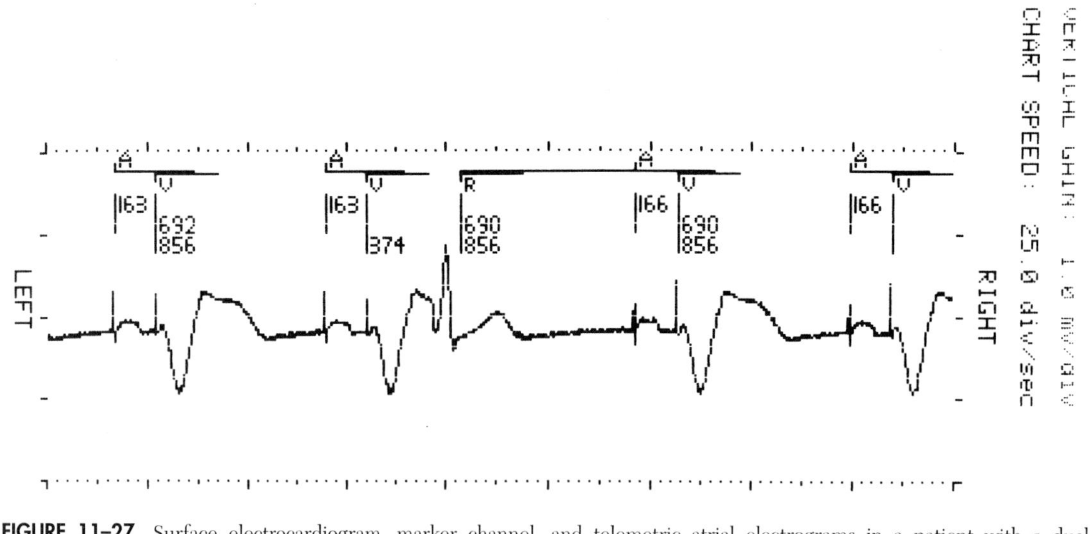

FIGURE 11–27. Surface electrocardiogram, marker channel, and telemetric atrial electrograms in a patient with a dual-chamber pacemaker and premature ventricular contractions (PVCs). The PVC promotes extension of the postventricular atrial refractory period to prevent pacemaker-mediated tachycardia.

that is higher than normal is chosen. In adolescents, that rate is usually 80 ppm because of its propensity to prevent tachycardia episodes.[68]

Other parameters that can be adapted to the individual patient's needs include AV intervals, rate adaptive parameters, and antitachycardia recognition and termination algorithms. Because the normal PR interval shortens with exercise,[79] a rate adaptive AV delay is preferable to a fixed AV delay in the majority of pediatric pacemaker patients. This parameter can be programmed to as low as 50 milliseconds without adverse sequelae. Rate adaptive parameters must be individualized for the type of sensor and to meet each patient's specific needs. In most cases, the various settings must be evaluated with exercise stress testing or twenty-four-hour ambulatory monitoring, or both.[80] Antitachycardia recognition and termination algorithms are programmed according to the tachycardia characteristics and are usually patient specific, but should be reassessed if any antiarrhythmic drug therapy is initiated.

TROUBLESHOOTING

Many patients will remain quite stable throughout the follow-up period, but some will require extra attention. Many of the problems encountered during this time can be alleviated with simple reprogramming of the implanted device. These problems include, but are not limited to, failure to capture, phrenic nerve stimulation, under- or oversensing, pacemaker-mediated tachycardia (PMT), atrial tachycardia recurrence in the patient with an implanted atrial antitachycardia device, and new-onset atrial tachycardia in a patient with a DDDCO pacemaker.

Failure to capture in the acute postoperative period requires prompt attention.[81] In most cases, programming the output to a higher value will correct the problem. Because this is only palliative and the pacing threshold normally rises to peak during this time, this could potentially become a greater problem. At the authors' institution, if the pacing threshold is greater than or equal to 0.2 millisecond at 5.0 V and there is no contraindication to steroid administration, oral prednisone is initiated at a dosage of 60 mg/m^2/day. The dosage is tapered by 10 mg/day over a 7 to 10-day period. This can be done on an outpatient basis if an adequate safety margin can be attained. Otherwise, the patient should be hospitalized for constant rhythm monitoring. Intravenous dexamethasone can be used for faster results.

Phrenic nerve stimulation, although rare, can present in the follow-up period. It is characterized by complaints of jerking or hiccupping. In the majority of cases, it can be reduced or even eliminated by programming a lower pulse amplitude coupled with a longer pulse width or duration. If it cannot be alleviated, one must consider, in conjunction with the patient and family, the frequency of occurrence and tolerability. If it is intolerable to the patient, lead repositioning or replacement may be necessary.

Sensing abnormalities can generally be corrected because of the broad range of sensitivity settings currently available in most pulse generators. As previously mentioned, for patients with bradycardia-tachycardia syndrome and congenital heart disease, it may be necessary to "accept" R-wave oversensing in those with atrial antitachycardia pacemakers. If the R-wave oversensing is alleviated, it generally results in undersensing of the intra-atrial re-entry tachycardia. A better effective rate can be achieved by increasing the lower rate of the device. Undersensing can occur with some bipolar leads because of a decrease in electrogram size; however, this can be corrected by reprogramming the sense configuration to unipolar, while allowing the pace configuration to be bipolar.

PMT is rare in the pediatric population; most of the patients who require device placement do not have intact retrograde conduction. PMT can be alleviated by lengthening the PVARP, decreasing the atrial sensitivity, and/or by eliminating PVCs, which often trigger episodes of PMT.

Atrial tachycardia may occur in children with implanted atrial antitachycardia devices with more than one arrhythmogenic substrate and in the presence of antiarrhythmic drugs that may have altered the tachycardia characteristics. Most recurrences can be treated by reprogramming the tachycardia detection and termination sequences. In rare cases, noninvasive programmed stimulation may offer some insight if the tachycardia is inducible.

Many postoperative patients with pacemakers for acquired AV block will subsequently experience atrial tachycardia in the follow-up period. Because these patients need AV synchrony for optimal hemodynamics, it is best not to reprogram the device to single-chamber mode. This lack of AV synchrony will often lead to tachycardia exacerbations. By programming the mode to DDICO or DDIRO, the atrium will not sense the tachycardia but will provide back-up ventricular pacing during the tachycardia episode. During periods without tachycardia, the device will pace AV sequentially. A more attractive option is that of mode switching, in which the device senses or averages a specific number of beats and reverts to an alternate mode until the episode has terminated.

SPECIAL CONSIDERATIONS

Special consideration is warranted in certain situations involving the patient with a permanently implanted cardiac pacemaker. These situations include pulse generator replacements for battery depletion, lead placement in patients with congenital heart disease, other medical procedures not associated with pacemaker implantation, and cardioversion-defibrillation in the patient with a permanent cardiac pacemaker.

PULSE GENERATOR REPLACEMENTS

When replacing a pulse generator that is at elective or imminent replacement, certain factors should be considered ahead of time. Because many older style leads are still implanted, the compatibility of these leads with the newer pulse generators must be taken into account. In most cases, the various manufacturers will provide pulse generators with headers that accept older lead pins, such as the 3.2-mm in-line with a long connector pin. Lead and pulse generator compatibility and availability must be verified before the implant procedure.

Pads for emergent temporary pacing should be placed on the patient in the event that the battery-depleted device completely fails. This is generally not the case, but one must always be prepared. A cardioverter-defibrillator with external pacing capabilities can be used in place of the former stand-alone external, transcutaneous pacemaker (Fig. 11–28). If this is not available, a temporary venous pacing catheter should be placed in those patients considered pacemaker dependent or hemodynamically vulnerable.

Electrocautery should be avoided with pulse generator replacements that are battery depleted, because the pacemakers will often cease to function when electrocautery is applied, sometimes permanently. Additionally, the risk of damaging the chronic lead is higher. Written reports of previous pacemaker procedures may be helpful in determining where the lead may have been placed (i.e., over or under the implanted pulse generator).

One should also be prepared for inadvertent damage to the lead during opening of the pocket or for previously undetected lead problems that materialize during intraoperative testing. Additional leads, stylets for the chronically implanted leads, and a tool to disconnent the pulse generator from the lead must be readily available.

LEAD PLACEMENT IN PATIENTS WITH CONGENITAL HEART DISEASE

In patients with congenital heart disease or cardiac malposition, the implanting physician must be able to adapt to the patient's underlying

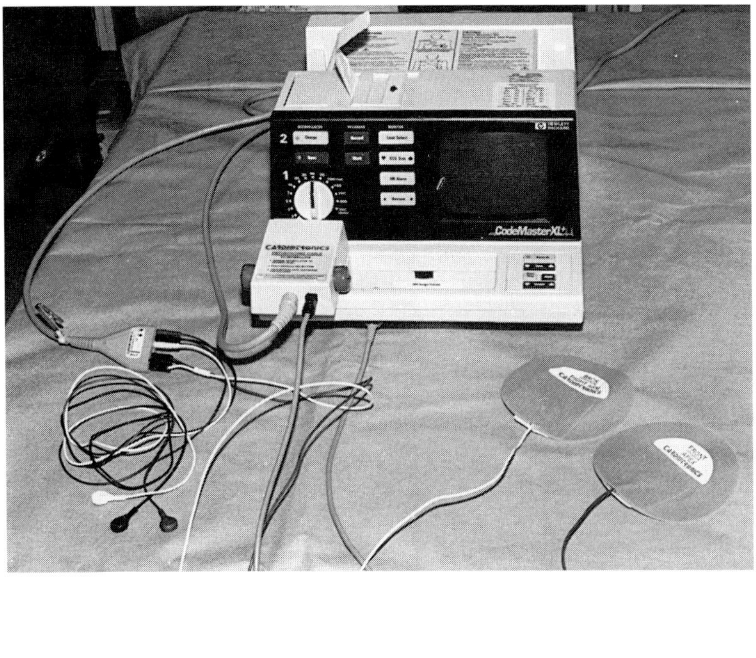

FIGURE 11–28. Combined external pacemaker-defibrillator. The same pads and patches are used for both purposes. The device is also capable of monitoring the electrocardiogram (ECG) (through the pads or via 3 ECG electrodes) and oxygen saturation.

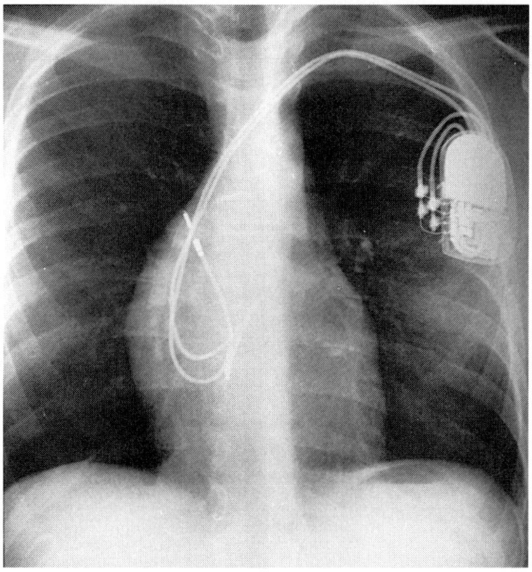

FIGURE 11–29. Lead position in a child who underwent repair of tetralogy of Fallot and who also has mesocardia. Note that the ventricular lead is pointing straight anterior and is placed in the right ventricular apex.

anatomy (Fig. 11–29). Angiography in these patients can be especially useful in further defining cardiovascular anatomy (Figs. 11–30 to 11–33). After the Fontan procedure, including the lateral tunnel-type operation, pacing can be accomplished by placing the atrial lead on the lateral wall (Fig. 11–34) or low in the atrium near the mouth of the coronary sinus (Fig. 11–35).

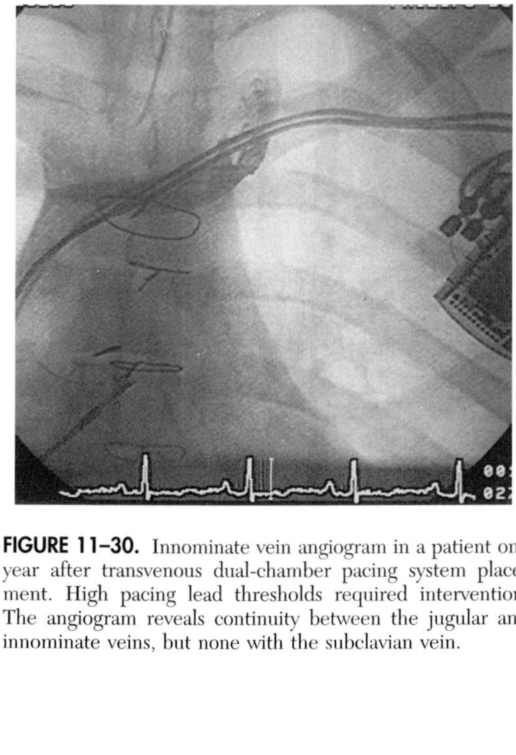

FIGURE 11–30. Innominate vein angiogram in a patient one year after transvenous dual-chamber pacing system placement. High pacing lead thresholds required intervention. The angiogram reveals continuity between the jugular and innominate veins, but none with the subclavian vein.

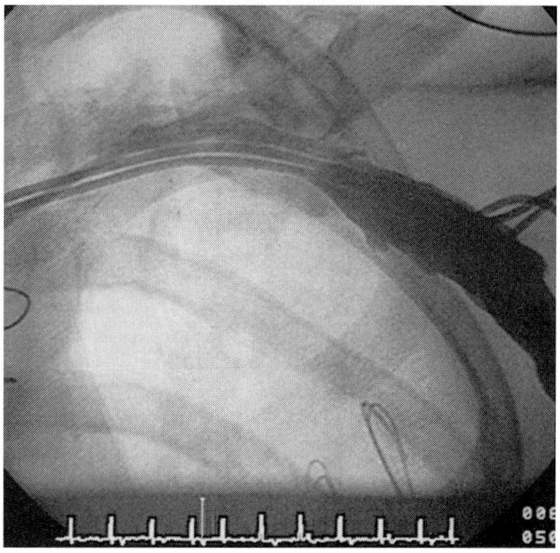

FIGURE 11–31. Axillary vein angiogram into the brachial vein indicating total thrombosis of the subclavian vein.

A team approach is often necessary in these patients. The skills of an interventionalist may be necessary for creating new venous channels or enlarging narrow ones, using balloon catheters or intravascular stents[82] (Figs. 11–36 to 11–38).

NONCARDIAC PROCEDURES ON THE CHILD WITH A PACEMAKER

Any time the child with a permanent cardiac pacemaker undergoes medical or surgical proce-

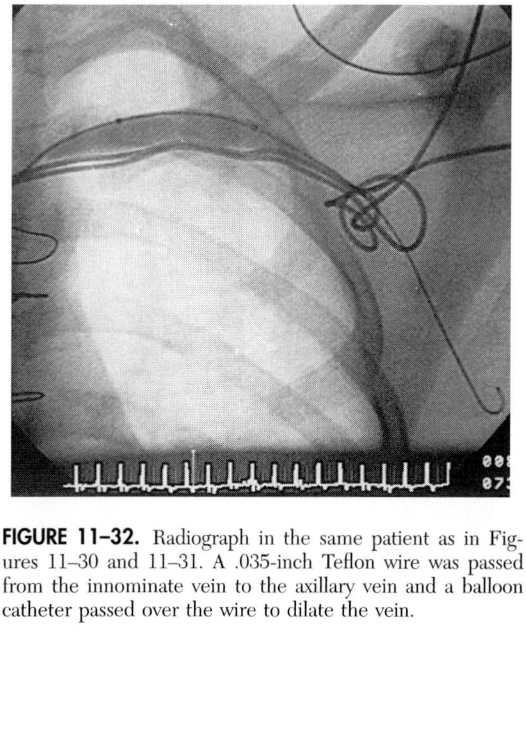

FIGURE 11–32. Radiograph in the same patient as in Figures 11–30 and 11–31. A .035-inch Teflon wire was passed from the innominate vein to the axillary vein and a balloon catheter passed over the wire to dilate the vein.

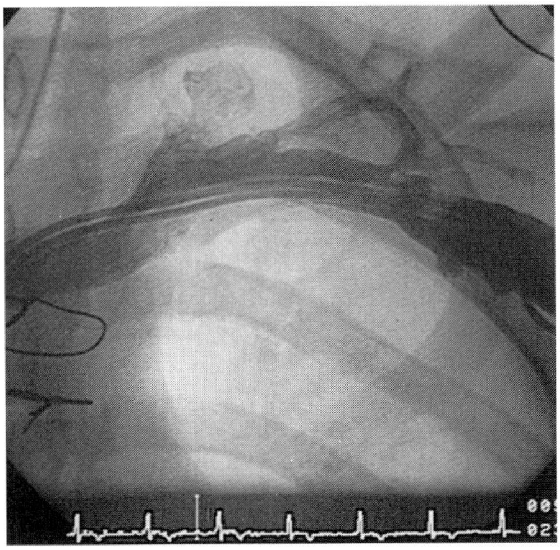

FIGURE 11–33. Angiogram in the same patient as in Figures 11–30 to 11–32. Axillary vein angiogram after balloon dilatation. The vein is now open, and the leads are repositioned without vein sacrifice.

dures, the pacemaker team should be made aware. This is often not the case but is the most desirable way of handling these patients. The physician performing the procedure should be aware of the patient's underlying rhythm, pacemaker indication, programmed settings of the device, and pocket location. When using electrocautery, care must be taken to avoid use directly over the implanted device. Ideally, it should be kept at least 4 to 6 inches from the pacemaker.[83]

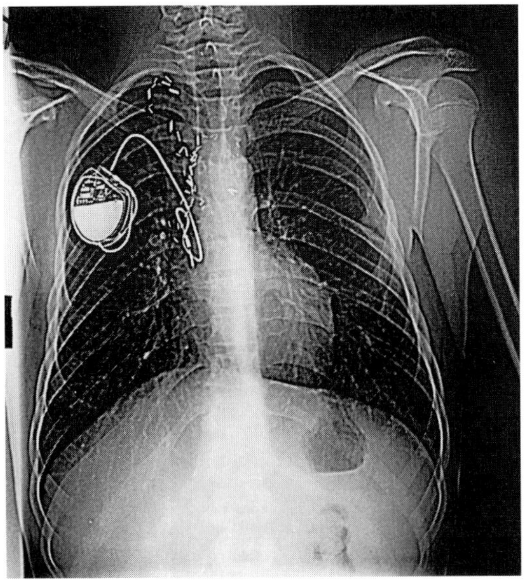

FIGURE 11–34. Lead position in a postoperative Fontan patient who underwent the lateral tunnel procedure. The lead is screwed into the atrial tissue near the cavopulmonary connection.

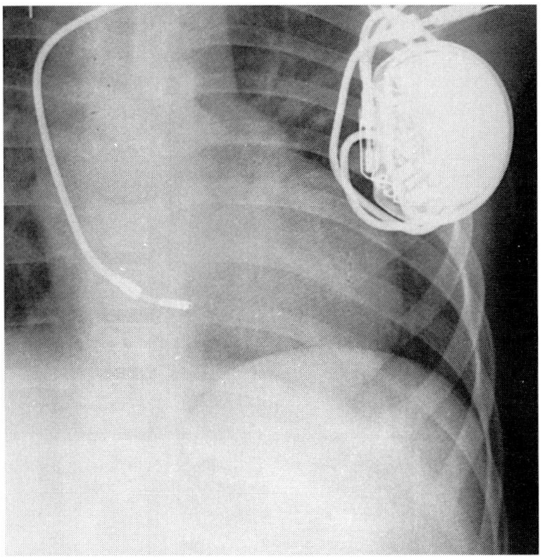

FIGURE 11–35. Posteroanterior chest radiograph of a transvenous atrial lead position in a patient with tricuspid atresia after Fontan procedure. The lead is positioned near the mouth of the coronary sinus.

The most common adverse effect of electrocautery is pacemaker inhibition, although other adverse effects can occur, including device reprogramming, reversion to a noise or fall-back mode,

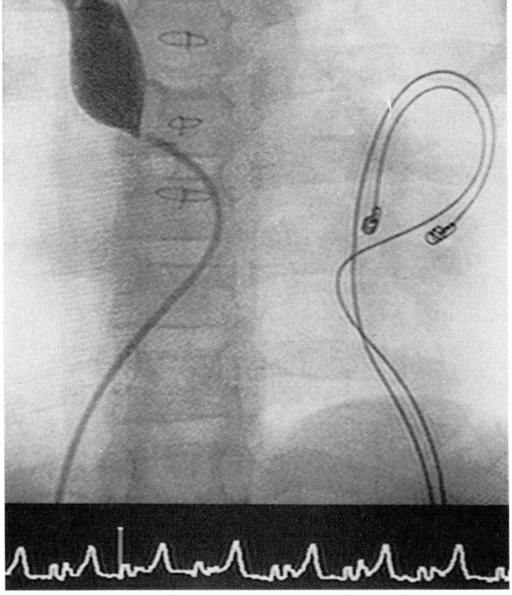

FIGURE 11–36. Depiction of the creation of a new superior vena cava for pacemaker lead implantation. This postoperative Mustard patient experienced exit block with epicardial pacing leads. A catheter was passed from the inferior vena cava to the right atrium at its junction with the superior vena cava. Contrast media demonstrating the atresia was injected via a catheter positioned from the jugular vein.

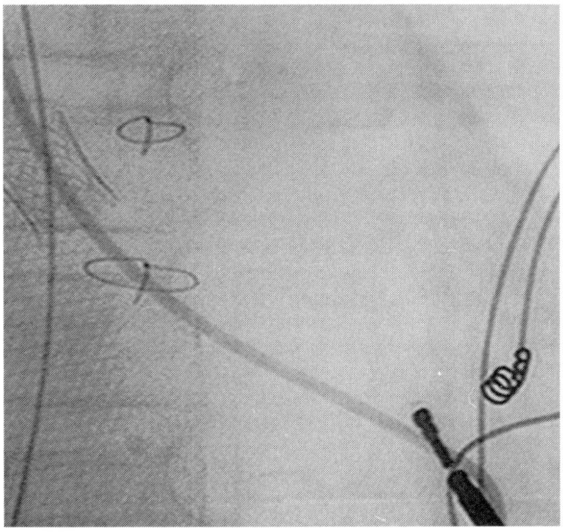

FIGURE 11–37. Magnified view of a stent placed in the superior vena cava–right atrial junction. A transseptal needle was used to puncture the narrowed area followed by placement of a sheath dilator set and wire. A balloon was used to dilate the vessel, and the stent was subsequently placed. The gridlike item in the background is a cutaneous defibrillation pad.

permanent damage to the pulse generator, and thermal damage to the myocardium resulting in myocardial infarction or ventricular fibrillation.[83] In adults, it is feasible to program to an asynchronous mode (by programming or magnet application), but this is not always feasible in children because of their ability to track the atrium at much higher rates than the adult. If feasible for a particular patient, this should certainly be undertaken. The use of a bipolar electrocautery system and multiple, short bursts during the procedure may help minimize permanent pacemaker damage. The grounding pad for the electrocautery should be placed as far away from the implanted device as possible and the pacing system evaluated by pacemaker personnel immediately after the procedure.

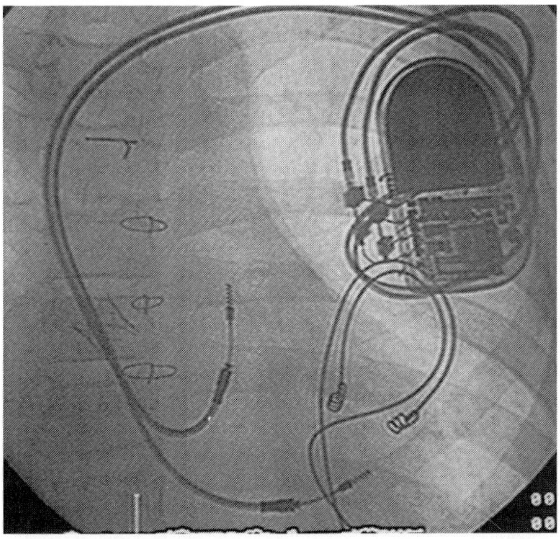

FIGURE 11–38. Final result of the same patient as in Figures 11–36 and 11–37. The old epicardial leads as well as the 2 new transvenous leads are seen; the latter are connected to a DDD pacemaker. Follow-up echocardiography reveals the channel to be open at 18 months followup. No evidence of lead insulation failure has been noted.

CARDIOVERSION-DEFIBRILLATION IN THE PACEMAKER PATIENT

Pacemaker patients rarely require cardioversion or defibrillation. If necessary, it can be performed using defibrillation paddles or multipurpose pads that attach directly to the patient's skin. It is crucial to be aware of the pulse generator's location to place the pads or paddles correctly. They should be placed as far away from the pulse generator as possible (Table 11–3). Adverse effects of cardioversion-defibrillation range from no change in pacemaker function to complete device destruction. Pacemaker function should be assessed immediately after cardioversion-defibrillation, including sensing and pacing thresholds and lead impedance assessment. Altamura and colleagues reported a significant rise in ventricular pacing threshold, including transient loss of capture in 50% of patients, worsening of sensing function, and generator failure (in 2 cases).[84] The lead impedance measurements may be increased or decreased immediately after cardioversion-defibrillation, but generally return to normal in several hours. It is not unusual after cardioversion-defibrillation for the device to exhibit elective replacement indicators or be in a

Table 11–3. Defibrillation Pad or Paddle Placement in the Permanent Pacemaker Patient

PACEMAKER POCKET LOCATION	PAD OR PADDLE PLACEMENT
Left subpectoral, subcutaneous	Left anterior apex (low) and right posterior (clavicular)
Right subpectoral, subcutaneous	Front and back on left side
Left rectus	Left anterior (high) and right anterior or posterior
Right rectus	Left anterior and right anterior or posterior

Adapted from Gillette PC, Zeigler VL (eds): Pediatric Cardiac Pacing. Armonk, NY, Futura, 1995, p 239. Used with permission.

back-up mode. This can usually be eliminated by simply reprogramming the device.

REFERENCES

1. Elmqvist R, Landegren J, Petterson SO, et al: Artificial pacemaker for treatment of Adams-Stokes syndrome and slow heart rate. Am Heart J 65:731–748, 1963.
2. Serwer GA, Dorostkar PC: Pediatric pacing. In Ellenbogen KA, Kay GN, Wilkoff BL (eds): Clinical Cardiac Pacing. Philadelphia, W.B. Saunders, 1995, pp 706–734.
3. Kugler JD, Danford DA: Pacemakers in children: An update. Am Heart J 117:665–679, 1989.
4. Karpawich PP, Perry BL, Farooki ZQ, et al: Pacing in children and young adults in nonsurgical atrioventricular block: Comparison of single-rate ventricular and dual-chamber modes. Am Heart J 113:316–321, 1987.
5. Serwer GA, Uzark K, Beekman R, et al: Optimal programming of rate altering parameters in children with rate-responsive pacemakers using graded treadmill exercise testing. Pacing Clin Electrophysiol 13:541, 1990 (abstract).
6. Yabek SM, Wernly J, Check TW, et al: Rate adaptive cardiac pacing in children using a minute ventilation biosensor. Pacing Clin Electrophysiol 13:2108–112, 1990.
7. Serwer GA, Dorostkar PC, LeRoy S, et al: Evaluation of rate variable pacemaker function at maximal exercise exertion in children and young adults. Pacing Clin Electrophysiol 16:899, 1991 (abstract).
8. Ross BA, Zeigler V, Zinner A, et al: The effect of exercise on the atrial electrogram voltage in young patients. Pacing Clin Electrophysiol 14:2092–2097, 1991.
9. Frye RL, Collins JJ, DeSanctis RW, et al: Guidelines for permanent cardiac pacemaker implantation, May 1984. A report of the Joint American College of Cardiology/American Heart Association Task Force on Assessment of Cardiovascular Procedures (Subcommittee on Pacemaker Implantation). Circulation 70:331A–339A, 1984.
10. Dreifus LS, Fisch C, Griffin JC, et al: Guidelines for implantation of cardiac pacemakers and antiarrhythmia devices. A report of the Joint American College of Cardiology/American Heart Association Task Force on Assessment of Cardiovascular Procedures. J Am Coll Cardiol 18:1–13, 1991.
11. Gregoratos G, Cheitlin MD, Conill A, et al: ACC/AHA guidelines for implantation of cardiac pacemakers and antiarrhythmia devices. J Am Coll Cardiol 31:1175–1209, 1998.
12. Gillette PC: Pacing indications and choosing the most appropriate generator. In Gillette PC, Zeigler VL (eds): Pediatric Cardiac Pacing. Armonk, NY, Futura, 1995, pp 9–22.
13. Boutjdir M, Chen L, Zhang ZH, et al: Serum and immunoglobulin G from the mother of a child with congenital heart block induce conduction abnormalities and inhibit L-type calcium channels in a rat heart model. Pediat Res 44:11–19, 1998.
14. Michaelsson M, Engle MA: Congenital complete heart block: An international study of the natural history. In Brest AN, Engle MA (eds): Cardiovascular Clinics. Philadelphia, FA Davis, 1972, pp 85–101.
15. Karpawich PP, Gillette PC, Garson A Jr, et al: Congenital complete atrioventricular block: Clinical and electrophysiological predictors of need for pacemaker insertion. Am J Cardiol 48:1098–1102, 1981.
16. Winkler RB, Freed MD, Nadas AS: Exercise-induced ventricular ectopy in children and young adults with complete heart block. Am Heart J 99:87–92, 1980.
17. Michaelsson M, Jonzon A, Riesenfeld T: Isolated congenital complete atrioventricular block: A prospective study. Circulation 92:283–285, 1995.
18. Rishi F, Hulse JE, Auld DO, et al: Effects of dual-chamber pacing for pediatric patients with hypertrophic obstructive cardiomyopathy. J Am Coll Cardiol 29:741–743, 1997.
19. Kappenberger L, Linde C, Daubert C, et al: Pacing in hypertrophic cardiomyopathy. A randomized crossover study. PIC Study Group. Eur Heart J 19:352–353, 1998.
20. Gillette PC, Wampler DG, Shannon C, et al: Use of cardiac pacing after the Mustard operation for transposition of the great arteries. J Am Coll Cardiol 7:138–141, 1986.
21. Fukushige J, Porter CB, Hayes DL, et al: Antitachycardia pacemaker treatment of postoperative arrhythmias in pediatric patients. Pacing Clin Electrophysiol 14:546–556, 1991.
22. Gillette PC, Zeigler VL, Case CL, et al: Atrial antitachycardia pacing in children and young adults. Am Heart J 122:844–849, 1991.
23. Gillette PC, Ross BA, Zeigler VL: Antitachycardia pacing. In Garson A Jr, Bricker JT, McNamara DG (eds): The Science and Practice of Pediatric Cardiology. Philadelphia, Lea & Febiger, 1990, pp 2156–2161.
24. Celiker A, Tokel K, Lenk MK, et al: Dual sensor pacemakers in children: What is the choice of sensor blending? Pacing Clin Electrophysiol 20:1301–1304, 1997.
25. Walsh CA, McAlister HF, Anders CA, et al: Pacemaker implantation in children: A 21-year experience. Pacing Clin Electrophysiol 11:1940–1944, 1988.
26. Till JA, Jones S, Rowland E, et al: Endocardial pacing in infants and children 15 kg or less in weight: Medium term follow up. Pacing Clin Electrophysiol 13:1385–1392, 1990.
27. Spotnitz HM: Transvenous pacing in infants and children with congenital heart disease. Ann Thorac Surg 49:495–496, 1990.
28. Serwer GA, Mericle JM, Armstrong BE: Epicardial ventricular pacemaker electrode longevity in children. Am J Cardiol 61:104–106, 1988.
29. Serwer GA, Uzark K, Dick M II: Endocardial pacing longevity in children. J Am Coll Cardiol 15:212A, 1990 (abstract).
30. Serwer GA, Dorostkar PC, LeRoy S, et al: Comparison of chronic thresholds between differing endocardial electrode types in children. Circulation 86:I-43, 1992 (abstract).
31. DeLeon SY, Ilbawi MN, Koster N, et al: Comparison of the sutureless and suture-type epicardial electrodes in pediatric cardiac pacing. Ann Thorac Surg 33:273–276, 1982.
32. Michalik RE, Williams H, Zorn-Chelten S, et al: Experience with a new epimyocardial pacing lead in children. Pacing Clin Electrophysiol 7:831–838, 1984.
33. Kugler J, Monsour W, Blodgett C, et al: Comparison of two myoepicardial pacemaker leads: Follow up in 80 children, adolescents, and young adults. Pacing Clin Electrophysiol 11:2216–2222, 1988.
34. DeLeon SY, Ilbawi MN, Backer CL, et al: Exit block in pediatric cardiac pacing. Comparison of the suture-type and fishhook epicardial electrodes. J Thorac Cardiovasc Surg 95:905–910, 1990.
35. Hoyer MH, Beerman LB, Ettedgui JA, et al: Transatrial lead placement for endocardial pacing in children. Ann Thorac Surg 58:97–101, 1994.
36. Hamilton R, Gow R, Bahoric B, et al: Steroid-eluting

epicardial leads in pediatrics: Improved epicardial thresholds in the first year. Pacing Clin Electrophysiol 14:2066–2072, 1991.
37. Karpawich PP, Hakimi M, Arciniegas E, et al: Improved chronic epicardial pacing in children: Steroid contribution to porous platinized electrodes. Pacing Clin Electrophysiol 15:1151–1157, 1992.
38. Cutler NG, Karpawich PP, Cavitt D, et al: Steroid-eluting epicardial pacing electrodes: Six year experience of pacing thresholds in a growing pediatric population. Pacing Clin Electrophysiol 20:2943–2948, 1997.
39. Johns JA, Fish FA, Burger JD, et al: Steroid-eluting epicardial pacing leads in pediatric patients: Encouraging early results. J Am Coll Cardiol 20:395–401, 1992.
40. Lau YR: Lead selection. In Gillette PC, Zeigler VL (eds): Pediatric Cardiac Pacing. Armonk, NY, Futura, 1995, pp 23–36.
41. Celiker A, Alehan D, Oto A, et al: Long-term clinical experience with a steroid-eluting active fixation ventricular electrode in children. Am J Cardiol 80:355–358, 1997.
42. Rosenthal E, Bostock J: VDD pacing in children with congenital complete heart block: Advantages of a single pass lead. Pacing Clin Electrophysiol 20:2102–2106, 1997.
43. Stojanov P, Velimirovic D, Hrnjak V, et al: Absorbable suture technique: Solution to the growth problem in pediatric pacing with endocardial leads. Pacing Clin Electrophysiol 21:65–68, 1998.
44. Friedman RA, Van Zandt H, Collins E, et al: Lead extraction in young patients with and without congenital heart disease using the subclavian approach. Pacing Clin Electrophysiol 19:778–783, 1996.
45. Case CL: Cardiac pacing in the infant and child with postoperative congenital heart disease. In Gillette PC, Zeigler VL (eds): Pediatric Cardiac Pacing. Armonk, NY, Futura, 1995, pp 95–113.
46. Gillette PC, Shannon C, Blair H, et al: Transvenous pacing in pediatric patients. Am Heart J 105:843–847, 1983.
47. Silka MJ, Rice MJ: Paradoxic embolism due to altered hemodynamic sequence following transvenous pacing. Pacing Clin Electrophysiol 14:499–503, 1991.
48. Zeigler VL: Intraoperative testing. In Gillette PC, Zeigler VL (eds): Pediatric Cardiac Pacing. Armonk, NY, Futura, 1995, pp 63–77.
49. Parsonett V, Furman S, Smyth NPD, et al: Optimal resources for implantable cardiac pacemakers. Circulation 68:227A–244A, 1983.
50. Winslow A: Nursing care of the pediatric pacemaker patient. In Gillette PC, Zeigler VL (eds): Pediatric Cardiac Pacing. Armonk, NY, Futura, 1995, pp 149–180.
51. Zeigler VL, Corbett KS: Psychosocial aspects of caring for pediatric pacemaker recipients and their families. In Gillette PC, Zeigler VL (eds): Pediatric Cardiac Pacing. Armonk, NY, Futura, 1995, pp 181–203.
52. Gillette PC: Implantation technique for pediatric cardiac pacing. In Gillette PC, Zeigler VL (eds): Pediatric Cardiac Pacing. Armonk, NY, Futura, 1995, pp 37–61.
53. Gillette PC, Edgerton J, Kratz J, et al: The subpectoral pocket: The preferred implant site for pediatric pacemakers. Pacing Clin Electrophysiol 14:1089–1092, 1991.
54. Sharma AD, Guiraudon GM, Klein GJ, et al: Pacemaker implantation techniques. In El-Sherif N, Samet P (eds): Cardiac Pacing and Electrophysiology, 3rd ed. Philadelphia, WB Saunders, 1998, pp 561–567.
55. Brenner JI, Gaines S, Cordier J, et al: Cardiac strangulation: Two-dimensional echo recognition of a rare complication of epicardial pacemaker therapy. Am J Cardiol 61:654–665, 1988.
56. Perry JC, Nihill MR, Ludomirsky A, et al: The pulmonary artery lasso: Epicardial pacing leads causing right ventricular outflow obstruction. Pacing Clin Electrophysiol 14:1018–1023, 1991.
57. Ott DA, Gillette PC, Cooley DA: Atrial pacing via the subxyphoid approach. Tex Heart Inst J 9:149–152, 1982.
58. Ulicny KS Jr, Detterbeck FC, Starek PJK, et al: Cojoined subrectus pocket for permanent pacemaker placement in the neonate. Ann Thorac Surg 53:1130–1131, 1992.
59. Robertson JM, Laks H: A new technique for permanent pacemaker implantation in infants and children. Ann Thorac Surg 44:209–211, 1987.
60. Shepard RB, Sand ME, Colvin EV: Cardiac pacing in children. In Grillo HC, Austen WG, Wilkins EW Jr, Mathison DJ, Vlahakes GJ (eds): Current Therapy in Cardiothoracic Surgery. Philadelphia, BC Decker, 1989, pp 564–567.
61. Rees PG: Use of pacemakers in children. In Stark J, deLeval M (eds): Surgery for Congenital Heart Defects. Philadelphia, WB Saunders, 1994, pp 139–153.
62. Kratz JM, Gillette PC, Crawford FA, et al: Atrioventricular pacing in congenital heart disease. Ann Thorac Surg 54:485–489, 1992.
63. Stokes K, Bornzin G: The electrode-biointerface: Stimulation. In Barold SS (ed): Modern Cardiac Pacing. Mt. Kisco, NY, Futura, 1985, pp 79–95.
64. Daubert C, Ritter P, Mabo P, et al: Rate modulation to the AV delay in DDD pacing. In Santini M, Pistolese M, Alliegro A (eds): Proceedings of the International Symposium on Progress in Clinical Pacing. Amsterdam, The Netherlands, Excerpta Medica, Medical Communications BV, 1990, pp 415–430.
65. Brownlee JR, Serwer GA, Dick M II, et al: Failure of electrocardiographic monitoring to detect cardiac arrest in patients with pacemakers. Am J Dis Child 143:105–107, 1989.
66. Gutgesell HP, Gessner IH, Vetter VL, et al: Recreational and occupational recommendations for young patients with heart disease. Circulation 74:1195A–1198A, 1986.
67. Vincent JA, Cavitt DL, Karpawich PP: Diagnostic and cost effectiveness of telemonitoring the pediatric pacemaker patient. Pediatr Cardiol 18:86–90, 1977.
68. Zeigler VL: Pacing system follow up. In Gillette PC, Zeigler VL (eds): Pediatric Cardiac Pacing. Armonk, NY, Futura, 1995, pp 205–242.
69. Cabrera ME, Hanisch DG, Cohen MH, et al: Cardiopulmonary responses to exercise in children with activity sensing rate responsive ventricular pacemakers. Pacing Clin Electrophysiol 16:1386–1393, 1993.
70. Bricker JT, Barison A, Traveek MS, et al: The use of exercise testing in children to evaluate abnormalities of pacemaker function not apparent at rest. Pacing Clin Electrophysiol 8:656–660, 1985.
71. Serwer GA, Kodali R, Eakin B, et al: Changes in pacemaker threshold with exercise in children and young adults. J Am Coll Cardiol 17:207A, 1991 (abstract).
72. Gillette PC, Zinner A, Kratz J, et al: Atrial tracking (synchronous) pacing in a pediatric and young adult population. J Am Coll Cardiol 9:811–815, 1987.
73. Frohlig G, Blank W, Schwerdt H, et al: Atrial sensing performance of AV universal pacemakers during exercise. Pacing Clin Electrophysiol 11:47–60, 1988.
74. Strathmore NF, Mond HG: Noninvasive monitoring and testing of pacemaker function. Pacing Clin Electrophysiol 10:1030–1035, 1987.
75. Janosik DL, Redd RM, Buckingham TA, et al: Utility of ambulatory electrocardiography in detecting dysfunction in the early postimplantation period. Am J Cardiol 60:1030–1035, 1987.

76. Stokes K, Bornzin G: The electrode-biointerface: Stimulation. In Barold SS (ed): Modern Cardiac Pacing. Mt. Kisco, NY, Futura, 1985, pp 33–77.
77. Brandt J, Attewell R, Fahraeus T, et al: Acute atrial endocardial P wave amplitude and chronic pacemaker sensitivity requirements: Relation to patient age and presence of sinus node disease. Pacing Clin Electrophysiol 13:417–424, 1990.
78. Chui CC, Gow RM, McCrindle BW, et al: Impact of programmed sensitivity safety factor on atrial sensing in children. Pacing Clin Electrophysiol 20:2163–2170, 1997.
79. Daubert C, Ritter P, Mabo P, et al: Physiological relationship between AV interval and heart rate in healthy subjects: Applications to dual chamber pacing. Pacing Clin Electrophysiol 9:1032–1039, 1986.
80. Zeigler VL, Gillette PC, Kratz J: Is activity sensored pacing in children and young adults a feasible option? Pacing Clin Electrophysiol 13:2104–2107, 1990.
81. Shepard RB, Kim J, Colvin EC, et al: Pacing threshold spikes months and years after implant. Pacing Clin Electrophysiol 14:1834–1841, 1991.
82. Ing FF, Mullins CE, Grifka RG, et al: Stent dilation of superior vena cava and innominate vein obstructions permits transvenous pacing lead implantation. Pacing Clin Electrophysiol 21:1517–1530, 1998.
83. Hayes DL: Electromagnetic interference, drug-device interaction, and other practical considerations. In Furman S, Hayes DL, Holmes DR Jr (eds): A Practice of Cardiac Pacing, 3rd ed. Mount Kisco, NY, Futura, 1993, pp 665–684.
84. Altamura G, Bianconi L, LoBianco F, et al: Transthoracic DC shock may represent a serious hazard in pacemaker dependent patients. Pacing Clin Electrophysiol 18:194–198, 1995.

CHAPTER 12

ADVANCED ELECTRICAL MANAGEMENT OF ATRIAL AND VENTRICULAR TACHYARRHYTHMIAS

Michael J. Silka and Paul C. Gillette

Conventional treatment strategies for pediatric patients with atrial or ventricular tachyarrhythmias include pharmacologic therapies for arrhythmia suppression and modification of the anatomic substrate of the arrhythmia, either with catheter or surgical ablation. Catheter ablation has become the preferred treatment for young patients with atrioventricular (AV) reciprocating tachycardia and AV node re-entrant tachycardia.[1] Other forms of tachycardia may not be amenable to definitive cure with catheter ablation and may not be effectively treated with antiarrhythmic drugs. In pediatric patients such arrhythmias most commonly are atrial muscle re-entrant tachycardia (atrial flutter) and various forms of ventricular tachycardia.[2, 3] A third treatment option for these arrhythmias is by advanced electrical or device therapy.

Device therapy may be relatively simple, such as atrial or ventricular pacing at physiologic rates for the suppression of ectopic beats or to alter the refractory periods of tissues involved in the arrhythmias. Device therapy more commonly requires the detection of a tachycardia followed by a series of electrical responses, ranging from antitachycardia pacing to synchronized cardioversion or defibrillation. These forms of electrical therapy are designed for the termination of a re-entrant tachycardia. Pharmacologic or ablative therapies are intended to prevent the initiation of tachycardia. This chapter specifically focuses on antitachycardia devices in children and patients with congenital heart disease. The current uses of these electrical devices for atrial and ventricular tachyarrhythmias differ and continue to evolve rapidly at this time. Thus, the indications, outcomes, and limitations of device therapies for atrial and ventricular tachyarrhythmias are considered separately.

BASIC CONSIDERATIONS IN DEVICE THERAPIES FOR ATRIAL TACHYARRHYTHMIAS

Electrophysiologic sequelae involving the atria are commonly observed after surgery for congenital heart disease and include both sinus bradycardia and re-entrant and/or automatic atrial tachycardias.[4, 5] These arrhythmias may occur after relatively simple procedures such as closure of an atrial septal defect, but are more common after complex repairs, such as atrial baffle procedures for transposition of the great arteries and various modifications of the Fontan procedure.

Postoperative atrial tachyarrhythmias are discussed in detail in Chapters 6 and 19. For the purposes of this chapter, these arrhythmias are referred to as atrial muscle re-entrant tachycardias,[6] although the terms *atrial flutter*, *intra-atrial re-entry*, and *primary atrial tachycardia* have also been known. As related to device therapy for these atrial arrhythmias, several considerations should be made:

A. Electrophysiologic aspects
   1. The anatomic basis of the tachycardia is confined to the atrium.
   2. The arrhythmias are usually but not always re-entrant, capable of onset and termination with programmed electrical stimulation.
   3. Multiple re-entrant circuits may be present, resulting in atrial tachycardias with differing cycle lengths and vectors of depolarization in the same patient.

B. Clinical aspects
   1. These arrhythmias require definitive therapy; a 20% 5-year mortality rate has been reported for young patients with chronic atrial flutter.[2]

2. Conventional antiarrhythmic drug therapy is of limited efficacy.
3. Catheter ablation may modify but not eliminate the substrate of tachycardia and has not been demonstrated to be of long-term efficacy.[6]
4. Approximately 33% of patients will not experience a recurrence of atrial muscle re-entrant tachycardia within 5 years of their first episode.

RATE SUPPORT FOR PREVENTION OF ATRIAL TACHYARRHYTHMIAS

One observation that has been apparent for several decades is the presence of a bradycardia-tachycardia syndrome in patients who have undergone the Mustard repair for transposition of the great arteries.[7] This has resulted in the proposal that bradycardia may predispose patients to the initiation of atrial tachycardias either by permitting subsidiary pacemaker sites to compete with the sinus node, resulting in competing wave fronts of atrial depolarization that initiate re-entry, or by prolonging the refractory period of atrial tissues, allowing the establishment of a functional re-entrant circuit.[8]

One option for patients with both recurrent atrial muscle re-entrant tachycardia and sinus bradycardia has been the use of atrial pacing for rate support with an option of back-up antitachycardia pacing. Several series[9–13] have been reported regarding the efficacy of atrial rate support in the prevention of clinically symptomatic arrhythmias in young patients with congenital heart disease (Table 12–1). These studies suggest that rate support alone (excluding patients who have used antitachycardia pacing) may eliminate episodes of tachycardia in up to 40% of patients with recurrent atrial muscle re-entrant tachycardia in conjunction with sinus node dysfunction. It has been specifically noted in several of these reports that a critical rate of atrial pacing (i.e., > 70/min) is required for the prevention of these tachycardias.[10, 11]

Regarding the indications for pacing in these patients, there is consensus that most patients with symptomatic bradycardia should undergo pacemaker implantation. It has been recommended (class IIa) that patients with bradycardia-tachycardia syndromes requiring therapy other than digoxin also should undergo pacemaker implantation.[14] Studies in adult patients have suggested improved outcomes in patients with atrial fibrillation when paced with physiologic modes (AAI or DDD) rather than VVI.[15] Thus, in young patients with sinus bradycardia and recurrent episodes of atrial re-entrant tachycardia, either atrial pacing with antitachycardia back-up or dual-chamber pacing should be considered among the therapeutic options. Although rate support may not be uniformly successful, it may benefit a substantial percentage of these patients and facilitate pharmacologic management in others.

Although less well described, rate support may also be an effective therapy for certain forms of automatic ectopic tachycardias. These unusual tachycardias are defined by pause dependency in their onset and irregular cycle lengths (Fig. 12–1). Pacing at physiologic rates does not represent an effective therapy for most forms of automatic ectopic tachycardia.

ANTITACHYCARDIA PACING FOR TERMINATION OF ATRIAL TACHYARRHYTHMIAS

Beyond atrial pacing with or without pharmacologic therapy, a second option for patients with atrial muscle re-entrant tachycardia is antitachycardia pacing. Although this modality is technically more complex than pacing at physiologic rates, it may improve the efficacy of pacing for

Table 12–1. Clinical Experience with Atrial Antitachycardia Pacing for Congenital Heart Disease

STUDY	PATIENTS	PATIENTS WITH SINUS BRADYCARDIA	AAI EFFECTIVE	AAI-T EFFECTIVE
McGoon et al[9]	4	4	2	2
Fukushige et al[10]	6	4	3	3
Silka et al[11]	14	12	7	—
Gillette et al[12]	20	18	4	16
Rhodes et al[13]	18	15	8	6
Total	62	53	24	27

AAI and AAI-T efficacy defined as no recurrences of tachycardia. AAI efficacy based on outcome for pacing at rates ≥ 70/min.

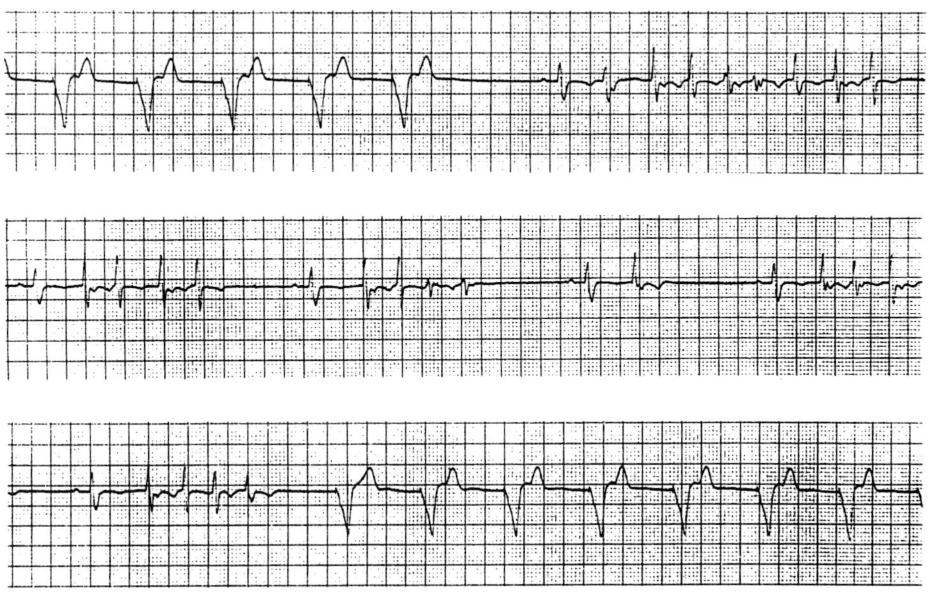

FIGURE 12–1. An example of tachycardia prevention by pacing at a physiologic rate. Top, The patient is VVI paced at a cycle length of 857 ms (70/min). With the pacemaker inhibited, there is a pause followed by the onset of an irregular narrow QRS tachycardia, which was demonstrated to be automatic junctional tachycardia by electrophysiologic study. Middle, There are recurrent salvos of tachycardia, with initiation following a pause after a single sinus capture beat. In the third panel, VVI pacing is restored, with complete suppression of the automatic junctional tachycardia.

either tachycardia prevention or termination to as many as 80% of patients.

The following considerations should be made regarding atrial antitachycardia pacing in young patients:

1. Most patients reported in the literature with this therapy have been carefully selected and tested for the reproducible termination of tachycardia.[9–13]
2. A number of problems have been recognized with atrial pacing in young patients with complex congenital heart disease.[16]
3. Sensing must be tested both during sinus rhythm and the atrial tachycardia because the electrogram amplitude may vary during different rhythms.
4. There is potential for acceleration, rather than termination, of the atrial tachycardia, which has been reported to degenerate into ventricular fibrillation.[13]

A number of algorithms for the detection as well as the termination of atrial muscle re-entrant tachycardias have been developed. Complex detection algorithms may be necessary to allow the differentiation of sinus from pathologic tachycardia. These include detection of high rate, sudden onset of high rate, stability of high rate, and combinations of these criteria.

One problem in tachycardia detection that has been observed in patients with congenital heart disease and atrial antitachycardia pacing is far-field sensing of the ventricular electrogram when high gain is required by the atrial lead. This may result in double counting of each beat and inappropriate antitachycardia responses. In the presence of a sinus or atrial rhythm, this may be avoided by extension of the refractory period. However, in patients with sinus node dysfunction, there may sensing of the junctional or ventricular rhythm by default (Fig. 12–2).

Similar considerations in pacing for the termination of tachycardia need to be made. Tachycardia termination algorithms include burst pacing at a specified cycle length, pacing at a cycle length that is a percentage of the tachycardia cycle length, pacing with atrial extra stimulation, and pacing at progressively shorter cycle lengths (ramp pacing). Several reports have noted the need for extensive testing and use of complex termination algorithms in postoperative Fontan patients.[12, 13]

At this time, the role of antitachycardia pacing versus radiofrequency catheter ablation for attempted definitive cure of atrial muscle re-entrant tachycardia remains to be defined. This is due, in part, to the uncertain availability of the current atrial antitachycardia device in the future. It appears that certain forms of atrial tachycardia (e.g., atrial flutter in the patient who is

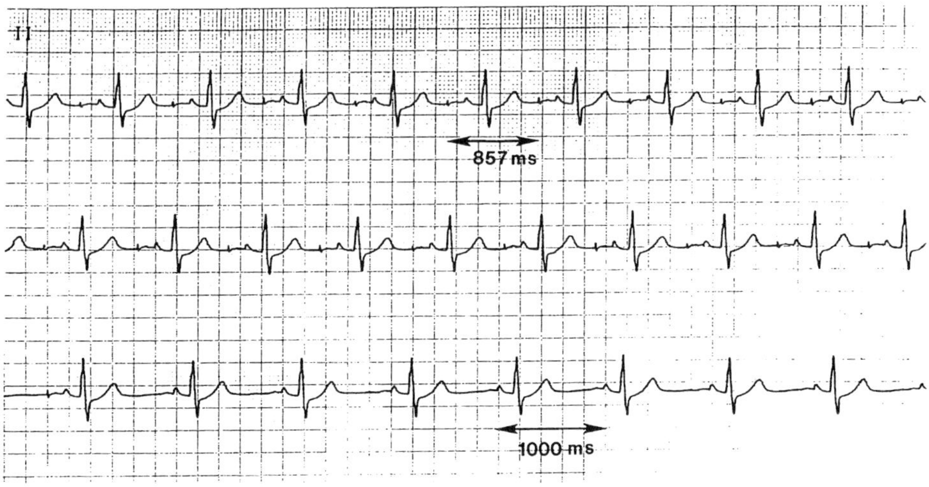

FIGURE 12–2. Atrial and ventricular "far-field" sensing by an atrial bipolar pacing lead. In this patient with a complex Fontan repair and atrial muscle re-entrant tachycardia, an antitachycardia pacemaker was implanted for control of arrhythmias. Because of the low amplitude of the atrial electrogram during tachycardia, the highest sensitivity was required during programming. Although the atrial pacing rate (AAI mode) was programmed to 857 ms (70/min), intermittent failure to pace at atrial cycle lengths of 1000 ms (bottom) were observed. This was due to sensing of the ventricular electrogram beyond the refractory period of 300 ms, with subsequent reset of the pacemaker detection interval.

postoperative for repair of an atrial septal defect) should be considered for attempted catheter ablation. Other patients who have undergone complex repairs, such as cavopulmonary modifications of the Fontan procedure, may have restricted atrial access and multiple re-entrant circuits, which may preclude catheter mapping and ablation. Thus, pacing with or without adjunctive pharmacologic therapy will remain a therapeutic option for these patients. Alternatively, atrial surgery has been reported in a few of these patients.[17] The long-term efficacy of a surgical approach and potential morbidity remain to be defined.

TRANSVENOUS ATRIAL COUNTERSHOCK FOR TERMINATION OF ATRIAL FLUTTER OR FIBRILLATION

The significant morbidity and risk of mortality associated with atrial flutter and fibrillation have resulted in investigation of laboratory and clinical methods for transvenous countershock for termination of these arrhythmias. The basic technology for tachycardia detection and termination represents an extension of concepts currently used in implantable cardioverter-defibrillators (ICDs), with several important modifications. This approach remains investigational at this time and is primarily focused on atrial defibrillation, although the same principles apply for termination of atrial muscle re-entrant tachycardias.

Preliminary studies of low-energy transvenous atrial defibrillation were largely unsuccessful because they were performed with electrodes placed in the right atrium and ventricle and did not incorporate the left atrium into the current path. Subsequent studies by Keane[18] and Cooper[19] and their colleagues demonstrated efficacy of low-energy termination of recent-onset atrial flutter or fibrillation when a right atrial to coronary sinus current path was used. With biphasic shock waveforms and optimal lead positions, atrial defibrillation thresholds averaged less than 1.5 J.

The risk of ventricular proarrhythmia has remained a major concern for shocks delivered in the atria (Fig. 12–3). R-wave shock synchronization appears to be the most effective method to limit this risk. In the case of atrial flutter or fibrillation with a rapid ventricular response, an R-wave synchronous shock may occur during the relative refractory period of the preceding beat in the RR interval. Several other concerns regarding an implantable atrial defibrillator have been cited and include failure of tachycardia detection and patient pain with transvenous shock, because loss of consciousness is unlikely to occur with acute-onset atrial flutter or fibrillation.[20]

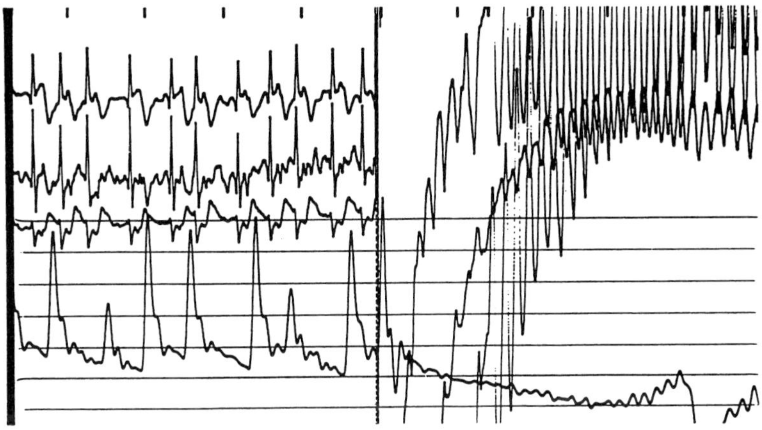

FIGURE 12–3. An example of the "proarrhythmic" potential of transvenous atrial countershock. During cardiac catheterization of a 10-year-old with Ebstein's anomaly, atrial muscle re-entrant tachycardia developed (left side of panel). A helical coil transvenous defibrillation lead was positioned in the right atrium, with a second external return electrode placed on the chest wall. The defibrillator was synchronized to the electrocardiogram. A 1-J countershock resulted in ventricular fibrillation (right side of panel), which then required a 10-J shock to restore sinus rhythm.

BASIC CONSIDERATIONS IN ANTITACHYCARDIA DEVICES FOR TREATMENT OF VENTRICULAR TACHYARRHYTHMIAS

Ventricular arrhythmias in the young patient may occur as sequelae of surgery for congenital heart disease or as manifestations of a primary electrophysiologic or structural abnormality of the ventricles. Because of the potential for sudden death, the development and clinical use of device therapies for ventricular arrhythmias have been accelerated compared with applications for atrial tachyarrhythmias.

One important difference between children and adults is the infrequency of sustained monomorphic ventricular tachycardia in younger patients. Limited reports have demonstrated ventricular fibrillation in young patients to be either a primary electrical event or the sequelae of atrial muscle re-entrant tachycardia or polymorphic ventricular tachycardia.[13, 21] Thus, the antitachycardia devices in young patients resuscitated from sudden cardiac arrest requires detection algorithms and responses that are different from those common in adults.

RATE SUPPORT FOR PREVENTION OF VENTRICULAR TACHYARRHYTHMIAS

One aspect of device therapy for ventricular arrhythmias that is similar to that for atrial arrhythmias is rate support with pacing in patients with bradycardia-mediated tachyarrhythmias. Historically, these were patients with congenital complete heart block or those in whom advanced atrioventricular block developed after surgical closure of a ventricular septal defect or related lesion. These patients have been observed to experience complex ventricular ectopy either associated with an inadequate escape rhythm or during states of increased physiologic demands. Because permanent pacing is now a standard recommendation in these patients, AV block as a cause of ventricular arrhythmias has been eliminated.[22]

Rate support for the prevention of ventricular arrhythmias in patients with congenital prolonged QT syndromes has gained increasing support during the past decade.[23] Several factors that support the logic of this treatment include the fact that many of these patients either have a low resting heart rate[24] or experience bradycardia during treatment with beta blockade. The long cycle lengths associated with the low resting heart rates favor prolongation and dispersion of refractoriness, which may be central to the mechanisms of arrhythmogenesis in these patients (Fig. 12–4). Although beta blockade remains primary therapy in patients with the long QT syndrome, pacing may need to be considered early as a secondary treatment, particularly in the presence of symptoms during beta blockade. The one exception to this rule is the newborn infant with 2:1 AV block in association with the prolonged QT syndrome. This form of the long QT syndrome represents one instance in which permanent pacing should be considered as primary therapy. However, concurrent treatment with beta blockade should be continued in these patients.[25]

ANTITACHYCARDIA PACING FOR TERMINATION OF VENTRICULAR TACHYARRHYTHMIAS

In most cases, ventricular tachycardia is due to re-entry and thus potentially may be termi-

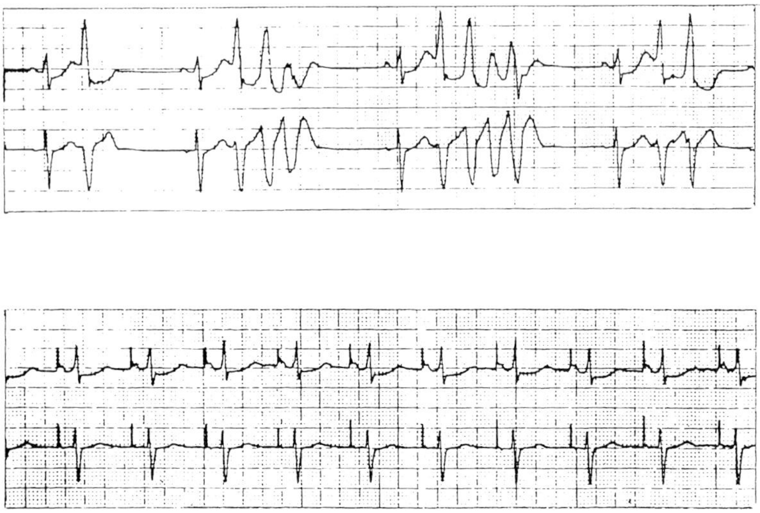

FIGURE 12–4. An example of atrial pacing for the suppression of polymorphic, nonsustained ventricular tachycardia associated with the long QT syndrome. Top, Recurrent episodes of complex ventricular ectopy in a 13-year-old with long QT syndrome and recurrent syncope. Bottom, AAI pacing at 700 ms (85/min) results in complete suppression of ventricular ectopy.

nated with programmed ventricular stimulation. Clinical experience with implantable antitachycardia pacemakers for patients with ventricular tachycardia has been minimal because of the potential for the degeneration of ventricular tachycardia to ventricular fibrillation during rapid pacing. In a few patients, antitachycardia pacemakers have been implanted in conjunction with first- or second-generation ICDs to limit the number of device shocks.[26]

Among the notable developments of third-generation ICDs is the capability of tiered therapies, with antitachycardia ventricular pacing using a number of programmable algorithms as a first option, followed by synchronized low-energy cardioversion and back-up defibrillation if other therapies fail. This heuristic approach to ventricular tachycardia therapy has permitted antitachycardia pacing to become an integral aspect of the therapies for patients with recurrent ventricular tachycardia.[27]

At this time, the percentage of pediatric patients with re-entrant ventricular tachycardia has not been established. Thus, it is not clear which patients are candidates for tiered therapy for ventricular tachycardia. Patients with a prior ventriculotomy or infarction appear most likely to have a macro–re-entrant tachycardia circuit and thus may be suitable for this therapy (Fig. 12–5).[28] Ventricular arrhythmias in other young patients may be polymorphic as a result of automaticity or may be primary ventricular fibrillation.[29] It has been recommended that formal electrophysiologic testing be performed in survivors of sustained ventricular tachycardia or sudden cardiac arrest to determine responses to tiered therapies, so that an ICD with appropriate tachycardia termination capabilities may be selected.[30]

ICDs IN YOUNG PATIENTS: CURRENT STATUS

After initial laboratory investigations of internal defibrillation during the 1970s, clinical trials with an automatic implantable defibrillator (AID) began in 1980. In the initial report of Mirowski et al,[31] the second patient to receive an AID was a 16-year-old boy with a cardiomyopathy. The overall clinical use of these devices in patients younger than 20 years has remained limited, representing 1% of all patients receiving these devices. This paucity of experience reflects both the infrequency of sudden cardiac arrest in young patients and the lower salvage rate of young patients who do experience sudden cardiovascular collapse.[32, 33]

In spite of the limited data, there is a gradually increasing experience with ICDs in young patients. This provides a basis for discussion of the use of these devices in context of the patient's cardiac disease and projected long-term prognosis. Several collaborative studies will be completed in the near future that may provide further guidance regarding the use of ICDs in young patients with diverse forms of cardiac disease.[34, 35]

In 1993, a comprehensive review of the clinical experience with ICDs in young patients was reported.[36] Although this study was based on a voluntary data registry, several salient points were established that have been validated during subsequent follow-up:

1. There are three distinct forms of cardiovascular disease in young patients in whom ICDs have been implanted: cardiomyopathies (hypertrophic and dilated); primary electrical diseases

(idiopathic ventricular fibrillation and long QT syndromes); and postoperative congenital heart disease.

2. Impaired ventricular function was the strongest predictor of sudden and total cardiac mortality after ICD implant.

3. The rates of acute implant complications and long-term morbidity were not different in children from those reported for adults during the same era (1980–1991).

4. The actuarial incidence of ostensibly appropriate ICD shocks was 50% at a mean follow-up of 24 months.

Several developments have resulted in a substantial increase in the use of ICDs, irrespective of patient age, since publication of this report. The first is that of advances in ICD technology, which have included the development of transvenous lead systems along with a reduction in device mass from 235 g to less than 100 g. The second has been the impact of the Cardiac Arrhythmia Suppression Trial (CAST) and a similar report by the Pediatric Electrophysiology Society, which have resulted in caution in the use of antiarrhythmic agents in patients with life-threatening cardiac arrhythmias as well as uncertainty regarding the ability to predict drug efficacy.[37, 38]

These developments have resulted in revised clinical standards and practices regarding these devices. Currently, three different clinical scenarios representing indications for ICD implantation may be anticipated in young patients:

1. The patient who is resuscitated from sudden cardiac arrest in whom either no arrhythmia is identified or a reliable treatment cannot be established (e.g., the resuscitated patient with hypertrophic cardiomyopathy or idiopathic ventricular fibrillation with no inducible ventricular arrhythmia during electrophysiologic testing).

2. The patient with recurrent symptomatic ventricular tachycardia who is identified at risk of sudden death and who is intolerant of antiarrhythmic treatment (e.g., the patient with recurrent ventricular tachycardia after repair of tetralogy of Fallot in whom pulmonary toxicity develops during amiodarone treatment).

3. The young patient who is asymptomatic but has known cardiovascular disease and a strong family history of sudden death (e.g., the sibling or child of a parent with long QT syndrome or hypertrophic cardiomyopathy who has died suddenly from the same disease); ICD implantation in this category is for "primary" prevention of sudden cardiac death and remains controversial at this time.[39]

It is important to emphasize that there are several areas of uncertainty regarding the use of ICDs in young patients. These may include but are not limited to:

1. The patient with long QT syndrome in whom cardiac arrest is the presenting symptom. The fundamental issue is whether treatment with beta blockade is adequate therapy or whether an ICD should be implanted.[40]

2. The patient with advanced ventricular dysfunction, syncope, and complex ventricular ectopy. The use of an ICD as a "bridge" to orthotopic heart transplantation has been advocated as a means to delay transplant in adults. However, the benefit and effectiveness of this approach remain to be demonstrated.[41]

3. The patient with known heart disease, syncope, and inducible ventricular arrhythmias during programmed stimulation. The relative bene-

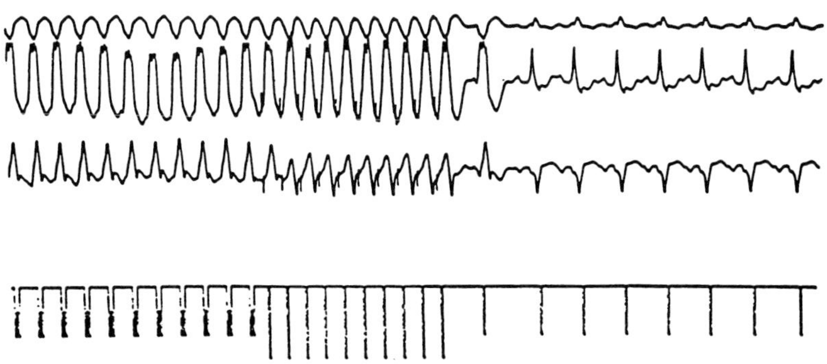

FIGURE 12–5. Antitachycardia pacing for the termination of ventricular tachycardia in a 15-year-old boy with prior anterolateral myocardial infarction associated with Kawasaki syndrome. Electrocardiogram leads I, aVF, and V_1 and a marker channel are displayed. The first 11 beats are ventricular tachycardia at a cycle length of 360 ms. Tachycardia detection is followed by 10 beats of ventricular pacing at 288 ms (80% of the detected tachycardia cycle length), with restoration of sinus rhythm. (Reproduced by permission Estes NAM III, Manolis AS, Wang PJ, eds: Implantable Cardioverter-Defibrillators: A Comprehensive Textbook. New York, Marcel Dekker, 1994.)

fits of antiarrhythmic drugs versus implantable defibrillator for these patients remain controversial.[42]

At this time, these issues remain unresolved but undoubtedly will be influenced by advances in ICD technology. The indications for ICD implant have evolved from secondary prevention in sudden cardiac arrest survivors to treatment of nonlethal ventricular arrhythmias and possible primary prevention in "high-risk" patients.

Once the decision to implant an ICD in a young patient has been made, the issues of device capability, implant site, and lead system along with lifestyle need to be considered. Current recommendations are that patients undergo electrophysiologic testing before ICD implantation to determine the inducibility of ventricular arrhythmias and responses to tiered therapies. Sustained monomorphic ventricular tachycardia is frequently inducible in adult survivors of sudden cardiac arrest, who thus are candidates for the tiered therapies of antitachycardia pacing, synchronized cardioversion, and defibrillation. However, polymorphic ventricular tachycardia or primary ventricular fibrillation are more probable in young patients resuscitated from sudden cardiac arrest. Thus, device selection and programming should be tailored to the underlying arrhythmic substrate in the young patient.

ICD lead configuration and device implant site represent areas where substantial progress has been made in ICD technology. One factor limiting ICD use for many years was the epicardial placement of defibrillator lead systems and the morbidity, cost, and duration of hospital stay associated with the surgical thoracotomy. These were particularly important considerations for patients with prior surgery for congenital heart disease or impaired ventricular function. Nonthoracotomy lead systems, composed of subcutaneous patch electrodes and multiple transvenous leads, represented efforts to avoid thoracotomy in these patients. Although these systems were complex, acceptable defibrillation thresholds (<20 J) could be achieved in 70 to 80% of patients.[43]

The Endotek lead systems (Cardiac Pacemakers Inc, St. Paul, MN) represented a significant development, combining within a 12-French tripolar transvenous lead the capabilities of bipolar sensing and pacing (distal tip cathode to distal spring electrode) and defibrillation (distal spring cathode to proximal spring anode). A similar advance has been provided by the 10.5-French Transvene lead systems (Medtronic Inc, Minneapolis, MN), which is based on defibrillation between a distal tip cathode and a patch in the pocket or a titanium electrode, which is incorporated into the defibrillator shell (Fig. 12–6).[44]

Lead position and configuration may be a difficult consideration for young patients, particularly when abnormal cardiac anatomy, chest wall deformities, or low-cardiac output are present. Limited current experience suggests that a transvenous system should be considered in the presence of normal cardiac anatomy. However, abnormal anatomy or size less than 40 kg may require use of an epicardial, subcutaneous, or hybrid (lead-patch) approach to ICD lead placement.

Concurrent with the development of transvenous ICD lead systems was the need for reduction in ICD size to allow pectoral implantation as with pacemakers. Some reduction in size has been achieved, primarily with the use of biphasic shocks, which have lowered the energy of defibrillation requirements compared with monophasic shocks.[45] Further reductions in size will be predicated on advances in battery and capacitor technologies, because these components currently account for two thirds of the total ICD mass.

A number of patient-specific issues must be considered after ICD implant in a young patient. These include driving, employment, athletics, and the differentiation of sinus from pathologic

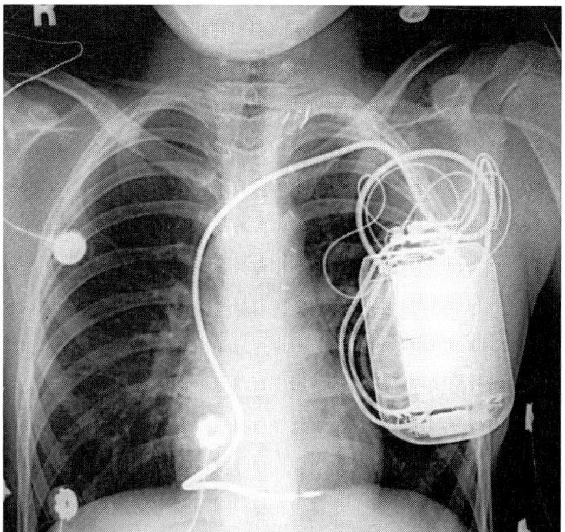

FIGURE 12–6. Posteroanterior chest radiograph from an 8-year-old boy with the long QT syndrome. He had transvenous implantation of a defibrillator using the coil and a patch in the subpectoral pocket. Sensing and pacing were accomplished from the distal electrodes of the defibrillator lead. Holter monitor leads can be seen on the chest wall.

tachycardia. Although the issues of driving and employment are debated in the medical literature, a consensus recommendation of medical experts does not appear probable in the near future.[46] Inappropriate responses to sinus tachycardia, either antitachycardia pacing or direct current countershock, may occur after ICD implant. For this concern, concurrent treatment with beta blockade may be required after defibrillator implant.

Advanced electrical therapies for cardiac arrhythmias will likely become more prevalent in the next decade. These will likely include atrial countershock and further reduction in ICD size to allow pectoral implantation in smaller patients. Further advances must continue to focus on prevention of arrhythmias and continued progress regarding the fundamental mechanisms of sudden cardiac death.

REFERENCES

1. Kugler JD, Danford DA, Deal BJ, et al: Radiofrequency catheter ablation for tachyarrhythmias in children and adolescents. N Engl J Med 330:1481, 1994.
2. Garson A Jr, Bink-Boelkens MT, Hesslein PS, et al: Atrial flutter in the young: A collaborative study of 380 cases. J Am Coll Cardiol 6:781, 1985.
3. Akhtar M: Clinical spectrum of ventricular tachycardia. Circulation 82:1561, 1990.
4. Peters NS, Sommerville J: Arrhythmias after the Fontan procedure. Br Heart J 68:199, 1992.
5. Flinn CJ, Wolff GS, Dick M, et al: Cardiac rhythm after the Mustard operation for transposition of the great arteries. N Engl J Med 310:1635, 1984.
6. Triedman JK, Saul JP, Weindling SN, et al: Radiofrequency catheter ablation of intra-atrial reentrant tachycardia after surgical palliation of congenital heart disease. Circulation 91:707, 1995.
7. Duster MC, Bink-Boelkens MT, Wampler D, et al: Long-term follow-up of dysrhythmias following the Mustard procedure. Am Heart J 109:1323, 1985.
8. Fisher JD, Johnston DR, Furman S, et al: Long-term efficacy of antitachycardia pacing for supraventricular and ventricular tachycardias. Am J Cardiol 60:1311, 1987.
9. McGoon MD, Maloney JD, McGoon DC: Long-term endocardial atrial pacing in children with bradycardia-tachycardia syndrome and limited ventricular access. Am J Cardiol 49:1750, 1982.
10. Fukushige J, Porter CB, Hayes DL, et al: Antitachycardia pacemaker treatment of postoperative arrhythmias in pediatric patients. Pacing Clin Electrophysiol 14:546, 1991.
11. Silka MJ, Manwill JR, Kron J, et al: Bradycardia-mediated tachyarrhythmias in congenital heart disease and responses to chronic pacing at physiologic rates. Am J Cardiol 65:488, 1990.
12. Gillette PC, Zeigler VL, Case CL, et al: Atrial antitachycardia pacing in children and young adults. Am Heart J 122:844, 1991.
13. Rhodes LA, Walsh EP, Gamble WJ, et al: Benefits and potential risks of atrial antitachycardia pacing after repair of congenital heart disease. Pacing Clin Electrophysiol 16:1005, 1995.
14. Gregoratos G, Cheitlin MD, Conill A, et al: ACC/AHA Guidelines for Implantation of Cardiac Pacemakers and Antiarrhythmia Devices. J Am Coll Card 31:1175, 1998.
15. Lamas GA, Estes NAM, Schneller S, et al: Does dual chamber or atrial pacing prevent atrial fibrillation? The need for a randomized controlled trial. Pacing Clin Electrophysiol 15:1109, 1992.
16. Case CL, Gillette PC, Zeigler V, et al: Problems with permanent atrial pacing in the Fontan patient. Pacing Clin Electrophysiol 12:92, 1989.
17. Balaji S, Johnson TB, Sade RM, et al: Management of atrial flutter after the Fontan procedure. J Am Coll Cardiol 23:1209, 1994.
18. Keane D, Sulke N, Cooke R, et al: Endocardial cardioversion of atrial flutter and fibrillation. Pacing Clin Electrophysiol 16:928, 1993.
19. Cooper RAS, Alferness CA, Smith WM, et al: Internal cardioversion of atrial fibrillation in sheep. Circulation 87:1673, 1993.
20. Levy S, Camm J: An implantable atrial defibrillator: An impossible dream? Circulation 87:1769, 1993.
21. Leenhardt A, Lucet V, Denjoy I, et al: Catecholaminergic polymorphic ventricular tachycardia in children: A seven year follow-up of 21 patients. Circulation 91:1512, 1995.
22. Michaelsson M, Jonzon A, Riesenfeld T: Isolated congenital complete atrioventricular block in adult life: A prospective study. Circulation 92:442, 1995.
23. Eldar M, Griffin JY, Abbott JA, et al: Permanent cardiac pacing in patients with the long QT syndrome. J Am Coll Cardiol 10:600, 1987.
24. Kugler JD: Sinus nodal dysfunction in young patients with long QT syndrome. Am Heart J 121:1132, 1991.
25. Van Hare GF, Franz MR, Roge C, et al: Persistent functional atrioventricular block in two patients with prolonged QT intervals: Elucidation of the mechanisms of block. Pacing Clin Electrophysiol 13:608, 1990.
26. Calkins H, Brinker J, Veltri EP, et al: Clinical interactions between pacemakers and automatic implanted cardioverter-defibrillators. J Am Coll Cardiol 16:666, 1990.
27. Saksena S, Chandran P. Shah Y, et al: Comparative efficacy of transvenous cardioversion and pacing in patients with sustained ventricular tachycardia: A prospective, randomized, crossover study. Circulation 72:153, 1985.
28. Misaki T, Tsubota M, Watanabe G, et al: Surgical treatment of ventricular tachycardia after repair of tetralogy of Fallot. Circulation 90:264, 1994.
29. Eisenberg SJ, Scheinman MM, Dullet NK, et al: Sudden cardiac death and polymorphous ventricular tachycardia in patients with normal QT intervals and normal systolic cardiac function. Am J Cardiol 75:687, 1995.
30. Zipes DP, DiMarco JP, Gillette PC, et al: Guidelines for clinical intracardiac electrophysiological and catheter ablation procedures: A report of the American College of Cardiology and American Heart Association task force on practice guidelines. Circulation 92:673, 1995.
31. Mirowski M, Reid PR, Mower MM, et al: Termination of malignant ventricular arrhythmias in man with an implanted automatic defibrillator. N Engl J Med 303:322, 1980.
32. Driscoll DJ, Edwards JE: Sudden unexpected death in children and adolescents. J Am Coll Cardiol 5:118B, 1985.
33. Eisenberg M, Bergner L, Hallstrom A: Epidemiology of cardiac arrest and resuscitation in children. Ann Emerg Med 12:672, 1983.
34. Groh WJ, Silka MJ, Oliver RP, et al: Use of implantable cardioverter-defibrillators in the congenital long QT syndrome. Am J Card 78:703–706, 1996.
35. Priori S, Borgreffe M, Camm AJ, et al: Role of the

implantable defibrillator in patients with idiopathic ventricular fibrillation (abstract). Pacing Clin Electrophysiol 18:799, 1995.
36. Silka MJ, Kron J, Dunnigan A, et al: Sudden cardiac death and the use of implantable cardioverter-defibrillators in pediatric patients. Circulation 87:800, 1993.
37. The Cardiac Arrhythmia Suppression Trial (CAST) Investigators: Preliminary report: Effect of encainide and flecainide on mortality in a randomized trial of arrhythmia suppression after myocardial infarction. N Engl J Med 321:406, 1989.
38. Fish FA, Gillette PC, Benson DW, et al: Proarrhythmia, cardiac arrest and death in young patients receiving encainide and flecainide. J Am Coll Cardiol 18:356, 1991.
39. Kuck KH: Value of prophylactic implantable cardioverter defibrillator therapy. Pacing Clin Electrophysiol 17:514, 1994.
40. Garson A Jr, Dick M II, Fournier A, et al: The long QT syndrome in children. An international study of 287 patients. Circulation 87:1866, 1993.
41. DEFIBRILAT Study Group: Actuarial risk of sudden death while awaiting cardiac transplantation in patients with atherosclerotic heart disease. Am J Cardiol 68:545, 1991.
42. Wever EFD, Hauer RNW, van Capelle FJL, et al: Randomized study of implantable defibrillator as first-choice therapy versus conventional strategy in postinfarct sudden death survivors. Circulation 91:2195, 1995.
43. Kron J, Silka MJ, Ohm OJ, et al: Preliminary experience with nonthoracotomy implantable cardioverter-defibrillators in young patients. Pacing Clin Electrophysiol 17:26, 1994.
44. Bardy GH, Johnson G, Poole JE, et al: A simplified, single-lead unipolar transvenous cardioversion-defibrillation system. Circulation 88:543–547, 1993.
45. Bardy GH, Ivey TD, Allen MD, et al: A prospective, randomized evaluation of biphasic versus monophasic waveform pulses of defibrillation efficacy in humans. J Am Coll Cardiol 14:728, 1989.
46. Stickberger SA, Cantillon CO, Friedman PL: When should patients with lethal arrhythmias resume driving? Ann Intern Med 115:560, 1991.

CHAPTER 13

MEDICAL ANTIARRHYTHMIC THERAPY

James C. Perry

The use of antiarrhythmic agents in children has undergone dramatic changes as a result of widespread catheter ablative techniques. As ablation has evolved to an exceptionally effective and safe procedure, a re-examination of the need for aggressive antiarrhythmic drug therapies has become necessary.

REGULATORY ISSUES AND "STANDARDS OF PRACTICE"

The only antiarrhythmic agent formally "approved" for use in children is digoxin.[1] The pharmaceutical industry has little financial imperative or incentive to perform drug trials in young patients to establish criteria acceptable to the Food and Drug Administration (FDA) when the market share from the pediatric population is so small. Several drugs have undergone extensive evaluation in the past 10 years without this work appearing in drug package inserts. In 1993, the FDA required that pediatric guidelines be issued for any new pharmaceutical agent. Two antiarrhythmic drugs (oral sotalol and intravenous amiodarone) with rigorously obtained pediatric data on efficacy, dosing, and safety have been approved and released subsequently without pediatric guidelines in their package inserts.

On a practical basis, an accrued volume of experience using the drugs by the pediatric cardiology community has brought about relatively well-recognized guidelines for dosing, efficacy, and safety outside the realm of formal approval by the FDA. Because it appears unlikely that pediatric use of antiarrhythmic agents will undergo wide-ranging approval by the FDA (unless under a "grandfather" clause), pediatric cardiologists are beholden to a "standard of practice" born primarily under the auspices of published material.

ANTIARRHYTHMIC AGENTS IN THE ABLATION ERA

DEGREE OF MEDICAL CONTROL VERSUS ABLATION SUCCESS

With the widespread application of ablative therapies, options for medical antiarrhythmic therapy are now based on the relative balance of efficacy rates, safety issues, and natural history data for arrhythmias in children compared with ablative therapy.[2–4] Medical efficacy rates for arrhythmia "control" vary considerably. Medical control of many supraventricular tachycardias (SVTs), consisting of elimination of episodes, may be achieved in 50 to 60% of patients over a given year.[5] Often this observation is confounded by the influence of the natural history aspects of arrhythmias. For many others, control may be deemed adequate if there are rare recurrences, shorter duration episodes, or diminution of symptoms. For more resistant arrhythmias, medical therapy can become quite complex. This situation is especially true for the patient in whom ablative therapy is not an option, when ablation has been attempted but proved unsuccessful, or when other antiarrhythmic interventional devices (e.g., defibrillators, pacemakers) are used in conjunction with drug therapy.

SIDE EFFECTS OF MEDICAL THERAPY VERSUS ABLATION COMPLICATIONS

Side effects of medical therapy can also influence both the complexity and duration of antiarrhythmic drug use. A spectrum of intolerable drug side effects and potential proarrhythmic effects can limit medical therapy. Combinations of two or more drugs now are rarely necessary and often bring about the examination of whether the arrhythmia being treated is amenable to ablation. Side effects may be transient, such as skin rashes and nausea, or more permanent, such as the pulmonary fibrosis reported with long-term amiodarone treatment and the potentially life-threatening proarrhythmias.

PHARMACOKINETICS

To use antiarrhythmic agents effectively in children, several factors need to be considered: the different profiles of absorption, distribution, metabolism, and excretion and the role of these variables in the dose and dosing schedule for each drug, including those of any active metabolites.

ABSORPTION AND DISTRIBUTION

The first two factors, absorption and distribution, are influenced by whether the drug is administered by an oral or intravenous route and the drug "vehicle." When a drug is given in a solution or suspension, it is readily available for absorption, but pill or capsule forms must be digested to release the active drug. So-called long-acting preparations tend to involve a cellulose matrix, resulting in slow absorption. Different preparations of a drug (pill, solution, suspension, matrix), therefore, result in different time-to-peak serum concentration and duration of effect.

For most agents, once absorbed, 75% to 90% may be available for drug action. A first-pass effect, whereby absorbed drug is metabolized in the liver or intestinal wall, occurs for a few drugs. Antiarrhythmic drugs given intravenously have rapid availability for action. Specific clinical settings may influence the bioavailability of orally administered drugs, including congestive heart failure, resulting in bowel wall edema and decreased absorption, and the chronic state of reduced absorption, which can occur in patients with high central venous pressures and liver enlargement (e.g., in the patient with single-ventricle physiology).

METABOLISM AND EXCRETION

The metabolism of drugs arises as an issue in two factors. The first is the age-related change in hepatic capabilities to metabolize drugs. Hepatic enzymes with a reduced ability to transform parent compounds to their metabolites can be saturated rapidly, leaving more drug unmetabolized. The second issue is the production of active metabolites. This is important for procainamide, quinidine, disopyramide, lidocaine, propafenone, amiodarone, and propranolol. Metabolites can be quite different in their antiarrhythmic activity. An example is the metabolite of the class IA drug procainamide, *N*-acetyl procainamide (NAPA). NAPA is classified as a class III drug.

Most antiarrhythmic drug excretion is renal, and renal failure will inhibit drug elimination, including low cardiac output states as well as those with selective low renal perfusion such as coarctation of the aorta. When the amount of drug excreted equals the amount given, "steady-state" kinetics exists. This state can truly exist only for drugs being given as a continuous intravenous infusion. Otherwise, the serum concentration of drugs will oscillate based on the frequency of administration and the pharmacokinetic characteristics. In practice, a clinical steady state is presumed to be present after five elimination half-lives (the $t_{1/2}$ beta) of a drug.

ANTIARRHYTHMIC DRUG CONCENTRATION

Drug concentrations need to be obtained as serum trough determinations before the sixth or seventh dose. This is important when drug dosing intervals are changed. When concentrations are in the "therapeutic" range, it implies neither a guarantee of efficacy nor safety, because serum concentrations do not reflect the drug concentrations at the target site and low serum concentrations may be correlated with antiarrhythmic efficacy if receptor sites are occupied. Erratic serum concentrations can be found for a number of agents (amiodarone, propafenone, sotalol) and may not reflect potential therapeutic dosing for the drug. Low serum trough levels obviously have no bearing on the peak concentration seen from 1 to 6 hours after the drug is given orally. Adverse effects, such as blurry vision with class IC drugs, may be more related to peak concentrations. In general, serum levels are important to check periodically for the class IA and IC drugs and intravenous lidocaine. Digoxin levels are helpful when there is lack of antiarrhythmic effect, when other drugs that can alter the digoxin concentration are given concurrently, when digoxin overdose is suspected, or to ascertain compliance.

PHARMACODYNAMICS AND DRUG CLASSIFICATION SCHEMES

Pharmacodynamics are the properties of the manner in which antiarrhythmic drugs interact with ionic channels and receptors, and they tend to be similar for children and adults. Some situations can alter pharmacodynamic principles, such as hypokalemia and myocardial infarction, but they are far more common in adults. Some changes may exist in the postoperative congenital heart defect patient, in whom the myocardial scar may resemble that after myocardial infarction.

The Vaughn Williams antiarrhythmic drug classification scheme groups drugs with similar antiarrhythmic effects.[6] Although it may be a useful means of teaching antiarrhythmic actions, the system has its flaws. Drugs' effects and metabolites often cross over into other classes, and drugs in the same class can have very different potentials for efficacy, side effects, and effects based on ion channel gating characteristics. Interactions with the autonomic nervous system, a major factor for some drugs, are not considered in the classification. Most important, drug classes are related to the cellular electrophysiologic responses of normal His-Purkinje tissue, which can be misleading for the clinician interested in atrial myocardial or atrioventricular (AV) nodal effects or the effects in diseased tissue.

In 1991, a task force of electrophysiologists treating adults met in Italy to develop a new scheme for classifying antiarrhythmic drugs based on the target tachyarrhythmia mechanism.[7] While the resulting "Sicilian gambit" was an effective means to force a reconsideration of drug classification schemes, its use in the clinical setting can be problematic. Many arrhythmia mechanisms remain unknown, and the vulnerable target (e.g., channels, receptors, use-dependent factors) is unclear.

Because the Vaughn Williams classification is most widely used, and because a number of the antiarrhythmic agents selected on the basis of a Sicilian gambit approach are eventually grouped by one of these standard classes, in this chapter

Table 13–1. Summary of Drug Use and Side Effects

DRUG	DOSING	WARNINGS
Quinidine	PO: 30–60 mg/kg/day	Torsades de pointes, "cinchonism"
Procainamide	PO: 40–100 mg/kg/day	Lupus-like syndrome
	IV: 7–15 mg/kg load, 40–100 mcg/kg/min infusion	Hypotension
Disopyramide	PO: 5–30 mg/kg/day (varies with age)	Anticholinergic effects
Lidocaine	IV: 1–2 mg/kg, 20–50 mcg/kg/min infusion	CNS side effects
Mexiletine	PO: 2–8 mg/kg/dose (varies with age)	Skin rash, nausea
Moricizine	PO: 200–600 mg/m²/day	Neurologic effects
Phenytoin	PO: 15 mg/kg load, chronic 5–6 mg/kg/day	CNS, gingival hyperplasia
	IV: 1–3 mg/kg load	Hypotension
Tocainide	PO: 200 mg bid/tid	Gastrointestinal, CNS
Flecainide	PO: 80–200 mg/m²/day (varies with age)	Avoid in abnormal hearts
	IV: 1–2 mg/kg	
Propafenone	PO: 150–600 mg/m²/day	Avoid in abnormal hearts
Propranolol	PO: 1–2 mg/kg/day	Fatigue, nightmares, bradycardia
	IV: 0.1–0.2 mg/kg	Bradycardia, hypotension
Atenolol	PO: 1–3 mg/kg/day	Postural hypotension, cool extremities
Metoprolol	PO: 50–200 mg bid (adult)	Similar to atenolol
Nadolol	PO: 1 mg/kg/day	Similar to atenolol
Esmolol	IV: 500 mcg/kg load, 50–200 mcg/kg/min infusion	Hypotension
Amiodarone	PO: 10–15 mg/kg load, 2–5 mg/kg chronic	Skin, liver, thyroid, pulmonary
	IV: 5 mg/kg load (in divided doses), 10–15 mg/kg/day infusion	Hypotension, bradycardia
Sotalol	PO: 90–200 mg/m²/day	Bradycardia, torsades de pointes
Bretylium	IV: 5 mg/kg push	Hypotension
Ibutilide	IV: 10–25 mcg/kg	Torsades de pointes
Verapamil	PO: 4–17 mg/kg/day	Bradycardia, constipation
		Bradycardia, hypotension
Diltiazem	PO: 30–120 mg tid (adult)	Headache
	IV: 0.15–0.45 mg/kg load, 3 mcg/kg/min infusion	Hypotension, AV block
Adenosine	IV: 100–300 mcg/kg push	Hypotension, flushing, bronchospasm
Digoxin	PO: 30–50 mcg/kg load, divided (see text)	Gastrointestinal, gynecomastia, proarrhythmia
	IV: ⅔–¾ of oral dose, divided (see text)	Proarrhythmia

CNS, central nervous system; bid, twice daily; tid, three times daily; PO, oral; IV, intravenous; AV, atrioventricular.

the drugs are reviewed on the basis of the Vaughn Williams class. Table 13–1 provides a summary of the drugs, doses, and comments on use and side effects.

VAUGHN WILLIAMS CLASSIFICATION

Class I Agents

The class I agents are the "local anesthetic agents" and block sodium channels. They are further subdivided (IA, IB, IC) on the basis of their effects on repolarization and effects at faster heart rates.

Class IA Agents

The class IA agents include quinidine, procainamide, and disopyramide. Repolarization is prolonged, antivagal effects play a major role, and these drugs have a greater effect at faster heart rates.

Quinidine. This is the oldest of the local anesthetic or membrane-active drugs in use. The drug is the D-isomer of quinine and is a cinchona derivative ("cinchonism" refers to overdose side effects).

Drug Action. Quinidine is a potent sodium and potassium channel blocker. Sodium channels blockade predominantly occurs in those channels with medium time constants and in the active state. Quinidine also has moderate potassium channel–blocking activity as well as low level effects on blocking alpha and muscarinic receptors.

Oral Administration, Kinetics, Metabolites. Quinidine is administered orally as quinidine sulfate or gluconate. In adults, the gluconate form is absorbed slowly, with a peak serum level 3 to 4 hours after administration. Its dosing schedule is generally every 8 hours. Quinidine sulfate reaches a serum peak concentration in 1 to 2 hours and is usually given every 6 hours. The drug is extensively bound to plasma proteins so that with hypoalbuminemia, serum levels may increase. Higher quinidine levels occur in congestive heart failure states as a result of changes in plasma proteins, but this finding varies because of the potential changes in absorption if bowel wall edema is present.

After absorption, quinidine is metabolized in the liver using the cytochrome P-450 system to a number of metabolites. Of these metabolites, 3-hydroxy quinidine is the most prevalent and most potent antiarrhythmic agent. Approximately 20% of the parent drug is eventually excreted unchanged in the urine. Like most antiarrhythmics, quinidine is a weak base, and alkaline urine can increase serum levels. The drug is poorly removed by dialysis techniques.[8] The elimination $t_{1/2}$ of quinidine is 6 to 8 hours, which dictates the dosing schedule. The presumed therapeutic range of quinidine at steady state is 2 to 6 μg/ml.

Side Effects. Side effects with quinidine are common; 25 to 30% of patients experience some difficulty. The most common problems are gastrointestinal. *Cinchonism* refers to central nervous system effects, including tinnitus, visual changes, headache, and mental status changes. Other noncardiac side effects are predominantly hematologic: thrombocytopenia, anemia, and agranulocytosis.

Cardiac side effects are those that may be expected and those that are unwanted and mostly proarrhythmic. Electrocardiographic effects include prolongation of the PR, QRS, and QT intervals, which need to be monitored at drug initiation in particular. Bradycardia can appear de novo or can be exacerbated. Bundle branch blocks may occur, and, with high levels of drug, AV block may result. The most dangerous side effect is drug-induced torsades de pointes ventricular tachycardia (VT), resulting in syncope and potential sudden death.[9] This phenomenon often occurs in the first several days of dosing and may be accompanied by slightly low serum potassium levels and by electrocardiographic evidence of significant QT prolongation. This possibility argues strongly for in-hospital initiation of quinidine. The drug may also be a negative inotropic agent and can worsen congestive heart failure.

Dosing and Interactions. Quinidine dosing depends on whether the sulfate or gluconate form is used. Quinidine sulfate is given in a dosage of 30 to 60 mg/kg/day, divided into a three or four times daily dose. Quinidine gluconate has 20% less quinidine base and needs to have the dose adjusted upward to compensate.

Drugs that increase microsomal enzyme activity, such as phenytoin, phenobarbital, and rifampin, can increase quinidine metabolism. In patients older than 5 years, administration of digoxin with quinidine has been shown to potentially increase digoxin levels.[10] Coadministration of warfarin with quinidine can result in prolongation of the prothrombin time, but effects on international ratio (INR) are unknown.

Procainamide. This is the most commonly

used class IA agent in pediatrics: as a single agent, in conjunction with digoxin, or less often in conjunction with other agents.

Drug Action. Procainamide is a potent sodium channel blocker (in the active state) and moderate potassium channel blocker. The drug delays repolarization and has greater effect at faster heart rates. The membrane effects of procainamide are greater on chronically infarcted cells.

Oral Administration, Kinetics, Metabolites. Procainamide is rapidly absorbed from the gastrointestinal tract, with approximately equal bioavailability of the standard and sustained release preparations (approximately 80%). Protein binding is not a factor. Sustained-release procainamide has a wax matrix. The parent drug is transformed in the liver to NAPA, which has mild to moderate class III antiarrhythmic effects. Levels of procainamide and NAPA are based on a genetic capability for hepatic acetylation. The standard formulation of the drug has a $t_{1/2}$ of 2.5 to 4 hours, whereas the sustained-release preparation has a longer $t_{1/2}$ of 6 to 8 hours.

Procainamide levels are in the range of 4 to 8 μg/ml. Infants often require slightly higher plasma levels. Therapeutic NAPA levels are similar. Procainamide and NAPA levels should never be added to reach a fictitious therapeutic combined level because the combined number could reflect inadequate concentration of the parent drug with exaggerated metabolism to NAPA or lack of acetylation and a subsequent high parent drug level. Procainamide crosses the placenta readily, with a fetal-maternal ratio of approximately 0.80.[11] After intravenous administration, procainamide is very rapidly distributed.

Dosing and Interactions. Chronic oral dosages range from 40 to 100 mg/kg/day. The amount is divided into six doses for administration every 4 hours in small patients and may be every 6 hours in most patients older than 1 to 2 years. In teenage patients, a schedule of every 8 hours is often possible. In the older patient who can swallow the fairly large pills, the sustained-release compound is administered every 8 hours. For patients with rare episodes of tachycardia, periodic therapy with procainamide has been advocated.[12] A single oral dose of procainamide (500–1500 mg) at home may terminate sustained tachyarrhythmia in older patients. Efficacy of this technique should be proved first in the hospital.

Intravenous administration of procainamide is somewhat more predictable. In patients younger than 1 year, a loading dose of 7 to 10 mg/kg, given over 30 to 45 minutes, is generally used. In older patients, the bolus dose is 15 mg/kg. The bolus is then followed by an infusion of procainamide, usually starting at 40 to 50 μg/kg/min. Top infusion rates of up to 100 μg/kg/min are occasionally necessary to maintain levels in infants. Plasma levels are obtained 4 hours after bolus during maintenance infusion. Procainamide does not elevate digoxin levels. Amiodarone, however, can elevate both procainamide levels and NAPA levels. Cimetidine will reduce renal clearance of procainamide and increase its $t_{1/2}$ by 25%.

Side Effects. The most common side effect is a drug-induced lupus-like syndrome. Fever, pericardial fluid accumulation, and arthralgia can be observed. During long-term procainamide therapy, more than half of patients will convert to a positive antinuclear antibody, but only 20% may show symptoms.[13] During intravenous administration, procainamide can have negative inotropic effects. Drug-induced ventricular arrhythmia is less common than sinus bradycardia as a result of procainamide administration.

Disopyramide. This agent has few antiarrhythmic applications in children. It has some use in the setting of vasodepressor syncope.[14]

Drug Action. Disopyramide has cellular channel effects similar to those of quinidine but without the added alpha receptor effects. The drug prolongs action potential duration in Purkinje tissue more than it does the effective refractory period. Disopyramide is available as a mixture of its D- and L-isomers. The D-isomer can prolong the QT interval, and the L-isomer can shorten it.

Oral Administration, Kinetics, Metabolites. Disopyramide is available in standard and sustained-release preparations. The standard form has a peak serum concentration at 0.5 to 3 hours. The drug is generally very protein bound. About 10% may be biotransformed to *N*-monoalkylated disopyramide, which has weak membrane effects. A slightly shorter $t_{1/2}$ (nearly 5 hours) may exist in children compared with adults. The therapeutic plasma range of disopyramide is 2 to 5 μg/ml, but there are very few data on the subject in children. Disopyramide crosses the placenta, but reaches fetal cord levels less than half that of maternal levels.

Dosing and Interactions. Dosing schedule has been as follows: younger than 2 years, 20 to 30 mg/kg/day; 2 to 10 years, 9 to 24 mg/kg/day;

older than 11 years, 5 to 13 mg/kg/day.[15] The maximum adult daily dose generally does not exceed 1200 mg. The $t_{1/2}$ of the preparations dictate the following schedules: every 6 hours for standard forms and every 12 hours for sustained-release forms. Coadministration of disopyramide with digoxin does not influence digoxin levels. Phenytoin can increase hepatic transformation, and atenolol can reduce renal clearance of disopyramide.

Side Effects. Many patients receiving disopyramide have anticholinergic side effects, which limit the drug's use. Up to 50% of patients can have urinary retention, constipation, nausea, anorexia, vomiting, blurred vision, or dry mouth. Exacerbation of AV block, sinus node disease, and new-onset VT are recognized clinical arrhythmic side effects.

Class IB Agents

The class IB agents are lidocaine, mexiletine, moricizine, phenytoin, and tocainide. These drugs generally block fast sodium channels, can shorten action potential duration and repolarization, and have somewhat greater effects at faster heart rates.

Lidocaine

Drug Action. Lidocaine blocks the fast sodium channel and shows frequency dependence. It has little or no effects on structures above the His bundle. Shortening of repolarization occurs most in cells with the longest initial action potential duration, resulting in an overall homogeneity of cardiac repolarization.

Intravenous Administration, Kinetics, Metabolites. Lidocaine has a rapid distribution phase. In congestive heart failure, metabolism is diminished, and the dose of lidocaine should be reduced. Kinetics for lidocaine show a $t_{1/2}$ of 2 hours, but $t_{1/2}$ may be slightly prolonged in newborns, up to 3 hours. Therapeutic lidocaine levels are in the range of 2 to 5 μg/ml.

Dosing and Interactions. Lidocaine is given as an intravenous bolus of 1 mg/kg and may be repeated in several minutes. Infusions of lidocaine are in the range of 20 to 50 μg/kg/min. Low cardiac output, common in critically ill patients requiring lidocaine infusions, often necessitates a reduction in the infusion rate because of decreased hepatic clearance and metabolism.

Because lidocaine undergoes extensive hepatic biotransformation, settings in which hepatic flow or microsomal enzyme activity are altered will influence lidocaine levels. Lower hepatic flow may occur with the drugs propranolol and cimetidine. Increased microsomal enzyme activity is seen with phenobarbital and phenytoin.

Side Effects. The major adverse drug reactions are related to the central nervous system: seizures, apnea, and altered mental status. Plasma concentrations are most often in excess of 6 to 7 μg/ml in this setting.[16] Rarely, in patients with atrial tachyarrhythmias or with variable degrees of AV block (especially when resulting from prolongation of the QT interval), lidocaine may increase the ventricular response rate.

Mexiletine. Although mexiletine's use is not widespread in pediatrics at this time, it may become the first-line drug used in the form of the congenital long QT syndrome resulting from a sodium channel defect.[17]

Drug Action. Mexiletine has primary effects on the fast sodium channel with greater effects at faster heart rates. Effects are exaggerated in diseased tissue and are dependent on the potassium concentration. In higher potassium states, effects on His-Purkinje tissue are more potent, with profound effects on the sodium channel. An additional action of mexiletine is suppression of early afterdepolarizations.

Oral Administration, Kinetics, Metabolites. Mexiletine is rapidly absorbed from the gastrointestinal tract, but cimetidine may slow absorption. Hepatic metabolism is extensive, with eight known metabolites, none of which have significant antiarrhythmic effects. Because metabolism is so extensive, alterations in hepatic flow and function can have important effects on mexiletine peak concentration and elimination.

The elimination $t_{1/2}$ of mexiletine is relatively long and variable, between 6 and 11 hours. Mexiletine levels are rarely checked, but may help when issues of absorption or metabolism are raised by inadequate clinical therapeutic effects. Effective concentrations tend to be in the range of 0.8 to 2.0 μg/ml.

Mexiletine crosses the placenta, but its use in fetal arrhythmias is rare. We have treated one fetus with apparent torsades de pointes VT successfully by maternal mexiletine administration. The fetus proved to have a congenital prolonged QT and intractable VT soon after birth.

Dosing and Interactions. The starting dosage

of mexiletine is 2 mg/kg every 8 hours. The dose may be increased up to approximately 5 mg/kg[18] and up to 7 to 8 mg/kg for infants. No loading dose is given. Antacids or cimetidine can slow mexiletine absorption. There are no reported interactions with digoxin.

Side Effects. Adverse side effects are fairly common during mexiletine administration. The most common ones are related to gastrointestinal upset and skin rash. Many of the gastrointestinal complaints can be avoided by giving the drug with food. The skin rash is a fine, sandpaper-like rash, mostly on the dorsum of the hands. Neurologic side effects are less common.

Moricizine. This drug was first investigated in the former Soviet Union in the 1960s as a phenothiazine agent. Its local anesthetic-like effects led to its later use for arrhythmias.[19] There are few pediatric applications.

Drug Action. Moricizine blocks fast sodium channels in the inactive state with both voltage and frequency-dependent effects. It also has effects on delayed afterdepolarizations and has been advocated for atrial ectopic arrhythmias.[20]

Oral Administration, Kinetics, Metabolites. Moricizine is absorbed rapidly from the gastrointestinal tract, is extensively bound to plasma proteins, and is nearly completely metabolized to more than 30 metabolites in the liver. The elimination $t_{1/2}$ is approximately 8 hours for chronic oral dosing.

Dosing and Interactions. The dose of moricizine has not been well established in children. Available data are based on body surface area with a starting dose of 200 mg/m^2/day divided every 8 hours.[20] The maximum is 600 mg/m^2/day. There are no known significant interactions of moricizine with digoxin. As with other drugs with extensive hepatic transformation, cimetidine may reduce clearance and prolong the elimination $t_{1/2}$.

Side Effects. At higher dose ranges, neurologic side effects include blurry vision, headache, paresthesia, and tingling. Gastrointestinal symptoms are also common and are often alleviated by coadministration with food.

Phenytoin. This is administered primarily as an anticonvulsive agent, but has found application in the treatment of postinfarction ventricular arrhythmias.[21]

Drug Action. Local anesthetic effects similar to lidocaine are observed, with both voltage and frequency dependence. Phenytoin binds predominantly to sodium channels in the inactivated state. High concentrations of phenytoin can have some calcium channel–blocking results and influence sinus and AV node automaticity. Elsewhere in the heart, phenytoin depresses phase 4 depolarization at standard concentrations, making the drug useful for treating digoxin-induced arrhythmias. There are also effects via the central nervous system, decreasing sympathetic effects in the ventricles.

Oral Administration, Kinetics, Metabolites. Peak serum concentrations are very variable, occurring 3 to 12 hours after dose administration. Dairy products may decrease absorption, whereas high protein or fatty diets can enhance absorption. The drug is metabolized extensively in the liver. None of the metabolites has significant antiarrhythmic effects. A number of drugs decrease phenytoin metabolism, including isoniazid, diazepam, methylphenidate, chlorpromazine, chlordiazepoxide, and disulfiram. Phenobarbital and carbamazepine enhance metabolism. Phenytoin has a unique metabolic feature among the antiarrhythmic agents: it saturates its metabolism at high doses, usually when doses are greater than 10 mg/kg/day. This is an important point, because levels can rise precipitously with small dose increases at the saturation point.

Despite more extensive metabolism in young patients, infants have a prolonged elimination $t_{1/2}$ of phenytoin, up to 24 hours. In patients older than 1 year, this drops to 8 hours and then rises again in the adult toward 24 hours. The usual therapeutic serum level range is 10 to 20 mg/ml.

Phenytoin crosses the placenta easily and has a high teratogenic capacity. Its use during pregnancy is contraindicated.

Intravenous Administration. Intravenous loading with phenytoin must be done carefully to avoid hypotension. The loading dose is on the order of 1 to 3 mg/kg given over 15 to 30 minutes, with a maximum daily load of 10 to 15 mg/kg.

Oral Dosing and Interactions. Oral loading with phenytoin avoids the risk of hypotension. The total loading dose (TLD) is 15 mg/kg, divided every 6 hours. Maintenance doses vary with age; those beyond the newborn period up to 5 to 6 years receive the drug every 12 hours, with a total daily dosage of 5 to 6 mg/kg.[21] Adults generally receive 300 to 600 mg/day.

One of the more important drug interactions with phenytoin involves warfarin, with an increase in the prothrombin time and INR. Phenytoin may displace verapamil from albumin and result in increased calcium blockade.

Side Effects. The most frequent side effect of phenytoin is hypotension associated with intravenous administration. For oral use, side effects are very rare and are related most to the central nervous system; nystagmus and ataxia are the most common when levels are high. Skin rashes are also common and may progress to Stevens-Johnson syndrome. Gingival hyperplasia is exacerbated by poor dental hygiene. Phenytoin has a high teratogenic capacity, leading to fetal hydantoin syndrome: midline facial clefts, hypertelorism, microcephaly with mental retardation, finger and nail hypoplasia, and congenital heart defects in 10%.[22]

Tocainide. There are no published data on experience with tocainide in children. It is available as an oral preparation in the United States.

Drug Action. Tocainide is similar to lidocaine in its electrophysiologic effects. Action potential duration and refractory periods are shortened. Blockade of sodium channels with fast time constants is the underlying mechanism of action, with some component of frequency dependence.

Administration, Kinetics, Metabolites. The drug is available as an enantiomer. The elimination $t_{1/2}$ is 10 to 11 hours. There are no significant metabolites. Peak concentrations are reduced when the drug is taken with a meal, but the total drug absorbed remains unchanged. Therapeutic plasma levels are from 3 to 9 μg/ml.

Dosing and Interactions. In adult patients, an initial dosage of 200 mg two or three times daily is common. Total adult dosages rarely exceed 2400 mg/day.[23] There are no significant drug interactions with tocainide.

Side Effects. Adverse effects are common, occurring in up to 50% of patients. The most common noncardiac complaints are nausea, vomiting, dizziness, and paresthesia. Pneumonitis has occurred. Side effects are more frequent when plasma concentrations exceed 10 μg/ml. Prolongation of the QT interval does not appear to happen, and torsades de pointes has not been reported.

Class IC Agents

The class IC agents are perhaps the most controversial and most extensively studied antiarrhythmic agents. They include flecainide, propafenone, and encainide. These drugs are potent sodium channel–blocking agents with a variable effect on repolarization and some frequency-dependent characteristics. Encainide was essentially eliminated from use in 1992 because of its proarrhythmic effects. Many studies have investigated the class IC drugs together as a group, including encainide in the past. The drugs are so different with respect to kinetics, metabolites, and drug effects that such studies become methodologically flawed. The impetus for extensive questioning of the use of class IC agents was a publication of the Cardiac Arrhythmia Suppression Trial (CAST).[24] These agents have widespread potential applications for atrial, junctional, and ventricular arrhythmias, both re-entrant and automatic.

Flecainide. This agent has been studied extensively,[22–28] but remains one of the more controversial antiarrhythmic agents in both children and adults with arrhythmias.[29–31]

Drug Action. Flecainide acetate blocks slow sodium channels in the activated state and has some mild potassium channel–blocking properties. Flecainide has a long time constant, in distinction from the class IA drugs, and therefore takes longer to dissociate from sodium channels. In specialized conduction tissue, refractory periods are shortened and automaticity decreased. Ventricular action potential duration and refractory periods are prolonged, leading to QRS widening.

Oral Administration, Kinetics, Metabolites. After an oral dose, flecainide reaches its maximum concentration in 1 to 2 hours. Milk products can block the absorption of flecainide such that, when patients are put on clear liquid diets (e.g., infants with gastroenteritis), flecainide levels can rise substantially.[32] Doses should be reduced, perhaps by 25 to 30%, in this setting.

Two metabolites of flecainide have weak membrane effects. Most of the drug is excreted unchanged in the urine. The elimination $t_{1/2}$ varies considerably with age. Newborns can have a $t_{1/2}$ as long as 27 hours in the first day,[26] but in general patients younger than 4 to 6 months of age have a $t_{1/2}$ of approximately 11 hours. In patients age 6 months to 10 years, the $t_{1/2}$ is approximately 8 hours and extends to 12 hours in those older than 10 to 11 years.[25]

Flecainide crosses the placenta readily, even in fetal hydrops. Its concentration in the fetus is approximately 70% that of maternal levels.[33]

Intravenous Parameters. Intravenous flecainide is available for use outside the United States. Its bolus dose is 1 to 2 mg/kg given over 5 to 10 minutes.

Dosing and Interactions. Flecainide dosing based on body surface area correlates better with serum flecainide concentrations than dosing based on weight.[25] The starting dosage in infants is often 80 to 90 mg/m^2/day, on a schedule of every 12 hours because of the prolonged $t_{1/2}$ at that age. The dosage for older patients is closer to 100 to 110 mg/m^2/day. This starting dosage tends to give trough levels of 200 to 400 ng/ml. A trough level of from 200 to 1000 ng/ml is considered therapeutic. Trough levels should be drawn 1 hour before the sixth or seventh maintenance dose. There is no loading dose. Older patients, 6 months to 10 years, may require a dosing schedule of every 8 hours with the same total daily dose because of the change in $t_{1/2}$. Dosages can be increased to as high as 200 mg/m^2/day, but caution is to be exercised for patients with documented low therapeutic levels on high-dose flecainide.[34] Often a dietary change can result in more extensive absorption of the drug, leading to serum levels more in keeping with the administered dose and a higher risk of adverse effects. Flecainide suspensions must be shaken vigorously to prevent inadvertent administration of drug doses that are too low or too high.

A rise in digoxin levels has been reported for adults on flecainide, but this experience has not been corroborated in pediatric patients. Flecainide can be used in combination with amiodarone for resistant arrhythmias[35] and with mexiletine for some infant ventricular tachyarrhythmias resulting from tumors.

Side Effects. On the basis of published data, side effects of flecainide are related to high levels and administration of the drug to patients with abnormal hearts. The drug is generally safe for those with normal cardiac anatomy.[29, 30] At peak concentration or with overdose, some patients may experience blurry vision and oral paresthesia. In patients with paroxysmal SVT, flecainide can result in slow conduction in more than one limb of a re-entrant circuit and bring about slower but incessant SVT.[25] This phenomenon is most often observed during the first 1 to 2 days of therapy and argues for in-hospital initiation of the drug. Proarrhythmic effects beyond this are rare, but they occur most commonly in the patient with an atrial tachyarrhythmia and abnormal anatomy (e.g., atrial flutter in a patient who has undergone a Mustard or Fontan procedure).

The results of the CAST study,[24] although identifying a subset of adult postinfarction patients at risk of serious proarrhythmia on flecainide, have limited application to the pediatric population. The exception may be related to the postoperative patient with right ventricular disease, such as tetralogy of Fallot, or left ventricular disease, such as aortic or subaortic stenosis.[31]

A mild negative inotropic effect, especially in adults with already depressed function, has been reported for flecainide. In children who present with incessant tachyarrhythmia, control with the drug was often achieved, and there were no noted adverse effects on echocardiographic indexes of function. An exacerbation of underlying conduction disturbances may occur.

Propafenone. Clinical applications of propafenone are similar to those of flecainide,[36] as are its potential adverse effects in postoperative patients.[37]

Drug Action. Propafenone blocks the sodium channel with a medium-range time constant for recovery. Propafenone also has mild beta-blocking properties. The drug has voltage and frequency-dependent effects. There are also effects on the slow inward calcium current and delayed outward potassium current, reflecting propafenone's relative clinical efficacy for control of automatic focus arrhythmias.

Oral Administration, Kinetics, Metabolites. Propafenone reaches maximum concentration 2 to 3 hours after an oral dose. Increases in the oral dose can result in significant elevations of the plasma level of the parent drug because of its saturation of the peripheral compartment. Propafenone is extensively metabolized in the liver. The major metabolite is 5-OH-propafenone.[38] Patients vary in their ability to oxidatively metabolize the drug. With extensive metabolism, the $t_{1/2}$ of propafenone is on the order of 4 hours. In patients who do not metabolize propafenone to 5-OH-propafenone to a great extent, the $t_{1/2}$ of propafenone is much longer, close to 14 to 16 hours. This has important clinical relevance with regard to dosing schedule and clinical efficacy.

Plasma levels of propafenone have an extremely wide range in clinical studies of the drug's efficacy and side effect profiles, from 100 to 5000 ng/ml. Most patients required levels of at least 150 to 200 ng/ml for clinical effect. There is no clear relationship between efficacy and level, likely because of the mixed population of metabolizers and nonmetabolizers.

Intravenous Administration. Intravenous propafenone is not commercially available in the

United States. After an intravenous dose, the drug has a distribution $t_{1/2}$ of 4 to 5 minutes and retains clinical effect for up to 1 hour.

Dosing and Interactions. The oral preparation is dosed on the basis of body surface area, starting at approximately 150 to 200 mg/m²/day on a schedule of every 8 hours. Dosing depends to a large extent on the ability of the patient to metabolize propafenone to 5-OH-propafenone. The upper dose range is 600 mg/m²/day. The intravenous preparation has been used in a dose of 0.2 to 1.0 mg/kg boluses, given slowly over 5 to 10 minutes each to a maximum of 2 mg/kg total load.[39] There are significant negative inotropic effects, often requiring intravascular volume expanding agents. An infusion of 4 to 10 μg/kg/min has been used. Elevation of serum digoxin levels has been reported with coadministration of digoxin with propafenone.

Side Effects. Like flecainide, propafenone should be provided with caution, if at all, in patients with a structurally abnormal heart, in particular those with atrial tachyarrhythmias. A higher risk of arrest and sudden death has been reported in this subpopulation.[37] Other side effects with oral therapy are similar to flecainide: blurry vision, paresthesia, and mild gastrointestinal discomfort. Rarely, propafenone may cause a lupus-like syndrome.

Conduction system disturbances are relatively common, including bundle branch blocks and intraventricular conduction delays. Highly concentrated sodium preparations such as sodium bicarbonate can rapidly reverse severe cardiac side effects of type IC agents.

Class II Agents

The class II agents are the beta-adrenergic blockers, with wide differences in $beta_1$, $beta_2$, and nonselective effects; drug $t_{1/2}$; and intrinsic sympathomimetic activity. Most selective beta blockers become nonselective at higher doses. Sotalol is discussed in the section on class III drugs. The most frequently used beta blockers in pediatrics are discussed here: propranolol, atenolol, metoprolol, nadolol, and esmolol.

Propranolol. Propranolol is the most commonly used beta-blocking agent. It is one of the few antiarrhythmic agents with a marketed liquid solution. There are at least two different concentrations: 20 mg/5 ml and 10 mg/ml. This lack of uniformity can result in erroneous overdosing or underdosing. The 20 mg/5 ml preparation is the more common of the two, and it is probably wise to make this concentration the standard, avoiding the 10 mg/ml solution.

Drug Action. Propranolol is the classic nonselective beta blocker. There are membrane effects on the sodium channel. At higher concentrations, propranolol can exert weak calcium channel blockade properties. There are no intrinsic sympathomimetic properties.

Oral Administration, Kinetics, Metabolites. Propranolol is completely absorbed after oral administration. Hepatic metabolism and clearance are extensive, and a higher oral dose is necessary to reach similar plasma concentrations than that with the intravenous preparation of the drug. The major metabolite is 4-OH-propranolol. The metabolite has a slightly longer $t_{1/2}$ and mild beta-blocking effects itself. As with most drugs with such significant hepatic metabolism, there are wide population variations in degree of metabolism of propranolol, and plasma levels vary widely.

In infants, propranolol has a slightly shorter $t_{1/2}$ (3–4 hours) than in children older than 1 to 2 years and adults (6 hours).[40] The plasma levels of propranolol range from 50 to 150 μg/ml, but appear helpful more in assaying absorption and compliance than in assessing therapeutic efficacy. Propranolol crosses the placenta easily such that fetal levels approximate maternal levels.[41] Fetal hypoglycemia is a concern.

Dosing and Interactions. Oral propranolol can be given as a liquid preparation, pill, or sustained-release preparation. Generally, the total daily doses are the same; starting dosages usually range from 1 to 2 mg/kg/day. In infants, the total dose is divided on a schedule of every 6 hours until age 6 to 8 months. By the time young children can swallow pills, a three times daily schedule of the standard propranolol is often effective. However, at this stage, a trial of once- or twice-a-day sustained-release propranolol could be considered. Intravenous propranolol is given as a 0.1 to 0.2 mg/kg dose over 1 to 5 minutes. Significant caution is advised, as discussed next.

As with other drugs that are extensively metabolized in the liver, all conditions that influence hepatic flow and biotransformation will affect propranolol levels. Coadministration of propranolol with calcium channel blockers is contraindicated because of the significant synergistic negative effects on contractility.

Side Effects. With intravenous administration, there can be bradycardia and hypotension.[42] This finding is particularly true in children younger than 1 year, and the drug probably needs to be avoided in intravenous form in these young patients. Tachyarrhythmias may be eliminated with a resultant sinus arrest and loss of vascular tone. The exception to this advice may be the use of intravenous propranolol in the young child with hypercyanotic spells, in whom the drug may be given with caution.

Propranolol has a number of potential adverse side effects besides bradycardia, AV block, and worsening congestive heart failure. The drug crosses the blood-brain barrier and can cause fatigue, depression, and nightmares. Because it is a beta blocker, it can exacerbate bronchospasm and increase the risk of hypoglycemia. A peripheral vasoreactive condition can cause discoloration and cool extremities.

Atenolol. Atenolol is a common, long-acting beta blocker in pediatrics.[43] It is provided in 25- and 50-mg pills, each of which is scored and can be broken in half while maintaining the sustained-release properties of the drug.

Drug Action. Atenolol is a selective beta blocker; it primarily affects $beta_1$-adrenergic receptors. There are no significant intrinsic sympathomimetic or membrane properties of atenolol, even at higher doses. The drug is hydrophilic and does not cross the blood-brain barrier.

Oral Administration, Kinetics, Metabolites. Atenolol reaches peak concentrations 2 to 3 hours after an oral dose and can be administered once or twice a day because of its $t_{1/2}$ of up to 9 to 10 hours. Atenolol has very little hepatic transformation and is excreted nearly entirely unchanged in the urine. There are no active metabolites. Atenolol does cross the placenta, but there are no reliable data on its concentration in the fetus.

Dosing and Interactions. The starting dosage of atenolol is 1 to 2 mg/kg/day, up to as high as 3 mg/kg/day. Because of the sustained-release nature of the agent, it can be given once a day or twice daily.[44] There are no reported significant drug interactions.

Side Effects. Because atenolol does not cross the blood-brain barrier, the side effect profile is considerably reduced compared with propranolol. Cardiovascular effects are similar to propranolol, and postural hypotension may occur. Although atenolol is a selective $beta_1$ agent, the risk of bronchospasm is not eliminated completely. Cool extremities can be a common complaint.

Metoprolol. Metoprolol is a beta blocker with a limited experience of use in pediatrics. It is gaining some favor in the therapy of autonomic dysfunction syndromes.[45]

Drug Action. Metoprolol is a selective $beta_1$-adrenergic blocker. It has no intrinsic sympathomimetic activity. The intravenous preparation is available outside the United States and may be useful for hypertension and thyrotoxicosis in addition to tachyarrhythmias.

Oral Administration, Kinetics, Metabolites. Extensive first-pass hepatic transformation occurs after oral administration. The elimination $t_{1/2}$ is 3 to 8 hours. There are no active metabolites. The drug crosses the placenta and can be metabolized by the fetal liver.

Dosing. There are no studies of dosing guidelines for metoprolol in children. In adults, a starting dosage of 50 mg twice daily may be used and increased to 150 to 200 mg twice daily.

Side Effects. Insufficient data exist for the side effect profile of metoprolol in children.

Nadolol. Nadolol is an oral sustained-release preparation. It has been administered to pediatric patients for SVT and for autonomic dysfunction syndromes.[46]

Drug Action. Nadolol is a nonselective beta-adrenergic blocking agent. There are no intrinsic sympathomimetic or membrane properties.

Oral Administration, Kinetics, Metabolites. Nadolol is poorly absorbed, and peak plasma levels occur 3 to 4 hours after administration. The drug is primarily excreted in the urine. The elimination $t_{1/2}$ is probably the longest of the sustained-release preparations, on the order of 20 to 24 hours. There are no active metabolites and no data on fetal use.

Dosing and Interactions. Nadolol is approximately 50% as effective a beta blocker as propranolol. Initial therapy is often recommended at 1 mg/kg/day. Because of its $t_{1/2}$, it can be given as a once-a-day dose. No significant drug interactions have been reported.

Side Effects. Effects on sinus rate and AV node conduction are similar to those of other nonselective beta-blocking agents.

Esmolol. Esmolol is given for therapy of a wide spectrum of tachyarrhythmias,[47] especially in the postoperative setting, and for control of blood pressure elevations, especially after cardiac transplantation.

Drug Action. Esmolol is an intravenous beta blocker with predominant $beta_1$ cardioselectivity. The predominant sites of action are the sinus and AV nodes.

Intravenous Administration, Kinetics, Metabolites. Esmolol has an elimination $t_{1/2}$ of 7 to 10 minutes. Any potentially deleterious effects, therefore, will be short lived.

Dosing. A loading dose of 500 mcg/kg is used, given over 1 to 2 minutes, followed by a maintenance infusion starting at 50 mcg/kg/min.[48] Additional bolus doses can be administered, with subsequent increases in the infusion rate up to 200 mcg/kg/min or higher.

Side Effects. The most frequent adverse effect is hypotension during bolus therapy. In small children and those with single-ventricle physiology, this effect can be profound, requiring volume and inotropic support.

Class III Agents

The class III agents in use include amiodarone, sotalol, bretylium, and ibutilide. The primary mode of action of all these agents is prolongation of refractoriness. There are many membrane and receptor effects, making the group of class III agents quite diverse.

Amiodarone. Amiodarone is a potent agent for control of a wide spectrum of cardiac tachyarrhythmias.[49, 50] Amiodarone was released in the United States for intravenous therapy, and a body of literature for its safety and effectiveness in resistant arrhythmias in children has been published.[51–53]

Drug Action. Amiodarone has a great number of cellular electrophysiologic effects. It is a sodium channel blocker with voltage and frequency dependence, a noncompetitive alpha- and beta-adrenergic receptor blocker, and an inhibitor of presynaptic norepinephrine release. The delayed outward potassium current is affected, resulting in amiodarone's prolongation of refractoriness. Sodium and calcium channel effects are predominant in the sinus node and refractory periods in the AV node.

Oral Administration, Kinetics, Metabolites. Amiodarone is lipid soluble and absorbed more slowly than any other antiarrhythmic agent; a peak plasma concentration occurs 3 to 7 hours after an oral dose. The drug is metabolized to an active agent, desethylamiodarone, in the liver. There is a very large volume of distribution; amiodarone and desethylamiodarone are stored in the peripheral compartment. Levels of either drug can remain substantial up to 3 months after amiodarone is discontinued. Therapeutic plasma levels range from 1.0 to 2.5 μg/ml, but they correlate poorly with clinical efficacy, partly because of the actions of the metabolite and the peripheral storage of both drugs. Although it takes several days to achieve a desired effect when initiating amiodarone, an electrophysiologic effect can be observed in 1 to 2 days with standard loading protocols.[54]

Amiodarone crosses the placenta poorly, with a 4:1 ratio of maternal to fetal levels. Although the drug is present in breast milk, its concentration there is low and should not be a contraindication to breast-feeding.

Intravenous Administration. In a multicenter trial of intravenous amiodarone for resistant, life-threatening pediatric tachyarrhythmias,[53] the drug showed a rapid onset of action; a clinical electrophysiologic effect often occurred during the initial bolus dose. The antiarrhythmic effect can persist for 1 to 6 hours. Amiodarone is mixed in 5% dextrose solution to prevent precipitation.

Dosing and Interactions. An oral loading protocol of 10 to 15 mg/kg/day is often provided for 5 to 10 days. During loading, this dosage is usually split in a twice-daily schedule to avoid gastrointestinal side effects. Some centers, particularly in Europe, advocate a higher dose loading for 3 to 5 days, using up to 50 mg/kg/day.[55]

The goal of long-term oral therapy is to use the lowest possible effective daily dosage. This is generally 2 to 5 mg/kg as a once-a-day dose. Amiodarone is only available as a 200-mg tablet. Although it can be broken into halves or quarters or even given every other day, a suspension is often made at a concentration of 10 mg/ml. Anecdotal experience from a number of institutions indicates that the suspension is stable for up to 1 month.

In the largest studies of intravenous amiodarone to date in young patients, a 5-mg/kg bolus was used and divided into five 1-mg/kg aliquots.[51, 53] Each was given over 5 minutes. No adverse effect was seen in the first 1- to 3-mg/kg bolus, so the drug can probably be given as two 2.5-mg/kg boluses. The average successful load was 6 mg/kg. Infusions of amiodarone were administered predominantly in those with ventricular tachyarrhythmias at 10 to 15 mg/kg/day.

The most frequently cited example of amiodarone interaction is digoxin coadministration, when digoxin levels may rise 25 to 100%. Decreasing the digoxin dose by 33 to 50% is prudent. Coadministration of amiodarone with most other antiarrhythmic agents, particularly procainamide, flecainide, quinidine, and phenytoin, also causes increased levels of these drugs. Excessive increases in prothrombin time and INR have been seen with amiodarone therapy for patients on warfarin. Therapy with beta blockers or calcium channel blockers with amiodarone is controversial because of the synergistic effects on sinus and AV node function.

Side Effects. The most commonly noted noncardiac side effects with oral amiodarone administration in children are skin photosensitivity, chemical hepatitis, hypothyroidism, hyperthyroidism, and corneal microdeposits. All patients should be advised to apply high-grade sunblock. Liver and thyroid function tests should be performed periodically. Amiodarone has a high iodine content, likely responsible for its effects on thyroid function. Therapy with thyroid replacement hormones, if necessary, does not seem to interfere with antiarrhythmic effect.

Cardiac side effects include sinus bradycardia, AV node blocks, and proarrhythmia. Torsades de pointes occurs rarely (<1%). In adult patients on long-term oral amiodarone, serious and irreversible pulmonary fibrosis can occur. This phenomenon has not been reported in the pediatric population, possibly because patients have not been on the drug long enough or in high enough maintenance doses for pulmonary abnormalities to appear. Pulmonary function testing has not been routinely advocated for most of these young patients, however, and the abnormalities may be present but undetected. A confounding variable is that many patients receiving long-term amiodarone therapy are postoperative patients with pre-existing abnormalities of pulmonary function because of either underlying cardiac defects or repeated surgical entry into the chest.

Side effects with intravenous therapy are predominantly related to hypotension. If intravenous amiodarone is given to a patient receiving high inspired oxygen concentrations, an adult respiratory distress syndrome may occur.[56]

Sotalol. Sotalol is generally available as a racemic mixture of D- and L-sotalol. In pediatrics, it is being given for a number of postoperative tachyarrhythmias that are difficult to control.[57, 58]

Drug Action. Sotalol is a nonselective beta-adrenergic blocking agent with class III effects as well. The beta-blocking action is approximately one third that of propranolol and tends to occur at lower doses of sotalol. The class III effects (prolongation of repolarization) are present more at higher sotalol doses. At higher concentrations, there are effects on the potassium delayed rectifier current and some effect on the sodium channel.

Oral Administration, Kinetics, Metabolites. Sotalol has excellent absorption, and peak plasma concentrations are present 2 hours after oral dosing. The elimination $t_{1/2}$ ranges from 7 to 12 hours and has not been studied extensively in children. There are no active metabolites, and the drug is excreted in the urine. Transplacental passage of the drug occurs, but the ratio of fetal to maternal concentrations is not established.

Dosing and Interactions. The starting sotalol dosage is generally 90 mg/m^2/day and can be given on a schedule of two or three times daily, up to 200 mg/m^2/day. The smallest unit dose is 80 mg, so that suspensions must be made up for small children. A concentration of 5 mg/ml is common. An intravenous preparation is available outside the United States, and doses are in the range of 0.2 to 1.5 mg/kg.

Side Effects. Sotalol has the usual side effect profile of beta-blocking agents, with mild negative inotropic effects. Unlike standard beta-blocking drugs, sotalol will prolong the QT interval because of its class III effects. The most serious adverse cardiovascular side effect is a drug-induced torsades de pointes, with an incidence approximating that of quinidine-induced torsades.

Bretylium. Bretylium has limited applications in the pediatric patient.[59] It is mostly utilized in resuscitative settings for polymorphic ventricular tachycardias or monomorphic ventricular tachycardias resistant to other standard forms of therapy.

Drug Action. Bretylium has significant effects in sympathetic ganglia, where it causes an initial release of norepinephrine stores but subsequently prevents further norepinephrine release and reuptake.

Intravenous Administration, Kinetics, Metabolites. The oral form of bretylium has very poor absorption, and the drug is, therefore, provided only as an intravenous agent. When given intravenously, there are electrophysiologic effects in minutes, allowing attempts at cardioversion or defibrillation. There are no established therapeutic levels and no significant metabolites. The electrophysiologic effects last for 30 to 120 minutes. Studies of bretylium in pediatric patients are nonexistent.

Dosing. The intravenous dose of bretylium is 5 mg/kg as a rapid push during ventricular fibrillation. There are hypotensive effects such that in patients with hemodynamically stable ventricular tachycardia, it should be diluted in 5% dextrose and given more slowly. The total dose should not exceed 30 mg/kg. A continuous infusion can be used at 15 to 30 μg/kg/min.

Bretylium may reverse the local anesthetic effect of quinidine and other sodium channel–blocking agents. This factor explains, to some degree, its application in quinidine-induced torsades de pointes. Although bretylium is given for digoxin-induced arrhythmias, the drug may worsen these rhythms initially because of the early release of norepinephrine. Tricyclic antidepressants block bretylium's synaptic effects.

Side Effects. The predominant adverse effect is hypotension, but during resuscitative measures this is rarely a concern if the rhythm being treated is ventricular fibrillation. The hypotensive effect is due to bretylium's peripheral adrenergic blocking properties.

Ibutilide. Ibutilide is an intravenous class III agent. The drug has not been studied in pediatric patients to date, and the adult data are not extensive, focusing primarily on the drug in acute termination of atrial fibrillation and atrial flutter.[60]

Drug Action. Action potentials are prolonged by an unknown mechanism. Refractoriness is prolonged in both atrial and ventricular myocardial cells. Rather than block potassium currents, ibutilide activates a slow, inward sodium current.

Intravenous Administration, Kinetics, Metabolites. The drug has extensive hepatic metabolism. The elimination $t_{1/2}$ of ibutilide is approximately 6 hours.

Dosing. Adult studies have used 10 to 25 μg/kg as a bolus over 10 minutes. The bolus may be repeated in 10 minutes.

Side Effects. About 8% of patients experience torsades de pointes ventricular tachycardia.[61] AV block can occur. The drug is teratogenic.

Class IV Agents

The class IV agents are calcium channel blockers. The predominant drug is verapamil, with limited experience and applications for nifedipine and diltiazem.

Verapamil. Verapamil is a papaverine derivative and was introduced as a coronary vasodilator. It is available in both standard and sustained-release oral preparations and in an intravenous preparation. It is useful for SVT, for verapamil-sensitive ventricular tachycardias,[62] and for hypertrophic cardiomyopathy.[63]

Drug Action. Verapamil has its greatest influence on cells in the sinus and AV nodes. The drug is an isomeric mixture and binds to the calcium channel in the inactive state. The calcium channel blockade becomes more apparent at faster rates. The D-isomer appears to have some mild capacity for sodium channel blockade. The drug is particularly effective in depressing enhanced automaticity and is a potent alpha-adrenergic blocker.

Oral Administration, Kinetics, Metabolites. Verapamil undergoes extensive first-pass metabolism and less than 25% is, therefore, bioavailable. Peak levels occur 2 hours after an oral dose, and elimination $t_{1/2}$ is from 4 to 7 hours. Because of a large volume of distribution, changes in verapamil dosing should be delayed for a true steady state at least 4 days.

There are many metabolites as a result of liver biotransformation. Less than 5% of the drug is excreted unchanged in the urine. None of the metabolites have relevant antiarrhythmic action. Hepatic dysfunction or low flow can have a dramatic effect on prolonging the elimination half-life.

Verapamil is available as both a standard form and a sustained-release preparation. The smallest sustained release dose is 120 mg. The elimination $t_{1/2}$ for the sustained preparation is 8 to 10 hours. Verapamil levels are not generally useful guidelines but range from 0.1 to 0.4 μg/ml. Although transplacental passage of verapamil occurs, it is fairly low, with a maternal to fetal concentration ratio of approximately 3:1.[64] The drug passes poorly in the presence of hydrops.

Intravenous Administration. Intravenous verapamil has a similar elimination $t_{1/2}$ to the oral preparation. This has important consequences when adverse effects are encountered in young children.

Dosing and Interactions. The oral preparation has been used with a wide range of reported effective daily doses, from 4 to 17 mg/kg/day. The drug is usually given on a schedule of three or four times daily. When the sustained-release preparation is given, the total daily dose is generally reduced slightly to account for the higher bioavailability. In adults, the standard daily dose is 80 to 360 mg divided three times a day or 120 to 240 mg once a day of the sustained release. The intravenous form of the drug should not be provided for patients younger than 1 year.

The use of concomitant calcium blockers with beta blockers is unwise because of the synergistic negative effects on ventricular function and sinus rate. A mild increase in digoxin levels has been reported.

Side Effects. With the oral preparation of verapamil, one of the more commonly reported adverse effects is constipation. Headaches, dizziness, rashes, and pruritus are other adverse reactions. Cardiovascular side effects include bradycardia, AV block, postural hypotension, and worsening of congestive heart failure.

The most significant side effect occurs with the intravenous preparation. Serious hypotension may occur, especially in young patients, resulting in asystole and cardiovascular collapse.[65] Intravenous administration should be considered as contraindicated in patients younger than 1 year. In either the oral or intravenous preparation, verapamil may increase the ventricular response rate of atrial fibrillation in patients with Wolff-Parkinson-White syndrome.

Diltiazem. Diltiazem for pediatric patients has been confined predominantly to control of hypertension.[66] The drug is available in both an oral and intravenous preparation, but no data are available from children, and few data are available from adults to extrapolate to children.

Drug Action. Diltiazem blocks the inward calcium channel. There are no significant sodium channel or alpha receptor effects. The predominant action, therefore, is on the sinus and AV nodes.

Administration, Kinetics, Metabolites. Diltiazem is available as both an oral and intravenous drug. After oral administration, it is rapidly absorbed, reaching peak levels within 1 hour. There is a wide range of variation in bioavailability because of first-pass metabolism. The elimination $t_{1/2}$ is 3 to 5 hours for both the intravenous and oral preparations. Therapeutic plasma levels have been in the range of 30 to 270 ng/ml, but there are no data on the clinical utility of levels.

Dosing. There are no clear guidelines on the oral dose of diltiazem in children. Adult doses are in the range of 30 to 120 mg three times a day. Intravenous doses are bolus doses of 0.15 to 0.45 mg/kg followed by an infusion rate of 0.003 mg/kg/min.

Side Effects. Therapy with diltiazem results in frequent but mild side effects, including headache and postural hypotension. Bradycardia and increased levels of AV block should be anticipated.

Other Agents

Adenosine. Adenosine is most widely used in the emergency room therapy of supraventricular tachyarrhythmias.

Drug Action. Adenosine is an endogenous purinergic agent. Its electrophysiologic effects are secondary to an increase in potassium channel conductance and depression of the slow inward calcium current, resulting in transient AV block and sinus bradycardia. It is also a peripheral vasodilator. The electrophysiologic effects are mediated by an A_1-purinergic extracellular receptor, which may be blocked by methylxanthines.

Intravenous Administration, Kinetics, Metabolites. The drug is given as a rapid intravenous bolus. Its effects are generally seen in 7 to 20 seconds. It is a very useful therapeutic and diagnostic agent.

Dosing and Interactions. Initial doses of 100 to 150 μg/kg are given as a rapid peripheral bolus, followed by a flush of saline. The dose may be doubled sequentially, up to a maximum of 300 μg/kg or the adult dose of 6 to 12 mg.[67] An adequate record of the electrocardiographic tracing is essential during adenosine administration. Aminophylline interferes with the actions of adenosine. Dipyridamole and diazepam can inhibit its cellular uptake and potentiate its effects.

Side Effects. Adenosine may cause hypotension, facial flushing, and mild bronchospasm.[68] Ventricular ectopy is not unusual and may be the mechanism of termination of some AV reciprocating tachycardias. Occasionally, atrial fibrillation results from adenosine administration during SVTs.

Digoxin. *Drug Action.* Digoxin has both direct and indirect properties. The indirect properties are autonomic effects mediated by the parasympathetic nervous system. These actions include the increase in responsiveness to acetylcholine, inhibition of norepinephrine release, augmentation of efferent parasympathetic output, and changes in the sensitivity of reflexogenic receptor systems.

The direct properties of digoxin are due to binding of the drug to the sodium-potassium adenosine triphosphatase transport complex, thereby inhibiting outward flux of sodium ions. The inotropic response of digoxin is due to intracellular calcium loading caused by the higher intracellular sodium concentration's enhancement of the sodium-calcium pump.

At standard concentrations of digoxin there are no significant effects in ventricular tissue, but at higher concentrations automaticity may be enhanced. A single study has shown that digoxin may shorten, lengthen, or leave the antegrade refractory period of accessory pathways unchanged.[69] Sudden death occurs in a small subset of patients with Wolff-Parkinson-White syndrome, and many believe that the use of digoxin in a patient with overt pre-excitation increases the risk.[70]

Oral Administration, Kinetics, Metabolites. A prolonged distribution phase of 6 to 8 hours follows oral intake of digoxin because of extensive binding to peripheral tissue proteins. Myocardial tissue concentrations of digoxin are higher in children than adults by a factor of three to six. Peak plasma levels occur in 1 to 2 hours, and the elimination $t_{1/2}$ is long: 1.5 to 2 days. Renal dysfunction has a direct influence on extending the $t_{1/2}$ to as long as 1 week. The drug is excreted unchanged in the urine.

Therapeutic plasma digoxin concentrations are in the range of 0.7 to 2.0 ng/ml. The need for routine screening of digoxin levels is somewhat controversial. In infants, the presence of a digoxin-like immunoreactive substance may complicate the assay. Digoxin crosses the placenta readily; fetal levels approximate maternal levels.[71] Digoxin remains an important drug for therapy of fetal SVT.

Intravenous Administration. The effects of digoxin in an intravenous vehicle are not different from those in an oral preparation. The onset of electrophysiologic effect is obviously more rapid, on the order of 5 to 10 minutes.

Dosing and Interactions. A loading protocol is generally followed for both oral and intravenous preparations. Usually, a TLD of 30 to 50 μg/kg is acceptable, with a slight decrease to 20 to 25 μg/kg for premature infants. This dose is divided as follows: 50% of the TLD initially, followed by two doses at 6-hour intervals of 25% of the TLD each. For intravenous loading, two thirds to three fourths of the TLD is used, divided in similar fashion. Oral liquid digoxin preparations are available in a 50-μg/ml concentration, and intravenous preparations are available as 100 μg/ml. For this reason, and because digoxin remains one of the most common drugs prone to prescription error, both the total dose and the volume of dose, whether oral or intravenous, should be written on all orders. Maintenance dosages of digoxin are 7 to 10 μg/kg/day. The dose of digoxin needs to be decreased in patients with renal dysfunction and in congestive heart failure.

Side Effects and Interactions. Side effects obviously include proarrhythmic effects, but also include gastrointestinal upset, visual changes, and drowsiness in small patients. Gynecomastia is a potential side effect with long-term use. Digoxin toxicity can occur at plasma levels as low as 2.0 ng/ml, but is more likely to occur at levels above 3.0 ng/ml.[72] The cardiac manifestations of digoxin toxicity are somewhat age dependent. Younger patients tend to have more supraventricular arrhythmias and conduction disturbances, whereas adult patients are prone to ventricular arrhythmias, junctional tachycardia, AV block, and premature ventricular contractions.

Any coadministered antiarrhythmic agent generally will require a reduction in the dose of digoxin, and levels should be monitored periodically.

SUMMARY

The safety and efficacy of radiofrequency ablation procedures have made complex drug therapy or use of agents with significant potential side effect profiles frequently unnecessary. Some drugs, such as quinidine, disopyramide, and moricizine, have either limited applications or significant risk of proarrhythmia, so that their use has become limited. Therapy of complicated atrial postoperative arrhythmias continues to require procainamide, sotalol, or amiodarone, but ablation remains an option for these patients as well. Short-term therapy of antiarrhythmic agents or combination therapies are now often considered while awaiting ablation scheduling or an anticipated resolution of arrhythmia because of natural history considerations.

REFERENCES

1. Physicians' Desk Reference: Montvale, NJ, Medical Economics, 1996.
2. Kugler JD, Danford DA, Deal BJ, et al: Radiofrequency catheter ablation for tachyarrhythmias in children and adolescents. N Engl J Med 330:1481–1487, 1994.
3. Perry JC, Iverson P, Kugler JD: Radiofrequency catheter ablation of tachyarrhythmias in young patients with structurally abnormal hearts. Pacing Clin Electrophysiol 19:579, 1996.
4. Schaffer MS, Silka MJ, Ross BA, Kugler JD: Inadvertent atrioventricular block during radiofrequency catheter ablation: Results of the Pediatric Radiofrequency Ablation Registry. Circulation 94:3214–3220, 1996.
5. Ludomirsky A, Garson A Jr: Supraventricular tachycardia. In Gillette PC, Garson A Jr (eds): Pediatric Arrhythmias: Electrophysiology and Pacing. Philadelphia, WB Saunders, 1990, pp 380–426.
6. Vaughn Williams EM: Classification of antiarrhythmic drugs. In Sandoe E, Flensted-Jensen E, Olsen KH (eds): Cardiac Arrhythmias. Sodertalje, Sweden, Astra, 1970, pp 449–472.
7. Task Force of the Working Group on Arrhythmias of the European Society of Cardiology: The Sicilian gambit. A new approach to the classification of antiarrhythmic drugs based on their actions on arrhythmogenic mechanisms. Circulation 84:1831–1851, 1991.
8. Kim SY, Benowitz NL: Poisoning due to class IA antiarrhythmic drugs. Quinidine, procainamide and disopyramide. Drug Safety 5:393, 1990.
9. Webb CL, Dick M II, Rocchini AP, et al: Quinidine syncope in children. J Am Coll Cardiol 9:1031–1037, 1987.
10. Marcus FI: Pharmacokinetic interactions between digoxin and other drugs. J Am Coll Cardiol 5:82A–90A, 1985.
11. Dumesic DA, Silverman NH, Tobias S, Golbus MS: Transplacental cardioversion of fetal supraventricular tachycardia with procainamide. N Engl J Med 307:1129–1131, 1982.
12. Benson DW Jr, Dunnigan A, Green TP, et al: Periodic procainamide for paroxysmal tachycardia. Circulation 72:147–152, 1985.
13. Woosley RL, Drayer DE, Reidenberg MM, et al: Effect of acetylator phenotype on the rate at which procainamide induces antinuclear antibodies and the lupus syndrome. N Engl J Med 298:1157–1159, 1978.
14. Milstein S, Buetikofer J, Dunnigan A, et al: Usefulness of disopyramide for prevention of upright tilt-induced hypotension-bradycardia. Am J Cardiol 65:1339–1344, 1990.
15. Tynan M, Keaton BR, Hayler AM, Holt D: The dosage of disopyramide in infants and children. Br J Clin Pract (Suppl 11):40–42, 1981.
16. Rosen MR, Hoffman BF, Wit AL: Electrophysiology and pharmacology of cardiac arrhythmias: V. Cardiac arrhythmic effects of lidocaine. Am Heart J 89:526–536, 1975.
17. Schwartz PJ, Priori SG, Locati EH, et al: Long QT syndrome patients with mutations of the SCN5A and HERG genes have differential responses to Na+ channel blockade and to increases in heart rate. Circulation 92:3381–3386, 1995.
18. Moak JP, Smith RT Jr, Garson A Jr: Mexiletine: An effective antiarrhythmic drug for treatment of ventricular arrhythmias in congenital heart disease. J Am Coll Cardiol 10:824–829, 1987.
19. Chazov EI, Shugushev KK, Rosenshtraukh LV: Ethmozine: I. Effects of intravenous drug administration on paroxysmal supraventricular tachycardia in the preexcitation syndrome. Am Heart J 108:475–482, 1984.
20. Evans VL, Garson A Jr, Smith RT, et al: Ethmozine (moricizine HCl): A promising new drug for "automatic" atrial ectopic tachycardia. Am J Cardiol 60:83F–86F, 1987.
21. Garson A Jr, Kugler JD, Gillette PC, et al: Control of late postoperative ventricular arrhythmias with phenytoin in young patients. Am J Cardiol 46:290–294, 1980.
22. Hanson JW, Smith DW: The fetal hydantoin syndrome. J Pediatr 87:285–290, 1975.
23. Roden DM, Woosley RL: Drug therapy: Tocainide. N Engl J Med 315:41–45, 1986.
24. The Cardiac Arrhythmia Suppression Trial (CAST) Investigators: Preliminary report: Effect of encainide and flecainide on mortality in a randomized trial of arrhythmia suppression after myocardial infarction. N Engl J Med 321:406–412, 1989.
25. Perry JC, McQuinn RL, Smith RT Jr, et al: Flecainide acetate for resistant arrhythmias in the young: Efficacy and pharmacokinetics. J Am Coll Cardiol 14:185–191, 1989.
26. van Engelen AD, Weijtens O, Brenner JI, et al: Management outcome and follow-up of fetal tachycardia. J Am Coll Cardiol 24:1371–1375, 1994.
27. Wren C, Campbell RWF: The response of paediatric arrhythmias to intravenous and oral flecainide. Br Heart J 57:171–175, 1987.
28. Priestley KA, Ladusans EJ, Rosenthal E, et al: Experience with flecainide in the treatment of cardiac arrhythmias in children. Eur Heart J 9:1284–1290, 1988.
29. Fish FA, Gillette PC, Benson DW Jr: Proarrhythmia, cardiac arrest and death in young patients receiving encainide and flecainide. J Am Coll Cardiol 18:356–365, 1991.
30. Perry JC, Garson A Jr: Encainide and flecainide: Separating the wheat from the chaff. J Am Coll Cardiol 18:366–367, 1991.
31. Case CL, Gillette PC: Treatment of ventricular arrhythmias in children without structural heart disease with class IC agents as guided by invasive electrophysiology. Am J Cardiol 66:1265--1266, 1990.
32. Russell GAB, Martin RP: Flecainide toxicity. Arch Dis Child 64:860–862, 1989.
33. Perry JC, Ayres NA, Carpenter RJ: Fetal supraventricular tachycardia treated with flecainide acetate. J Pediatr 118:303–305, 1991.
34. Till JA, Herxheimer A: Death of a child with supraventricular tachycardia. Lancet 339:8809, 1992.
35. Fenrich AL, Perry JC, Friedman RA: Flecainide and amiodarone: Combined therapy for refractory tachyarrhythmias in infancy. J Am Coll Cardiol 25:1195–1198, 1995.

36. Janousek J, Paul T, Reimer A, Kallfelz HC: Usefulness of propafenone for supraventricular arrhythmias in infants and children. Am J Cardiol 72:294–300, 1993.
37. Erickson C, Perry J, Marlow D, Garson A Jr: Sudden death during propafenone therapy for atrial flutter in young postoperative heart patients. Pacing Clin Electrophysiol 16:939, 1993.
38. Kates RE, Yee YG, Winkle RA: Metabolite cumulation during chronic propafenone dosing in arrhythmia. Clin Pharmacol Ther 37:610–614, 1985.
39. Garson A Jr, Moak JP, Smith RT Jr, Norton JB Jr: Usefulness of intravenous propafenone for control of postoperative junctional ectopic tachycardia. Am J Cardiol 59:1422–1424, 1987.
40. Pickoff AS, Zies L, Ferrer PL, et al: High-dose propranolol therapy in the management of supraventricular tachycardia. J Pediatr 94:144–146, 1979.
41. Kleinman CS: Prenatal diagnosis and management of intrauterine arrhythmias. Fetal Ther 1:92–95, 1986.
42. Shand DG: State of the art: Comparative pharmacology of the beta adrenoceptor blocking drugs. Drug (Suppl 2):92–99, 1983.
43. Trippell DL, Gillette PC: Atenolol in children with ventricular arrhythmias. Am Heart J 119:1312–1316, 1990.
44. Trippell DL, Gillette PC: Atenolol in children with supraventricular tachycardia. Am J Cardiol 64:233–236, 1989.
45. O'Marcaigh AS, MacLellan-Tobert SG, Porter CJ: Tilt-table testing and oral metoprolol therapy in young patients with unexplained syncope. Pediatr 93:278–283, 1994.
46. Mehta AV, Chidambaram B: Efficacy and safety of intravenous and oral nadolol for supraventricular tachycardia in children. J Am Coll Cardiol 19:630–635, 1992.
47. Esmolol Research Group: Intravenous esmolol for the treatment of supraventricular tachyarrhythmia: Results of a multicenter, baseline controlled safety and efficacy study in 160 patients. Am Heart J 112:498–505, 1986.
48. Trippel DL, Wiest DB, Gillette PC: Cardiovascular and antiarrhythmic effects of esmolol in children. J Pediatr 119:142–147, 1991.
49. Garson A Jr, Gillette PC, McVey P, et al: Amiodarone treatment of critical arrhythmias in children and young adults. J Am Coll Cardiol 4:749–755, 1984.
50. Coumel P, Fidelle J: Amiodarone in the treatment of cardiac arrhythmias in children: 135 cases. Am Heart J 100:1063–1069, 1980.
51. Perry JC, Knilans TK, Marlow D, et al: Intravenous amiodarone for life-threatening tachyarrhythmias in children and young adults. J Am Coll Cardiol 22:95–99, 1993.
52. Figa FH, Gow RM, Hamilton RM, Freedom RM: Clinical efficacy and safety of intravenous amiodarone in infants and children. Am J Cardiol 74:573–577, 1994.
53. Perry JC, Fenrich AL, Hulse JE, et al: Pediatric use of intravenous amiodarone: Efficacy and safety in critically ill patients from a multicenter protocol. J Am Coll Cardiol 27:1246–1250, 1996.
54. Escoubet B, Coumel P, Poirer J, et al: Suppression of arrhythmias within hours after a single oral dose of amiodarone and relation to plasma and myocardial concentrations. Am J Cardiol 55:696–702, 1985.
55. Mostow ND, Vrobel TR, Noon D, Rakita L: Rapid suppression of complex ventricular arrhythmias with high-dose oral amiodarone. Circulation 6:1231–1238, 1986.
56. Donica SK, Paulsen W, Simpson BR, et al: Danger of amiodarone therapy and elevated inspired oxygen concentrations in mice. Am J Cardiol 77:109–110, 1996.
57. Maragres P, Tipple M, Fournier A: Effectiveness of oral sotalol for treatment of pediatric arrhythmias. Am J Cardiol 69:751–754, 1992.
58. Pfammatter JP, Paul T, Lehmann C, Kallfelz HC: Efficacy and proarrhythmia of oral sotalol in pediatric patients. J Am Coll Cardiol 26:1002–1007, 1995.
59. Heissenbuttel RH, Bigger JT: Bretylium tosylate: A newly available antiarrhythmic drug for ventricular arrhythmias. Ann Intern Med 91:229–238, 1979.
60. Ellenbogen KA, Stambler BS, Wood MA, et al: Efficacy of intravenous ibutilide for rapid termination of atrial fibrillation and atrial flutter: A dose-response study. J Am Coll Cardiol 28:130–136, 1996.
61. Ibutilide. Med Lett 38:38–39, 1996.
62. Ohe T, Shimomura K, Aihahra N, et al: Idiopathic sustained left ventricular tachycardia: Clinical and electrophysiologic characteristics. Circulation 77:560–568, 1988.
63. Spicer RL, Rocchini AP, Crowley DC, et al: Hemodynamic effects of verapamil in children and adolescents with hypertrophic cardiomyopathy. Circulation 67:413–420, 1983.
64. Wolff F, Breuker KH, Schlensker KH, Bolte A: Prenatal diagnosis and therapy of fetal heart rate anomalies: With a contribution on the placental transfer of verapamil. J Perinat Med 8:203–208, 1980.
65. Epstein ML, Kiel EA, Victorica BE: Cardiac decompensation following verapamil therapy in infants with supraventricular tachycardia. Pediatrics 75:737–740, 1985.
66. Dougherty AH, Jackman WM, Naccarelli GV, et al: Acute conversion of paroxysmal supraventricular tachycardia with intravenous diltiazem. Am J Cardiol 70:587–592, 1992.
67. Overholt ED, Rheuban KS, Gutgesell HP, et al: Usefulness of adenosine for arrhythmias in infants and children. Am J Cardiol 61:336–340, 1988.
68. Till J, Shinebourne EA, Rigby MC, et al: Efficacy and safety of adenosine in the treatment of supraventricular tachycardia in infants and children. Br Heart J 62:204–211, 1989.
69. Wellens HJJ, Durrer D: Effect of digitalis on atrioventricular conduction and circus-movement tachycardias in patients with Wolff-Parkinson-White syndrome. Circulation 47:1229–1233, 1973.
70. Byrum C, Wahl RA, Behrendt DM, Dick M: Ventricular fibrillation associated with the use of digitalis in a newborn infant with Wolff-Parkinson-White syndrome. J Pediatr 101:400–403, 1982.
71. Kleinman CS, Copel JA, Weinstein EM, et al: In utero diagnosis and treatment of fetal supraventricular tachycardia. Semin Perinatol 9:113–129, 1985.
72. Smith TW: Digitalis toxicity: Epidemiology and clinical use of serum concentration measurements. Am J Med 58:470–476, 1975.

SECTION IV

Common Clinical Problems

CHAPTER 14

SYNCOPE

Ronald J. Kanter

Syncope is a common complaint in the older pediatric patient. It is often disruptive to the family or school life out of proportion to the severity of the problem. *Syncope* is sudden in onset, results in loss of consciousness and loss of postural tone, and is transient in duration. If there is sensory and postural impairment but not complete loss of consciousness, the term *presyncope* is used. Most causes of syncope do not represent potentially fatal conditions; however, some patients have a life-threatening disease, but the initial episodes are self-limited, fulfilling the definition of syncope. Identification of this group of children (from among the much larger group having more benign causes) before they suffer an irreversible event challenges the primary care physician and specialist alike. Irrespective of etiology, syncope is caused by interruption of essential energy substrates to the brain. Some conditions, notably certain seizure types and conversion reactions, do not fit this definition, but are included in this discussion because of the similarity in clinical presentation.

In this chapter, the epidemiology, pathophysiology, and etiology of syncope are discussed, with emphasis on cardiac causes and on neurally mediated reflexes. Essentials of the patient evaluation follow, with special consideration of head-up tilt table testing. Treatment options are then considered, especially of neurally mediated syncope.

EPIDEMIOLOGY

The incidences of syncope in the general pediatric population are unknown, but among young adult populations of undergraduate and postgraduate students[1] and military inductees[2] the incidences were 15.5% and 22.3%, respectively. The occurrence of the common forms of syncope begins to increase during adolescence. The single exception is the pallid breath-holding spell of the toddler years, which is physiologically similar to the cardioinhibitory form of neurally mediated syncope. Menkes estimated that 5% of children 6 months to 6 years of age demonstrate some form of breath-holding spell, some of which are of this type.[3] These youngsters have an increased risk of having neurally mediated syncope as adults as well.[4] Syncope in adults recurs in about 30% of cases.[1, 5, 6] About 60% of adult cases are neurally mediated syncope[7]; 10 to 40% have a cardiac basis. Despite being a tertiary referral center for cardiac disease, about 80% of children and teenagers referred to us for syncope have neurally mediated syncope as the diagnosis.

There is a familial tendency to faint. Among 30 consecutive children seen by Camfield and Camfield[8] with syncope as the primary diagnosis, 27 had at least one first-degree relative with a history of syncope compared with only 8 of 24 control children ($P < .01$). The physiologic versus behavioral components of this tendency are unknown.

The incidence of syncope as a symptom of primary arrhythmia is unknown, but given the important incidence of sudden death after repair of some congenital heart diseases (from 0–4% after repair of ventricular septal defect[9, 10] to 18% after repair of double-outlet right ventricle[11]), its occurrence in a postoperative patient must be taken very seriously. Among patients having hypertrophic cardiomyopathy, syncope may also be a harbinger of sudden death. Among 29 adults with this condition, age younger than 30 years was an independent risk factor for syncope.[12] In a 5-year follow-up of 287 patients younger than 21 years having the long QT syndrome, 4% had syncope and 1% had seizures.[13] Syncope in this group is a clear indication for more aggressive treatment to prevent sudden death. The actual incidence of syncope in young people with the Wolff-Parkinson-White (WPW) syndrome is unknown, because the exact prevalence of asymptomatic WPW syndrome is not certain. In two large series, the high incidences of resuscitated sudden death (11%)[14] and syncope (19%)[15] and WPW syndrome in children are related to referral bias.

PATHOPHYSIOLOGY

The healthy young person maintains cerebral blood flow at about 60 ml/min/100 g tissue or about 11.4 ml of oxygen at a normal hemoglobin of 14 g/dl. This is maintained by autoregulation of flow over a wide range of perfusion pressures.[16] Cerebral vasodilatation occurs with critical reduction in partial pressure of arterial oxygen (PaO_2) or elevation of partial pressure of arterial carbon dioxide ($PaCO_2$). Perfusion pressure is also supported by baroreceptor-related changes in peripheral vascular resistance and heart rate and by complex barorecepter-related and chemoreceptor-related neurohumoral mechanisms that maintain intravascular volume. Oxygen delivery is also maintained during sudden drops in hemoglobin concentration by augmentation of cardiac output and cerebral blood flow. When cerebral oxygen delivery drops below 3.5 ml O_2/min/100 g tissue for longer than 8 seconds, syncope may ensue. This will occur in the presence of sudden cerebrovascular tone dysregulation (basilar migraine, hyperventilation), overwhelming drop in perfusion pressure on a cardiac basis (cardiac arrhythmia, cardiac inflow impairment, cardiac outflow impairment, neurally mediated asystole), overwhelming drop in cardiac preload (primary hypovolemia, autonomic neuropathy), or overwhelming drop in arteriolar resistance (autonomic neuropathy, neurally mediated vasodepression).

Cerebrovascular autoregulation is impaired in the presence of chronic hypertension,[17] a not uncommon problem in older adolescents in the United States and in some children after coarctation of the aorta repair. Among children and teenagers with chronic congestive heart failure, adrenergic receptors are typically down-regulated, and their intravascular volume may be reduced by diuretics, also making them prone to syncope.

ETIOLOGIES OF SYNCOPE

In this section I discuss the causes of syncope, the specific pathophysiologies when appropriate, clinical presentations, and—in certain instances—treatment considerations. Table 14–1 includes a categorical listing of disorders associated with syncope.

CARDIAC ARRHYTHMIAS

Cardiac arrhythmias result in syncope by causing a sudden fall in cardiac output. Bradycardias do this when the stroke volume cannot be augmented sufficiently to compensate for the lower heart rate, and tachycardias result in sufficiently short diastolic filling time that the stroke volume is insufficient. In some patients suffering acute cardiac arrhythmias while upright, assumption of a recumbent position results in resumption of consciousness despite persistence of the arrhythmia. However, in some patients suffering from rapid ventricular tachycardia or sudden severe bradycardia, persistence of the arrhythmia will result in death irrespective of body position.

Cardiac Arrhythmias in the Abnormal Heart

When a patient known to have congenital heart disease presents with syncope, an arrhythmic cause must be sought. Tables 14–2 and 14–3 list the incidences of arrhythmia types most frequently seen in patients with preoperative and postoperative congenital heart defects, respectively.

Tachy-Brady Syndrome (Sick Sinus Syndrome)

Children with the "tachy-brady syndrome" usually have marked sinus arrhythmia, severe sinus bradycardia, or junctional rhythm. However, syncopal episodes may occur despite pacemaker implantation, suggesting the need for tachycardia prevention as well.

The Mustard or Senning operation for d-transposition of the great arteries frequently results in damage to the sinus node, perinodal structures and their blood supplies,[18] and to atrial pacemaking tissue throughout the atrium. Although symptomatic bradycardia usually presents as exercise intolerance or chronic fatigue, syncope may be the presenting complaint. Investigators have reported that between 5 and 11% of patients require pacemakers over 4.5 to 8.3 years follow-up, usually for chronic fatigue or syncope.[19, 20] Syncope may also be caused by atrial flutter in these patients, either because of 1:1 atrioventricular (AV) conduction during atrial flutter or by marked overdrive suppression of all subsidiary pacemakers with resultant asystole after spontaneous termination of flutter. Syncope is a serious symptom in these patients, because the presence of atrial flutter on electrocardiogram (ECG) may increase the risk of sudden death 4.7-fold.[21] Syncope may also result from ventricular tachycardia, especially in the presence of reduced right ventricular function and after additional ventricular surgery for ventricular septal defect or for left ventricular outflow tract obstruction.

After the Fontan operation, Driscoll et al

Table 14–1. Classification of Etiologies of Syncope

I. Cardiac arrhythmias
   A. Postoperative tachycardias
      1. Atrial surgery: Mustard, Senning, Fontan, ASD, TAPVR-PAPVR, AV valve replacement
         Atrial flutter/re-entry tachycardia
         Atrial fibrillation
         Atrial ectopic tachycardia
      2. Ventricular surgery: tetralogy of Fallot, left ventricular outflow tract repair, above with VSD closure
         Ventricular tachycardia
         Ventricular fibrillation
   B. Postoperative bradycardias
      1. Atrial surgery: Mustard, Senning, Fontan, ASD, TAPVR-PAPVR
         Sinus bradycardia or standstill
         Junctional rhythm
      2. AV valve surgery: mitral or tricuspid valve replacement
         Complete AV block
      3. Ventricular surgery: AVSD, VSD (especially with l-TGA)
         Complete AV block
   C. Associated with congenital heart disease
      1. Atrioventricular re-entry tachycardia: Ebstein's anomaly, l-TGA, AVSD, tricuspid atresia, d-TGA
      2. WPW syndrome: Ebstein's anomaly, l-TGA, AVSD, tricuspid atresia
      3. Severe sinus bradycardia or atrial standstill: Holt-Oram syndrome (ASD), familial ASD, polysplenia
      4. Atrial fibrillation: familial ASD, Ebstein's anomaly
      5. Complete AV block: polysplenia, asplenia, l-TGA, Holt-Oram syndrome (ASD), familial ASD, pulmonic stenosis (LEOPARD syndrome)
   D. Other sinus bradycardia or standstill
      1. Familial
      2. Associated with neuromuscular disorders, muscular dystrophies
   E. Other atrial fibrillation-flutter
      1. Familial sinus node disease–atrial standstill
      2. Secondary to IHSS
      3. WPW syndrome
      4. Vagally mediated
      5. Drug related
      6. Thyrotoxicosis
      7. Associated with neuromuscular disease
   F. Other AV conduction system abnormalities
      1. Congenital complete AV block
      2. Familial AV block (may include atrial standstill, atrial fibrillation)
      3. Secondary to IHSS
      4. Associated with neuromuscular disease
      5. Familial bifascicular block or LBBB
      6. Acquired in myocarditis, rheumatic carditis
      7. Drug related
   G. Other ventricular tachycardias
      1. Dilated cardiomyopathy
      2. IHSS
      3. Congenital long QT syndrome
      4. Acquired long QT syndrome
      5. Arrhythmogenic right ventricular dysplasia
      6. Catecholamine-sensitive VT
      7. VT in otherwise normal heart
      8. WPW syndrome
      9. Drug related
   H. Artificial pacemaker related
      1. Myopotential oversensing
      2. Ventricular noncapture
      3. Ventricular lead fracture
      4. Battery depletion
      5. Pacemaker syndrome
      6. Pacemaker-mediated tachycardia
      7. AICD induced

II. Structural cardiac disease
   A. Hypertrophic cardiomyopathy
   B. Aortic valve stenosis
   C. Pulmonic stenosis
   D. Unoperated tetralogy of Fallot
   E. Dilated cardiomyopathy
      1. Idiopathic
      2. Familial
   F. Restrictive cardiomyopathy
      1. Acquired
      2. Familial
   G. Pulmonary hypertension
      1. Primary
      2. With Eisenmenger's syndrome physiology
   H. Pericardial effusion
   I. Constrictive pericarditis
   J. Atrial myxoma
   K. Coronary artery (occlusion)
      1. Anomalous coronary (especially left)
      2. Coronary spasm
      3. Cocaine related
   L. Pulmonary embolus
   M. Congenital partial absence of pericardium
   N. After heart transplant
   O. Associated with mitral valve prolapse

III. Neurally mediated reflexive syncope
   A. Postural
   B. Emotional (including pallid breath holding)
   C. Cough syncope
   D. Swallow syncope
   E. Micturition syncope
   F. Defecation syncope
   G. Stretch and hair groomers' syncope
   H. Hypersensitive carotid sinus

IV. Orthostatic and peripheral neurologic
   A. Primary orthostasis
   B. Drug induced
   C. Pregnancy
   D. Systemic mastocytosis
   E. Hyperbradykininism
   F. Autonomic neuropathy
      1. Secondary (diabetes mellitus)
      2. Primary dysautonomia
      3. Brain stem related (syringomyelia, Arnold-Chiari malformation)
   G. Addison's disease
   H. Burn related
   I. Deconditioning related
   J. Other causes of dehydration
   K. Familial dysautonomia
   L. Acute intermittent porphyria
   M. Guillain-Barré and other neuropathies

V. Central neurologic or neurovascular
   A. Basilar migraine
   B. Seizures
   C. Hydrocephalus
   D. Ventriculoperitoneal or ventriculoatrial shunt malfunction
   E. Cerebral vasculitis (SLE-PAN)
   F. Narcolepsy
   G. Subclavian steal syndrome (and other vertebral artery compression syndromes)
   H. Subarachnoid hemorrhage

VI. Metabolic
   A. Hypoglycemia
   B. Hypercalcemia

VII. Behavioral and psychiatric
   A. Cyanotic (hypoxic) breath-holding spells
   B. Panic attacks (hyperventilation)
   C. Secondary hyperventilation
   D. Conversion reaction
   E. Malingering

ASD, atrial septal defect; TAPVR, total anomalous pulmonary venous return; PAPVR, partial anomalous pulmonary venous return; AV, atrioventricular; VSD, ventricular septal defect; AVSD, atrioventricular septal defect; TGA, transposition of the great arteries; IHSS, idiopathic hypertrophic subaortic stenosis; LBBB, left bundle branch block; WPW, Wolff-Parkinson-White; AICD, automatic implantable cardioverter-defibrillator; SLE, systemic lupus erythematosus; PAN, polyarteritis nodosa.

From Kanter RJ: Syncope and sudden death in children. In Garson A, Bricker JT, Fisher DJ, Neish SR (eds): The Science and Practice of Pediatric Cardiology, 2nd ed. Baltimore, Williams & Wilkins, 1998. Used with permission.

Table 14–2. Incidence of Arrhythmias in Patients With Preoperative Congenital Heart Defects

CARDIAC DEFECT	ATRIAL FLUTTER-FIBRILLATION	PSVBs	SINUS BRADYCARDIA–JUNCTIONAL RHYTHM	WOLFF-PARKINSON-WHITE SYNDROME	SUPRAVENTRICULAR TACHYCARDIA	AV BLOCK	PVBs	VENTRICULAR TACHYCARDIA–SUDDEN DEATH
Sinus venosus and secundum ASD	+ – + + +,°		+ – + +	°°	°°	0– +,°		
Ebstein's anomaly	+ – + +,°			+ +	+ +			°°,†
Pulmonary valve stenosis		+ +						
VSD		+ +		°°	°°		+ +	+
AVSD				°°	°°			
PDA	0– + + + +,°			°°	+	°°	+	
Tetralogy of Fallot				°°	+		0– + + +,° (PVBs and ventricular tachycardia–sudden death together)	
Aortic valve stenosis	0– + + +,°	+		°°	+ – + +		+,†	°°,†
Coarctation of the aorta				°°		°°/°°,†		°°,†
d-TGA	0 – +	0 – +	+ – + + + (intermittent)		°°		+ – + +	0– +
l-TGA	‡			°°	+ +	+ – + +	+ + – + + + (PVBs and ventricular tachycardia–sudden death together)	
Polysplenia	‡		+ – + + + +,°	°°	°°	+ +		
Asplenia	‡		+	°°	°°	°°		
Tricuspid atresia	‡			+	+			
Eisenmenger's syndrome physiology			°°,† (paroxysmal)				+ + + +	+ +

PSVBs, premature supraventricular beats exceeding normal for age; PVBs, premature ventricular beats exceeding normal for age; +, up to 10% incidence; + +, 10–40% incidence; + + +, 40–60% incidence; + + + +, 60–90% incidence; °, progressive incidence with age; °°, reported but incidence not established; †, progressive incidence with advancement of hemodynamic abnormality; ‡, related to highly prevalent associated abnormalities; ASD, atrial septal defect; VSD, ventricular septal defect; AVSD, atrioventricular septal defect; PDA, patent ductus arteriosus; TGA, transposition of the great arteries.

From Kanter RJ, Garson A: Arrhythmia in congenital heart disease. In Podrid PJ, Kowey PR (eds): Cardiac Arrhythmias: Mechanisms, Diagnoses, and Management. Baltimore, Williams & Wilkins, 1995. Used with permission.

Table 14–3. Incidence of Arrhythmias After Congenital Heart Defects

VARIABLE	ATRIAL FLUTTER-FIBRILLATION	SINUS-JUNCTIONAL BRADYCARDIA	SVPBs	COMPLETE AV BLOCK	PACEMAKER REQUIREMENT	VPBs	VENTRICULAR TACHYCARDIA	SUDDEN DEATH
Mustard-Senning operation	1–10%	10–60%	25%	0–5%	5–10%	5–15%	1–5%	1–20%
Fontan operation	10–20%	10–20%	20%	1–5%	5–20%	5%	5–10%	1–5%
Tetralogy of Fallot	1–5%	1–5%	1%	5–10%	5%	20–60%	10–20%	5%
Ebstein's anomaly	5–10%	1–5%						5–10%
Pulmonic stenosis			10–20%			5–10%	5–10%	+
Atrial septal defect	10–60%		1–5%	5–10%				
Ventricular septal defect							5–10%	1–5%
Aortic stenosis						20–60%	5–20%	1–10%

SVPBs, supraventricular premature beats; VPBs, ventricular premature beats; *, related to time since surgery; **, reported but incidence not established; †, highest with hemodynamic compromise; ‡, highest with longer time since surgery; #, includes ventricular tachycardia inducibility during electrophysiology study; ##, related to presence of preoperative arrhythmia; +, 0–1% incidence; + +, 1–5% incidence; + + +, 5–10% incidence; + + + +, 10–20% incidence; + + + + +, 20–60% incidence.

From Kanter RJ, Garson A: Arrhythmia in congenital heart disease. In Podrid PJ, Kowey PR (eds): Cardiac Arrhythmias: Mechanisms, Diagnoses, and Management. Baltimore, Williams & Wilkins, 1995. Used with permission.

found that 20% of 352 patients had sufficient signs or symptoms of sick sinus syndrome to require antiarrhythmic drugs or pacemaker implantation at 5- to 15-year follow-up.[22] Right atrial stretch, impaired ventricular function, and AV valve regurgitation were considered causative for symptomatic tachy-brady syndrome. The incidence of pacemaker requirement after this operation ranges from 5 to 15%,[22–24] but includes congenital postoperative AV block as well as sinus node disease.

In Murphy's report of the natural history of 123 patients who had undergone secundum or sinus venosus atrial septal defect (ASD) repair, 5 (4%) had required pacemakers and 2 (2%) experienced complete AV block.[25] Late follow-up (27–32 years) also revealed that the incidence of atrial flutter or fibrillation increased with increase in age at repair from 4% if operated on at 11 years of age or younger up to 59% if operated on when older than 41 years. The incidence of symptomatic sinus node dysfunction after ASD repair was even higher at 7.5% among 269 patients at Texas Children's Hospital.[26]

The occurrence of dizziness, presyncope, or syncope among children with certain other unoperated congenital heart defects should also raise suspicion of sudden severe sinus bradycardia or atrial tachycardia. These include familial ASD, ASD as part of Holt-Oram syndrome, polysplenia syndrome, and Ebstein's anomaly. Atrial flutter or fibrillation may also occur in the presence of AV valve disease, hypertrophic cardiomyopathy, dilated cardiomyopathy, restrictive cardiomyopathy, and rheumatic carditis.

The workup of children with any of these defects and suffering dizzy spells, presyncope, or syncope should include careful evaluation of cardiac function and documentation of their rhythm during symptoms using an ambulatory event monitor. Invasive electrophysiologic studies should be strongly considered when these symptoms occur after Mustard operation or Fontan operation or in the presence of abnormal ventricular function because of the increased risk of ventricular tachycardia. Documentation of the rhythm type is crucial because elimination of atrial flutter by ablation or suppression by antiarrhythmic drugs may be as lifesaving for these patients as pacing is for those with bradycardia. Indeed, we generally recommend prophylactic digoxin in all patients after these operations, hoping to reduce the risk of 1:1 AV conduction, should atrial flutter develop. Presyncope or syncope are class I indications for pacing in children whose symptoms are bradycardia related.[27] Most clinicians now routinely implant pacemakers in patients with sick sinus syndrome who are receiving antiarrhythmic drugs other than digoxin and phenytoin, because of the negative chronotropic or dromotropic effects of these agents.

Atrioventricular Block

Syncope after certain cardiac operations may be caused by sudden third-degree AV block. Children undergoing aortic, mitral, or tricuspid valve replacement; ventricular septal defect closure (especially with corrected transposition of the great arteries); or AV septal defect repair may be at such risk. A pacemaker should be implanted in any child with type II second-degree or complete AV block lasting more than 14 days after heart surgery.

In the presence of new right bundle branch block and left axis deviation or right bundle branch block, left axis deviation, and first-degree AV block after a period of postoperative complete AV block that lasted less than 14 days, 24-hour ECG monitoring should be performed before discharge and then regularly. In all other patients who have undergone ventricular septal defect surgery (especially near the crux of the heart), 24-hour ECG monitoring should be performed every 2 to 5 years. In any such child, symptoms of dizziness, presyncope, or syncope are deserving of Holter or ambulatory event monitoring or possible electrophysiologic study. Type II second-degree AV block during ambulatory monitoring, demonstration of severe HV interval prolongation, or evidence of block below the His bundle with atrial pacing rates below 120 bpm deserves consideration of pacemaker placement, especially in the absence of inducible ventricular tachycardia. This recommendation is in part based on limited data from Friedli and Bolens, who showed that two of five postoperative patients who demonstrated infra-Hisian block at atrial rates below 120 bpm later experienced complete AV block.[28]

The occurrence of syncope in patients with certain other congenital or acquired heart defects should also arouse suspicion of intermittent complete AV block. Corrected transposition of the great arteries is usually associated with an anterior AV node giving rise to an elongated His bundle, which encircles the pulmonary valve. The His bundle may undergo fibrous degeneration or complete disruption.[29] Surprisingly, in a report by Huhta et al of 107 patients with corrected transposition,[30] 4 of whom had congenital AV block and 19 others in whom it later developed, there was only one sudden death, in a 28-year-old who died suddenly during exercise 4 years after onset of AV block. Data analysis showed an approximately 2%/year risk of AV block after diagnosis. Children with the heterotaxia syndromes may also have congenital or acquired AV block. Momma et al showed that by age 15 years two thirds of those with left atrial isomerism had junctional rhythm,[31] although this generally follows gradual loss of atrial pacemaker rate, and syncope is rarely observed.

Such developmental or acquired cardiac conditions as hypertrophic cardiomyopathy, myocarditis, rheumatic carditis, and endocarditis with perivalvular abscess may present with syncope resulting from sudden AV block. Lyme disease, in particular, has an 87% incidence of some degree of AV block as the manifestation of carditis, and carditis occurs in 4 to 10% of patients, usually about 5 weeks after disease onset.[32] The AV block may have associated bundle branch block pattern, and in reported adults with complete AV block there was syncope with an escape rate greater than 40 bpm in an important minority. AV block is always self-limited in this disease.

Supraventricular Tachycardia

As regards risk of syncope, supraventricular tachycardia (SVT) is of greater concern in children with coexisting heart disease than in those without. Intuitively, a heart having marginal cardiac output will be more adversely affected by reduction in ventricular filling time and coronary perfusion time. The occurrence of syncope in patients with hemodynamically significant congenital heart disease should suggest the need for careful provocation of SVT as part of their electrophysiologic study. This is particularly pertinent in children with Ebstein's anomaly and corrected transposition because of the relatively high association of accessory AV connections in these lesions and, hence, risk of AV reciprocating tachycardia.

Ventricular Tachycardia

In a report by Rocchini et al, among 38 children with ventricular tachycardia, the association of syncope or dizziness was more frequently found in patients with underlying heart disease than in those without.[33] Dreyer et al showed, using a dog model of repaired tetralogy of Fallot, that the presence of elevated right ventricular pressure resulted in higher plasma norepinephrine levels and lower right ventricular myocardial blood flow during rapid ventricular pacing than in control dogs.[34] They concluded that this could potentiate the occurrence of ventricular fibrillation and sudden death.

After ventricular surgery, the cause of sudden death is virtually always ventricular arrhythmias.[35–37] Syncope in such a patient should always be assumed to represent ventricular tachycardia, mandating appropriate investigation. Although there is a relationship between complex ventricular arrhythmias by 24-hour ECG monitoring and inducible ventricular tachycardia during electrophysiologic study,[38] the role of invasive electrophysiologic testing is not yet completely defined in this population. After repair of tetralogy of Fallot, the presence and severity (by Lown grade) of ventricular ectopy during ambulatory testing are reported most frequently to be related to older age at repair,[37, 39] elevation of right ventricular systolic pressure,[36, 39] and longer periods of follow-up since surgery.[36, 39] The most recent predictor of risk for life-threatening ventricular tachycardia after tetralogy repair is a QRS duration (180 ms on resting ECG).[40] However, there are no established independent risk factors that are predictive for risk of sudden death in this group of patients.[41]

Cardiac Arrhythmias in the Apparently Normal Heart

Tachy-Brady Syndrome

Familial congenital sinus node anomalies, sometimes associated with atrial fibrillation[42] or with progressive AV block,[43] may cause syncope. The existence of a family history of this disease or of atrial fibrillation in a patient with syncope and ECG evidence for sinus node dysfunction should prompt a more thorough evaluation of sinus node function and possible pacemaker placement. Additional noncardiac diseases that may include sinus bradycardia or atrial standstill and atrial fibrillation include fascioscapulohumeral dystrophy,[44, 45] Emery Dreifuss dystrophy,[44] myotonic dystrophy,[46] Kugelberg-Welander syndrome, and Guillain-Barré syndrome.

Atrioventricular Block

Congenital AV block in the absence of coexisting heart disease was probably first recognized in 1901 when Morquio reported familial incidence of children with very low heart rates and syncope.[47] The international cooperative study by Michaelsson and Engle showed that early infancy was the highest risk period for Adams-Stokes attacks, and identified a ventricular rate less than 55 bpm, an atrial rate greater than 140 bpm, and cardiomegaly as specific risk factors.[48] In older children, syncope occurred during what was thought to be periods of excessive vagal stimulation. Michaelsson reported that, among 102 patients who had been asymptomatic for their first 15 years with congenital AV block (mean age at follow-up, 38 years), 27 later suffered Adams-Stokes attacks, 8 of whom had a fatal outcome.[49] All 7 patients with additional prolonged QT interval had Adams-Stokes attacks. Eight of the 27 patients were younger than 20 years. These important observations suggest the need for routine prophylactic pacemaker implantation during adolescence. We have liberalized our criteria for pacemaker implantation, and do so in any child with this entity and syncope or presyncope; a resting awake heart rate less than 50 bpm (or older child or teenager with rates less than 40 bpm); prolonged QTc interval; wide QRS escape rhythm; chronic fatigue or exercise intolerance; pauses greater than 3 to 4 seconds; signs of congestive heart failure; or more than occasional ventricular ectopy.

Other noncardiac medical conditions that may eventually cause AV block with associated syncope include X-linked Becker's muscular dystrophy,[44] limb-girdle muscular dystrophy,[44] myotonic dystrophy, Kugelberg-Welander syndrome, McArdle's disease, and Kearns-Sayre syndrome.[50] In Kearns-Sayre syndrome, the presence of intraventricular conduction delay or new-onset bundle branch block should prompt consideration of elective pacemaker implantation because of the known progression to complete AV block.

The occurrence of syncope in a young patient with no history of heart disease or neuromuscular disease but bundle branch block on ECG is a difficult problem. Isolated or familial right bundle branch block is usually nonprogressive,[51, 52] and probably does not merit further conduction system evaluation. However, its association with other conduction system abnormalities, including left axis deviation, justifies more invasive evaluation of the conduction system because of the risk of progression to complete AV block. The occurrence of nonsurgical left bundle branch block mandates further evaluation because of its association with myocarditis, endocarditis, hemochromatosis, and myocardial infarction.[53, 54] A familial form associated with cardiomyopathy may progress to complete AV block.[55] AV block at any anatomic level may result from endocarditis or myocarditis and can result in syncope.

Supraventricular Tachycardia

Garden-variety SVT in otherwise healthy children occasionally causes presyncope and rarely results in syncope. Factors that may predispose to syncope include elevated activity level and hence metabolic demands, relative dehydration, and unusually fast SVT. However, in an adult study (mean patient age, 38 years), syncope from induced SVT during tilt table testing was not related to heart rate but to vasomotor factors.[56]

The presence of antegrade AV conduction through an accessory connection, the WPW syndrome, usually either is an isolated finding on ECG or is associated with a clinical history of SVT. Rarely, however, the antegrade refractory periods of the accessory connection and the AV node are such that spontaneous atrial fibrillation will result in ventricular tachycardia or fibrillation (Fig. 14–1). Hence, the finding of WPW syndrome in a young person, usually a teenager, who has suffered a syncopal spell requires electrophysiologic evaluation and potential radiofrequency ablation of the accessory connection. During electrophysiologic study, a shortest interval between consecutively pre-excited beats of less than 200 milliseconds or an average cycle length of less than 330 milliseconds during induced atrial fibrillation accurately identified all 12 children having WPW syndrome and who had suffered resuscitated sudden cardiac death in one report.[14] Paul et al also found that inducibility of sustained atrial fibrillation and a shortest consecutively pre-excited interval of less than 230 milliseconds identified young people who had a history of syncope from among a larger group of WPW patients.[15]

Atrial fibrillation is a rare arrhythmia in the absence of heart disease in children and teenagers. It has been reported immediately after classic neurally mediated syncope in persons as young as 18 years.[57] In this instance, paroxysmal atrial fibrillation accompanied, but did not cause, syncope. Chronic atrial fibrillation is reported to cause syncope in older adults related to intermittent ventricular standstill as a result of increased parasympathetic tone.[58]

Ventricular Tachycardia

In the absence of known heart disease, ventricular tachycardia as a cause for syncope or presyncope may be considered if symptoms are preceded by palpitations, symptoms occur with exertion, or there is complex ventricular ectopy on resting ECG or 24-hour ambulatory ECG.[59] Ventricular tachycardia may then be demonstrated by ambulatory event monitor or invasive electrophysiologic study. The differential diagnosis of ventricular tachycardia in young persons is discussed elsewhere, but the finding of this

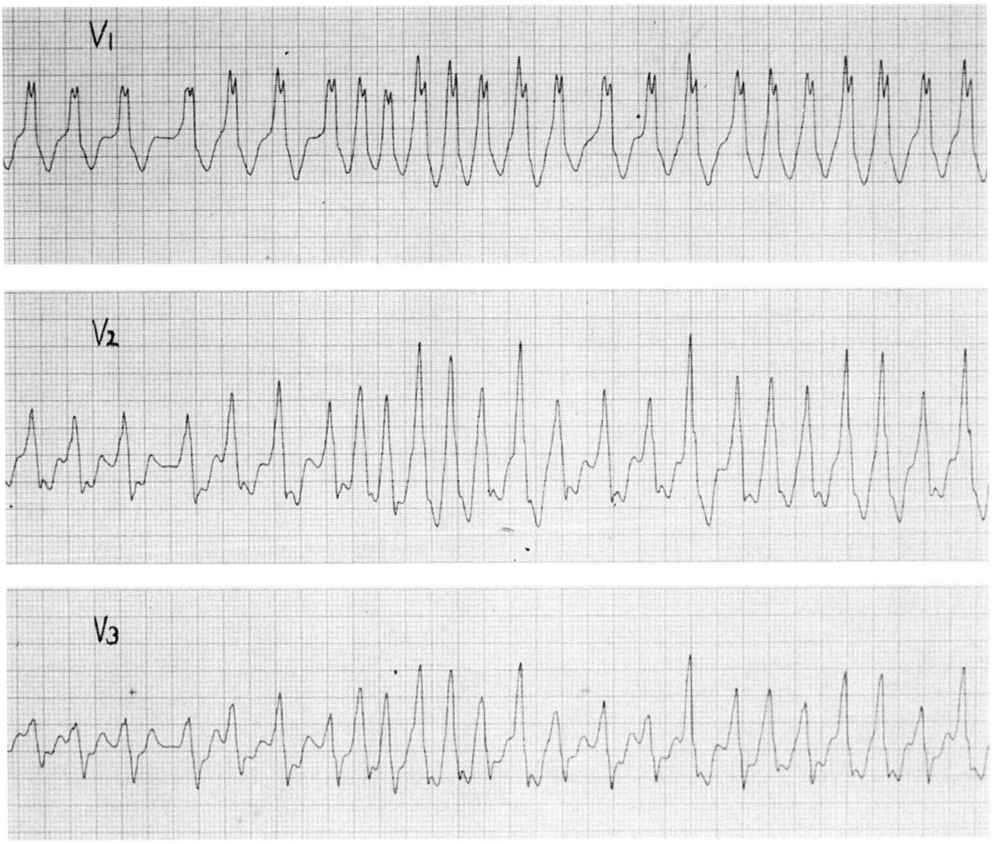

FIGURE 14–1. A three-lead rhythm strip from a 16-year-old who presented with syncope. The rhythm is atrial fibrillation in the presence of Wolff-Parkinson-White syndrome and a left lateral accessory pathway. The shortest consecutively pre-excited RR interval is 190 ms.

arrhythmia in a child with syncope necessitates evaluation for more occult disorders, including coronary artery abnormality, long QT syndrome, myocardial tumors, arrhythmogenic right ventricular dysplasia, myocarditis, hypertrophic cardiomyopathy, or other types of cardiomyopathy. Once these are successfully ruled out, "ventricular tachycardia in a normal heart" becomes the diagnosis. It is usually one of three morphologies: left bundle branch block and inferior axis from the right ventricular outflow tract; right bundle branch block and left axis deviation from the left side of the ventricular septum; and polymorphic ventricular tachycardia, which is catecholamine dependent.[60, 61] The first two types may respond to calcium- or beta-blocking agents and may be eliminated by catheter ablation, and catecholaminergic polymorphic ventricular tachycardia is responsive to beta blockers. It should be emphasized that right ventricular outflow tract and left ventricular septal tachycardias in the normal heart more often present with palpitations alone or even incidentally on the sports physical examination.

Children with congenital long QT syndrome are at risk for sudden death from a very rapid polymorphic ventricular tachycardia, called torsades de pointes. If nonsustained, it will result in dizziness, presyncope, or syncope, sometimes with seizures. In the international study by Garson et al, of 287 patients younger than 21 years with long QT syndrome, 26% presented with syncope.[13] Symptoms were preceded by exercise in 67%, although sudden emotional events may also trigger episodes. Besides a prolonged QTc interval, the patient's routine ECG also demonstrated second- or third-degree AV block in 5% and ventricular arrhythmias in 16% of patients. Evidence of sinus node dysfunction may also be present.[62] The QTc interval was normal in 6%, representing a subgroup of children at risk who may be missed by routine screening. Nevertheless, it is this entity among only a few others that justifies obtaining an ECG on almost any child who faints. In unclear cases, measuring the QTc interval immediately after exercise or during isoproterenol[63] or epinephrine infusions may be of value. The treatment of this disorder is discussed elsewhere.

Acquired prolongation of the QTc interval may also predispose to torsades de pointes ventricular tachycardia and syncope, particularly in the presence of bradycardia or hypokalemia. Unlike congenital long QT syndrome, symptoms do not occur after a catecholamine surge but tend to be pause related. Correction of the underlying condition, chronotropic support if necessary, treatment of coexisting hypokalemia, and acute administration of magnesium sulfate constitute treatment for this cause of syncope and potential sudden death.

Pacemaker Malfunction

When a young person has a pacemaker, especially if he or she is pacemaker dependent, and suffers sudden dizziness, presyncope, or syncope, it must first be assumed that the symptoms are due to a drop in cardiac output related to either pacemaker malfunction or inappropriate programmed parameters. For example, some children with AV block and dual-chamber pacing are very sensitive to the dropped beat at higher sinus rates caused by pacemaker Wenckebach, a normal pacemaker phenomenon and one that may be prevented by reprogramming.

Myopotential oversensing is primarily a problem in patients having systems using unipolar sensing. This may result in rapid ventricular pacing in cases of oversensing by a unipolar atrial lead in a patient with AV block and a dual-chamber pacemaker, or it may result in ventricular asystole in the case of oversensing by a ventricular lead. It is important to inquire as to the patient's body and arm positions when they had symptoms and to try to reproduce symptoms during clinic evaluation. In-house telemetry may be necessary and will usually demonstrate at least subclinical periods of oversensing and thereby guide therapy: reprogramming sensitivity or switching to bipolar sensing.

Ventricular noncapture may be intermittent and not readily apparent when it is caused by lead fracture that is not obvious by radiograph. The diagnosis my be suggested by a sudden change in lead impedance, sensitivity, or pacing threshold, but often a prolonged period of rhythm monitoring is necessary. When noncapture is due to exit block, there will be an increase in pacing threshold. The programmed output at the time of presentation is usually close to that threshold with inconsistent ventricular capture. Battery depletion occurs in the setting of noncompliance with outpatient monitoring in the presence of a previously well-functioning pacing system or in the instance of lead insulation fracture and rapid current drain. In either case, if the patient survives, he or she will usually report syncope or presyncope followed by obvious symptoms of low cardiac output caused by a slow escape rate.

Pacemaker syndrome refers to a constellation of symptoms, including presyncope, syncope, dizziness, easy fatigability, orthopnea, and dyspnea, that occur in patients receiving ventricular pacing and who have intact ventriculoatrial conduction. This results in jugular venous pulsations, reflex vasodilatation,[64] diminished cardiac output,[65] and, in adults, increased risk of atrial fibrillation.[66] Children and teenagers with ventricular pacemakers for sick sinus syndrome are most prone to this problem. Once diagnosed, changing to atrial pacing, if antegrade AV conduction is adequate, or dual-chamber pacing will alleviate symptoms.

Pacemaker-mediated tachycardia may be caused by ventricular tracking of appropriately sensed paroxysmal atrial tachyarrhythmias in the presence of a dual-chamber pacemaker or by pacemaker sensing of a retrograde P wave in the presence of a premature ventricular beat and intact ventriculoatrial conduction, also in the presence of a dual-chamber pacemaker. Because these young patients invariably have coexisting heart disease, the sudden acceleration of rate may result in at least presyncope. Mode switching, pharmacologic suppression of atrial tachyarrhythmias, and extension of the post ventricular atrial refractory period will treat this problem.

Once all of these considerations have been ruled out, consideration of intrinsic tachycardias as the cause of symptoms must be considered, depending on the underlying heart disease. Despite the emphasis on pacemaker malfunction, the cause of syncope in paced adult patients is not usually arrhythmia related but is neurally mediated syncope or orthostatic hypotension.[67] This has even been demonstrated in a teenager with congenital AV block and a dual-chamber pacemaker.[68]

HYPERTROPHIC CARDIOMYOPATHY

Syncope may be a harbinger of sudden death in children having hypertrophic cardiomyopathy, and the screening evaluation of young persons who faint should consider this diagnosis. Independent predictors of syncope in a group of adults (mean age, 44.8 years) having this disease included younger age (< 30 years) and nonsustained ventricular tachycardia during ambulatory ECG monitoring.[12] However, among children and teenagers with this entity who have survived cardiac arrest, ambulatory ECG monitoring has demonstrated only infrequent ectopy.[69, 70] Dilsizian et al[71] demonstrated myocardial ischemia by exercise thallium scintigraphy in all 15 young patients (6–23 years) with hypertrophic cardiomyopathy and previous cardiac arrest or syncope. Only 27% of those with symptoms had inducible ventricular tachycardia during electrophysiologic study. The authors proposed that myocardial ischemia may be the major cause of severe symptoms in these patients. The mechanisms for myocardial ischemia could include compression of the coronary microcirculation by impaired left ventricular relaxation, intrinsic abnormalities of the intramural coronary arteries causing reduced vasodilator response, and increase in oxygen demand by myocardial hypertrophy and outflow tract obstruction. The well-known efficacy of beta blockers and calcium channel blockers to prevent syncope recurrences in young persons with hypertrophic cardiomyopathy is consistent with these pathophysiologic postulates.

A proposed algorithm for the evaluation and management of the child or teenager with hypertrophic cardiomyopathy and syncope or sudden death appears in Figure 14–2. After ruling out myocardial ischemia and ventricular tachycardia as causes for syncope, this schematic takes into account the observation in some adults that neurally mediated syncope may occur in this disease.[72] In 1994, however, Sneddon et al suggested that tilt table testing is only of limited value in these patients because of its poor predictive accuracy.[73] The occasional coexistence of AV block or of WPW syndrome with hypertrophic cardiomyopathy makes investigation of these rhythm abnormalities also part of the workup, especially after ischemia has been evaluated.[74, 75] Finally, paroxysmal atrial fibrillation may occur in teenagers with hypertrophic cardiomyopathy and may cause syncope or presyncope.

OTHER CAUSES OF OUTFLOW TRACT OBSTRUCTION

Aortic valve stenosis may cause exercise-induced syncope by several proposed mechanisms: inadequate stroke volume, subendocardial ischemia causing low output or ventricular arrhythmia, or reflex peripheral vasodilatation from excessive left ventricular mechanoreceptor stretch. The latter mechanism has been demonstrated in adults with only mild resting outflow tract gradients[76] and yet results in secondary ischemic changes caused by coronary hypoperfusion. When syncope occurs in the presence of exercise-induced ST-segment abnormalities or in the presence of an excessive outflow tract gradient, valvotomy or valve replacement should be considered.

Hypercyanotic spells evolving to syncope may occur in children having unoperated tetralogy of Fallot, tricuspid atresia, or transposition of the great arteries and left ventricular outflow tract obstruction. The current trend toward repair of these lesions in infancy has resulted in a lower prevalence of such events, except in infants. So called "tetralogy spell" typically begins with crying, with associated prolonged expiration, and results in increased intrathoracic pressure, reduced pulmonary blood flow, and increased right-to-left intracardiac shunting. Hypoxemia increases the infant's high catecholamine state, and metabolic acidosis causes peripheral vasodilatation, all serving to promote the cycle of right-to-left shunting. If left unattended, low output, syncope, and death may ensue. Calming the infant and forcing a knee-chest position are appropriate initial maneuvers, but supplemental oxygen and parenteral morphine sulfate are often required. Intravenous phenylephrine or propranolol have also been used to "break the cycle" and restore pulmonary blood flow.

Children and especially teenagers with Eisenmenger's syndrome are at increased risk of syncope or sudden death. The mechanism for symptoms may involve ventricular tachyarrhythmias or lethal hypercyanotic spells.[77] Of 20 patients with ventricular septal defects and Eisenmenger's syndrome in the Natural History Study-2, during 24-hour ECG monitoring, 89% had multiform ventricular premature beats (VPBs), and 20% had more than one episode of ventricular tachycardia.[78] Sudden severe cyanosis with syncope has been noted in many patients without apparent arrhythmia, suggesting near cessation of pulmonary blood flow.

Patients with these lesions, even if previously unknown to the health care provider, will have physical findings suggestive of the defect responsible for the symptoms. More difficult to diagnosis is the child with primary pulmonary hypertension. This entity may present with increasing fatigue, but exercise-induced chest pain or syncope may be the first symptom. Appreciation of an increased and narrowly split S_2 is a valuable sign of elevated pulmonary artery pressure. The

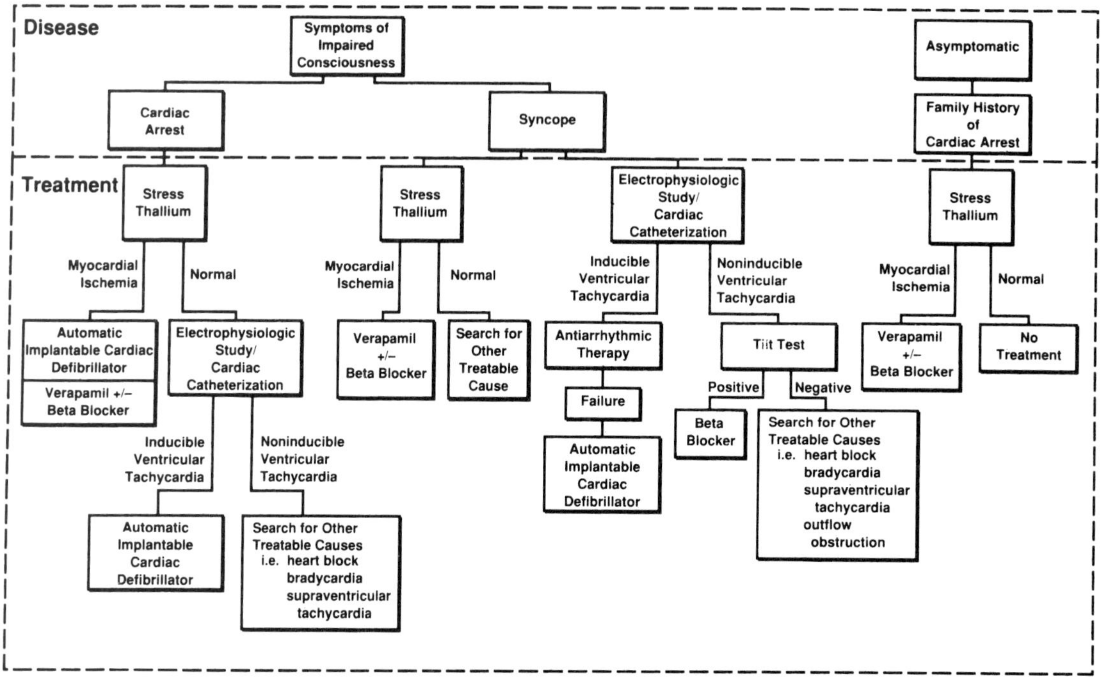

FIGURE 14–2. Management algorithm of young patients with hypertrophic cardiomyopathy and symptoms of impaired consciousness or family history of cardiac arrest. From Dilsizian V, Bonow RO, Epstein SE, Fananapazir L: Myocardial ischemia detected syncope in young patients with hypertrophic cardiomyopathy. J Am Coll Cardiol 22:796–804, 1993. Used with permission.

screening ECG will be useful if it shows right ventricular hypertrophy. This is an ECG diagnosis, but cardiac catheterization will ultimately be required to determine pulmonary vascular reactivity to oxygen and pharmacologic agents. Syncope in children with pulmonary hypertension is a grave symptom because it represents loss of cardiac output resulting from restrictive right ventricular outflow. In preparation for lung transplantation or newer pharmacologic therapies, some such patients have benefited short term from the creation of an atrial-level communication by blade and balloon septostomy.[79] The ASD created allows right-to-left shunting and preservation of cardiac output during sudden exacerbations of pulmonary hypertension.

OBSTRUCTION TO CARDIAC FILLING

Restriction to atrial filling occurs during pericardial tamponade. Any syncopal child or teenager known to have a chronic illness that may have associated pericardial effusion should be examined for jugular venous distention, muffled heart sounds, and pulsus paradoxus. The risk of syncope is increased when there is reduced intravascular volume. The diagnosis is made echographically, and pericardiocentesis provides immediate restoration of stroke volume.

Obstruction to ventricular filling must be considered as the cause of a syncopal event in any patient known to have a replaced AV valve. The diagnosis may be suspected in the patient with a long-standing tissue valve who has a murmur of AV valve stenosis and a high diastolic flow gradient by Doppler evaluation. If a prosthetic valve is present, its closure sound may be less crisp than usual, the inflow velocity by Doppler will be greater than what is normal for that valve type, and its mobility will be limited when viewed fluoroscopically. Thrombolytic agents may restore valve function if recent thrombosis has occurred. Otherwise, and especially if the patient has outgrown the valve, this constitutes a surgical urgency.

Tumors may obstruct AV valve inflow. The most common atrial tumors are myxomas. Left atrial and mitral valve myxomas[80, 81] may present with recurrent syncope, and severe symptoms from such tumors have been reported in patients as young as 18 years.[81]

A rare cause of recurrent syncope is partial

absence of the pericardium.[82] This usually involves the left pericardium with herniation and potential strangulation of the left atrial appendage. If the clinical scenario is not typical neurally mediated syncope, this entity may be considered. A chest radiograph and fluoroscopy will show an atypical heart border and pulsatile nature of the left atrial appendage. The defect may be easily repaired surgically. Finally, constrictive pericarditis or restrictive cardiomyopathy may present with syncope with exertion or periods of dehydration. Clues to these diagnoses include abnormal ventricular filling sounds, hepatojugular reflex, Kussmaul's sign, and pulsus paradoxus. Echocardiography and cardiac catheterization are then necessary to discriminate these entities.

CORONARY ARTERY ANOMALIES

A patient suffering a syncopal event who is then demonstrated to have one of several types of coronary artery anomalies should be presumed to be at risk of sudden death. Symptoms are usually exercise related and in several instances have been shown to be caused by ischemia-related ventricular tachycardia.[83]

The left main coronary artery may arise from the right sinus of Valsalva,[84] or, less frequently, the right may arise from the left sinus.[85–87] In either instance, the aberrantly arising coronary artery tends to have a partial intramural course, may have a narrowed origin, and may be prone to compression between the ascending aorta and pulmonary artery during exercise. Symptoms of exercise-induced syncope preceded sudden death in approximately 50% of affected individuals.

Other coronary abnormalities presumed to be causative of syncope include myocardial overbridges in association with hypoplasia of the posterior descending coronary artery, coronary-cameral fistulas, coronary artery-to-main pulmonary artery fistulas,[88] and coronary artery spasm. Myocardial overbridges have been identified in 0.5 to 2.7% of otherwise normal coronary angiograms,[89] making those with associated hypoplasia of the coronary arteries either a small subset of those with overbridges or a different disease altogether.

The most important discriminatory factor in deciding whether to consider coronary abnormality as a cause for a syncopal event is if it is exercise related. When syncope occurred during the physical motion of a high intensity activity, we recommend careful evaluation, including echocardiography, exercise testing, and selective coronary arteriography. We know of several instances in which even radionuclide perfusion scans with exercise were normal, but selective arteriograms demonstrated an intramural anomalously arising left coronary artery. Surgical intervention in such a case may restore a normal lifestyle.

MITRAL VALVE PROLAPSE

Mitral valve prolapse (MVP) is present in 4 to 5% of the adult population[90, 91] but is less common in children. In older teenagers and adults, it is associated with reduced blood pressure,[92] orthostatic hypotension,[93] and symptomatic palpitations and syncope.[94] These patients are characteristically asthenic and may have associated pectus excavatum, scoliosis, or straight back. Case–control family studies do not support a true association between MVP and atypical chest pain, dyspnea, or panic attacks as previously thought.[91, 94]

Age appears to be an important factor in the development of complications of MVP. Bisset et al found no progression of mitral regurgitation and no sudden deaths among 119 children monitored for a mean of 7 years starting at mean age of 10 years.[95]

In patients with MVP, the relationship of palpitations, orthostatic hypotension, or syncope with autonomic dysfunction is a controversial subject. Gaffney et al found decreased vagal responsiveness and increased alpha-adrenergic response in 19 women with MVP compared with controls.[96] In another report, among 20 symptomatic patients with MVP, including 6 with syncope or presyncope, there were greater levels of excretion of epinephrine and norepinephrine compared with controls.[97]

The incidence of sudden death in patients with MVP ranges from 0% in children[95] to 0.5% yearly in adults,[98] and thus older teenagers having MVP and syncope may be an at-risk group. Although selection bias influences reported series, it is concluded that some subgroups of adults with MVP are at high risk for refractory ventricular arrhythmias, and identification of which older teenagers will be at risk is becoming a task of the pediatrician and pediatric cardiologist. It is clear that sudden death in this group most frequently is arrhythmia related. In adult studies, important mitral regurgitation[99, 100] and repetitive ventricular arrhythmias[101] are positively related to this risk.

Teenagers with MVP and significant regurgitation should undergo periodic ambulatory ECG monitoring. The presence of multiform VPBs, couplets, or nonsustained ventricular tachycardia, or the presence of long QTc interval during ECG or exercise testing should merit consideration of beta-blocker therapy. Presyncope or syncope in the adolescent with MVP should include consideration of an arrhythmic cause, orthostatic hypotension, or neurally mediated syncope. An accurate cause may be obtained by ambulatory event recorder and tilt table study so that directed therapy may be applied. The role for invasive electrophysiologic study in this patient group is unclear. In Bissett's series, one child suffered a cerebrovascular accident related to MVP, so nonarrhythmic causes of syncope may also rarely occur.[95]

EXTRACRANIAL CEREBROVASCULAR DISEASE

Isolated syncope is an uncommon manifestation of extracranial cerebrovascular disease, but may occur in response to embolic events during endocarditis, as a complication of cardiac catheterization or cardiac surgery, or in the presence of a cardiac tumor or ventricular aneurysm, diverticulum, or mural thrombus.

The subclavian steal syndrome refers to several phenomena that have in common impaired proximal subclavian artery flow causing reversal of ipsilateral vertebral artery flow into the distal subclavian artery. Symptoms most frequently occur during ipsilateral arm exercise and may include dizziness as well as syncope or presyncope. Symptoms may occur in children who underwent a subclavian artery-to-pulmonary artery anastomosis for congenital heart disease or a congenital anomaly of the proximal subclavian artery[102] or may be due to costoclavicular or cervical rib compression as in Klippel-Feil syndrome.[103] Among our newer technologies, venoarterial extracorporeal membrane oxygenation (ECMO) in neonates requires cannulation of the right carotid artery. Subclavian steal occurred in 31% of infants during ECMO in a report by Graziani,[104] but vertebral artery flow returned to normal after arterial decannulation. Unintended damage to the proximal innominate artery could theoretically result in long-term symptoms. Symptoms of syncope, especially if accompanied by dizziness in a child who had undergone any such procedure, should prompt imaging and functional studies of the posterior cerebral circulation. Balloon dilatation or surgical bypassing, if necessary, may eliminate symptoms.

SYNCOPE AFTER HEART TRANSPLANTATION

There is a wide range of intermittent ECG changes that occur from the donor heart after transplantation,[105] most of which do not have clinical implications. Addonizio et al reported on 2 of 29 pediatric transplant recipients requiring permanent pacing as a result of severe sinus bradycardia or sinus arrest.[106] They also described 2 patients having atrial fibrillation and 1 having ventricular tachycardia, all during rejection episodes.[106] Hence, syncope after transplantation may have an arrhythmic source and, if present, should suggest that rejection may be occurring.

A vasodepressor form of neurally mediated syncope has been demonstrated by head-up tilt table testing in 7 of 10 patients (the youngest was 18 years old) from 6 to 38 months after transplantation[107] and in 1 patient during infusion of sodium nitroprusside and sympathetic nerve activity monitoring.[108] Whereas cardiac sympathetic reinnervation has been demonstrated after transplantation,[109–111] 3 patients in Fitzpatrick's series who manifested a vasodepressor response also experienced donor atrial bradycardia, suggesting parasympathetic reinnervation as well.[107] In the others who experienced no change in heart rate during hypotension and during atropine infusion and in Scherrer et al's case report,[108] it is implied that an afferent limb of the neurally mediated syncopal reflex other than the cardiac vagus nerve may be operational.

SYNCOPE PREDICTING SUDDEN DEATH: OTHER ETIOLOGIES

Although many of these cardiac causes of syncope could also be fatal, syncope related to two other entities is an especially important harbinger of sudden death: advanced congestive heart failure and pulmonary embolism.

In a study by Middlekauff et al,[112] 491 consecutive adult patients with advanced heart failure, New York Heart Association (NYHA) Class III or IV, were evaluated for the presence and origin of syncope and the relationship of the occurrence of syncope with that of sudden death. Comparing the 60 patients (12%) having syncope with all others, the actuarial incidence of sudden death by 1 year was greater in those having prior syncope (45%) than in those not having syncope (12%, $P < 0.00001$). The cause of syncope, cardiac versus noncardiac, did not influence that risk. The incidence of cardiac syncope, mostly ventricular tachycardia, was equal to that of noncardiac syncope, mostly orthostatic hypotension. Similar data from children are lacking.

Pulmonary embolism in children and teenagers occurs during periods of immobilization, after long bone fractures or surgery, or in the presence of uncommon hypercoagulable states. A minority of adults having pulmonary embolism present with syncope,[113] and we have seen presyncope in an adolescent Fontan patient before fatal pulmonary embolism. Although it may have other pathophysiologic mechanisms, defecation syncope,[114] in particular, in a young person otherwise at risk for pulmonary embolism suggests the need for thorough evaluation of this problem.

NEURALLY MEDIATED REFLEXIVE SYNCOPE

These conditions are the most common causes of syncope in young persons, and are also referred to as "vasovagal episodes," "neurocardiogenic syncope," the "common faint," and, in toddlers, "pallid breath-holding spells." They have in common disturbances in autonomic control of heart rate and blood pressure in response to emotional events, pain, postural change, or a variety of normal vegetative functions that involve cranial nerve and spinal cord stimulation (Fig. 14–3). At all other times, the patient's autonomic nervous system function seems to be normal. Children who suffer from these conditions usually have normal cardiac structure and conduction systems.

Pathophysiology of Emotional and Postural Forms

During lower body venous pooling or periods of hypovolemia, normal arterial pressure is maintained by arterial and cardiopulmonary reflex responses. The sensors for these reflexes include baroreceptors in the aortic arch and carotid sinus and mechanoreceptor C fibers in the atria, pulmonary arteries, and especially the inferoposterior left ventricle. Afferent signals from these receptors travel to nuclei in the medulla, including the nucleus ambiguous and dorsal motor nucleus of the vagus nerve (parasympathetic activity) and the costal ventromedial and ventrolateral me-

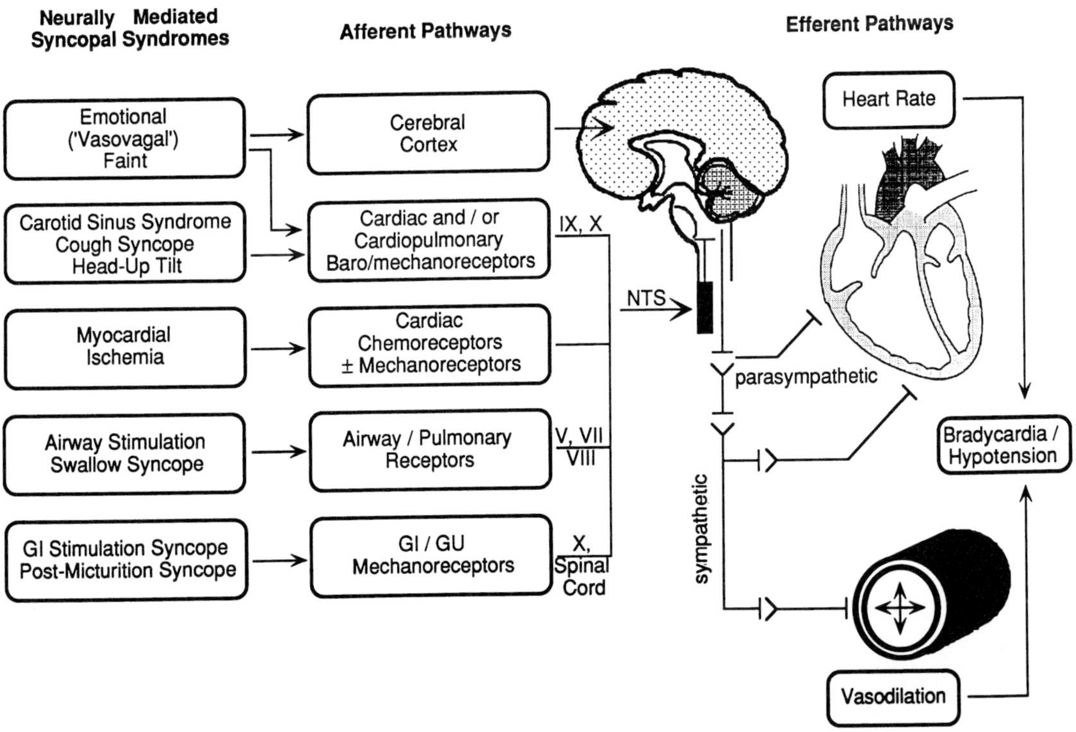

FIGURE 14–3. Schematic depiction of current concepts of mechanisms of neurally mediated syncope. (NTS, nucleus tractus solitarius; GI, gastrointestinal; GU, genitourinary.) From Benditt DB: Pathophysiology and causes of syncope. In Podrid PJ, Kowey PR (eds): Cardiac Arrhythmia: Mechanisms, Diagnoses, and Management. Baltimore, MD, Williams & Wilkins, 1995. Used with permission.

dulla (sympathetic activity).[115] The C fibers travel within the vagus nerve primarily to the dorsal vagus nerve.[116] Receptor stretch (increased firing) in any of these regions results in a reduction of sympathetic stimulation and an increase in parasympathetic stimulation causing vasodilatation and reduced heart rate; reduction in intravascular volume causes reduced firing of these receptors with resultant increase in sympathetic activity and vasoconstriction and tachycardia.

In persons with neurally mediated syncope secondary to postural changes, the major efferent event is vasodilatation caused by profound sympathetic withdrawal, probably resulting from a paradoxic increase in afferent traffic from peripheral receptors, especially cardiac mechanoreceptors. Evidence for this in children includes the observations by Balaji et al[117] and by Perry and Garson[118] that children with positive tilt studies had lower blood norepinephrine concentrations and beta-adrenergic hypersensitivity compared with controls. Cardiac mechanoreceptor stimulation is presumably due to the exaggerated contractile state, which is related to beta-adrenergic hypersensitivity. This is supported by the observation during upright tilt that patients demonstrate a reduction in left ventricular end-systolic and end-diastolic dimensions, an increase in ejection fraction, and cavitary obliteration compared with controls.[119] Studies of heart rate variability have shown a pronounced sympathetic surge during upright tilt, followed by paradoxical parasympathetic input.[120]

The primary abnormality initiating these events is unclear, but may include beta-adrenergic hypersensitivity[118] to mild reduction in blood pressure as is normally seen immediately on arising or abnormalities in venous tone,[121] although total vascular volume is not reduced in affected adults.[122] More direct evidence for impaired peripheral vasoconstriction comes from Sneddon et al's report of reduced forearm vascular resistance in adults during neurally mediated syncope.[123] In children, unlike adults, the renin-angiotensin system responds normally to hypotension and does not appear to have an important role.[124]

Central nervous system mediators of peripheral vasodilatation are more uncertain. Animal studies of hemorrhagic shock have shown that serotonin mediates a reduction in renal sympathetic nerve activity and an increase in adrenal nerve activity.[125] Successful clinical trials of serotonin-reuptake inhibitors in human adults and children with neurally mediated syncope support the role of serotonin in the pathogenesis of syncope.[126] The role of a central opiate receptor mechanism is also suggested by the observation that plasma beta endorphins are very elevated during vasodepressor syncope.[127] That the brain stem is central to this disorder is also suggested by the coexistence of neurally mediated syncope in a boy with central hypoventilation syndrome (Ondine's curse).[128]

Enhanced parasympathetic activity is the major efferent response in some patients with neurally mediated syncope. Heart rate variability studies in adults have shown a paradoxical increase in parasympathetic input during positive tilt studies.[120] This mechanism may be primary in about 10 to 15% of children[117, 129] who are described as having the "malignant cardiodecelerator" form of neurally mediated syncope, with up to many seconds of asystole, and in most toddlers having pallid breath-holding spells.

Finally, there is evidence for derangement of cerebral autoregulation in adults during episodes of tilt table–induced hypotension.[130] Whereas the expected response of the cerebral circulation to hypotension is vasodilatation, these patients showed a vasoconstrictor response. This may result in symptoms at relatively higher mean peripheral arterial pressure.

In summary, the reflex resulting in neurally mediated syncope in young persons seems to begin with beta-adrenergic hypersensitivity after subtle changes in postural tone or circulating volume. This results in increased baroreceptor and left ventricular mechanoreceptor firing, followed by an efferent response consisting of peripheral alpha-adrenergic withdrawal and enhanced parasympathetic tone (Fig. 14–4).

A syncopal response to the sight of blood, pain, or anticipated pain may be due to a true phobia or to a nonphobic fear.[131] This may occur while supine[132] and, therefore, does not necessarily involve a primary hypovolemic phase. The pathophysiologic mechanism may involve beta-adrenergic hypersensitivity to direct catecholamine release from higher cerebral centers without postural and baroreflex changes. Whereas postural changes usually require a few to several minutes to cause syncope, blood or injury syncope is usually instantaneous after a stimulus.

Clinical Aspects of Emotional and Postural Forms

Symptoms immediately preceding syncope in the older child or teenager include weakness, light-headedness, a sensation of being tired, repeated yawning or sighing, or a general feeling of being hot. Visual changes include blurring, bright or dark spots, or peripheral restriction of the visual field. Sounds and voices may become

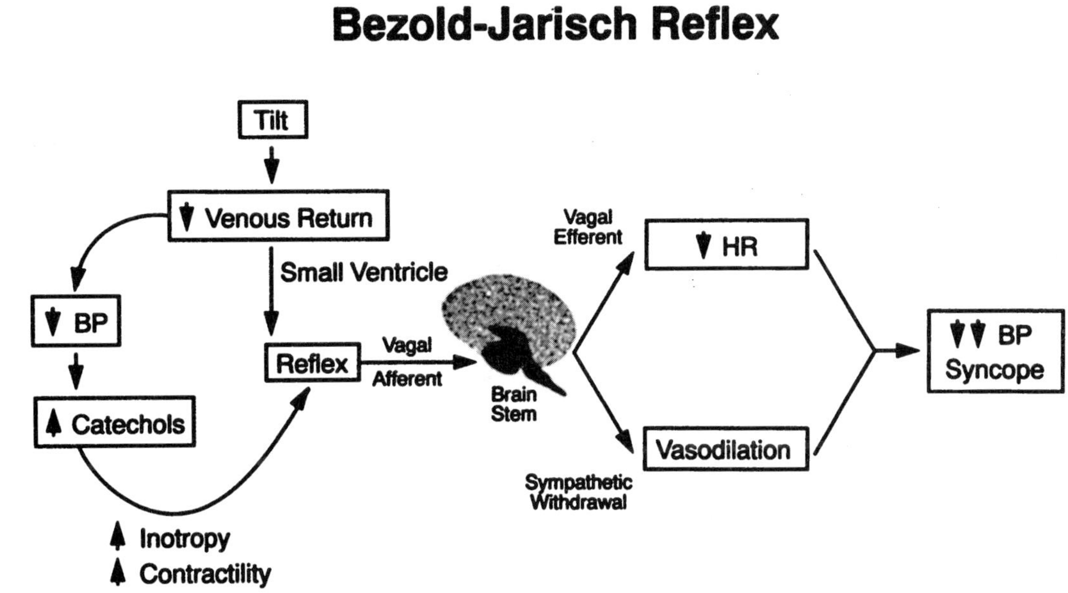

FIGURE 14–4. A summary of the reflex initiated by release of catecholamines or decreased circulating volume and resulting in bradycardia and/or hypotension. (BP, blood pressure; HR, heart rate.) From Kanter RJ: Syncope and sudden death in children. In Garson A, Bricker T, Fisher D, Neish S (eds): The Science and Practice of Pediatric Cardiology, 2nd ed. Baltimore, Williams & Wilkins, 1998. Used with permission.

distant or have a ringing quality. This is generally unpleasant to most patients, but fear or apprehension is inconstant. Nausea or dizziness may also occur but, if prominent, should raise the suspicion of a migraine variant. Less specific symptoms that may confuse the picture are headache or palpitations. Although palpitations usually represent the sinus tachycardia caused by cardiac sympathetic hypersensitivity, we usually will lend such a patient an event recorder that has "memory" to be certain a pathologic tachycardia is not occurring. Symptoms may occur while sitting or standing, but characteristically occur after at least minutes of a change in posture. Similar symptoms that occur within seconds of standing represent orthostatic hypotension and usually requires only reassurance and the recommendation that the patient arise more slowly and near a supportive object.

Some patients faint without warning, and this will more likely lead to head injury. When this occurs while in a sitting position, the physician must be particularly careful to disallow driving by the teenager until the problem has been completely controlled for a significant period; we recommend 6 months.

After the patient has fainted, the observation of tonic posturing or clonic jerks within 10 seconds suggests the occurrence of the "malignant asystolic or cardiodecelorator form" of neurally mediated syncope. Assumption of a reclined position results in spontaneous resumption of consciousness, even in these patients. Although they may experience continued fatigue, weakness, or nausea because of ongoing parasympathetic effects, they are usually lucid and appropriate almost immediately. Patients with epilepsy will often have an aura before losing consciousness, and they are more likely to have a period of confusion after the seizure. The observation by a parent or schoolmate that the child appeared dazed or had a "blank look on their face" before fainting strongly suggests a primary seizure. The occurrence of a headache after the event is a nonspecific finding, although migraine disease would then become a greater consideration.

The nomenclature used to describe the cardiovascular changes observed refers to the "cardioinhibitory" form of neurally mediated syncope as primary severe bradycardia, "vasodepressor" form as primary hypotension with minimal drop in heart rate, and mixed form as having features of both cardiodecelerator and vasodepressor forms. Although Sutton et al provided specific heart rate and blood pressure values for classifying the different cardiovascular responses in adults,[133] such criteria may not be appropriate for children. Using head-upright tilt study data from 20 young patients 7 to 22 years old, Pongiglione et al defined the cardioinhibitory form based on 3 patients with maximum pauses of 6.5 to 11 seconds, the vasodepressor form based on 2 patients with a mean blood pressure less than or equal to 38 mm Hg but a heart rate no less than 135 bpm during isoproterenol infusion, and the mixed form based on 11 patients with a mean blood pressure of less than or equal to 54 mm Hg and a heart rate of 50 to 103 bpm.[129] Differentiating one form from the other does not seem to be of great clinical importance.

Breath-holding spells of the toddler age group deserves additional comments. Most first episodes occur before 18 months, and all by 3½ years. Anger, pain, fear, or frustration initiates the spell. As initially described by Lombroso and Lermana[134] and Laxdol et al,[135] two types of breath-holding spells exist: so-called cyanotic type and pallid type. In cyanotic spells, a period of intense crying precedes apnea and cyanosis, and there is associated sinus tachycardia.[134] In pallid spells, there is usually only a brief cry or startle followed by syncope, often with tonic postural changes or clonic jerks. Given the history alone, long QT syndrome–related ventricular tachycardia must be considered. In pallid breath-holders, there is usually associated asystole (Fig. 14–5); this is an infantile form of cardioinhibitory neurally mediated syncope. This is almost always a self-limited event, although status epilepticus has been reported in a few children in whom a family history of epilepsy also existed.[136] Pallid breath-holders are more likely to grow up and have neurally mediated syncope[4] but are not at increased risk of developmental delay.[135] Therefore, therapy is only of value in these youngsters if events are frequent enough to disrupt family dynamics or day care provisions or if injury occurs. Belladonna has been used[135]; we have experienced success with fludrocortisone and with beta-adrenergic blocking agents; and there is a report of toddlers successfully treated with artificial pacing.[137]

Insight into the personal profiles of young persons prone to faint at the sight or thought of injury or blood was provided by Kleinknecht.[138] On the basis of data from 429 college students (average age, 19.45 years), 14.5% had a history of such an event. Affected individuals were more likely to have a positive family history. Fainters were more likely to acknowledge such a fear; they had greater anxiety sensitivity; and they had overall greater personal distress than nonfainters.

ECG correlates in children with neurally mediated syncope reflect the extent of parasympathetic influence. The cardioinhibitory form is associated with sinus arrest, high-grade AV block, complete AV block, and junctional bradycardia. Salim and DiSessa showed that the QTc interval prolongs more during upright tilt in tilt-positive versus tilt-negative children, but that it shortens appropriately during and after exercise.[139] They concluded that the QTc interval prolongation is vagally mediated and only during postural change.

Other Forms of Neurally Mediated Reflexive Syncope

Swallow or deglutition syncope is a well-established entity in adults and is usually related to esophageal pathology, parapharyngeal space lesions, or glossopharyngeal neuralgia, but may exist in the absence of other abnormalities. Although it is uncommon in the young, it has even been described in a normal infant.[140] Swallow syncope manifests as presyncope or syncope associated with swallowing and with swallowing exceptionally warm or cold substances or even at the sight of food. The afferent limb of this reflex is probably cross-talk within the medulla from esophageal afferent fibers, and the efferent response is mostly vagal with sinus bradycardia, sinus arrest, or varying degrees of AV block.[140–142] In one report, it was suggested that there is a hereditary component.[140] This is not a self-limited disorder in children and has been successfully treated with parasympatholytic drugs, surgical selective cardiac vagotomy, or permanent cardiac pacing.[141, 143]

Paroxysms of coughing may be accompanied by giddiness, dizziness, or syncope. "Cough syncope" usually occurs in middle-aged patients with chronic lung disease, but may occur in children with asthma or croup. There have been several proposed mechanisms for syncope: increased cerebrospinal fluid pressure and diminished cerebral blood flow caused by sudden high intrathoracic and intracerebral pressures; reflex peripheral vasodilatation; a "super-Valsalva maneuver," which briefly diminishes cardiac output; and reflex hypervagotonia, as suggested by cases of associated intranodal type II second-degree and complete AV block.[144]

Micturition syncope is defined as syncope occurring just before, during, or just after voiding. It occurs in persons of all ages from adolescents to the elderly.[145] Younger patients tend to be male, and predisposing factors include reduced food intake, recent upper respiratory infection, fatigue, and alcohol ingestion.[146] Events usually occur in the early evening or when voiding after awakening from sleep and, hence, immediately after a recumbent position. In the younger patients, syncope has little or no warning and oc-

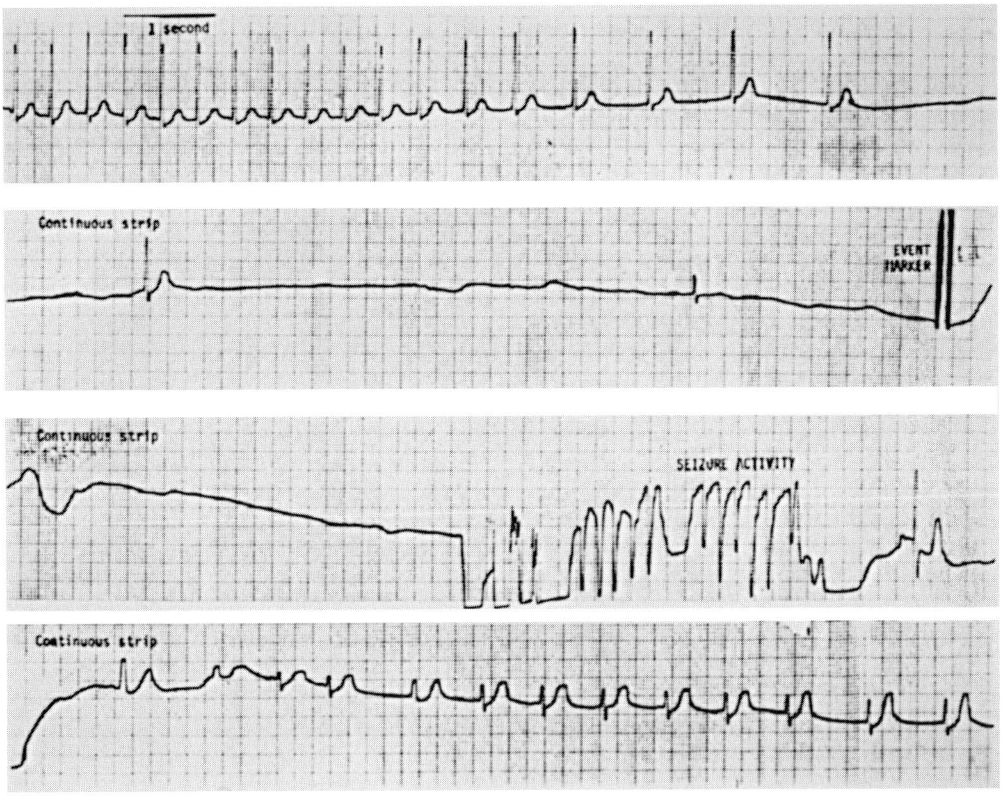

FIGURE 14–5. A continuous rhythm strip from an ambulatory event recorder in an 18-month old during a pallid breath-holding spell. Illustrated is a period of asystole, followed by motion artifact from seizure activity and resumption of a supraventricular escape rhythm.

curs during or just after completion of the void.[146] Recurrences are uncommon, and patients rarely have other forms of syncope.[146] The causes for micturition syncope are unknown and perhaps differ at different ages. Proposed mechanisms include vagal stimulation with cardioinhibition, visceral afferent stimulation by a full bladder, and postural hypotension to name a few. Treatment is seldom necessary because episodes in teenagers tend to be solitary.

Syncope or presyncope during defecation has multiple potential causes, including gastrointestinal, cardiovascular, and cerebrovascular. To our knowledge, its repeated occurrence beginning in childhood has only been described in one instance: in a 25-year-old woman whose symptoms began at 6 years of age and in whom recurrences abated after resection of Meckel's diverticulum.[147]

"Hair-grooming syncope" occurs mostly in girls while combing, brushing, or blow drying their hair. It is mentioned separately from postural neurally mediated syncope because other mechanisms have also been suggested, including stimulation of the trigeminal nerve during scalp stimulation, compression of carotid baroreceptors, or impedance of vertebrobasilar blood flow during neck flexion or extension.[148] In our experience, this simply represents a common clinical setting for neurally mediated syncope in patients who usually just stepped out of a warm bath or shower and are already vasodilated. When tested, they generally have a positive tilt study. Therapy may be limited to better hydration and "cooling off" before hair grooming.

Carotid sinus hypersensitivity is estimated to occur in 10% of mostly older adults.[149] Syncope results from vagally mediated sinus bradycardia or arrest or AV block in response to sometimes minimal pressure on the carotid sinus. Three cases of carotid sinus hypersensitivity in teenagers have been reported, including a wrestler during competition[150] and in another boy during tightening of an orthodontic cervical appliance.[151]

Other less common scenarios for syncope include "stretch-yawn syncope" and "weight lifter's blackout." Syncope induced by stretching with the neck extended occasionally occurs in teenagers. The proposed mechanism of so-called stretch-yawn syncope has been thought to be reduced venous return during the Valsalva maneuver portion of the stretch. However, Pelekanos et al reported the results of autonomic evaluations, including quantitative Valsalva maneuver, from six affected teenagers at rest and during a controlled stretch.[152] Only when the stretch was performed with neck extended was there a difference between patients and controls. The authors concluded that impaired posterior cerebral circulation during neck hyperextension is at least part of the pathophysiology leading to syncope. In all patients, subsequent symptoms were avoided by stretching without neck extension. Weight lifter's blackout refers to presyncope or syncope during squatting and the clean and jerk lift. On the basis of intraesophageal and intra-arterial pressure monitoring during lifting by national representative weight lifters from New Zealand,[153] a transient but severe fall in arterial pressure follows marked intrathoracic pressure elevation, comprising a "super-Valsalva maneuver" and easily accounting for risk of syncope.

Finally, iatrogenic syncope results from severe sinus bradycardia or AV block secondary to visceral stretch and vagal afferent stimulation. This typically occurs during oro- or nasotracheal intubation, placement of a nasogastric tube or esophageal pacing catheter, pleural or peritoneal effusion or irritation, sudden distention of viscera, and even placement of vascular catheters or pressure over the femoral vessels. The immediate circumstances surrounding the loss of consciousness help make the diagnosis. This may be treated or prevented with intravenous atropine, 0.01 mg/kg.

ORTHOSTATIC SYNCOPE AND THE DYSAUTONOMIAS

When a person stands, the cardiac output and cerebral arterial blood pressure are normally maintained by a combination of mechanical pumping action by skeletal muscles on venous return, one-way venous valves favoring return to the right atrium, baroreflex-mediated arterial constriction, and cerebral autoregulation. If stroke volume is still not maintained, reflex sinus tachycardia will occur. In orthostatic hypotension, compensatory responses are inadequate, and, despite sinus tachycardia, there is reduction in brain perfusion, resulting in symptoms. Before loss of consciousness, these symptoms include a sensation of fullness in the head, weakness, and visual changes. Many of the other symptoms associated with neurally mediated syncope are absent in these patients. Orthostatic hypotension as a cause for syncope is suggested by an inappropriate drop in blood pressure with compensatory rise in heart rate during supine-to-standing vital signs. During tilt table testing, the sinus tachycardia coinciding with hypotension is proportionately greater than the heart rate changes occurring in the vasodepressor form of neurally mediated syncope.

Hypovolemia is the most frequent predisposing condition for orthostatic hypotension, and may be caused by severe and ongoing diarrhea or vomiting, marked diaphoresis, primary adrenal insufficiency, hemorrhage, overuse of diuretics, diabetes insipidus, hemodialysis, or heat injury. In these patients, the tendency to faint is made worse by the coexistence of chronic anemia.

Impairment of vascular tone with syncope may occur as a sign of rare conditions, such as hyperbradykininism[154] or systemic mastocytosis.[155] In these diseases, concomitant signs and symptoms, including characteristic rashes, are of diagnostic value.

Diseases of the spinal cord or peripheral nerves may interfere with sympathetic reflex mechanisms and are uncommon causes of orthostatic syncope. They include syringomyelia, Arnold-Chiari malformation,[156] autonomic neuropathy of poorly controlled diabetes mellitus,[157] acute intermittent porphyria, Guillain-Barré syndrome, and other peripheral neuropathies. Patients with syringomyelia may have other sometimes subtle neurologic defects, and syncope caused by mild forms of Arnold-Chiari malformation is usually associated with coughing or certain head movements.[156] Familial dysautonomia, or Riley-Day syndrome, is characterized by abnormal sweating, labile hypertension, postural hypotension, absent lacrimation, and episodic fevers. Signs of this disease begin in infancy, and patients rarely survive to adulthood.

Many drugs interfere with sympathetic vasomotor response or cause direct vasodilatation or excessive venous pooling with hypotension. These include calcium channel blockers, angiotensin-converting enzyme inhibitors, nitrates and nitroglycerin, guanethidine, hydralazine, and phenothiazines. Centrally acting antihypertensive drugs such as methyldopa and clonidine produce only mild orthostatic hypotension. Beta-blocking agents do not produce postural hypotension, although one patient with idiopathic orthostatic hypotension was made worse by atenolol.

Idiopathic orthostatic hypotension may occasionally occur in teenagers. This diagnosis is made only after all other causes of orthostatic hypotension have been ruled out. Treatment options include volume expansion with fludrocortisone and a high-fluid, high-sodium diet; moderate pressure support stockings; and alpha-sympathetic drugs such as pseudoephedrine.

Finally, prolonged bed rest and cachexia predispose patients to orthostatic hypotension.

NORMOTENSIVE SYNCOPE FROM CENTRAL NERVOUS SYSTEM EVENTS

Transient loss of consciousness as part of a seizure or as part of a migraine attack may be difficult to discriminate from neurally mediated syncope. Conversely, symptoms of headache, dizziness, nausea, and visual field changes from neurally mediated syncope can mimic migraine disease; and brief but severe cerebral hypoxia during the cardioinhibitory form of neurally mediated syncope can cause a seizure. Hence, discriminating these entities may challenge the pediatric neurologist and cardiologist.

Hoafnegels et al compared the signs and symptoms from 41 patients with seizures and loss of consciousness with those from 53 patients with other causes of syncope.[158] The best discriminatory finding was normal orientation after the event in the syncope but not the seizure patients. Nausea or sweating before the event tended to exclude seizure patients. Incontinence and fall-induced trauma were nondiscriminatory findings. An auditory, visual, olfactory, or gustatory sensation; vague abdominal discomfort; or automatism may precede a seizure. A prolonged clonic seizure after the patient is recumbent is not expected in a primary syncopal event. The blood pressure and heart rate tend to be elevated during seizures, although sinus bradycardia with syncope has been reported as part of otherwise typical partial epilepsy.[159] Finally, an abnormal electroencephalogram may be abnormal during the postictal period in seizure but not in syncope patients.[160]

Migraine disease, when it affects the vertebrobasilar arterial system, occasionally causes loss of consciousness as a result of impaired circulation to the reticular activating system. Proximate involvement of the eighth cranial nucleus may cause tinnitus, vertigo, or other "aura" just before the faint. Vital signs do not change during the syncopal period. Occipital or lateral headache is the rule after the event, but this is a particularly nonspecific symptom. A family history of migraine disease is of value. The clinical spectrum of syncope in migraine appears to overlap neurally mediated syncope. In a series of 500 migraine patients, Lance and Anthony found that 12.2% suffered presyncope or syncope with attacks,[161] and Raskin and Knittle found that 40 of 59 migraine patients presented with hypotensive symptoms related to upright posture.[162] Cortelli et al[163] observed that norepinephrine levels rose less than for controls during tilt testing of patients during migraine episodes, similar to children with neurally mediated syncope, but tilt testing increased norepinephrine levels normally between attacks in these patients. Hence, there is increasing evidence for a defective noradrenergic nervous system in migraine patients.

Narcolepsy is an uncommon condition that usually begins in the second decade and presents as excessive and inappropriate periods of sleep during the day. This may be associated with sudden fright- or emotion-induced loss of postural tone, known as cataplexy. Although this may closely mimic syncope, there is no loss of consciousness. Periods of sleepiness without cataplexy, a family history of narcolepsy, response to verbal stimuli during attacks, and certain human leukocyte antigen types make this diagnosis.

Other diseases that affect the brain may cause loss of consciousness and are suggested by the history, physical exam, and coexisting signs. They include head trauma, intracranial hemorrhage, cerebral vasculitis, and hydrocephalus with shunt malfunction.

DRUGS

Pharmacologic agents cause syncope by causing cardiac arrhythmias, vasodilatation, direct central nervous system depression, or a combination of these. Drugs that prolong the QT interval may predispose to torsades de pointes ventricular tachycardia and cause sudden death. "Quinidine syncope" in children has been well researched and is especially hazardous with coexisting bradycardia and hypokalemia.[164] Proarrhythmic effects of other antiarrhythmic drugs include other kinds of ventricular tachycardia and various types of conduction block. Agents causing severe sinus bradycardia or AV block include overdose of digoxin, beta-adrenergic blocking drugs, or carbamazepine.[165] Fluoxetine is a nontricyclic antidepressant and has caused bradycardia-induced syncope in young adults.[166] This is of special importance because of current interest in its therapeutic effects in neurally mediated syncope.

Hallucinogens, barbiturates, and opiates may cause syncope with or without hypotension. In adolescents, cocaine use has been reported to cause loss of consciousness in 2% of light users, 7% of intermediate users, and 27% of heavy users.[167]

PSYCHIATRIC ETIOLOGIES FOR SYNCOPE

Hyperventilation syndrome, sometimes as part of panic disorder, is characterized by rapid and often deep breathing with chest tightness, a smothering sensation, and palpitations. When hypocapnia ensues, there will be circumoral and hand paresthesias and eventually syncope because of cerebral vasoconstriction. Episodes last up to 30 minutes with mild sinus tachycardia and fluctuation in blood pressure. The coexistence of other signs of panic attacks and the ability to reproduce these symptoms during voluntary hyperventilation help make the diagnosis. Although teenagers with hyperventilation syndrome sometimes require psychiatric intervention, we have observed this entity secondary to neurally mediated presyncope; successful management of the primary problem has usually been sufficient.

Epidemic hysteria has been reported many times in the literature of this century. It characteristically involves adolescent girls, generally during a state of stress, and usually when they are in close proximity with others. It has been reported several times among high school marching band members.[168] Associated signs before syncope among affected patients have inconsistently included hyperventilation.[168, 169] Whether these events represent mass hysteria (implying conversion reaction) or mass hyperventilation is unclear.

Conversion reactions also affect females more than males and, to the observer, appear similar to syncopal episodes. The patient tends to not injure herself and usually has episodes only in the presence of others. Patients typically have no premonitory symptoms and usually provide an unemotional and unconcerned description of the event. Episodes may occur many times in succession during a single day. They may be reproduced during tilt table testing, during which time heart rate, blood pressure, and electroencephalogram are normal.[170] Unresponsiveness continues despite return to supine position and may persist for many minutes. Affected teenagers require psychiatric intervention.

Finally, patients with malingering and Munchausen syndrome may choose apparent syncope as their method of health care access.

METABOLIC ETIOLOGIES FOR SYNCOPE

Impairment of substrates to the brain despite a normal cardiovascular system occurs in the presence of hypoxia, acute anemia, or hypoglycemia. Individuals who move to a high altitude are at risk of hypoxia-related syncope until they acclimate. Hypoglycemic syncope is preceded by weakness, pallor, diaphoresis, hunger, and palpitations. This is an overdiagnosed cause of syncope, except in patients receiving hypoglycemic agents, such as children with diabetes mellitus, and in individuals with rare inborn errors of metabolism.

Intrinsic or extrinsic toxins may cause loss of consciousness, although this is usually not sudden. Hyperammonemia may cause loss of consciousness, usually after nausea and vomiting, in certain older individuals with mild forms of urea cycle defects. Any cause of metabolic acidosis or hypercalcemia will reduce the level of consciousness, although this is gradual. Consideration of these entities should be reserved for discussions of coma, not syncope.

SYNCOPE IN YOUNG ATHLETES

Young persons who faint during physical exertion require a comprehensive evaluation because of the relatively high likelihood that this symptom represents a severe drop in cardiac output resulting from a condition that could at some time be fatal. The conditions that tend to cause symptoms during physical stress and that may present with episodes of syncope before a fatal event include hypertrophic cardiomyopathy, congenital coronary artery malformations, arrhythmogenic right ventricular dysplasia, and primary conduction system abnormalities.[171–173] In our institution, the evaluation of such a patient includes a complete history and physical examination, 12-lead ECG, treadmill exercise test, 24-hour ambulatory ECG, signal-averaged ECG, echocardiogram, electrophysiologic study, selective coronary angiography, and, if warranted, ventriculography and endomyocardial biopsy.

There are ECG and echocardiographic changes that normally occur in some conditioned adolescent and young adult athletes. Understanding that these adaptations are not pathologic will prevent unnecessary additional testing or withholding the athlete from sports participation. ECG changes may include tall, notched, or elongated P waves[174]; first-degree AV block (8–45%)[175–177]; type I second-degree AV block (6–40%)[178–181]; left ventricular hypertrophy[182]; incomplete right bundle branch block (16%)[183]; elevation or depression of ST segments and peaking or inversion of T waves[184, 185]; QTc interval prolongation[181]; sinus bradycardia and pauses up

2.8 seconds[178–180]; atrial premature depolarizations (41–100%)[178–181]; complex ventricular premature depolarizations (12.5–20%)[178–181]; and ventricular tachycardia (2–7.5%).[178, 179, 181] Most of these ECG changes, especially repolarization changes, normalize during treadmill testing or isoproterenol infusion. Presyncope during second-degree AV block, even if it is only due to high vagal tone, may require attention. Episodes of ventricular tachycardia, even if asymptomatic, are worthy of further evaluation.

The left ventricular mass and chamber dimensions, as determined echocardiographically, is increased in dynamically trained athletes.[186] Discrimination of the trained heart from that of someone with hypertrophic cardiomyopathy is the task of the cardiologist. Unlike the heart with pathologic hypertrophic cardiomyopathy, the normally adapted heart will have symmetry of the septum and posterior wall (ratio 1.3), an interventricular septal-to-early systolic diameter ratio of less than 0.5, normal Doppler mitral inflow, and normalization of ventricular wall thickness (< 1.3 cm) after deconditioning.[187] Except for isometrically trained athletes, the left ventricular cavity will usually not be small, unlike the reduced cavity seen in patients with hypertrophic cardiomyopathy.

Once potentially dangerous conditions have been ruled out, consideration of autonomically mediated cardiovascular changes is appropriate. Normally, during early exercise, vagal withdrawal precedes a gradual increase in sympathetic tone. On discontinuation of exercise, a relatively sudden return of vagal influences occurs with only gradual reduction of catecholamine levels. Variability of these responses is based on loading conditions and degree of fitness. Heart rate recovery is generally faster after exercise in athletes because of enhanced vagal tone.[188] Extreme vagotonia immediately on discontinuation of exercise has been shown to cause asystolic syncope in young adult athletes.[189–191] The possible contribution of catecholamine-mediated ventricular mechanoreceptor stimulation has also been suggested as a mechanism.[192] In otherwise asymptomatic teenage athletes whose symptoms start immediately after discontinuation of activity, one generally proceeds first to tilt table testing and not to more invasive studies.

Exercise-induced pure vasodepressor syncope has been demonstrated in two teenagers by reproduction of symptoms with an associated drop in blood pressure during treadmill testing.[193] Grubb et al[194] reported on 24 young athletes (mean age, 18 years) with recurrent exercise-induced syncope. Nineteen experienced syncope with associated hypotension during head-upright tilt table testing compared with none of 10 asymptomatic athletes.[194] They concluded that this test was useful in the diagnosis of vasovagal syncope in young athletes with recurrent exercise-related syncope.

Treatment of autonomically mediated hypotension or asystole during or immediately after exercise may consist of fludrocortisone with an increase in sodium and fluid intake, because beta-adrenergic blocking agents are poorly tolerated by athletes. Some marathon runners have opted for pacemaker implantation so that they may continue to compete.

In a case report of an adult with exercise-induced high-grade AV block, Hurwitz et al[195] illustrated the point that conditioning-related vagotonia may unmask underlying cardiac conduction system abnormalities. This may occasionally occur in adolescents who underwent successful congenital heart surgery in early childhood and are later able to compete in high level sports.

EVALUATION OF THE PATIENT WITH SYNCOPE

HISTORY

A careful history from the child or teenager who has had a syncopal episode and from family members and witnesses of the event is usually of great value. A practitioner with a busy practice who does not see the patient promptly will usually lose valuable historic information, because recall by observers diminishes greatly over time. The existence of known medical problems must be sought first, especially cardiac disease, neurologic disease, diabetes mellitus, hematologic disease, psychiatric conditions, and the use of drugs that may cause dehydration, heart rhythm disturbances, hypotension, or mental status changes.

All symptoms before and after the event and any witnessed signs during the event should be determined. The patient and family should be questioned about his or her recent fluid, drug, and food intake; emotional upset or discord with a family member or friend; and whether the episode occurred during or just after exertion. The practitioner should try to ascertain the patient's body position at the time of the faint, whether there was recent head trauma, and whether the patient injured him- or herself during the faint. He or she should be specifically asked whether the episode was associated with stretching, coughing, swallowing, urination, or defecation. The older teenager must be specifically asked whether these symptoms have ever occurred while driving or otherwise seated. Premonitory symptoms of palpitations, lightheadedness, headaches, visual changes, hearing deficits, tinnitus, vertigo, nausea, a sensation of warmth, diaphoresis, hyperventilation, and any aura (visual, gustatory, auditory, or vague abdominal sensations) should be questioned. Observers of the event should be asked several key questions. Did the patient lose postural tone forcefully or more gracefully? Was there associated pallor, tonic posturing, clonic jerking, eye deviation, facial expressions representing automatisms, or incontinence? What was the exact sequence of the events? After the event, the patient and observers should describe the time course of recovery of mental orientation; the presence of neurologic symptoms or signs or bodily injury; and the occurrence (or recurrence) of headaches, weakness, fatigue, nausea, diaphoresis, or perception of bradycardia or tachycardia. Repetition of syncopal events should be specifically determined, because conversion reactions may occur in rapid sequence over a day's time. During the interview, the patient's overall level of concern as well as mood and affect should also be assessed. Other medical history questions should include the presence of chronic disease, occurrence of palpitations, chest pain, head trauma, chest trauma, headaches, illicit drug use, and dietary pattern. The clinical signs and symptoms surrounding syncope associated with selective causative entities appear in abridged form in Table 14–4.

Cardiopulmonary resuscitation is sometimes started by persons who witness an individual having the asystolic form of reflexive syncope (some episodes of vasovagal, deglutition, or micturition syncope). Although these episodes are nearly always self-limited once the patient becomes supine, the label of "resuscitated sudden death" sometimes is applied anyway. In these individuals, the history surrounding the event is especially important, so that an extensive and potentially unnecessary workup may be avoided. The duration of asystole, even in these patients, may be important because an occasional young person has such prolonged vagally mediated asystole-bradycardia that permanent pacing may be advisable. If the history is not completely compatible with one of the reflexive causes of syncope mentioned previously, and a reliable witness has seen fit to initiate cardiopulmonary resuscitation for pulselessness or for marked tachycardia, then a comprehensive evaluation is mandated. A family history of syncope, seizures, or sudden death is also critically important.

PHYSICAL EXAMINATION

The heart rate, blood pressure, and respiratory rate should be noted, and the heart rate and respiratory rate counted for 1 minute. If a patient is being seen immediately after a syncopal event, supine and upright vital signs will demonstrate orthostatic changes if dehydration is present. The physical examination should concentrate on the cardiovascular and neurologic components. Abnormalities of the heart rhythm, presence of any murmurs, changes in the quality of murmurs with handgrip and Valsalva maneuvers, very reduced heart sounds, a loud S_2, or any focal neurologic signs are especially valuable findings. However, most children and teenagers who faint will have a normal physical examination between episodes.

LABORATORY EXAMINATION

The laboratory examination should be guided by the results of the history and physical examination. Clinical intuition will dictate a logical sequence of testing when the syncopal patient is known to have a specific condition. For example, the young diabetic should undergo scrupulous blood glucose testing; the pregnant teenager should have orthostatic blood pressures measured; and postmenarchal females should have a hemoglobin concentration measured to rule out unsuspected anemia. Further evaluation and definitive treatment are required in children known to have structural cardiac disease or arrhythmias and who faint, because they represent the highest risk patients. Definitive therapy for each condition appears elsewhere in this textbook.

An ECG should be obtained in all patients with new-onset syncope. This inexpensive test is most definitive in the presence of WPW syndrome, long QT syndrome, high-grade ventricular ectopy, complete AV block, left bundle branch block, and extremes of sinus, atrial, or junctional rates. However, moderate sinus arrhythmia, moderate sinus bradycardia, simple junctional rhythm, unifocal ventricular premature beats, and right bundle branch block are relatively nonspecific and may not be related to the syncopal event. In Table 14–5, a logical approach to the child with one of these common and less specific ECG findings is offered. If the screening ECG is normal but the history still suggests an arrhythmic source for syncope, or the relationship of a nonspecific ECG abnormality to symptoms is unclear, an ambulatory ECG event recorder should be lent to the patient. Pocket-sized mod-

Table 14–4. Clinical Presentation of Selected Causes of Syncope

DIAGNOSIS	CIRCUMSTANCES	OTHER DISEASES	PREMONITORY SYMPTOMS	SYNCOPE: Description	SYNCOPE: HR	SYNCOPE: BP	SYNCOPE: Risk of SD	POST EVENT SYMPTOMS
Neurally Mediated								
Postural-emotional	Emotional stress; upright for minutes	None	Light-headedness; dizziness; weakness; vision changes; palpitations; diaphoresis	Pallor; seizure (late); incontinence	↓; NC	↓	0	Weakness; nausea; headache; diaphoresis
Deglutition	Swallowing	None in children	Light-headedness or none	Pallor; seizure (late)	↓	↓	0	Occasional weakness; nausea
Cough	Paroxysm of coughing	Asthma; croup	Light-headedness or none	No other signs	NC	NC	0	Rare
Micturition	During or after void; evening	None	None; light-headedness	Pallor	↓	↓	0	Occasional weakness; nausea
Orthostatic	Standing	Addison's disease; pregnancy; drugs; bed rest	Light-headedness; vision changes; palpitations	Pallor	↑	↓	0	Recur if upright
Neurologic								
Seizure	Flashing lights; music; any	Neurologic; after trauma	Aura; déjà vu; none	Seizure (early); incontinence; cyanotic; stertorous breathing	↑; NC; (↓)	↑; NC; (↓)	+	Confusion; headache; neurologic defect
Migraine	Any	None	Headache; vertigo; none	No other signs	NC	NC	0	Headache

Table continued on following page

Table 14–4. Clinical Presentation of Selected Causes of Syncope *Continued*

DIAGNOSIS	CIRCUMSTANCES	OTHER DISEASES	PREMONITORY SYMPTOMS	SYNCOPE				POST EVENT SYMPTOMS
				Description	**HR**	**BP**	**Risk of SD**	
Psychiatric								
Hyperventilation	Anxiety; sports	None; neuroses	Chest tightness; feeling of suffocation; paresthesias; palpitations	Continued hyperpnea; tachypnea	NC; ↓	NC; ↓	0	Lethargic; none
Conversion	In presence of audience	Psychiatric	None; or any	No response to pain; avoidance eye movements to light	NC	NC	0	None
Cardiac								
HCM	Exercise; any		Chest pain; palpitations; shortness of breath; light-headedness; none	Pallor; seizure (late)	NC; ↑	↓	+	Lethargic or none
Coronary artery abnormality	Exercise		Chest pain; shortness of breath; none	Pallor; seizure (late)	↑	↓	+	Lethargic or none
Inflow obstruction	Dehydration		Light-headedness; palpitations; none	Pallor	↑	↓	+	Lethargic or none
Arrhythmic	Exercise; emotional stress; any	R/O structural heart disease; myocarditis; none	Palpitations; shortness of breath; chest pain; light-headedness; none	Pallor; seizure (late)	↑; ↓	↓	+	Lethargic or none
Metabolic								
Hypoglycemia	Lack of food; too much insulin	Diabetes mellitus; nonketotic in toddlers	Diaphoresis; weakness; hunger; palpitations	Pallor; seizure	↑	NC	+	Not relieved by reclined position
Hypoxia	Breath holding; altitude	None; chronic lung disease	Shortness of breath; light-headedness; palpitations	Cyanotic	↑	↑; ↓	+	Lethargic or none

HCM, hypertrophic cardiomyopathy; NC, no change; ↓, decrease; ↑, increase; +, positive; HR, heart rate; SD, sudden death; BP, blood pressure.

From Kanter RJ: Syncope and sudden death in children. In Garson A, Bricker JT, Fisher DJ, Neish SR (eds): The Science and Practice of Pediatric Cardiology, 2nd ed. Baltimore, Williams & Wilkins, 1998. Used with permission.

Table 14–5. Management of Children with Non-Specific Electrocardiographic Abnormalities

REST ECG FINDING	CONCERN FOR THIS ARRHYTHMIA	SCREENING TEST	OUTCOME SUGGESTING BENIGN RHYTHM	OUTCOME SUGGESTING NEED FOR DEFINITIVE TEST OR TREATMENT
Marked sinus or junctional bradycardia (or marked sinus arrhythmia)	Sinus node dysfunction	Loop monitor when symptomatic Exercise test	Acceptable rate when symptomatic Adequate rate response	Severe sinus bradycardia when symptomatic Inadequate rate response (especially with symptoms)
Type I second-degree AV block	Intermittent third-degree AV block	Loop monitor when symptomatic	Normal AV conduction	Higher grade AV block
Frequent unifocal PVCs	Ventricular tachycardia	Exercise test	Suppression of ectopy	Higher grade of ectopy or ventricular tachycardia
Mild prolongation QTc interval (0.44–0.48 s)	Torsades de pointes ventricular tachycardia	Exercise test	Shortening QTc during early recovery; normal sinus rate response	Longer QTc during early recovery; inadequate sinus rate response

AV, atrioventricular; ECG, electrocardiogram; PVCs, premature ventricular contractions.
From Kanter RJ: Syncope and sudden death in children. In Garson A, Bricker JT, Fisher DJ, Neish SR (eds): The Science and Practice of Pediatric Cardiology, 2nd ed. Baltimore, Williams & Wilkins, 1998. Used with permission.

els may be conveniently carried by older children and teenagers and applied to the bare chest during premonitory symptoms or by a companion during syncope. Continuously attached "loop recorders" provide even higher yield to rule in or rule out an arrhythmic source.[196] These are less well tolerated by children because they are continuously attached but will record data from a period of time before activation. Therefore, late activation by a recovering patient or by a companion will still permit reliable rhythm acquisition.

An echocardiogram should be reserved for patients with previously known heart disease, pathologic heart murmurs, evidence of chamber enlargement by ECG or chest radiograph, repolarization abnormalities consistent with ischemia or "strain," ventricular ectopy, or historic features compatible with cardiomyopathy or myocarditis.

Treadmill or other exercise tests have limited application for the syncopal child. We use such tests for the conditioned athlete who faints while at rest and who has nonspecific ECG abnormalities to determine whether they will normalize with exercise. Children with borderline prolonged QTc interval (0.44–0.46 seconds) may have characteristic changes during exercise testing if they do have the long QT syndrome: subnormal sinus rate response to maximum effort and prolongation of QTc interval in early recovery (when it should normally be shorter than it was at baseline because of persistent beta-adrenergic influence). Ventricular ectopy of a benign nature ordinarily suppresses with exercise, but may worsen if it is catecholamine dependent, uses a triggered mechanism, or is related to myocarditis or cardiomyopathy. Exercise testing may be of value in children with first-degree, second-degree, or variable AV block to determine what their ventricular rate response is to higher sinus rates. Despite vagolysis and a high catecholamine state, some such patients worsen their degree of block and even produce symptoms of syncope or presyncope. Finally, children with pacemakers may demonstrate atrial undersensing, myopotential sensing, or ventricular noncapture during exercise testing.

Thoughtful application of these outpatient tests to the previously healthy child who faints will identify nearly all cardiac causes of syncope, except for those with an anomalous coronary artery and those with mild forms of arrhythmogenic right ventricular dysplasia and a normal baseline ECG. Children with coronary artery anomalies, in particular, generally have symptoms only during exertion.

The role of invasive electrophysiologic testing for adult patients with syncope has evolved over the last 10 years. Denes and Ezri[197] and Olshansky et al[198] originally reported that electrophysiologic testing uncovered inducible supraventricular and ventricular tachycardia in 20% and 35% of adults with unexplained syncope, respectively. More recently, however, Bachinsky et al[199] identified the presence of organic heart disease, VPBs, sinus bradycardia, first-degree AV block, bundle branch block, and nonsustained ventricular tachycardia by Holter monitoring as the only pretest findings that predicted a high yield from electrophysiologic testing. Similar reports on children are not available. We reserve electrophysiologic testing for children and teenagers with syncope during exertion or syncope at rest plus (1) known cardiac disease that has any associated risk of tachyarrhythmia; (2) nonsustained or sustained wide-complex tachycardia by ambulatory monitoring or regular ECG; (3) nonsustained or sustained SVT (including atrial flutter) for radiofrequency ablation; or (4) WPW syndrome. It may also be of value to elucidate further conduction characteristics in children with AV block or sick sinus syndrome in preparation for pacemaker implantation, but ambulatory event monitoring is required to correlate syncope with a bradycardiac rhythm. Finally, there is the rare patient who ultimately requires electrophysiologic testing after complete cardiac, neurologic, and psychiatric evaluations are negative, and the patient either does not have typical neurally mediated syncope or does not respond to therapy for that condition.

Because of advances in ambulatory ECG monitoring plus a trend toward reduced inpatient management of diagnostic problems, fewer children with the primary complaint of syncope are currently hospitalized. Hospitalization is required if there is a high suspicion that syncope is from a cardiac cause or drug effect; if there is any risk that known hypoglycemia or a seizure may recur; if the patient required resuscitation; if the patient is potentially suicidal; or if the patient's neurologic status does not return to baseline.

TILT TABLE TESTING

Controlled passive assumption of upright posture to 60 to 80° increases the yield of the diagnostic evaluation of syncope by identifying most patients prone to experience postural neurally mediated syncope. The sensitivity of this test improves from 0 to 27% to 73 to 87% in adults by adding isoproterenol infusion.[200, 201] Among teenagers, the sensitivity of this test ranges from 43 to 57% without isoproterenol, with an excellent specificity of from 83 to 100%.[202–204] In uncontrolled studies during which isoproterenol was added after a negative baseline study, the sensitivity ranged from 70 to 100%.[205–207] Adult data suggest that specificity suffers from the addition of isoproterenol. Other catecholamines, including epinephrine,[208] have not enhanced the vasodepressor response to orthostatic tilt as has isoproterenol.

By studying 26 children (mean age, 14.8 years) with unexplained syncope using 60° of upright tilt table testing, my colleagues and I have shown that those having reproduction of symptoms without requiring isoproterenol will do so at a mean time of 7 minutes, and all will have done so by 15 minutes.[209] Fish et al showed that this test is reproducible 30 minutes after the original test in two thirds of cases but often with a different hemodynamic response (cardioinhibitory vs. vasodepressor).[210] Excellent reproducibility of the results of tilt table testing after longer time intervals has also been shown in adults, allowing reasonable interpretation of tilt table studies after the addition of therapeutic interventions.

Tilt table studies have been used to differentiate primary epilepsy,[211] recurrent vertigo,[212] and psychiatric causes[170] of apparent loss of consciousness from neurally mediated syncope.

Our indications to perform tilt table testing include (1) three or more syncopal episodes while at rest during a 12-month period and no indications of heart disease by history, physical exam, or ECG; (2) a single syncopal episode while driving or resulting in body injury and no evidence of heart disease; (3) a seizure not thought by neurologic consultation to represent epilepsy and not thought to be related to heart disease; (4) syncope during physical exertion and demonstrated by comprehensive evaluation to not be caused by heart disease; and (5) recurrent syncopal episodes thought to represent primary psychiatric disease. Strieper et al[205] showed that an extensive workup is not routinely necessary in syncopal children whose histories are consistent with neurally mediated syncope. In those patients, we limit the laboratory component of the patient's evaluation to a 12-lead ECG and tilt table study. Furthermore, if a patient's history is classic for neurally mediated syncope and the cardiovascular and neurologic examination and ECG are normal, empiric therapy without tilt table testing is well within the standard of medical care. However, we have found that such testing often demystifies the problem to patients and their families. It may also serve as a control study if follow-up tilt testing is later necessary during drug therapy.

A sensitively and carefully performed tilt table study using an indwelling arterial catheter and intravenous catheter can be performed in most children as young as 10 years. Our studies are performed in a low-stimulation, low-light environment at about noontime, 4 hours after a light breakfast. The child is placed supine on an electrical tilt table with footplate, and electrocardiographic leads are placed first. Vascular access is then obtained; local infiltration with lidocaine is always used for the arterial catheter, and EMLA (eutetic mixture of local anesthetics) cream is sometimes used for both venous and arterial sites. Next, the patient is comfortably secured to the cushioned table with the feet together and flush onto the footplate. Straps are placed above the knees, across the pelvis, and across the shoulders. An automated noninvasive blood pressure device is applied to the arm contralateral to the arterial catheter. A 15-minute period of equilibration ensues with the patient supine. Upright tilt to 70° follows with continuous rhythm and blood pressure monitoring. The table is returned to the supine position when there is reproduction of symptoms even without change in vital signs; there is asystole, severe bradycardia, or severe systolic hypotension corroborated by noninvasive blood pressure cuff; or 20 minutes has elapsed.

The heart rate or blood pressure changes that constitute a positive test in children depend on the baseline values and the values just before observed changes. A heart less than 40 bpm always represents a cardioinhibitory response, but such a response may also be said to occur if the rate drops from 130 to 90, for example, and the rhythm becomes junctional. A vasodepressor response generally requires a drop in systolic pressure to less than 80 mm Hg. If the baseline test is negative, isoproterenol at 1.0 μg/min (or 0.025 μg/kg/min for children weighing less than 40 kg) is started, and the patient is returned to upright position. This dose is doubled every 10 minutes, up to a maximum of 4.0 μg/min (or 0.10 μg/kg/min), until symptoms occur or until the maximum dose is reached. Other laboratories exclusively use noninvasive blood pressure monitoring, including fingertip plethysmographic sensors in cooperative patients. This study may be modified for younger children by eliminating the arterial catheter. We always have an external transthoracic pacemaker available, but do not place the patches on the patient in advance unless there is a history of cardiopulmonary resuscitation.

The only hemodynamic changes that may be discriminated by this methodology are hypotension with minimal change in heart rate (vasodepressor response), marked bradycardia or asystole (cardioinhibitory response), mixed vasodepressor and cardioinhibitory forms, and hypotension with sinus tachycardia resulting from orthostatic hypotension. A more critical evaluation of the autonomic nervous system is occasionally clinically valuable, for example, in teenagers with long-standing diabetes mellitus or in children with peripheral neuropathies. Table 14–6 lists commonly used tests of cardiovascular responses to autonomic nervous system control, those components of the autonomic nervous system being tested, and normal responses.

TREATMENT OF SELECTED CONDITIONS

The three most popular therapeutic options for children and teenagers with neurally mediated syncope are 1) augmentation of water and dietary salt intake; (2) fludrocortisone and a high-sodium, high-fluid diet; and (3) beta-adrenergic blocking drugs. Controlled trials comparing the efficacy of these interventions in children are lacking.

The use of tilt table testing as a way to guide medical therapy is controversial. There are contradictory data regarding the value of response to intravenous beta-blocker administration during tilt table testing in children as a means to predict clinical response to orally administered agents.[213, 214] Leor et al[215] reported that beta-blocking agents among a group of adults were more likely to be efficacious in persons having sinus tachycardia before actual syncope during tilt table testing compared with those who did not.[215] Morrillo et al[216] could not demonstrate predictive value of tilt table testing in adults, using a placebo-controlled cross-over trial with disopyramide. In their patients, there was a striking decrease in the incidence of positive tilt tests over time regardless of intervention. However, Natale et al[217] reported only a 6% recurrence of symptoms from 210 adult patients receiving head-up tilt-guided therapy versus 36% of 44 patients receiving empiric therapy ($P < .01$). My colleagues and I require follow-up tilt table testing therapy in children who have injured themselves and in teenagers whose syncope has no warning, especially while sitting, and who wish to drive.

Therapy should be individualized. The patient who states that symptoms are related to periods of inadequate hydration may only require dietary counseling, but the individual who suffers repeated episodes or episodes with accompanying seizures or bodily injury requires more definitive therapy. General guidelines include avoidance of fludrocortisone and high-sodium diet as first-line therapy in children with resting hypertension and avoidance of beta-blocking agents in children with asthma, diabetes mellitus, or, perhaps, depression. Failure of one agent necessitates add-

Table 14–6. Examples of Cardiovascular Autonomic Nervous System Tests

TEST	MEASUREMENT OF INTEREST	NORMAL RESPONSE	INTERPRETATION OF ABNORMAL RESPONSE
Baroreflex sensitivity (graded phenylephrine boluses)	Slope of RR intervals ÷ corresponding systolic BP	Log (reflex sensitivity slope) = 2.47 − (0.0164 × age) − (0.086 × mean arterial BP)	Defect in reflex arc involving SNS alpha-receptors, carotid and aortic arch baroreceptors, brain stem, cardiac vagal efferents
Cold pressor test	BP rise HR rise	20 mm Hg systolic BP rise 10 bpm HR rise	Defect in reflex arc involving sensory nerves, spinothalamic tracts, suprapontine and intrathalamic relays, descending SNS pathways, SNS alpha-receptors, cardiac SNS efferents and beta-receptors
Cuff occlusion test	BP drop	Systolic BP drop by < 10 mm Hg	Defect in reflex response involving cardiac chamber volume sensors and carotid and aortic arch baroreceptors, brain stem, efferent SNS nerves and alpha-receptors
Isoproterenol test (graded boluses)	HR rise	25 bpm rise after 1.0 μg (adolescent response)	Hypersensitive response: reduced circulating catecholamines (beta-receptor up-regulation) Reduced response: beta-receptor down-regulation
Neuronal norepinephrine stores (graded tyramine boluses)	BP rise	<20 mm Hg systolic BP rise after 1.0 g	If reduced response, neuronal stores of NE reduced by drugs or peripheral SNS neuronal destruction
		>25 mm Hg systolic BP rise after 6.0 g (usual adult response: 25 mm Hg rise after 2.0–3.0 g)	Exaggerated response if excessive neuronal NE stores (pheochromocytoma)
Sinus arrhythmia (controlled breathing for 1 min)	HR variation	>15 bpm	Dysfunction of vagus nerve, thoracic afferent fibers, or the vasomotor center
Valsalva maneuver	Phase IV-II RR ratio	>1.2	Defect in baroreceptor, brain stem, cardiac vagal efferent (IV) reflex; or cardiac SNS efferent or beta-receptor (II) reflex
	Phase II HR rise	>20 bpm	Defect in baroreceptor, brain stem, or cardiac SNS efferent or beta-receptor
	Phase IV HR drop		Defect in baroreceptor, brain stem, or cardiac vagal efferent
	Phase IV BP rise	>10 mm Hg (mean)	SNS dysfunction (as in CHF)

BP, blood pressure; HR, heart rate; CHF, congestive heart failure; NE, norepinephrine; SNS, sympathetic nervous system.

Adapted from Robertson D: Assessment of autonomic function. In Baughman KL, Green BM (eds): Clinical Diagnostic Manual for the House Officer. Baltimore, Williams & Wilkins, 1981. Used with permission.

ing or switching to the other. Among patients started on fludrocortisone and a high-sodium diet, my colleagues and I request follow-up blood pressure and serum electrolyte measurements after 2 and 4 weeks of therapy and then every 6 months thereafter.

If these first-line measures fail, singly or in combination, disopyramide is a popular drug for adults with this problem. Unlike Morrillo et al's report,[216] its efficacy has been shown in a tilt-guided clinical trial in 10 patients 16 to 74 years of age.[218] The rationale for its effectiveness includes its vagolytic and negative inotropic properties. We have found the anticholinergic side effects, especially the blurred vision, to be prohibitive in nearly all the children who have used it. Other agents reported to be of value in children and adolescents include pseudoephedrine[219] for its blood pressure–raising effect, sertraline[126] (presumably because of its central nervous system effects), and theophylline.

Young children having documented cardioinhibitory, neurally mediated syncope, including toddlers with pallid breath-holding spells, have been reported to benefit from permanent cardiac pacing.[137] However, if there is a vasodepressor component to their symptoms, pacing will not be sufficient therapy.[220] Cardiac pacing is, therefore, not generally accepted as first-line therapy for pediatric patients having neurally mediated syncope. In our experience of more than 100 patients, first-line medical or dietary therapy is successful in preventing syncope recurrences in 70% and the addition of second or third medications in another 25%. (Morrillo et al's placebo-controlled report from adults[216] even suggests that no therapy is necessary in many patients.) Pacing has been a successful adjunct to medical therapy in only one of our teenagers. Nevertheless, patients having recurrent, probably pure hypervagotonia exist and may be best treated with artificial pacing. These especially include some patients having deglutition syncope or some athletes with postexercise asystolic syncope.

REFERENCES

1. Dermksian G, Lamb LE: Syncope in a population of healthy young adults. JAMA 168:1200–1207, 1958.
2. Collins TA: Evaluation of current USAF policy in regards to management of disturbances of consciousness [thesis]. Randolph Air Force Base, TX, USAF School of Aviation Medicine, 1956.
3. Menkes JH: Textbook of Child Neurology, 2nd ed. Philadelphia, Lea and Febiger, 1980.
4. Prazar GE: Temper tantrums and breath-holding spells. In Hoekelman RA (ed): Primary Pediatrics, 3rd ed. Melbourne, Churchill Livingtone, 1994.
5. Savage DD, Corwin L, McGee DL, et al: Epidemiologic features of isolated syncope: The Framingham study. Stroke 16:626–629, 1985.
6. Kapoor WN, Karpf M, Wieand S, et al: A prospective evaluation and follow-up of patients with syncope. N Engl J Med 309:197–204, 1983.
7. Wayne HH: Syncope: Physiological considerations and an analysis of the clinical characteristics in 510 patients. Am J Med 30:418–438, 1961.
8. Camfield PR, Camfield CS: Syncope in childhood: A case control clinical study of the familial tendency to faint. Can J Neurol Sci 17:306–308, 1990.
9. Fournier A, Young M-L, Garcia OL, Tamer DF, Wolff GS: Electrophysiologic cardiac function before and after surgery in children with AV canal. Am J Cardiol 57:1137–1141, 1986.
10. Moller JH, Patton C, Varco RL, et al: Post-operative ventricular septal defect: 24–30 years follow-up of 232 patients. In Proceedings of the Second World Congress of Pediatric Cardiology. New York, Springer-Verlag, 1985, p 20.
11. Shen W-K, Holmes DR, Porter CJ, et al: Sudden death after repair of double-outlet right ventricle. Circulation 81:128–136, 1990.
12. Nienaber CA, Hiller S, Spielman RP, et al: Syncope in hypertrophic cardiomyopathy: Multivariate analysis of prognostic indicators. J Am Coll Cardiol 15:948–955, 1990.
13. Garson A, Dick M, Fournier A, et al: The long QT syndrome in children: An international study of 287 patients. Circulation 87:1866–1872, 1993.
14. Kanter RJ, Raines KH, Wharton JM, Packer DL: Characterization of sudden cardiac death risk in pediatric patients with the Wolff-Parkinson-White syndrome. J Am Coll Cardiol 15:212A, 1990.
15. Paul T, Guccione P, Garson A: Relation of syncope in young patients with Wolff-Parkinson-White syndrome to rapid ventricular response during atrial fibrillation. Am J Cardiol 65:318–321, 1990.
16. Rowell LB: Human Circulation. Regulation During Physical Stress. New York, Oxford University Press, 1986.
17. Scheinberg P, Blackburn I, Rich M, Saslow M: Effects of aging on cerebral circulation and metabolism. Arch Neurol Psychiatry 70:77–85, 1953.
18. Martin TC, Smith L, Hernandez A, Weldon CS: Dysrhythmias following the Senning operation for dextrotransposition of the great arteries. J Thorac Cardiovasc Surg 85:928–932, 1983.
19. Turina M, Siebenmann R, Nussbaumer P, Senning A: Long-term outlook after atrial correction of transposition of great arteries. J Thorac Cardiovasc Surg 95:828–835, 1988.
20. Turley K, Hanley FL, Verrier ED, et al: The Mustard procedure in infants (less than 100 days of age): Ten year follow-up. J Thorac Cardiovasc Surg 96:849–853, 1988.
21. Gewillig M, Cullen S, Mertens B, et al: Risk factors for arrhythmia and death after Mustard operation for simple transposition of the great arteries. Circulation 84:III-187–III-192, 1991.
22. Driscoll DJ, Offord KP, Feldt RH, et al: Five- to fifteen-year follow-up after Fontan operation. Circulation 85:469–496, 1992.
23. Weber HS, Hellenbrand WE, Kleinman CS, et al: Predictors of rhythm disturbances and subsequent morbidity after the Fontan operation. Am J Cardiol 64:762–767, 1989.
24. Mair DD, Hagler DJ, Julsrud PR, et al: Early and late results of the modified Fontan procedure for double-inlet left ventricle: The Mayo Clinic experience. J Am Coll Cardiol 18:1727–1732, 1991.
25. Murphy JG, Gersh BJ, McGoon MD, et al: Long-term outcome after surgical repair of isolated atrial septal defect. N Engl J Med 323:1645–1650, 1990.
26. Bricker JT, Gillette PC, Cooley DA, McNamara DG: Dysrhythmia after atrial septal defect repair. Tex Heart Inst J 13:203–208, 1986.
27. Dreifus LS, Fisch C, Griffin JC, et al: Guidelines for implantation of cardiac pacemaker and antiarrhythmia devices. J Am Coll Cardiol 18:1–13, 1991.
28. Friedli B, Bolens M: Intraventricular conduction disturbances after correction of tetralogy of Fallot: Can bifascicular and trifascicular block be diagnosed from the surface ECG? Pediatr Cardiol 6:133–136, 1985.
29. Anderson RH, Becker AE, Arnold R, Wilkinson JL: The conducting tissues in congenitally corrected transposition. Circulation 50:911–923, 1974.
30. Huhta JC, Maloney JD, Ritter DG, et al: Complete atrioventricular block in patients with atrioventricular discordance. Circulation 67:1374–1377, 1983.
31. Momma K, Takao A, Shibata T: Characteristics and natural history of abnormal atrial rhythms in left isomerism. Am J Cardiol 65:231–236, 1990.
32. McAlister HF, Klementowicz PR, Andrews C, et al: Lyme carditis: An important cause of reversible heart block. Ann Intern Med 110:339–345, 1989.
33. Rocchini A, Chun P, Dick M: Ventricular tachycardia in children. Am J Cardiol 47:1091–1097, 1981.
34. Dreyer WJ, Paridon SM, Fisher DJ, Garson A Jr: Rapid

ventricular pacing in dogs with right ventricular outflow tract obstruction: Insights into a mechanism of sudden death in postoperative tetralogy of Fallot. J Am Coll Cardiol 21:1731–1737, 1993.
35. Quattlebaum TG, Varghese PJ, Neill CA, Donahoo JS: Sudden death among postoperative patients with tetralogy of Fallot. A follow-up study of 243 patients for an average of twelve years. Circulation 54:289–293, 1975.
36. Garson A Jr, Gillette PC, Gutgesell HP, McNamara DG: Stress-induced ventricular arrhythmia after repair of tetralogy of Fallot. Am J Cardiol 46:1006–1012, 1980.
37. Katz NM, Blackstone EH, Kirklin JW, et al: Late survival and symptoms after repair of tetralogy of Fallot. Circulation 65:403–410, 1982.
38. Chandar JS, Wolff GS, Garson A, et al: Ventricular arrhythmias in postoperative tetralogy of Fallot. Am J Cardiol 65:655–661, 1990.
39. Kobayashi J, Hirose H, Nakano S, et al: Ambulatory electrocardiographic study of the frequency and cause of ventricular arrhythmia after correction of tetralogy of Fallot. Am J Cardiol 54:1310–1313, 1984.
40. Gatzoulis MA, Till JA, Somerville J, et al: Mechanoelectrical interaction in tetralogy of Fallot. Circulation 92:231–237, 1995.
41. Bricker JT: Sudden death and tetralogy of Fallot. Circulation 92:158–159, 1995.
42. Bharati S, Surawicz B, Vidaillet HJ, Lev M: Familial congenital sinus rhythm anomalies: Clinical and pathological correlations. Pacing Clin Electrophysiol 15:1720–1729, 1992.
43. Schneider MD, Roller DH, Morganroth J, Josephson ME: The syndromes of familial atrioventricular block with sinus bradycardia: Prognostic indices, electrophysiologic and histopathologic correlates. Eur J Cardiol 7:337–351, 1978.
44. Perloff JK: The heart in neuromuscular disease. In O'Rourke RA (ed): Current Problems in Cardiology. Chicago, Year Book Medical, 1986, p 11.
45. Baldwin AJ, Talley RC, Johnson C, et al: Permanent paralysis of the atrium in a patient with fascioscapulohumeral muscular dystrophy. Am J Cardiol 31:649, 1973.
46. Moorman RJ, Coleman RE, Packer DL, et al: Cardiac involvement in myotonic muscular dystrophy. Medicine 64:6, 1985.
47. Morquio L: Sur une maladie infantile et familiale caracteristique et la mort subite. Arch Med Enfantes 4:467–475, 1901.
48. Michaelsson M, Engle MA: Congenital complete heart block: An international study of the natural history. In Brest AN, Engle MA (eds): Cardiovascular Clinics. Philadelphia, FA Davis, 1972, pp 85–101.
49. Michaelsson M, Jonzon A, Riesenfeld T: Isolated congenital complete atrioventricular block in adult life. Circulation 92:442–449, 1995.
50. Charles R, Holt S, Kay JM, et al: Myocardial ultrastructure and the development of atrioventricular block in Kearns-Sayre syndrome. Circulation 63:214, 1980.
51. Husson GS, Blackman MS, Rogers MC, et al: Familial congenital bundle branch system disease. Am J Cardiol 32:365–369, 1973.
52. Esscher E, Hardell L, Michaelsson M: Familial isolated complete right bundle branch block. Br Heart J 37:745–747, 1975.
53. Garson A: Interventricular conduction disturbances. In The Electrocardiogram in Infants and Children. Philadelphia, Lea & Febiger, 1983, pp 119–142.
54. Josephson ME: Intraventricular conduction disturbances. In Clinical Cardiac Electrophysiology. Philadelphia, Lea & Febiger, 1979, pp 103–118.
55. Fuhrman BP, Bass JL, Laurence C, et al: Progressive cardiac conduction defect and cardiomyopathy in siblings with syncope. Pediatr Cardiol 2:57–62, 1982.
56. Leitch JW, Klein GJ, Yee R, et al: Syncope associated with SVT. Circulation 85:1064–1071, 1992.
57. Leitch J, Klein G, Yee R, et al: Neurally mediated syncope and atrial fibrillation [letter]. N Engl J Med 324:495–496, 1991.
58. Rebello R, Brownlee WC: Intermittent ventricular standstill during chronic atrial fibrillation in patients with dizziness or syncope. Pacing Clin Electrophysiol 10:1271–1276, 1987.
59. Seliem MA, Benson W, Strasburger JF, et al: Complex ventricular ectopic activity in patients <20 years of age with or without syncope, and the role of ventricular extrastimulus testing. Am J Cardiol 68:745–750, 1991.
60. Leenhardt A, Lucet V, Denjoy I, et al: Catecholaminergic polymorphic ventricular tachycardia in children: A 7-year follow-up of 21 patients. Circulation 91:1512–1519, 1995.
61. Coumel P: Polymorphous ventricular tachyarrhythmias in the absence of structural heart disease [editorial]. Pacing Clin Electrophysiol 18:633–636, 1995.
62. Kugler J: Sinus node dysfunction in young patients with long QT syndrome. Am Heart J 121:1132, 1991.
63. Shimizu W, Ohe T, Kurita T, et al: Early afterdepolarizations induced by isoproterenol in patients with congenital long QT syndrome. Circulation 84:1915–1923, 1991.
64. Noll B, Irappe J, Goke B, Maisch B: Influence of pacing mode and rate on peripheral levels of atrial natriuretic peptide. Pacing Clin Electrophysiol 12:1763, 1989.
65. Dicarlo LA, Morady F, Krol RB, et al: The hemodynamic effects of ventricular pacing with and without atrioventricular synchrony in patients with normal and diminished left ventricular function. Am Heart J 114:746–752, 1987.
66. Langerfeld H, Grimm W, Marsch B, Kochsiek K: Course of symptoms and spontaneous ECG in pacemaker patients: A 5-year follow-up study. Pacing Clin Electrophysiol 11:2198–2206, 1988.
67. Pavlovic SV, Kocovic D, Djordjevic M, et al: The etiology of syncope in pacemaker patients. Pacing Clin Electrophysiol 14:2086–2091, 1991.
68. Dikkala V, Sreeram N: Congenital complete heart block and vasodepressor syncope. Int J Cardiol 43:319–320, 1994.
69. McKenna WJ, Deanfield J, Faruqui A, et al: Prognosis in hypertrophic cardiomyopathy: Role of age and clinical, electrophysiologic, and hemodynamic features. Am J Cardiol 47:535–538, 1981.
70. McKenna WJ, Deanfield JE: Hypertrophic cardiomyopathy: An important cause of sudden death. Arch Dis Child 59:971–975, 1984.
71. Dilsizian V, Bonow RU, Epstein, S, et al: Myocardial ischemia detected by thallium scintigraphy is frequently related to cardiac arrest and syncope in young patients with hypertrophic cardiomyopathy. J Am Coll Cardiol 22:796–804, 1993.
72. Gilligan DM, Nikohannopoulos P, Chan WL, et al: Investigation of a hemodynamic basis for syncope in hypertrophic cardiomyopathy. Circulation 85:2140–2148, 1992.
73. Sneddon JF, Slade A, Seo H, et al: Assessment of the diagnostic value of head-up tilt testing in the evaluation of syncope in hypertrophic cardiomyopathy. Am J Cardiol 73:601–604, 1994.
74. Khair GZ, Bamrah VS: Syncope in hypertrophic cardiomyopathy: I. Association with atrioventricular block. Am Heart J 110:1081–1083, 1985.
75. Khair GZ, Soni JS, Bamrah VS: Syncope in hypertrophic

cardiomyopathy: II. Coexistence of atrioventricular block and Wolff-Parkinson-White syndrome. Am Heart J 110:1083–1086, 1985.
76. Grech ED, Ramsdale DR: Exertional syncope in aortic stenosis: Evidence to support inappropriate left ventricular baroreceptor response. Am Heart J 121:603–606, 1991.
77. Brammell H, Vogel J, Pryor R, et al: The Eisenmenger syndrome: A clinical and physiologic reappraisal. Am J Cardiol 28:679–692, 1971.
78. Wolfe RR, Driscoll DJ, Gersony WM, et al: Arrhythmias in patients with valvar aortic stenosis, valvar pulmonary stenosis, and ventricular septal defect. Circulation 87(Suppl):I-89–I-101, 1993.
79. Rich S, Lam W: Atrial septostomy as palliative therapy for refractory primary pulmonary hypertension. Am J Cardiol 51:1560–1561, 1983.
80. Peterson DI: Syncope due to right atrial myxoma. Bull Clin Neurosci 49:63–66, 1984.
81. Puff M, Taff ML, Spitz WV, et al: Syncope and sudden death caused by a mitral valve myxoma. Am J Forensic Med Pathol 7:84–86, 1986.
82. Hoorntje JCA, Mooyaart EL, Meuzelaar KJ: Left atrial herniation through a partial pericardial defect: A rare cause of syncope. Pacing Clin Electrophysiol 12:1841–1845, 1989.
83. Amarasena NL, Pillai RP, Forfar JC: Atypical ventricular tachycardia and syncope with left coronary artery origin from the right coronary sinus. Br Heart J 70:391–392, 1993.
84. Liberthson RR, Dinsmore RE, Bharati S, et al: Aberrant coronary artery origin from the aorta: Diagnosis and clinical significance. Circulation 50:774–779, 1974.
85. Roberts WC, Siegel RJ, Zipes DP: Origin of the right coronary artery from the left sinus of Valsalva and its functional consequences: Analysis of 10 necropsy patients. Am J Cardiol 49:363–368, 1982.
86. Liberthson RR, Gang DL, Custer J: Sudden death in an infant with aberrant origin of the right coronary artery from the left sinus of Valsalva of the aorta: Case report and review of the literature. Pediatr Cardiol 4:45–48, 1983.
87. Berdoff R, Haimowitz A, Kupersmith J: Anomalous origin of the right coronary artery from the left sinus of Valsalva. Am J Cardiol 58:656–657, 1986.
88. Bartorelli AL, Pepi M, Sganzerla P, et al: Syncope with cardiac arrest as the first manifestation of two congenital left coronary artery-to-main pulmonary artery fistulae. Am Heart J 127:207–209, 1994.
89. Morales AR, Romanelli R, Boucek RJ: The mural left anterior descending coronary artery, strenuous exercise, and sudden death. Circulation 62:230–237, 1980.
90. Devereux RB, Perloff JK, Reichek N, Josephson ME. Mitral valve prolapse. Circulation 54:3–14, 1976.
91. Devereux RB, Kramer-Fox R, Kligfield P: Mitral valve prolapse: Causes, clinical manifestations, and management. Ann Intern Med 111:305–317, 1989.
92. Devereux RB, Brown WT, Lutas EM, et al: Association of mitral valve prolapse with low body-weight and low blood pressures. Lancet 2:792–795, 1982.
93. Santos AD, Mathew PK, Hilal A, Wallace WA: Orthostatic hypotension: A commonly unrecognized cause of symptoms in mitral valve prolapse. Am J Med 71:746–750, 1981.
94. Devereux RB, Kramer-Fox R, Brown WT, et al: Relation between clinical features of the mitral prolapse syndrome and echocardiographically documented mitral valve prolapse. J Am Coll Cardiol 8:763–772, 1986.
95. Bisset GS, Schwartz DC, Meyer RA, et al: Clinical spectrum and long term follow-up of isolated mitral valve prolapse in 119 children. Circulation 62:423–429, 1980.
96. Gaffney F, Karlsson E, Campbell W, et al: Autonomic dysfunction in women with mitral valve prolapse syndrome. Circulation 59:894–901, 1979.
97. Boudoulas H, Reynolds J, Mazzaferri E, et al: Metabolic studies in mitral valve prolapse syndrome. Circulation 61:1200–1205, 1980.
98. Duren DR, Becker AE, Dunning AJ: Long-term follow-up of idiopathic mitral valve prolapse in 300 patients: A prospective study. J Am Coll Cardiol 11:42–47, 1988.
99. Kligfield P, Levy D, Devereux RB: Arrhythmias and sudden death in mitral valve prolapse. Am Heart J 113:1298–1307, 1987.
100. Kligfield P, Devereux RB: Is the patient with mitral valve prolapse at high risk for sudden death identifiable? In Cheitlin MD (ed): Dilemmas in Clinical Cardiology. Cardiovascular Clinics. Philadelphia, FA Davis, 1990, pp 143–157.
101. Kligfield P, Hochreiter C, Niles N, et al: Relation of sudden death in pure mitral regurgitation, with and without mitral valve prolapse, to repetitive ventricular arrhythmias and right and left ventricular ejection fractions. Am J Cardiol 60:397–399, 1987.
102. Yamakawa H, Nishikawa M, Nakahara I, et al: Congenital subclavian steal syndrome with anomaly of the aortic arch. Surg Neurol 39:133–137, 1993.
103. Brill CB, Peyster RG, Keller MS, et al: Isolation of the right subclavian artery with subclavian steal in a child with Klippel-Feil anomaly. Am J Med Genet 26:933–940, 1987.
104. Graziani LJ, Streletz LJ, Mitchell DG, et al: Electroencephalographic, neuroradiologic, and neurodevelopmental studies in infants with subclavian steal during ECMO. Pediatr Neurol 10:97–103, 1994.
105. Shreve MR, Crosson JE, Eusebio EJ, Braunlin EA: Electrocardiographic changes during long-term follow-up of pediatric heart transplant recipients. Am J Cardiol 71:1253–1256, 1993.
106. Addonizio LJ, Hsu DT, Smith CR, et al: Late complications in pediatric cardiac transplant recipients. Circulation 82(Suppl IV):IV-295–IV-301, 1990.
107. Fitzpatrick AP, Banner N, Cheng A, et al: Vasovagal reactions may occur after orthotopic heart transplantation. J Am Coll Cardiol 21;1132–1137, 1993.
108. Scherrer U, Vissing S, Morgan BJ, et al: Vasovagal syncope after infusion of a vasodilator in a heart-transplant recipient. N Engl J Med 322:602–604, 1990.
109. Kaye DM, Esler M, Kingwell B, et al: Functional and neurochemical evidence for partial cardiac sympathetic reinnervation after cardiac transplantation in humans. Circulation 88:1110–1118, 1993.
110. Burke MN, McGinn AL, Homans DC, et al: Evidence for functional sympathetic reinnervation of left ventricle and coronary arteries after orthotopic cardiac transplantation in humans. Circulation 91:72–78, 1995.
111. De Marco T, Dae M, Yuen-Green MSF, et al: Iodine-123 metaiodobenzylguanidine scintigraphic assessment of the transplanted human heart: Evidence for late reinnervation. J Am Coll Cardiol 25:927–931, 1995.
112. Middlekauff HR, Stevenson WG, Stevenson LW, et al: Syncope in advanced heart failure: High risk of sudden death regardless of origin of syncope. J Am Coll Cardiol 21:110–116, 1993.
113. Thames MD, Alpert JS, Dolen JE: Syncope in patients with pulmonary embolism. JAMA 238:2509–2511, 1977.
114. Kollef MH, Schachter DT: Defecation syncope caused by pulmonary embolism [letter]. Ann Intern Med 113:86, 1990.

115. Rea R, Thames MD: Neural control mechanisms and vasovagal syncope. J Cardiovasc Electrophysiol 4:587–595, 1993.
116. Thoren P: Role of cardiac vagal C-fibers in cardiovascular control. Rev Physiol Biochem Pharmacol P6:2–92, 1979.
117. Balaji S, Oslizlok PC, Allen MC, et al: Neurocardiogenic syncope in children with a normal heart. J Am Coll Cardiol 23:779–785, 1994.
118. Perry JC, Garson A Jr: The child with recurrent syncope: Autonomic function testing and beta-adrenergic hypersensitivity. J Am Coll Cardiol 17:1168–1171, 1991.
119. Nwosu EA, Rahko PS, Hanson P, et al: Hemodynamic and volumetric response of the normal left ventricle to upright tilt testing. Am Heart J 128:106–113, 1994.
120. Pruvot E, Vesin JM, Schlaepfer J, et al: Autonomic imbalance assessed by heart rate variability analysis in vasovagal syncope. Pacing Clin Electrophysiol 17(II):2201–2206, 1994.
121. Hargreaves AD, Muir AL: Lack of variation in venous tone potentiates vasovagal syncope. Br Heart J 67:486–490, 1992.
122. Jaeger FJ, Maloney JD, Castle LW, Fouad-Tarazi FM: Is absolute hypovolemia a risk factor for vasovagal response to head-up tilt? Pacing Clin Electrophysiol 16:743–750, 1993.
123. Sneddon JF, Counihan PJ, Bashir Y, et al: Impaired immediate vasoconstrictor responses in patients with recurrent neurally mediated syncope. Am J Cardiol 71:72–76, 1993.
124. Uchiyama M, Otsuka T, Sakai K: Response of plasma renin activity to postural change in vasovagal syncope in children, with observations on syncope. Hormone Res 23:147–150, 1986.
125. Morgan DA, Thoren P, Wilczysnski EA, et al: Serotonergic mechanisms mediate moderate renal sympathoinhibition during severe hemorrhage in rats. Am J Physiol 255:H496–H502, 1988.
126. Grubb BP, Samoil D, Kosinski D, et al: Use of sertraline hydrochloride in the treatment of refractory neurocardiogenic syncope in children and adolescents. J Am Coll Cardiol 24:490–494, 1994.
127. Perna GP, Ficola V, Salvatori MP, et al: Increases of plasma beta endorphin in vasodepressor syncope. Am J Cardiol 65:929–930, 1990.
128. O'Sullivan J, Cottrell AJ, Wren C: Ondine's curse and neurally mediated syncope—A new and important association. Eur Heart J 14:1289–1291, 1993.
129. Pongiglione G, Fish FA, Strasburger JF, Benson DW: Heart rate and blood pressure response to upright tilt in young patients with unexplained syncope. J Am Coll Cardiol 16:165–170, 1990.
130. Grubb BP, Gerard G, Roush K, et al: Cerebral vasoconstriction during head-upright tilt-induced vasovagal syncope: A paradoxic and unexpected response. Circulation 84:1157–1164, 1991.
131. Kleinknecht RA, Lenz J, Ford G, DeBerard S: Types and correlates of blood/injury-related vasovagal syncope. Behav Res Ther 28:289–295, 1990.
132. Paul DL, McKeown DW: Supine faints. Anaesthesia 42:1120–1121, 1987.
133. Sutton R, Petersen M, Brignole M, et al: Proposed classification for tilt induced vasovagal syncope. Eur J Cardiac Pac Electrophysiol 3:180–183, 1992.
134. Lombroso CT, Lerman P: Breathholding spells (cyanotic and pallid infantile syncope). Pediatrics 39:563–581, 1967.
135. Laxdol T, Gomez MR, Reiker J: Cyanotic and pallid syncopal attacks in children (breath-holding spells). Dev Med Clin Neurol 11:755–763, 1969.
136. Emery S: Status epilepticus secondary to breath-holding and pallid syncopal spells. Neurology 40:859, 1990.
137. Sapire DW, Casta A, Safley W, et al: Vasovagal syncope in children requiring pacemaker implantation. Am Heart J 106:1406–1411, 1983.
138. Kleinknecht RA: Specificity and psychosocial correlates of blood/injury fear and fainting. Behav Res Ther 26:303–309, 1988.
139. Salim MA, DiSessa TG: QT interval response to exercise in children with syncope. Am J Cardiol 73:976–977, 1994.
140. Golf S, Forfang K: Congenital swallowing-induced symptomatic heart block: a case report of a probably hereditary disorder. Pacing Clin Electrophysiol 9:602–605, 1986.
141. Wood RC, Kiel EA: Swallowing syncope in a child. Pediatrics 78:507–509, 1986.
142. Engelhardt W, Kotlarek F, Von Bernuth G: Deglutition syncope in childhood with complete atrioventricular block. Am J Cardiol 58:1113–1114, 1986.
143. Keningsberg K, Boris M, Joseph P, et al: Reflex bradycardia after tracheoesophageal fistula repair. Surgery 71:125–129, 1972.
144. Baron SB, Huang SK: Cough syncope presenting as Mobitz type II atrioventricular block—An electrophysiologic correlation. Pacing Clin Electrophysiol 10:65–69, 1987.
145. Kapoor WN, Peterson JR, Karpf M: Micturition syncope: A reappraisal. JAMA 253:796–798, 1985.
146. Lyle CB, Monroe JT, Flinn DE, et al: Micturition syncope: Report of 24 cases. N Engl J Med 265:982–986, 1961.
147. Kapoor WN, Peterson J, Karpf M: Defecation syncope: A symptom with multiple etiologies. Arch Intern Med 146:2377–2379, 1986.
148. Lewis DW, Frank LM: Hair-grooming syncope seizures. Pediatrics 91:836–837, 1993.
149. Morley CA, Sutton R: Carotid sinus syncope. Int J Cardiol 6:287–293, 1984.
150. Berger TM, Porter CJ: Carotid sinus syndrome and wrestling. Mayo Clin Proc 68:366–369, 1993.
151. Achiron A, Regev A: Carotid sinus syncope induced by an orthodontic appliance [letter]. Lancet 8675:1339, 1989.
152. Pelekanos JT, Dooley JM, Camfield PR, et al: Stretch syncope in adolescence. Neurology 40:705–707, 1990.
153. Compton D, Hill PN, Sinclair JD: Weight-lifters blackout. Lancet 2:1234–1237, 1973.
154. Streeten DHP, Kerr LP, Kerr CB, et al: Hyperbradykininism: A new orthostatic syndrome. Lancet 7786:1048–1053, 1972.
155. Roberts LJ: Recurrent syncope due to systemic mastocytosis. Hypertension 6:285–294, 1984.
156. Weig SG, Buckthal PE, Choi SK, et al: Recurrent syncope as the presenting symptom of Arnold-Chiari malformation. Neurology 41:1673–1674, 1973.
157. Bernstein RK: Severe diabetic cardiac autonomic neuropathy in a 14-year-old girl, normalized after 15 months of improved glycemic control. Diabetes Care 9:310–312, 1986.
158. Hoefnagels WAJ, Padberg GW, Overweg J, et al: Transient loss of consciousness: The value of the history for distinguishing seizure from syncope. J Neurol 238:39–43, 1991.
159. Constantin L, Martins JB, Fincham RW, et al: Bradycardia and syncope as manifestations of partial epilepsy. J Am Coll Cardiol 15:900–905, 1990.
160. Hoefnagels WAJ, Padberg GW, Overweg J, et al: Syncope or seizure? The diagnostic value of the EEG and hyperventilation test in transient loss of consciousness. J Neurol Neurosurg Psychiatry 54:953–956, 1991.
161. Lance JW, Anthony M: Some clinical aspects of migraine. Arch Neurol 15:356–361, 1966.

162. Raskin NH, Knittle SC: Ice cream headache and orthostatic symptoms in patients with migraine. Headache 16:222–225, 1976.
163. Cortelli P, de Carolis P, Sturani A, et al: Cardiovascular and biochemical assessment in migraine patients submitted to tilt test. Functional Neurol 1:285–290, 1986.
164. Webb CL, Dick M, Rocchini AP, et al: Quinidine syncope in children. J Am Coll Cardiol 9:1031–1037, 1987.
165. Stone S, Lange LS: Syncope and sudden unexpected death attributed to carbamazepine in a 20-year-old epileptic [letter]. J Neurol Neurosurg Psychiatry 49:1460–1461, 1986.
166. Ellison JM, Milofsky JE, Ely E: Fluoxetine-induced bradycardia and syncope in two patients. J Clin Psychiatry 51:385–386, 1990.
167. Schwartz RH: Seizures and syncope in adolescent cocaine abusers [letter]. Am J Med 85:462, 1988.
168. Levine R: Epidemic faintness and syncope in a school marching band. JAMA 238:2373–2376, 1977.
169. Ruiz MT, Lopez JM: Mass hysteria in a secondary school [letter]. Int J Epidemiol 17:475–476, 1988.
170. Grubb BP, Gerard G, Wolfe DA, et al: Syncope and seizures of psychogenic origin: Identification with head-upright tilt table testing. Clin Cardiol 15:839–842, 1992.
171. Corrado D, Thriene G, Nava A, et al: Sudden death in young competitive athletes: Clinicopathologic correlations in 22 cases. Am J Med 89:588–596, 1990.
172. Burke AP, Farb A, Virmani R, et al: Sports-related and non-sports-related sudden cardiac death in young adults. Am Heart J 121:568–575, 1991.
173. Thiene G, Pennelli N, Rossi L: Cardiac conduction system abnormalities as a possible cause of sudden death in young athletes. Hum Pathol 14:705–709, 1983.
174. Ikaheimo M, Ilkka JP, Takkunen JT: Noninvasive evaluation of the athletic heart: Sprinters versus endurance runners. Am J Cardiol 44:24–30, 1979.
175. Beswick FW, Jordan RC: Cardiological observations at the Sixth British Empire and Commonwealth Games. Br Heart J 23:113–130, 1960.
176. Northcote RJ, Canning GP, Ballantyne D: Electrocardiographic findings in male veteran endurance athletes. Br Heart J 61:155–160, 1988.
177. Vitasolo MT, Kala R, Eisalo A: Ambulatory electrocardiographic findings in young athletes between 14–16 years of age. Eur Heart J 5:2–6, 1985.
178. Brodsky M, Wu D, Denes P, et al: Arrhythmias documented by 24 hour continuous electrocardiographic monitoring in 50 male medical students without apparent heart disease. Am J Cardiol 39:390–395, 1977.
179. Sobotka PA, Moyer JH, Bauerenfeind RA, et al: Arrhythmias documented by 24 hour continuous ambulatory electrocardiographic monitoring in young women without apparent heart disease. Am Heart J 6:753–759, 1981.
180. Talan DA, Bauerenfeind RA, Ashley W, et al: Twenty-four hour continuous ECG recordings in long distance runners. Chest 82:19–24, 1982.
181. Palatini P, Maraglino G, Sperti G, et al: Prevalence and possible mechanisms of ventricular arrhythmias in athletes. Am Heart J 110:560–567, 1985.
182. Sokolow M, Lyon TP: The ventricular complex in left ventricular hypertrophy as obtained by unipolar precordial and limb leads. Am Heart J 37:161–186, 1949.
183. Lichtman J, O'Rourke RA, Klein A, Karliner J: Electrocardiogram of the athlete. Arch Intern Med 132:763–770, 1973.
184. Gibbons LW, Cooper KH, Martin RP, Pollock ML: Medical examination and electrocardiographic analysis of elite distance runners. Ann NY Acad Sci 301:283–396, 1977.
185. Zeppilli P, Pirrani M, Sassara M, Fenici R: T wave abnormalities in top ranking athletes: Effects of isoproterenol, atropine and physical exercise. Am Heart J 100:213–222, 1980.
186. Roeske WR, O'Rourke RA, Klein A, et al: Noninvasive evaluation of ventricular hypertrophy in professional athletes. Circulation 53:286–292, 1975.
187. Maron BJ: Structural features of the athlete heart as defined by echocardiography. J Am Coll Cardiol 7:190–203, 1986.
188. Imai K, Sato H, Hori M, et al: Vagally mediated heart rate recovery after exercise is accelerated in athletes but blunted in patients with chronic heart failure. J Am Coll Cardiol 24:1529–1535, 1994.
189. Tamura Y, Onodera O, Kodera K, et al: Atrial standstill after treadmill exercise test and unique response to isoproterenol infusion in recurrent postexercise syncope. Am J Cardiol 65:533–535, 1990.
190. Oswald S, Brooks R, O'Nunain SS, et al: Asystole after exercise in healthy persons. Ann Intern Med 120:1008–1011, 1994.
191. Kapoor WN: Syncope with abrupt termination of exercise. Am J Med 87:597–599, 1989.
192. Arad M, Solomon A, Roth A, et al: Postexercise syncope: Evidence for increased activity of the sympathetic nervous system. Cardiology 83:121–123, 1993.
193. Sneddon JF, Scalia G, Ward DE, et al: Exercise induced vasodepressor syncope. Br Heart J 71:554–557, 1994.
194. Grubb BP, Temesy-Armos PN, Samoil D, et al: Tilt table testing in the evaluation and management of athletes with recurrent exercise-induced syncope. Med Sci Sports Exerc 25:24–28, 1993.
195. Hurwitz JL, Conley MJ, Wharton JM, et al: Syncope secondary to paroxysmal high grade AV block in a heavily trained man. Pacing Clin Electrophysiol 14:994–999, 1991.
196. Linzer M, Pritchett ELC, Pontinen M, et al: Incremental diagnostic yield of loop electrocardiographic recorders in unexplained syncope. Am J Cardiol 66:214–219, 1990.
197. Denes P, Ezri MD: The role of electrophysiologic studies in the management of patients with unexplained syncope. Pacing Clin Electrophysiol 8:424, 1985.
198. Olshansky B, Mazuz M, Martins JB: Significance of inducible tachycardia in patients with syncope of unknown origin: A long-term follow-up. J Am Coll Cardiol 5:216, 1985.
199. Bachinsky WB, Linzer M, Weld L, et al: Usefulness of clinical characteristics in predicting the outcome of electrophysiologic studies in unexplained syncope. Am J Cardiol 69:1044–1049, 1992.
200. Almquist A, Goldenberg IF, Milstein S, et al: Provocation of bradycardia and hypotension by isoproterenol and upright posture in patients with unexplained syncope. N Engl J Med 320:346–351, 1989.
201. Waxman MB, Yao L, Cameron DA, et al: Isoproterenol induction of vasodepressor-type reaction in vasodepressor-prone persons. Am J Cardiol 63:58–65, 1989.
202. Fouad FM, Sitthisook S, Vanerio G, et al: Sensitivity and specificity of the tilt test in young patients with unexplained syncope. Pacing Clin Electrophysiol 16:394–400, 1993.
203. Ross BA, Hughes S, Anderson E, et al: Abnormal responses to orthostatic testing in children and adolescents with recurrent unexplained syncope. Am Heart J 122:748–754, 1991.
204. Lerman-Sagie T, Rechovia E, Strassberg B, et al: Head-up tilt for the evaluation of syncope of unknown origin in children. J Pediatr 118:676–679, 1991.

205. Strieper JM, Auld DO, Hulse E, et al: Evaluation of recurrent pediatric syncope: Role of tilt table testing. Pediatrics 93:660–662, 1994.
206. Grubb BP, Temesy-Armos P, Moore J, et al: The use of head-upright tilt table testing in the evaluation and management of syncope in children and adolescents. Pacing Clin Electrophysiol 15:742–748, 1992.
207. Thilenius OG, Quinones JA, Husayni TS, et al: Tilt test for diagnosis of unexplained syncope in pediatric patients. Pediatrics 87:334–338, 1991.
208. Calkins H, Kadish A, Sousa J, et al: Comparison of responses to isoproterenol and epinephrine during head-up tilt in suspected vasodepressor syncope. Am J Cardiol 67:207–209, 1991.
209. Kanter RJ, Pressley JC, Greenfield R, et al: Duration of tilt table testing in pediatric patients [abstract]. Circulation 84:II–224, 1991.
210. Fish FA, Strasburger JF, Benson W: Reproducibility of a symptomatic response to upright tilt in young patients with unexplained syncope. Am J Cardiol 70:605–609, 1992.
211. Grubb BP, Gerard G, Roush K, et al: Differentiation of convulsive syncope and epilepsy with head-up tilt testing. Ann Intern Med 115:871–876, 1991.
212. Grubb BP, Rubin AM, Wolfe D, et al: Head-upright tilt-table testing: A useful tool in the evaluation and management of recurrent vertigo of unknown origin associated with near-syncope or syncope. Otolaryngol Head Neck Surg 107:570–576, 1992.
213. Ovadia M, Thoele D: Esmolol tilt testing with esmolol withdrawal for the evaluation of syncope in the young. Circulation 89:228–235, 1994.
214. O'Marcaigh AS, MacLellan-Tobert SG, Porter CJ: Tilt-table testing and oral metoprolol therapy in young patients with unexplained syncope. Pediatrics 93:278–283, 1994.
215. Leor J, Rotstein Z, Vered Z, et al: Absence of tachycardia during tilt test predicts failure of β-blocker therapy in patients with neurocardiogenic syncope. Am Heart J 127:1539–1543, 1994.
216. Morillo CA, Leitch JW, Yee R, et al: A placebo-controlled trial of intravenous and oral disopyramide for prevention of neurally mediated syncope induced by head-up tilt. J Am Coll Cardiol 22:1843–1848, 1993.
217. Natale A, Sra J, Dhala A, et al: Efficacy of different treatment strategies for neurocardiogenic syncope. Pacing Clin Electrophysiol 18(Pt I):655–662, 1995.
218. Milstein S, Buetikofer J, Dunnigan A, et al: Usefulness of disopyramide for prevention of upright tilt-induced hypotension-bradycardia. Am J Cardiol 65:1339–1344, 1990.
219. Strieper MJ, Campbell RM: Efficacy of alpha-adrenergic agonist therapy for prevention of pediatric neurocardiogenic syncope. J Am Coll Cardiol 22:594–597, 1993.
220. Sra JS, Jazayeri MR, Avitali B, et al: Comparison of cardiac pacing with drug therapy in the treatment of neurocardiogenic (vasovagal) syncope with bradycardia or asystole. N Engl J Med 328:1085–1090, 1993.

CHAPTER 15

ARRHYTHMIAS AND SUDDEN DEATH

Arthur Garson, Jr.

Specific data on the individual arrhythmias and their likelihood to lead to sudden death are discussed in other chapters of this book. In order to provide an indication of what the pediatric cardiologist might encounter in practice, I examined the factors present in a large number of pediatric cardiology patients who had died suddenly, with specific reference to the presence of chronic arrhythmias in these patients. In the first section, data are presented on the entire patient group. In the second and third sections, the differences between the diagnostic classes and the individual diagnoses are discussed. Finally, each of the arrhythmias are discussed with specific reference to this patient population and sudden death.

PATIENT DATA AND METHOD OF STUDY

The charts of all patients seen in the Pediatric Cardiology Section at Texas Children's Hospital who died in the 24-year period between 1959 and 1983 were reviewed. Patients were included in the study if the following criteria were met:

1. Patient older than 1 year at the time of death.
2. A sudden event occurred that rendered the patient unconscious, with the patient never regaining consciousness before death.
3. Occurrence of this sudden event outside the hospital.
4. Absence of acute illness in the patient shortly before sudden death.

Patients were excluded from this study if they had had cardiac catheterization or cardiac surgery within 1 month before death.

Certain definitions were used in the gathering of the data. The New York Heart Association criteria for clinical status were used. Cardiac catheterization hemodynamic findings were classified as excellent (normal hemodynamics), fair (unoperated or postoperative without the need for medical or surgical treatment), or poor (hemodynamics that would require eventual operative intervention or, if inoperable, subpulmonary ventricular pressure two-thirds that of systemic pressure, or end-diastolic pressures greater than 1.5 times normal), or as pulmonary hypertension (pulmonary artery systolic pressure beyond and stenoses of at least two thirds that of systemic pressure). The presence of arrhythmias was ascertained from a review of routine resting electrocardiograms taken during two time periods: 1 week to 1 year before sudden death and 1 year to 2 years before sudden death. Holter electrocardiograms were not used because there were insufficient data on these patients to permit adequate comparison. In defining the cause of death, a "probable arrhythmia" was said to be present if indicated on an electrocardiogram obtained at the time of the sudden event, or if the event leading to sudden death had a similar history to a previous episode of a documented arrhythmia causing syncope. A "possible arrhythmia" was said to be present if a history of arrhythmia in a high-risk category could be obtained in a patient in whom the exact arrhythmia at the time of death was not known: for example, a patient with postoperative tetralogy of Fallot with prior ventricular arrhythmia or a patient with prior bradyarrhythmia who had undergone Mustard repair.

RESULTS

DIAGNOSTIC CATEGORIES

Of the 981 patients seen in the Pediatric Cardiology Section at Texas Children's Hospital who died between 1959 and 1983, 101 (10.3%) died suddenly. We have divided the diagnoses of these 101 patients into five categories (Table 15–1). The largest two groups consisted of patients with unoperated congenital heart disease and patients

Table 15–1. Diagnoses in 101 Patients Who Were Treated at Texas Children's Hospital Between 1959 and 1983 and Who Subsequently Died Suddenly

DIAGNOSIS (TOTAL)	NUMBER OF PATIENTS
Unoperated congenital heart disease (n = 36)	
Left-to-right shunt with pulmonary hypertension	11
Tetralogy of Fallot/pulmonary atresia + VSD	7
Cardiomyopathy	5
Aortic insufficiency	3
Hypertrophic cardiomyopathy	3
L transposition of the great arteries	2
Aortic stenosis	2
Aortic aneurysm	1
Hypoplastic coronary arteries	1
Myxomatous mitral + tricuspid	1
Unoperated, acquired heart disease (n = 7)	
Primary pulmonary hypertension	4
Acquired cardiomyopathy	3
Prolonged QT interval (n = 5)	
No congenital heart disease	4
With congenital heart disease	1
Palliated congenital heart disease (n = 17)	
Right-to-left shunt PO AP anastomosis	12
Transposition PO Blalock-Hanlon	4
Left-to-right shunt PO PA banding	1
Postoperative repair: congenital heart disease (n = 36)	
Tetralogy of Fallot: pulmonary atresia/VSD	11
AV canal/VSD	5
Transposition: PO Mustard	5
Transposition + VSD: PO Mustard + VSD	4
Aortic valve replacement	4
Mitral valve replacement	3
Tricuspid valve replacement	1
Ostium primum ASD	1
Hypertrophic obstructive cardiomyopathy: PO myotomy	1
Patent ductus arteriosus (with CCAVB)	1

AP, aorticopulmonary; ASD, atrial septal defect; AV, atrioventricular; CCAVB, congenital complete AV block; PA, pulmonary artery; PO, postoperative; VSD, ventricular septal defect.

with postoperative repair of congenital heart disease. These were followed by patients with palliated congenital heart disease, those with unoperated acquired heart disease, and those with a prolonged QT interval. Of note is the fact that no patient in this group who died suddenly had a normal heart. All of these patients, by the fact that they were seen in a pediatric cardiology clinic at least once, were thought to have heart disease. Nonetheless, no patient discharged from the clinic with a diagnosis of normal heart later died suddenly.

CLINICAL INFORMATION

The male:female ratio was 1.5:1 (62 male, 39 female). Although this indicated a trend, it did not achieve statistical significance. Of the 101 patients, 86% had been seen in the Pediatric Cardiology Clinic within 1 year before death. The clinical status (using New York Heart Association criteria) was Class I–II in 28%, Class III in 49%, and Class IV in 23%. Therefore, 72% of the patients were thought to be in fair or poor condition at the time of their last clinic visit. On chest radiography at this last visit, 85% were found to have cardiac enlargement. Hemodynamics had been assessed at cardiac catheterization in 75 of the 101 patients. This was done an average of 2.3 years before the patient's death; 89% of these patients had catheterization performed less than 5 years before death. The hemodynamics were excellent in 6%, fair in 5%, and poor in 46%, with pulmonary hypertension in 43%. Therefore, in 89% of the patients, a severe hemodynamic abnormality was present. Overall, more than three quarters of the patients who died suddenly in this series were severely symptomatic, had an abnormal chest roentgenogram, or had poor hemodynamics at cardiac catheterization.

ELECTROCARDIOGRAPHIC FINDINGS

Arrhythmias

A routine electrocardiogram taken between 1 week and 1 year before the patient's death was available in 86 patients. Of these patients, 49 (57%) had an arrhythmia, and 37 (43%) had no arrhythmia on routine electrocardiogram (Table 15–2).

The arrhythmias present on electrocardiogram 2 years before death were compared with those present within 1 year before death. In electrocardiograms taken 2 years before death, arrhythmias were present in 1 in 42 of the patients. Therefore, a significantly higher ($p < 0.05$) proportion of patients had arrhythmias in the year before their death than had arrhythmias 2 years before death. In 6 patients, the change in arrhythmia resulted from an operation that occurred in the year before death. It appears that in a certain number of patients, arrhythmias develop in the year before sudden death. This does not necessarily imply that the arrhythmia caused the death, only that the development of an arrhythmia was associated with later sudden death.

Table 15–2. Arrhythmias on ECG 1 Week to 1 Year Before Death (N = 86)

ARRHYTHMIA	PERCENTAGE OF PATIENTS
PVC	20
Atrial flutter	8
Sinus bradycardia	7
Junctional rhythm	7
Complete AV block	6
Complete AV block with pacemaker	5
JR + PVC	5
CAVB + PM + PVC	2
AFL + PVC	2
SVT	1
VT	1
Total	64

AFL, atrial flutter; AV, atrioventricular; CAVB, complete AV block; JR, junctional rhythm; PM, pacemaker; PVC, premature ventricular contraction; SVT, supraventricular tachycardia; VT, ventricular tachycardia. Some patients had more than one arrhythmia.

Other Findings

On the electrocardiogram taken less than 1 year before death, 9 additional patients without arrhythmias had a severe abnormality on the electrocardiogram: 3 had a prolonged QT interval, 3 had old myocardial infarction, 1 had left ventricular strain in hypertrophic cardiomyopathy, 1 had left ventricular strain after aortic valve replacement, and 1 had complete right bundle branch block after a left septal myotomy for hypertrophic obstructive cardiomyopathy. If these 9 patients are added to the 49 with arrhythmias before sudden death, then 67% of patients had an electrocardiographic abnormality other than the one that might be expected for their underlying lesion (e.g., the usual abnormality for tetralogy of Fallot is right ventricular hypertrophy; this was not included).

TREATMENT

Medical treatment had been prescribed for only a small number of these patients who died suddenly. Drug treatment at the time of death included digoxin (79%), diuretics (49%), quinidine (7%), propranolol (3%), isoproterenol (2%), mexiletine (1%), and belladonna (1%). Three patients being treated with quinidine for atrial flutter were noted at the time of their sudden episode to have a slow rate; in one, this was high grade AV block, and in the other two, slow junctional rhythm. An additional patient with junctional rhythm and premature ventricular contractions treated with quinidine was found at the time of his death to have extremely slow junctional rhythm. Propranolol had been prescribed for three patients. In one, this had been prescribed for atrial flutter and had been ineffective. The other two patients had a prolonged QT interval and were known to be noncompliant in taking their propranolol. Only one patient had been prescribed phenytoin at the time of his death. Phenytoin was effective in treating his premature ventricular contractions, but he was noncompliant. This was also the case for one patient who had been prescribed mexiletine. Therefore, four patients who died from ventricular arrhythmias were known to be noncompliant. Isoproterenol had been given to two patients with complete atrioventricular (AV) block, and belladonna had been prescribed for one patient with junctional rhythm. Three of these four patients had documented ventricular arrhythmias.

CIRCUMSTANCES OF DEATH

The activity of the patient immediately preceding death was known in 46 of the 101 cases. Sudden death occurred during sports in 22% of patients, with the patient awake but not active in 50%, and with the patient asleep in 28%. The mean age at death was 12.4 years (range, 1 year to 30 years). In postoperative patients, sudden death occurred an average of 4.5 years after surgery (2 months to 18 years). A presumed cause of death was known in 53 of the 101 patients (Table 15–3).

CLINICAL FINDINGS

Differences Among Diagnostic Categories

Among the five diagnostic classes (unoperated congenital heart disease, unoperated acquired

Table 15–3. Known Cause of Death (N = 53)

CAUSE		PERCENTAGE OF PATIENTS
Arrhythmia		
Probable	32	
Possible	21	
Pacemaker	9	
Total		62
SBE		11
CVA		9
Pulmonary embolus		8
Aspiration		4
Penicillin anaphylaxis		2
Hemoptysis		2
Aortic aneurysm dissection		2
		100

CVA, cerebrovascular accident; SBE, subacute bacterial endocarditis.

heart disease, palliated congenital heart disease, postoperative congenital heart disease, and long QT interval) the clinical findings differed in four major areas. With respect to clinical status, the unoperated patients were more limited than the palliated or postoperative congenital heart disease patients: 95% of the unoperated patients were in class III–IV compared with 62% of those with congenital heart disease that had been palliated or repaired ($p < 0.001$).

There was a marked difference in the presence of preceding arrhythmia. An arrhythmia was present in the year before sudden death in 88% of those who had undergone repair of congenital heart disease compared with 35% of those in the unoperated or palliated group ($p < 0.0001$). Premature ventricular contractions in the year preceding sudden death were significantly higher in the postoperative repair group (88%) than in the unoperated or palliated group (34%) ($p < 0.01$).

The activity preceding death also varied with the group. Those patients who died during sports were in the following three groups: (1) unoperated congenital heart disease, (2) prolonged QT interval, or (3) postoperative congenital heart disease. None of the patients with palliated congenital heart disease died during sports, perhaps because these patients were not physically capable of participating in vigorous sports. Death occurred during sleep in patients in all of the groups except the prolonged QT interval group.

With respect to the cause of death, patients after repair of congenital heart disease had significantly more known or suspected arrhythmias (78%) compared with the unoperated or palliated patients (31%) ($p < 0.001$).

Most Common Cardiac Diagnoses

The eight most common diagnoses in these patients were, in descending order, right-to-left shunt postoperative anastomosis (12%), left-to-right shunt with pulmonary hypertension (Eisenmenger's syndrome) (11%), postoperative tetralogy of Fallot (11%), tetralogy of Fallot unoperated (7%), cardiomyopathy (5%), postoperative AV canal (5%), postoperative Mustard operation for transposition of the great arteries (5%), and prolonged QT interval (5%). These eight diagnoses made up 61% of the patients. Other diagnoses were present in 4% or less of the patients.

Presence of Arrhythmias

There were significant differences among the diagnoses with respect to the presence of arrhythmias within 1 year preceding sudden death (Table 15–4). There was a low incidence of arrhythmias (less than 25%) in the patients with left-to-right shunt and pulmonary hypertension (Eisenmenger's syndrome) and in those with unoperated or palliated tetralogy of Fallot. In all the other diagnoses, more than 50% of the patients had arrhythmias in the year before death. The only diagnoses in which premature ventricular contractions occurred in 25% or more of the patients were postoperative tetralogy of Fallot and long QT interval. Atrial flutter was uncommon except in postoperative Mustard patients. Sinus bradycardia and junctional rhythm occurred in less than 25% of the patients except those with a prolonged QT interval and postoperative Mustard. AV block was uncommon except in patients who had undergone repair of complete AV canal or ventricular septal defect.

Circumstances of Death

The majority of patients died while at rest, not during sports or while asleep (Table 15–5). The only deaths that occurred during sports were in

Table 15–4. Arrhythmias Present 1 Week to 1 Year Before Death

DIAGNOSIS	NUMBER OF PATIENTS	% ANY ARRHYTHMIA	% PVC	% AFL	% JR	% AVB	% COMPLEX
L-to-R shunt PH	11	14	14				
TOF	7	17				17	
CM	5	60	20	20			20
LQTS	5	75	25		50		
R-to-L anas	12	10	10				
PO TOF	11	100	70		10	10	10
PO canal	5	75				75	
POM	5	100		50	25		25

AFL, atrial flutter; AVB, atrioventricular block; CM, cardiomyopathy; JR, junctional rhythm; LQTS, long QT syndrome; L-to-R, left to right; PH, pulmonary hypertension; PO canal, postoperative AV canal repair; POM, postoperative Mustard procedure; PO TOF, postoperative tetralogy of Fallot; PVC, premature ventricular contractions; R-to-L anas, right-to-left shunt postoperative anastomosis; TOF, tetralogy of Fallot.

Table 15–5. Circumstances of Death

DIAGNOSIS	NUMBER OF PATIENTS	ACTIVITY AT TIME OF DEATH		ARRHYTHMIA CAUSE (%)	AGE AT DEATH ± SEM (years)	PO INTERVAL ± SEM (years)
		Active (%)	**Sleep (%)**			
L-to-R shunt PH	11	0	0	33	15.9 ± 2.0	—
TOF	7	0	67	25	10.6 ± 3.4	—
CM	5	50	50	100	10.6 ± 3.1	—
LQTS	5	67	0	100	11.4 ± 2.5	—
R-to-L anas	12	0	0	30	10.4 ± 2.5	4.2 ± 1.5
PO TOF	11	28	14	100	16.2 ± 2.2	4.2 ± 1.3
PO canal	5	0	0	100	8.6 ± 2.9	1.7 ± 0.5
POM	5	60	40	100	11.5 ± 3.8	7.1 ± 2.6

CM, cardiomyopathy; LQTS, long QT syndrome; L-to-R, left to right; PO canal, postoperative AV canal repair; POM, postoperative Mustard procedure; PO TOF, postoperative tetralogy of Fallot; R-to-L anas, right-to-left shunt postoperative anastomosis; SEM, standard error of mean; TOF, tetralogy of Fallot.

patients with a prolonged QT interval or cardiomyopathy and in postoperative Mustard or tetralogy patients. The only patients who died during sleep were those who had unoperated tetralogy of Fallot or cardiomyopathy or were postoperative Mustard or tetralogy of Fallot patients. Either a probable arrhythmia or a possible arrhythmia was present in the majority of these diagnoses. However, an arrhythmia did not appear to be involved in patients with a left-to-right shunt and pulmonary hypertension, with unoperated tetralogy of Fallot, or with a right-to-left shunt postoperative anastomosis.

There were two groups in which patients were significantly older at the time of death than in other groups: postoperative tetralogy of Fallot and left-to-right shunt with pulmonary hypertension ($p < 0.01$). Patients who had undergone repair of AV canal died at a significantly younger age than the rest of the group. From examination of the postoperative interval, it is apparent that the postoperative AV canal patients died at a young age because they died relatively early postoperatively. The postoperative Mustard patients actually died significantly longer after surgery than did other patients but at an earlier age than postoperative tetralogy patients. Postoperative tetralogy patients died at an older age because, presumably, reparative surgery occurred at an older age than did the Mustard operation.

ARRHYTHMIA FINDINGS

Diagnostic Differences

Specific arrhythmias found in the year preceding sudden death differed among the diagnoses. Premature ventricular contractions were found in 50% or more of patients with acquired cardiomyopathy, ostium primum atrial septal defect, transposition of the great arteries, or ventricular septal defect or following Mustard or tetralogy of Fallot repair. Atrial flutter was found in 50% or more of those with aortic insufficiency or acquired cardiomyopathy and in those who had undergone Mustard repair. Sinus bradycardia or junctional rhythm was found in more than 50% of patients with transposition of the great arteries, ventricular septal defect, or prolonged QT interval or in postoperative Mustard patients. Complete AV block was found in more than 50% of patients with L transposition of the great arteries and following patent ductus arteriosus (congenital complete AV block) surgery or tricuspid valve replacement.

The presence of arrhythmia was related to poor hemodynamics at cardiac catheterization in these patients. An arrhythmia was found in 11% of those with good hemodynamics compared with 50% of those with poor hemodynamics ($p < 0.01$). Each of the individual arrhythmias (e.g., premature ventricular contractions) was significantly related to poor hemodynamics, with the exception of junctional rhythm. Junctional rhythm was significantly related to good hemodynamics ($p < 0.01$); good hemodynamics were found in 56% of those with junctional rhythm compared with 5% of the patients without junctional rhythm ($p < 0.01$). This indicates that the postoperative patients with junctional rhythm (largely postoperative Mustard patients) who died suddenly had good hemodynamics.

The presumed direct cause of death was significantly related to the presence of arrhythmia in the year before death. However, there were some exceptions. Among the 17 patients without

Table 15–6. Number of Patients Seen at Texas Children's Hospital, Pediatric Cardiology Section, from 1959 to 1983, and Frequently of Sudden Death

VARIABLE	1959–1963	1964–1968	1969–1973	1974–1978	1979–1983
Number of patients	2330	1716	4668	6562	8126
Number of sudden deaths	3	27	21	37	22
Percentage of total patients	0.13	0.92	0.43	0.54	0.27

previous arrhythmia noted on routine electrocardiogram within 1 year before death, 4 had a probable arrhythmia at the time of death, and 13 died of other causes. Of the 28 patients with an arrhythmia in the year preceding death, only 4 had another known cause for their death, leaving 24 of 28 with either a probable or possible arrhythmia responsible for their death.

HISTORICAL COMPARISON

Between 1959 and 1983, 23,402 patients were seen in the Pediatric Cardiology Section at Texas Children's Hospital; 981 (4.2%) of these patients are known to have died. Sudden death, by our criteria, occurred in 101, nonsudden death in 730, and accidental death in 10; there was insufficient information for 140 of the patients. Since 1968, each 5-year period has seen an increase in the total number of patients seen (Table 15–6). Between 1978 and 1983, there were two major changes in arrhythmia management, with aggressive drug treatment of premature ventricular contractions and aggressive pacemaker treatment of bradydysrhythmias. During those years, none of the 18 sudden deaths occurred in patients with prior ventricular arrhythmias; however, 16 of the 69 patients who died suddenly in the previous 20 years had ventricular arrhythmias ($p < 0.05$). Since 1978, there has been one sudden death; this was caused by a documented pacemaker failure in a postoperative tetralogy patient with surgical complete AV block. Since 1977, there has been no sudden death in a patient after a Mustard procedure for transposition of the great arteries.

SUMMARY

In this study of sudden death in patients previously seen in a pediatric cardiology clinic, we attempted to identify factors that might have been associated with later sudden death. The true denominator of these factors is unknown. For example, the number of patients with these defects who have arrhythmias and do not die is not known in all cases. Further studies are planned to document the incidence of these factors in patients with similar lesions who did not die. The following conclusions can be drawn from the study:

1. More than three quarters of the patients who died suddenly had severe limitation of activity, cardiac enlargement on chest radiograph, and poor hemodynamics at cardiac catheterization.
2. The majority of patients who died suddenly had an arrhythmia in the 12-month period preceding death. A significant number of these arrhythmias developed for the first time in the year preceding death.
3. The presence of arrhythmias was generally related to poor hemodynamics in patients who died suddenly.
4. Approximately one quarter of the patients with arrhythmias received therapy that would currently be thought to be appropriate.
5. Most sudden deaths occurred with the patient at rest, and only approximately one quarter occurred during sports participation.
6. Specific arrhythmias are present in association with specific conditions and appear to be correlated with the risk of sudden death in that group.
7. Conspicuously absent from the list of patients and diagnoses are children with a normal heart and children with mitral valve prolapse.
8. With improvement in treatment practices (i.e., more aggressive drug treatment of ventricular arrhythmias and more aggressive pacemaker treatment in bradyarrhythmias), the incidence of sudden death at our institution has been reduced significantly from previous years.

ACKNOWLEDGMENTS

Research was supported in part by grants HL24916, HL07190, and RR00188 from the National Institutes of Health, Bethesda, Maryland, and by a grant from the J.S. Abercrombie Foundation.

CHAPTER 16

FETAL ARRHYTHMIAS

John M. Clark and Christopher L. Case

The diagnosis and treatment of arrhythmias in the fetus have been the latest frontiers encountered in the field of pediatric electrophysiology (EP). Widespread use of electronic fetal monitoring by obstetricians as well as technologic advances in fetal echocardiography have been instrumental in elucidating the incidence and natural history of rhythm disturbances in the fetus. The purpose of this chapter is to summarize current concepts in the diagnosis and treatment of commonly encountered antenatal rhythm problems.

ELECTROPHYSIOLOGY AND HEMODYNAMICS OF THE NORMAL FETUS

An appreciation of normal in utero cardiac development, EP, and hemodynamics facilitates understanding aberrations of fetal heart function. The conduction system of the fetal heart is fully mature by the 16th week of gestation. The atrioventricular (AV) node and the His bundle form separately and unite in approximately the 8th week of gestation. The sinus node is fully formed by 10 weeks' gestation, and by 16 weeks sinus rhythm of the normal fetus can be adequately characterized by fetal echocardiography.

Gestational changes in fetal heart rate have been studied. At six menstrual weeks, mean heart rate was 100 bpm. This increased to 143 bpm by 9 menstrual weeks and to 149 bpm by 20 menstrual weeks. Thereafter, heart rate declines to a mean of 135 bpm at term.[1, 2] Normal fetal heart rate in the third trimester varies between 110 and 150 bpm.

Hemodynamics of the normal fetus have been studied extensively both in animals and in humans. The ventricular compliance characteristics of the fetus are very similar to those of the newborn. Both right and left ventricles are less compliant than their adult counterparts.[3] However, like the adult, the Frank-Starling relationship has been demonstrated to be a very important determinant of fetal cardiac output.[4] The effect of fetal heart rate on cardiac output is a more controversial subject. Rudolph and Heymann demonstrated that there was a direct relationship between spontaneous fetal heart rate and right and left ventricular output.[5] However, with artificial right or left atrial pacing, the effects of heart rate on fetal cardiac output are not simple. It seems that with pacing, cardiac output either correlates negatively or does not change. Doppler echocardiography has also aided in evaluating hemodynamics of the fetus. This is discussed in more detail later.

Developmental aspects of the cellular EP in the fetus have also been studied in various animal models. The cardiac action potential and the ionic currents responsible for the various phases of the action potential go through developmental changes as the fetus matures in utero.[6] The sensitivity of the myocardial cells to various drugs also shows gestational changes. However, these changes appear to be more species specific.[7–9] Understanding the developmental aspects of fetal drug sensitivity on the cellular and molecular level may form the basis for future advances in the pharmacologic treatment of fetal arrhythmias.

FETAL ARRHYTHMIAS: GENERAL CONCEPTS

During the second and third trimester, fetal heart rate varies between 110 and 150 bpm. The predominant rhythm is regular, with an undulatory pattern of variability. Fetal arrhythmias can be defined as any irregularity to the predominant rhythm or any prolonged rate less than 110 or greater than 160 bpm not associated with uterine contractions. Of 3882 obstetric ultrasounds, Calvin et al reported that 162 patients (or 4%) were referred for evaluation of suspected arrhythmia.[10] Of those, 80 (49%) had a documented arrhythmia by fetal echocardiography. Thus, the incidence of fetal arrhythmias overall is 1 to 2%.[10]

Fetal arrhythmias can be divided into three main types. The first are premature beats, which may originate from either the atrium or the ventricle; the second are tachycardias, either supraventricular (SVT) or ventricular (VT); and the third are bradycardias, either sinus or caused by some degree of AV block. For SVT, the predominant mechanism is thought to be AV re-entry, although atrial flutter is not rare. Atrial fibrillation and chaotic atrial tachycardia have also been reported. Ventricular arrhythmias in the fetus may be either re-entrant or the result of an automatic focus. Bradycardia can be caused either by a sick sinus node or by some degree of functional or structural AV block. The majority (80–90%) of fetal arrhythmias are premature beats. Re-entrant SVT constitutes approximately 5% of fetal arrhythmias. Complete heart block accounts for about 2.5%, and atrial flutter-fibrillation occurs in approximately 1 to 2% of fetal arrhythmias.[10, 11] Documented VT is rare in the fetus. Junctional ectopic tachycardia has been diagnosed at least once in a fetus.[12]

The evaluation of the fetus with a suspected or documented arrhythmia must include an investigation for associated fetal or maternal conditions that may alter arrhythmia management. Approximately one half of fetuses with congenital complete AV block have an associated structural cardiac anomaly, usually AV septal defect and left atrial isomerism.[13–16] Those fetuses with isolated complete heart block and structurally normal hearts have a near 100% association with maternal anti-Ro (SS-A) antibody and connective tissue disorders, specifically systemic lupus erythematosus (SLE) and Sjögren's syndrome.[14, 17] The incidence of structural cardiac anomalies in fetuses with SVT is 1 to 5%.

The hemodynamic consequences of fetal arrhythmias are varied. Isolated premature contractions in a fetus with a structurally normal heart are generally hemodynamically insignificant. Congestive heart failure and hydrops fetalis are a common consequence of sustained fetal arrhythmias. Nonimmune hydrops seems to be the common pathophysiologic expression of many fetal disease states, but its association with fetal arrhythmias is strong. In a fetus with a structurally normal heart, hydrops is a common consequence of SVT. Bradycardia secondary to AV block may cause hydrops in a fetus with a normally structured heart, although cardiac compromise is more common with structural heart disease.

DIAGNOSTIC EVALUATION

ON WHOM?

The indications for fetal echocardiography for arrhythmia diagnosis are still evolving. Most fetal arrhythmia evaluations are prompted by an irregularity of the fetal heart tone noted on routine prenatal evaluation by the obstetrician. When hydrops is suspected on the basis of a routine obstetric sonogram, evaluation of the fetal rhythm should also be done because of the high association between these two entities. In the United States, generally only pregnant women with suspected fetal heart disease or whose fetuses are at high risk are examined by fetal echocardiography. In general, it is part of the routine complete fetal echocardiography exam to assess fetal heart rate and rhythm. Risk factors, such as those proposed by Reed and Sahn, are generally utilized as indications for fetal echocardiography,[18] although the most predictive risk factor to date is a positive screening obstetric ultrasound.

WHEN?

The most advantageous time for fetal examination is between 16 and 32 weeks' gestation. This happens to coincide with the time period when most (75%) fetal arrhythmias are first detected.[19] At 14 weeks, the heart can be imaged but is inconsistently examinable. After 32 weeks, high-quality imaging is more difficult, but examination can be performed until term.

WHY?

The importance of diagnosing the cause of fetal arrhythmias (whether they are intrinsic or extrinsic alterations of rhythm) has been well studied. Since the early 1970s, antenatal variations of the fetal heart rate in response to uterine contraction or fetal movement (stress and nonstress tests) have been used to assess fetal well-being. Obstetricians have also used fetal heart rate and variability monitored during labor to predict outcome and guide therapy. Sustained fetal tachycardia and bradycardia have been well correlated with perinatal morbidity and mortality. Fetal bradycardia, coinciding with the end of uterine contraction (type 2 pattern of deceleration), has been used as a sign of fetal distress. Also a study by Hager and Pauly has confirmed an increased risk of neonatal complications in association with intrapartum fetal tachycardia.[20]

In a study of 113 cases of intrinsic fetal bradycardias and tachycardias, Lingman et al demonstrated an increased incidence of fetal distress in labor, perinatal and neonatal mortality, and congenital malformations in the arrhythmia group compared with the general population.[21] Fetal heart rate abnormalities are also correlated with gross congenital malformations. Biale et al noted abnormal fetal heart rates (the most common being bradycardia and variable decelerations) in 54% of fetuses with congenital malformations versus 16% in a control group.[22] The highest rate of pathologic heart rate tracings was found in the group with multiple malformations, chromosomal aberrations, and central nervous system lesions. Therefore, when an abnormal heart rate or rhythm is diagnosed by auscultation of fetal heart tones, characterization of the arrhythmia may be important in predicting fetal outcome and in aiding in treatment planning.

BY WHOM?

It is important to realize that the diagnosis and treatment of fetal arrhythmias require a team effort. Interaction among the primary obstetrician, perinatologist, pediatric cardiologist, and neonatologist is of utmost importance to ensure proper treatment planning. Many times, the initial impetus for the evaluation comes from the primary care obstetrician. Many obstetric ultrasonographers are adept at performing four-chamber views of the fetal heart and beginning an initial assessment of fetal rhythm. To characterize fully the exact cause and mechanism of the fetal rhythm, the pediatric cardiologist may readily provide the needed expertise. When the rhythm has been defined and the possibility of associated cardiac anomalies evaluated, interaction between the entire team is again needed to formulate treatment strategies.

HOW?

Electrocardiography currently is of minimal use in assessing the nature of fetal arrhythmias. Its inability to display clearly both the P wave and the QRS makes it ill suited for fetal rhythm diagnosis. Fetal echocardiography is the mainstay of evaluation. Three modes of ultrasonography—two dimensional, M mode, and Doppler—are used in the assessment of fetal rhythm problems. Two-dimensional examination is used mainly to characterize the structure of the fetal heart and associated abnormalities, such as pleural or pericardial effusions, seen with hydrops fetalis.

M mode is most useful in defining the relationship of AV electrical events. The M-mode probe may be positioned in such a way as to image simultaneously (1) both the atrium or atrial septum and the ventricle; (2) the AV valve and the ventricle; or (3) the semilunar valve and the atrium. Timing between the atrial and ventricular events and their interaction in the AV node is made by the timing of (1) atrial and ventricular contraction; (2) AV valve opening and closing; or (3) atrial contraction and semilunar valve opening.

Doppler echocardiography is also extremely helpful in characterizing fetal arrhythmias. Pulse Doppler echocardiography is used to define AV contraction sequences as well as atrial and ventricular rates. By using a large Doppler sample volume, which is positioned in the ventricle, to sample ventricular inflow (atrial contraction) and outflow (ventricular contraction) simultaneously, AV relationship can be delineated.[23]

Hemodynamic assessment of the severity of the fetal arrhythmia can be performed with analysis of Doppler waveform and color flow Doppler patterns. Premature beats and tachycardia result in flow reversal in the inferior vena cava. The faster the tachycardia rate, the greater the degree of flow reversal. With Doppler wave form analysis or color flow Doppler, this flow reversal can be seen as venous pulsations in the umbilical vein.[24, 25] In the fetus with sustained SVT, AV valve incompetence may be a sign of SVT-induced "cardiomyopathy." A semiquantitative analysis of the degree of regurgitation, using color flow Doppler to measure the length and the width of the regurgitant jet, may be useful in assessing the degree of ventricular dysfunction induced by the SVT.[26] It may also be useful to monitor the response to therapy.

GENERAL PRINCIPLES OF THERAPY

Before dealing with the treatment of specific fetal arrhythmias, it is important to review some general principles that are applicable to all rhythm disturbances. First, similar to therapy in pediatric or adult patients, fetal rhythm disturbances should be treated "in their clinical context." In other words, the mere presence of a fetal arrhythmia may not, in itself, be an indication for treatment. The decision to treat should be based on the hemodynamic consequences of the arrhythmia and its implications to fetal well-being, the gestational age of the fetus, and the possible consequences of in utero therapy on maternal health. Formulation of a risk-benefit ratio is the basis of good treatment planning. Once the specific treatment plan is established, careful follow-up in all situations is mandatory. It has been shown clinically as well as in experimental animals that hydrops can develop within 48 hours in the fetus with tachycardia.[27–29] Thus, benign arrhythmias, such as premature contractions, that are of no hemodynamic consequence at one time within a few days may result in a severely compromised fetus should tachycardia be provoked.

When a hemodynamically significant fetal arrhythmia is present in a near-term fetus, the treatment of choice, if possible, is delivery. Thus, fetal maturity and the possibility of perinatal morbidity and mortality resulting from prematurity must be weighed against the risks of in utero treatment. These decisions can be made only in conjunction with both a perinatologist and neonatologist. Clinical and laboratory assessment of maturity is not exact, and must be weighed against the hazards of in utero arrhythmia therapy.

SPECIFIC ARRHYTHMIAS

RE-ENTRANT SVT

The diagnosis of AV re-entrant SVT requires a one-to-one relationship between atrial and ventricular contractions, with a corresponding heart rate generally in the range of 240 to 260 bpm. This arrhythmia is usually not associated with structural heart disease; however, there is a frequent association with hydrops fetalis. In the fetus, the vast majority of re-entrant AV SVT is caused by an anomalous AV accessory connection. The tachycardia circuit is antegrade down the AV node and retrograde up the accessory connection. In 1969, Silber and Durnin reported the first case of nonimmune hydrops fetalis associated with fetal SVT.[30] Since then, Friedman et al evaluated 984 fetal arrhythmias, 89% of which were isolated premature contractions and 5% were re-entrant SVT.[11] Van Engelen[31] and Maxwell[32] and their colleagues reported that between 40 and 50% of fetuses with re-entrant SVT will have some degree of hydrops.

The hemodynamic consequences of fetal SVT depend, in part, on the rate of tachycardia as well as the duration. In addition, there are certainly some as yet undefined factors that make some fetuses more prone to hydrops than others. On ultrasonography, what may be seen are venous pulsations in the umbilical vein and flow reversal in the IVC as well as signs of congestive heart failure, including ventricular dilatation, decreased cardiac function, AV valve insufficiency, pericardial or pleural effusions, ascites, skin edema, and decreased fetal movements. The most critical issue when diagnosing an arrhythmia by echocardiography is to document that a tachycardia is supraventricular and not ventricular in origin. This is because digoxin is the first-line drug of choice for SVT, whereas it is contraindicated in VT because it can exacerbate the rhythm disturbance.

Re-entrant SVT is the most common fetal arrhythmia requiring treatment. Digoxin has historically been the first-line drug of choice. Lingman reported its first successful use in utero to treat fetal SVT in 1980.[33] Since that time, it has been used extensively during pregnancy with both safety and efficacy. The dose and route of administration vary depending on the clinical scenario. Digoxin has been administered maternally by both oral and intravenous routes. It has also been administered directly to the fetus by intramuscular, intraperitoneal, and intraamniotic routes as well as intravenously, with direct injection into the umbilical vein.[34–37] In general, maternal doses are in the high range, with the total loading dose of 1 to 2 mg and maintenance dose of 0.5 to 0.75 mg daily. Maternal levels should be kept in the high therapeutic range (1.5–2.0 ng/ml).

Placental transfer of digoxin is excellent; fetal levels are 80 to 100% of maternal levels. Placental transfer is decreased, however, in the hydropic fetus; fetal levels are 10 to 50% of maternal levels.[38] It is in this situation that direct fetal therapy may be indicated. In the hydropic fetus with SVT, Friedman et al recommended direct fetal therapy with intraumbilical adenosine and intraumbilical digoxin at a dose of 10 μg/kg estimated fetal weight, followed by oral maternal maintenance digoxin.[11] If this regimen fails, they then add flecainide or procainamide.

Flecainide is currently the second-line drug of choice for fetal SVT. However, in several series, it has been used safely and effectively as a first-line treatment.[31, 39, 40] Some of the positive aspects of flecainide therapy are (1) more rapid conversion to sinus rhythm with a mean time to conversion of 48 hours with flecainide versus 2 to 3 weeks with digoxin[40]; (2) ease of administration, most commonly given by maternal oral route; (3) good placental transfer with fetal levels 65 to 95% of maternal levels[40–42]; and (4) no known teratogenic or noncardiac side effects to the fetus.[43] Some of the concerns about flecainide use in pregnancy are that it (1) may be proarrhythmic in adults with ambient ectopy and myocardial infarctions (whether this is of significance when used in a healthy pregnant female is unknown)[44]; and (2) decreases heart rate variability.[45] This second issue seems to be dose dependent and is noted in the absence of any change in fetal movements. It, therefore, appears to be a side effect of the medication and not an indication of fetal distress. Allan et al reported one fetal death 3 days after conversion to sinus rhythm with flecainide.[40] However, the fetus had also undergone cordocentesis 24 hours before death. Whether the fetal death was due to flecainide therapy, cordocentesis, or some other factor is unknown. It seems prudent, however, that if flecainide is used as a first-line therapy for fetal SVT, once sinus rhythm is achieved, it could be gradually discontinued or tapered to the lowest dose that maintains sinus rhythm. The usual starting dose for flecainide is 200 to 300 mg/day in two to three divided doses given by maternal oral route. It is then tapered by 50-mg increments over 1 to 2 weeks. Therapeutic levels are 400 to 800 μg/L.

Amiodarone is also an effective, second-line drug for the therapy of fetal SVT. Because of known maternal and fetal side effects, it will not likely become a drug of first choice. In published series, amiodarone was more commonly given by direct fetal routes than was digoxin or flecainide. This is probably due to the more desperate clinical status of the fetus as well as the poor placental transfer of amiodarone (fetal levels approximately 12% of maternal levels). Flack reported administering 10 mg/kg intraumbilically and, in the same procedure, 10 mg/kg intraperitoneally, followed by maternal oral dosing of 200 mg orally every 8 hours.[46] This regimen achieved sinus rhythm in 3 days. Arnoux reported achieving sinus rhythm in 14 days with an oral regimen of 1600 mg/day for 4 days, then 1200 mg/day for 4 days, followed by 800 mg/day for 6 weeks given by the maternal oral route.[47]

The most common side effect of amiodarone therapy is thyroid dysfunction, either hyper- or hypothyroidism, in either the mother or the fetus.[47–51] Occasionally, the hypothyroidism requires transient therapy with L-thyroxine. However, there have been no reports to date of permanent thyroid dysfunction in an infant or child with fetal exposure to amiodarone. Less common, but more concerning, are potential neurologic side effects to the fetus exposed to amiodarone. Magee et al reported that of 12 infants with known in utero exposure to amiodarone, 1 had developmental delay, 1 had congenital nystagmus, and 2 had transient thyroid dysfunction.[48] Three of these infants were exposed from the first trimester onward. Plomp et al reported one patient with motor delay and speech impairment and one transient hypothyroidism out of five children exposed in utero.[50] De Wolf et al reported one other case of an infant with severe transient hypothyroidism and psychomotor retardation who was exposed to amiodarone from 13 weeks' gestation on.[51] Many other authors reported successful use of amiodarone in utero with normal neurologic development afterward.[47, 49, 52–54]

Other medications that have been used to treat fetal SVT include sotalol, procainamide, propranolol, quinidine, verapamil, and adenosine.[43, 55–60] Sotalol is currently gaining wider usage, whereas verapamil is used less often because of its inhibitory effects on myocardial function. Adenosine may play a greater role in the future for rapid conversion of hydropic fetuses that either have already been loaded with an antiarrhythmic medication or will be loaded concurrently with the adenosine. Adenosine is limited in that it can be given only by the intraumbilical route.

ATRIAL FLUTTER-FIBRILLATION

Atrial flutter-fibrillation is about one third as common as re-entrant SVT as a cause of fetal tachycardia. It constitutes 1 to 2% of all fetal arrhythmias. The echocardiographic diagnosis is usually made on the basis of an atrial contraction rate in the 400- to 460-bpm range with varying degrees of AV block. The ventricular response can be fixed and regular or variable and irregular. The incidence of associated structural heart disease is greater than that for re-entrant SVT, with approximately 20% of patients having a coexistent heart defect. Those patients with structural defects have the worst prognosis.

Treatment for atrial flutter-fibrillation is similar to that for re-entrant SVT; digoxin and flecainide are first- and second-line drugs, respectively. In theory, flecainide could increase the ventricular response to atrial flutter and worsen hemodynamics. In practice, however, flecainide has had good success in converting atrial flutter into sinus rhythm. Van Engelen[31] and Allan[40] and their colleagues published their successful results using flecainide as a first-line drug. Friedman et al suggested maternal intravenous digoxin as first-line therapy.[11] Oral quinidine can be added, if needed, but the digoxin dose should be decreased by one half the initial dose. If this regimen fails, they recommended adding amiodarone.

Overall, drug therapy is successful in converting SVT to sinus rhythm in 82% of patients. Van Engelen et al[31] found that patients with re-entrant-type SVT are slightly more likely to convert than patients with atrial flutter (88% vs. 67%, respectively). They were almost as likely to convert hydropic fetuses compared with nonhydropic fetuses (80% vs. 84%). However, hydropic fetuses took more days (mean, 12 days vs. 3 days) and more medications (mean, 2 vs. 1) to control. All of the nonhydropic fetuses survived the neonatal period, whereas 86% of the hydropic fetuses survived (18 of 21). Fifty percent of the fetuses successfully converted had their tachycardia reappear at birth. Overall, 78% of the patients were on some medication at 1 month of age. Fourteen percent were still on an antiarrhythmic medication at 3 years of age.

VENTRICULAR TACHYCARDIA

VT is a rare arrhythmia in the fetus. Friedman et al[11] reported 4 patients with VT of 984 fetuses with an arrhythmia. The usual rate for VT is between 220 and 280 bpm. The diagnosis is usually made by demonstrating AV dissociation on fetal echocardiography. It is important to exclude the possibility that a fetal tachycardia is ventricular in origin to avoid digoxin therapy, which could potentially exacerbate this arrhythmia. The agents usually used for the treatment of fetal VT are propranolol, quinidine, procainamide, and phenytoin.

SINUS BRADYCARDIA

Fetal bradycardia may be caused by a persistently low sinus rate between 80 and 100 bpm. It is important to exclude fetal hypoxia and distress as the primary cause of the bradycardia. A nonstress test can be used to assess fetal heart rate variability and, thus, fetal well-being. If normal variability exists, then the fetus can be followed and delivery performed vaginally.

GROUP BEATING

Other mechanisms of fetal bradycardia have been termed *group beating*. There are two potential mechanisms of grouped beating. The first is 2:1 AV block. The second, and most common, is blocked atrial ectopy. This is usually blocked atrial bigeminy but can also be trigeminy or quadrigeminy. Grouped beating is easily diagnosed on fetal echocardiography by simultaneous recording of atrial and ventricular contractions. It is important to distinguish these arrhythmias from complete AV block because these types of arrhythmias have a benign course and require no intervention, unlike many cases of complete AV block.[61]

ATRIOVENTRICULAR BLOCK

Congenital complete heart block is diagnosed on echocardiography by the finding of complete AV dissociation in a fetus with ventricular bradycardia. Its incidence is about 1 to 10 in 20,000 live births.[13] It accounts for approximately 2.5% of all fetal arrhythmias diagnosed. Slightly less than half of these patients have a structurally normal heart. The remainder of the fetuses usually have a major structural cardiac anomaly. Of those with a structurally normal heart, virtually all are associated with a maternal connective tissue disease.

In 1977 McCue et al reported an association of congenital complete heart block and maternal SLE.[62] Since that time, studies have shown that, in 1% of pregnancies in females with SLE, the fetus is affected with complete heart block.[14, 17] Virtually all of the affected fetuses in children are born to mothers who are positive for the anti-Ro (SS-A) antibody. Overall, complete heart block affects 1% of pregnancies in women with SLE, but 5% of those who are anti-Ro positive.[63, 64] Another maternal disease that is commonly associated with congenital complete heart block is Sjögren's syndrome. It is important to note, however, that in the majority of pregnancies in which the fetus has congenital complete AV block, the mother is asymptomatic, with no clinical evidence of connective tissue disease.[14, 65] The maternal diagnosis, therefore, is often made after the fetal diagnosis.

The pathophysiologic mechanism of heart block in the fetus is most likely transplacental transfer of antibodies, which then initiate an immune-mediated destruction of the AV conduction system with resultant replacement of the AV node by fibrous tissue. This theory is supported by the fact that greater than 50% of all cases are diagnosed between 16 and 24 weeks' gestation. This time period coincides with the time period when antibody transport across the placenta is increasing. Olah and Gee[66] identified four factors that place the fetus at increased risk for fetal heart block: (1) previous affected pregnancy; (2) high titers of anti-SS-A (>1:16); (3) presence of anti-SS-B (La) in addition to anti-SS-A antibodies; and (4) positive HLA-DR3 haplotype. A previously affected child is the single greatest risk factor; 15 to 30% of subsequent pregnancies are affected.[65, 66] The risk of congenital complete heart block in anti-SS-A–negative females is almost nonexistent.[17]

The hemodynamic consequences in a well-compensated fetus with complete heart block are ventricular dilatation and increased stroke volume.[67] These adaptive mechanisms allow the fetus to maintain a cardiac output adequate to meet metabolic demands. However, 25% of fetuses with isolated complete heart block show signs of congestive heart failure and hydrops fetalis.[14, 19] At least two factors may play a role in the development of hydrops. First, bradycardia may become severe enough to prohibit an adequate cardiac output. Eighty-five percent of fetuses with heart rates less than 55 bpm have hydrops fetalis and fetal or neonatal death.[13] Second, there may be an associated inflammatory myocarditis that results in myocardial dysfunction.

There are two goals of therapy for congenital complete heart block. The first is to ameliorate heart failure and improve survival in those fetuses with complete heart block and nonimmune hydrops fetalis. The second, more recent aim of therapy is to prevent or, in some instances, reverse heart block in a fetus at risk.

The current medicines that have shown some efficacy in treating hydrops in a fetus with complete heart block are digoxin and steroids. Digoxin is given to improve cardiac function, although it has a theoretic possibility of worsening bradycardia. Steroids are given to treat associated myocarditis. The preferred drugs are betamethasone or dexamethasone because these cross the placenta in active form. This regimen has shown favorable results in eliminating effusions and ascites,[63, 68–71] and has also shown occasional improvement in the degree of AV block.[71, 72] Complete heart block, once established, is irreversible. However, there may be a window of opportunity early in the development of complete heart block when it can be either partially or totally reversed.

Furosemide (Lasix) has also been used in addition to the medications just mentioned.[68] Sympathomimetic drugs have also been administered maternally, with some improvement in heart rate but variable results in terms of hydrops. Medicines that have been reported as effective in increasing fetal heart rate include terbutaline, isoproterenol, ritodrine, and salbutamol.[19, 73] Groves et al reported a 20% increase in both heart rate and fractional shortening in bradycardic fetuses after maternal administration of salbutamol. In the severely hydropic fetus with absent fetal movement and at imminent risk of fetal death, transuterine, transthoracic fetal ventricular pacing as well as transuterine, transvenous fetal pacing have been performed, which have proven to be technically feasible.[74, 75]

The alternative to in utero therapy is delivery and immediate pacing. There is high morbidity and mortality associated with premature delivery of a hydropic fetus in addition to the risks and difficulties associated with pacing of a premature infant. This approach requires the greatest amount of cooperation among the perinatologist, neonatologist, and pediatric cardiologist. Case reports have shown some success of premature delivery and placement of temporary pacing wires, either transvenous or epicardial, until the infant is big enough for placement of a permanent pacemaker.[76, 77]

The second goal of therapy—prevention of heart block in a fetus at risk—is a much better goal if it can be achieved. Various therapeutic regimens have been recommended, including plasmapheresis three times a week, starting before the 20th week of gestation, in addition to prednisone to decrease maternal antibodies and dexamethasone to inhibit fetal myocarditis.[63] Kaaja et al[78] reported a single case in which a patient with one previously affected infant was given gamma globulin, 1 g/kg intravenously, at 14 and 18 weeks' gestation in addition to prednisone. After the second dose of gamma globulin, anti-Ro antibody was no longer detectable in the maternal serum. The infant was born without heart block. Azathioprine has also been suggested, although not yet tried, to prevent fetal heart block.[66] It has been used safely in pregnancies in patients with inflammatory bowel disease and a renal transplant recipient. It may be useful in suppressing maternal antibodies.

The other, slightly more common group of patients with congenital complete heart block are those with an associated structural heart defect. These patients have no association with maternal connective tissue disease. The majority of these patients have AV septal defects and left atrial isomerism.[13, 14] Congenitally corrected transposition of the great arteries is also a commonly associated lesion. In general, these patients do much worse than those with isolated complete heart block. Of those with no structural heart defects, 20 to 30% will die in utero or in the first year of life.[14, 19, 79] Of those patients with complete heart block and structural heart disease, 80 to 90% die in utero or within the first year.[13, 14] In both groups, development of hydrops and a fetal heart rate less than 55 bpm are associated with a very high rate of mortality. Given the current therapeutic options, a hydropic fetus with complete heart block and structural heart disease almost never survives. This is the group of patients who stand to benefit the most if in utero pacing becomes clinically applicable.

RESEARCH AND FUTURE DEVELOPMENTS

In utero epicardial pacemaker techniques are progressing in animal models.[80] In addition, an animal model has been developed for fetal complete heart block.[81] These investigations may one day make fetal pacing for complete heart block a viable option. Also transuterine fetal pacing may play a bridging role.[74, 75] Various therapeutic alternatives look hopeful for preventing complete heart block in a fetus at risk. These include steroids, gamma globulin, immunosuppressive agents, and plasmapheresis or plasma exchange. Clinical trials are necessary before definite benefit can be proven.

In the treatment of tachycardias, there are several new medicines as well as routes of administration that offer hope for improved outcomes. Flecainide, sotalol, and amiodarone are newer antiarrhythmics in the early stages of clinical usage. In addition, adenosine may prove to be a useful adjunct to therapy. Under ultrasonographic guidance, medications can now be given directly to the fetus by intravenous, intramuscular, intraperitoneal, and intra-amniotic routes. The exact indications for these approaches will take time and experience to elucidate.

REFERENCES

1. Hertzberg BS, Mahony BS, Bowie JD: First trimester fetal cardiac activity: Sonographic documentation of a progressive early rise in heart rate. J Ultrasound Med 7:573–575, 1988.
2. Swartjes JM, van Geijn HP, Mantel R, Schoemaker HC: Quantitated fetal heart rhythm at 20, 32 and 38 weeks of gestation and dependence on rest-activity patterns. Early Hum Dev 28:27–36, 1992.
3. Romero T, Covell J, Friedman WF: A comparison of pressure-volume relations of the fetal, newborn and adult heart. Am J Physiol 5:1285–1290, 1972.
4. Kirkpatrick SE, Pitlick PT, Naliboff J, et al: Frank-Starling relationship as an important determinant of fetal cardiac output. Am J Physiol 231:495–500, 1976.
5. Rudolph AM, Heymann MA: Cardiac output in the fetal lamb: The effects of spontaneous and induced changes of heart rate on right and left ventricular output. Am J Obstet Gynecol 124:183–192, 1976.
6. Danilo P: Electrophysiology of the fetal and neonatal heart. In Legato MJ (ed): Developing Heart. Boston, Martinus Nijhoff, 1984, pp 21–38.
7. Danilo P, Reder RF, Binah O, et al: Fetal canine cardiac Purkinje fibers: Electrophysiology and ultrastructure. Am J Physiol 15:H250–260, 1984.
8. Bernard C: Establishment of ionic permeabilities of myocardial membrane during embryonic development of the rat. In Liberman M, Sano T (eds): Developmental and Physiological Correlates of Cardiac Muscle. New York, Raven Press, 1976, pp 169–184.
9. Shigenobu K, Sperelakis N: Development of sensitivity to terodotoxin of chick embryonic hearts with age. J Mol Cell Cardiol 3:271–286, 1971.
10. Calvin SE, Gaziano EP, Bendel RP, et al: Evaluation of fetal cardiac arrhythmias. Ultrasound findings and neonatal outcome. Minn Med 75:29–31, 1992.
11. Friedman AH, Copel JA, Kleinman CS: Fetal echocardiography and fetal cardiology: Indications, diagnosis and management. Sem Perinatol 17:76–88, 1993.
12. Gillette PC, Garson A Jr, Porter CJ, et al: Junctional automatic ectopic tachycardia: New proposed treatment by transcatheter His bundle ablation. Am Heart J 106:619–623, 1983.
13. Schmidt KG, Ulmer HE, Silverman NH, et al: Perinatal outcome of fetal complete atrioventricular block: A multicenter experience. J Am Coll Cardiol 91:1360–1366, 1991.
14. Machado MVL, Chita SC, Allan DL: Acceleration time in the aorta and pulmonary artery measured by Doppler echocardiography in the midtrimester normal human fetus. Br Heart J 58:15–18, 1987.
15. Gembruch U, Hansmann M, Redel DA, et al: Fetal complete heart block: Antenatal diagnosis, significance and management. Eur J Obstet Gynecol Reprod Biol 31:9–22, 1989.
16. Shenker L, Reed KL, Anderson CF, et al: Congenital heart block and cardiac anomalies in the absence of maternal connective tissue disease. Am J Obstet Gynecol 157:248–253, 1987.
17. Buyon JP, Winchester RJ, Slade SG, et al: Identification of mothers at risk for congenital heart block and other neonatal lupus syndromes in their children: Comparison of enzyme-linked immunosorbent assay and immunoblot for measurement of anti-SS-A/Ro and anti-SS-B/La antibodies. Arthritis Rheum 36:1263–1273, 1993.
18. Reed KL, Sahn DJ: A proposal for referral patterns for fetal cardiac studies. Semin Ultrasound CT MR 5:249, 1984.
19. Buyon JP, Waltuck J, Kleinman C, Copel J: In utero identification and therapy of congenital heart block. Lupus 4:116–121, 1995.
20. Hager DW, Pauly TH: Fetal tachycardia as an indicator of maternal and neonatal morbidity. Obstet Gynecol 66:191–194, 1985.
21. Lingman G, Lundstrom NR, Marsal K, et al: Fetal cardiac arrhythmia: Clinical outcome in 113 cases. Acta Obstet Gynecol Scand 65:263–267, 1986.
22. Biale Y, Brawer-Ostrosky Y, Insler V: Fetal heart rate tracings in fetuses with congenital malformations. J Reprod Med 30:43–47, 1985.
23. Strasburger JF, Huhta JC, Carpenter RJ Jr, et al: Doppler echocardiography in the diagnosis and management of persistent fetal arrhythmias. J Am Coll Cardiol 7:1386–1391, 1986.
24. Reed KL, Appleton CP, Anderson CF, et al: Doppler studies of vena cava flows in human fetuses: Insights into normal and abnormal cardiac physiology. Circulation 81:498–505, 1990.
25. Indik JH, Chen V, Reed KL: Association of umbilical venous with inferior vena cava blood flow velocities. Obstet Gynecol 77:551–557, 1991.
26. Gembruch U, Redel DA, Bald R, Hansmann M: Longitudinal study in 18 cases of fetal supraventricular tachycardia: Doppler echocardiographic findings and patho-

physiologic implications. Am Heart J 125:1290–1301, 1993.
27. Kleinman CS, Copel JA, Weinstein EM, et al: In utero diagnosis and treatment of fetal supraventricular tachycardia. Semin Perinatol 9:113–129, 1985.
28. Stevens DC, Hilliard J, Schreiner RL, et al: Supraventricular tachycardia with edema, ascites, and hydrops in fetal sheep. Am J Obstet Gynecol 142:316–322, 1982.
29. Nimrod C, Davies D, Harder J, et al: Ultrasound evaluation of tachycardia-induced hydrops in the fetal lamb. Am J Obstet Gynecol 157:655–659, 1987.
30. Silber DL, Durnin RE: Intrauterine atrial tachycardia. Am J Dis Child 117:722–726, 1969.
31. Van Engelen AD, Weijtens O, Brenner JI, et al: Management outcome and follow-up of fetal tachycardia. J Am Coll Cardiol 24:1371–1375, 1994.
32. Maxwell DJ, Crawford DC, Curry PVM, et al. Obstetric importance, diagnosis, and management of fetal tachycardias. BMJ 297:107–110, 1988.
33. Lingman G, Ohrlander S, Ohlin P: Intrauterine digoxin treatment of fetal paroxysmal tachycardia. Br J Obstet Gynaecol 87:340–342, 1980.
34. Wiggins JW, Bowes W, Clewell W, et al: Echocardiographic diagnosis and intravenous digoxin management of fetal tachyarrhythmias and congestive heart failure. Am J Dis Child 140:202–204, 1986.
35. Weiner CP, Thompson MIB: Direct treatment of fetal supraventricular tachycardia after failed transplacental therapy. Am J Obstet Gynecol 158:570–573, 1988.
36. Gembruch U, Hansmann M, Redel DA, Bald R: Intrauterine therapy of fetal tachyarrhythmias: Intraperitoneal administration of antiarrhythmic drugs to the fetus in fetal tachyarrhythmias with severe hydrops fetalis. J Perinat Med 16:39–44, 1988.
37. Hallak M, Neerhof MG, Perry R, et al: Fetal supraventricular tachycardia and hydrops fetalis: Combined intensive, direct, and transplacental therapy. Obstet Gynecol 78:523–525, 1991.
38. Younis JS, Granat M: Insufficient transplacental digoxin transfer in severe hydrops fetalis. Am J Obstet Gynecol 157:1268–1269, 1987.
39. Smoleniec JS, Martin R, James DK: Intermittent fetal tachycardia and fetal hydrops. Arch Dis Child 66:1160–1161, 1991.
40. Allan LD, Chita SK, Sharland GK, et al: Flecainide in the treatment of fetal tachycardias. Br Heart J 65:46–48, 1991.
41. Wren C, Hunter S: Maternal administration of flecainide to terminate and suppress fetal tachycardia. BMJ 296:249, 1988.
42. Bourget P, Pons J-C, Delouis C, et al: Flecainide distribution, transplacental passage, and accumulation in the amniotic fluid during the third trimester of pregnancy. Ann Pharmacother 28:1031–1034, 1994.
43. Wagner X, Jouglard J, Moulin M, et al: Coadministration of flecainide acetate and sotalol during pregnancy: Lack of teratogenic effects, passage across the placenta, and excretion in human breast milk. Am Heart J 119:700–701, 1990.
44. The Cardiac Arrhythmia Suppression Trial (CAST) Investigators: Preliminary report: Effect of encainide and flecainide on mortality in a randomized trial of arrhythmia suppression after myocardial infarction. N Engl J Med 321:406–412, 1991.
45. Van Gelder-Hasker MR, de Jong CL, de Vries JI, van Geijn HP: The effect of flecainide acetate on fetal heart rate variability: A case report. Obstet Gynecol 86:667–669, 1995.
46. Flack NJ, Zosmer N, Bennett PR, et al: Amiodarone given by three routes to terminate fetal atrial flutter associated with severe hydrops. Obstet Gynecol 82:714–716, 1993.
47. Arnoux P, Seyral P, Llurens M, et al: Amiodarone and digoxin for refractory fetal tachycardia. Am J Cardiol 59:166–167, 1987.
48. Magee LA, Downar E, Sermer M, et al: Pregnancy outcome after gestational exposure to amiodarone in Canada. Am J Obstet Gynecol 172:1307–1311, 1995.
49. De Catte L, De Wolf D, Smitz J, et al: Fetal hypothyroidism as a complication of amiodarone treatment for persistent fetal supraventricular tachycardia. Prenat Diagn 14:762–765, 1994.
50. Plomp TA, Vulsma T, de Vijlder JJ: Use of amiodarone during pregnancy. Eur J Obstet Gynecol Reprod Biol 43:201–207, 1992.
51. De Wolf D, De Schepper J, Verhaaren H, et al. Congenital hypothyroid goiter and amiodarone. Acta Paediatr Scand 77:616–618, 1988.
52. Gembruch U, Manz M, Bald R, et al: Repeated intravascular treatment with amiodarone in a fetus with refractory supraventricular tachycardia and hydrops fetalis. Am Heart J 118:1335–1338, 1989.
53. Valensise H, Civitella C, Garzetti GG, Romanini C: Amiodarone treatment in pregnancy for dilatative cardiomyopathy with ventricular malignant extrasystole and normal maternal and neonatal outcome. Prenat Diagn 12:705–708, 1992.
54. Widerhorn J, Bhandari AK, Bughi S, et al: Fetal and neonatal adverse effects profile of amiodarone treatment during pregnancy. Am Heart J 122:1162–1166, 1991.
55. Wolff F, Breuker KH, Schlensker KH, Bolte A: Prenatal diagnosis and therapy of fetal heart rate anomalies: With a contribution on the placental transfer of verapamil. J Perinatol 8:203–208, 1980.
56. Teuscher A, Bossi E, Imhof P, et al: Effect of propranolol on fetal tachycardia in diabetic pregnancy. Am J Cardiol 1978;42:304–307, 1978.
57. Spinnato JA, Shaver DC, Flinn GS, et al: Fetal supraventricular tachycardia: In utero therapy with digoxin and quinidine. Obstet Gynecol 64:730–735, 1984.
58. Blanch G, Walkinshaw SA, Walsh K: Cardioversion of fetal arrhythmia with adenosine. Lancet 344:1646, 1994.
59. Kohl T, Tercanli S, Kececioglu D, Holzgreve W: Direct fetal administration of adenosine for the termination of incessant supraventricular tachycardia. Obstet Gynecol 85(5,Pt 2):873–874, 1995.
60. Dumesic DA, Silverman NH, Tobias S, Bolbus MS: Transplacental cardioversion of fetal supraventricular tachycardia with procainamide. N Engl J Med 307(18):1128–1131, 1982.
61. Friedman DM, Borg M, Rutkovsky L, Buyon JP: Benign fetal bradycardias diagnosed by echocardiography. Am J Perinatol 12:87–90, 1995.
62. McCue CM, Mantakas ME, Tingelstad JB, Ruddy S: Congenital heart block in newborns of mothers with connective tissue disease. Circulation 56:82–90, 1977.
63. Le Thi Huong D, Wechsler B, Piette JC, et al: Pregnancy and its outcome in systemic lupus erythematosus. Q J Med 87:721–729, 1994.
64. Jones WR: Autoimmune disease and pregnancy. Aust N Z J Obstet Gynaecol 34:251–258, 1994.
65. Waltuck J, Buyon JP: Autoantibody-associated congenital heart block: Outcome in mothers and children. Ann Intern Med 120:544–551, 1994.
66. Olah KS, Gee H: Fetal heart block associated with maternal anti-Ro (SS-A) antibody: Current management. A review. Br J Obstet Gynaecol 98:751–755, 1991.
67. Veille JC, Covitz W: Fetal cardiovascular hemodynamics

in the presence of complete atrioventricular block. Am J Obstet Gynecol 170:1258–1262, 1994.
68. Harris JP, Alexson CG, Manning JA, Thompson HD: Medical therapy for the hydropic fetus with congenital complete atrioventricular block. Am J Perinatol 10:217–219, 1993.
69. Watson WJ, Katz VL: Steroid therapy for hydrops associated with antibody-mediated congenital heart block. Am J Obstet Gynecol 165:553–554, 1991.
70. Carreira PE, Gutierrez-Larraya F, Gomez-Reino JJ: Successful intrauterine therapy with dexamethasone for fetal myocarditis and heart block in a woman with systemic lupus erythematosus. J Rheumatol 20:1204–1207, 1993.
71. Silverman ED: Congenital heart block and neonatal lupus erythematosus: Prevention is the goal. J Rheumatol 20:1101–1104, 1993.
72. Ishimaru S, Izaki S, Kitamura K, Morita Y: Neonatal lupus erythematosus: Dissolution of atrioventricular block after administration of corticosteroid to the pregnant mother. Dermatology 189:92–94, 1994.
73. Groves AMM, Allan LD, Rosenthal E: Therapeutic trial of sympathomimetics in three cases of complete heart block in the fetus. Circulation 92:3394–3396, 1995.
74. Carpenter RJ, Strasburger JF, Garson A Jr, et al: Fetal ventricular pacing for hydrops secondary to complete atrioventricular block. J Am Coll Cardiol 8:1434–1436, 1986.
75. Walkinshaw SA, Welch CR, McCormack J, Walsh K: In utero pacing for fetal congenital heart block. Fetal Diagn Ther 9:183–185, 1994.
76. Martin TC, Arias F, Olander DS, et al: Successful management of congenital atrioventricular block associated with hydrops fetalis. J Pediatr 112:984–986, 1988.
77. Weindling SN, Saul JP, Triedman JK, et al: Staged pacing therapy for congenital complete heart block in premature infants. Am J Cardiol 74:412–413, 1994.
78. Kaaja R, Julkunen H, Ämmälä, et al: Congenital heart block: Successful prophylactic treatment with intravenous gamma globulin and corticosteroid therapy. Am J Obstet Gynecol 165:1333–1334, 1991.
79. Julkunen H, Kaaja R, Wallgren E, Teramo K: Isolated congenital heart block: Fetal and infant outcome and familial incidence of heart block. Obstet Gynecol 82:11–16, 1993.
80. Scagliotti D, Shimokochi DD, Pringle KC: Permanent cardiac pacemaker implant in the fetal lamb. Pacing Clin Electrophysiol 10:1253–1261, 1987.
81. Assad RS, Jatene MB, Moreira LFP, et al: Fetal heart block: A new experimental model to assess fetal pacing. Pacing Clin Electrophysiol 17:1256–1263, 1994.

CHAPTER 17

PALPITATIONS

Arthur Garson, Jr

Palpitations, defined as feelings of a rapid or irregular heartbeat, are neither sensitive nor specific in children.[1] Bizarre rhythms may result in no symptoms. In fact, the most common presentation of nonsustained ventricular tachycardia is when a Holter monitor is obtained after a physician hears an irregular heartbeat. The child with incessant supraventricular tachycardia (SVT) is also generally asymptomatic and does not report palpitations.[2] In contrast, children may report a rapid heartbeat at times when the Holter examination reveals normal sinus rhythm or sinus tachycardia.[1] I have also seen children who complained of rapid heartbeats but who, in fact, had transient bradycardia (in one case resulting from paroxysmal AV block) but who felt the sinus tachycardia after resumption of normal rhythm.

The purpose of this chapter is to attempt to differentiate, on the basis of the history, whether the child who presents with palpitations needs further workup. The first question to be asked is whether the child's heart is otherwise normal. If the child has an underlying known cardiac abnormality, palpitations of any kind should be taken seriously. It is likely that further workup involving testing such as Holter monitor, telephone transmitter, exercise test, or even electrophysiology study may be necessary depending on the severity of the heart disease and severity of symptoms.

The remainder of this discussion centers on the child who is thought to have an otherwise normal heart by history, physical examination, and electrocardiogram. In general, the patient who has a normal history and physical examination and who does not have Wolff-Parkinson-White Syndrome or long QT syndrome on electrocardiogram is extremely unlikely to have sudden death from an arrhythmia. In this situation, the consequences of palpitations, no matter what their underlying cause, are not likely to be disastrous; therefore, it seems reasonable to classify patients clinically as either those who are likely not to have a pathologic arrhythmia (need further workup) or those who are likely to have a pathologic arrhythmia (need further follow-up). Because ventricular tachycardia in children with a normal heart generally does not present with palpitations, and atrial flutter usually does not present in a child with a normal heart, the main differential diagnosis in the child presenting with rapid palpitations is either SVT or sinus rhythm. The answers to the following seven questions may help classify these patients. It should be emphasized that these questions refer only to the child who has palpitations, and not to the individual with severe presyncope or syncope.

HOW MANY TIMES HAVE THE PALPITATIONS OCCURRED?

The typical child with palpitations from SVT reports to his parents that "My heart is beating fast." It seems that the normal familial response is to tell the child to do some quiet work or to lie down. The episodes of palpitations usually occur several times or last long enough so that the child becomes increasingly symptomatic with pallor and light-headedness to draw the attention of the parents. On presentation to the physician, therefore, most children with SVT have had several episodes. The parents of children without SVT seem to make an appointment to see the physician the very next day after the first episode.

HOW OFTEN HAVE THE EPISODES OCCURRED?

The individual with SVT rarely has daily episodes. It is more common for attacks of SVT to occur every few weeks to months. This is compared with episodes in the child without SVT who seems to complain that the episodes occur daily or several times per day. As one would imagine, in an individual whose episodes are thought to occur "daily," application of a 48-hour Holter monitor may result in a "cure," because that "happens to be the first 48 hours in the past several weeks that the individual had no episodes." This is perhaps the one time that a Holter examination is indicated, because one can "rule in" or "rule out" a pathologic diagnosis in the individual who reports daily symptoms.

HOW LONG DID THE EPISODES LAST?

It is not clear whether individuals with SVT at the onset of their course have very brief episodes, but by the time most children present to the physician, they have usually had at least one episode lasting longer than 5 minutes, some up to 30 minutes. The patient without a pathologic arrhythmia generally reports the episode lasting only several seconds.

WHAT BRINGS ON THE EPISODE?

It seems that SVT can occur at almost any time. The most typical time for presentation is when the child is watching television. It is uncertain whether this is a commentary on how the typical American child spends most of his or her time. The episodes may occur during a meal or even when sitting quietly. Occasionally, episodes occur during sports. It is extremely unusual for SVT to awaken a child at night. On the other hand, it seems that patients without SVT will frequently complain that their heart beats fast after they run (so does mine). In those individuals in whom a number of factors would point toward true SVT, a formal exercise test may be helpful if symptoms can be reproduced.

WHAT DOES THE CHILD LOOK LIKE DURING AN EPISODE?

Most children who have an episode of SVT are not red in the face. A red face is more typical in the child who simply overexerts during exercise and has sinus tachycardia. On the other hand, the child with SVT (certainly in those who have episodes lasting more than a few minutes) is typically pale and diaphoretic and may be nauseated.

WHERE DO YOU FEEL THE PALPITATIONS?

Most children with palpitations, when asked this question, point to the middle of their chest. However, occasionally children with SVT will report, without undue prompting, that they feel the tachycardia in their neck.

WHAT MAKES THE TACHYCARDIA DISAPPEAR?

By the time a child with SVT sees a physician, generally several episodes have occurred, and the child may have developed a method for stopping the episodes. Some children recognize that if they gag, swallow, yawn, or drink cold water, occasionally the episodes may stop. It is clearly helpful if the child tells you that he or she gets extremely sick to the stomach and vomits and the tachycardia stops. On the other hand, although some children with SVT will report that the palpitations disappear with rest, it is almost a universal finding among those who do not have a pathologic arrhythmia that it disappears with lying down.

CONCLUSIONS

When the answers to these seven questions are tallied, the physician can generally get an idea of whether SVT is likely or not (Table 17–1). Unfortunately, it is rare for the answers to all

Table 17–1. Palpitations in Children With a Normal Heart

QUESTION	PROBABLE SVT	PATHOLOGIC ARRHYTHMIA NOT LIKELY
How many times?	Several	Once
How often?	Monthly	Daily
How long is each episode?	5–30 minutes	Seconds
Circumstances	Anytime (watching TV)	Immediately after exercise, at night
Appearance	Pale, sweaty	Red
Where felt?	Chest, neck	Chest
What makes it disappear?	Gag, swallow, vomit	Rest

SVT, Supraventricular tachycardia.

seven questions to fall consistently in the same column. Nonetheless, an overall impression can be developed. For the individual who seems to fall into the category of "no pathologic arrhythmia," I provide reassurance that, in the presence of an otherwise normal history, physician examination, and electrocardiogram, even if there is a pathologic arrhythmia, it is unlikely to be dangerous. I ask the patient to keep a diary and if the episodes more frequently and consistently last longer than 5 to 10 minutes, or if they are associated with presyncope or syncope, then I see the patient again. On the other hand, for the child who falls into the category of likely SVT, I issue him or her a recording telephone transmitter and ask him or her to return after the ECG has been recorded during typical palpitations; if sinus rhythm is documented, no further follow-up is necessary. However, if there are no tracings, or the child was unable to "catch" an episode, I ask him or her to return in 3 months.

REFERENCES

1. Porter CJ, Gillette PC, McNamara DG: Twenty-four hour ambulatory ECGs in the detection and management of cardiac dysrhythmias in children. Pediatr Cardiol 1:203–208, 1980.
2. Garson A Jr, Gillette PC, McNamara DG: Supraventricular tachycardia in children: Clinical features, response to treatment and long-term follow-up in 217 patients. J Pediatr 98:875–882, 1981.

CHAPTER 18

ARRHYTHMIAS IN LONG QT AND WPW SYNDROMES

Brian K. O'Connor

Arrhythmias resulting from primary disorders of automaticity, conduction, and repolarization may occur in patients with structurally normal hearts and may carry a risk of sudden cardiac death. Two relatively common disorders in children that predispose to a risk of life-threatening arrhythmias and sudden cardiac death are long QT syndrome (LQTS) and Wolff-Parkinson-White (WPW) syndrome. This chapter focuses on the approach to diagnosis and management of each of these syndromes.

LONG QT SYNDROME

The congenital LQTS is a genetically determined abnormality of ventricular repolarization. The syndrome frequently manifests as QT-interval prolongation on the surface electrocardiogram (ECG) and carries an increased risk of life-threatening ventricular arrhythmias, often triggered by physical or emotional stress (Fig. 18–1).

The syndrome was first described in 1957 by Jervell and Lange-Nielsen, who reported a Swedish family in whom four of six children with congenital deafness experienced recurrent syncope and manifested QT-interval prolongation on surface ECG.[1] Three of the children died suddenly. The mode of inheritance was determined to be autosomal recessive. Romano et al,[2] in 1963, and Ward,[3] in 1964, independently described similar findings in children without the congenital hearing deficit with an autosomal dominant inheritance pattern. Since these early reports, there has been much work describing the clinical and ECG features of prolonged QT, along with the probable electrophysiologic mechanisms underlying the syndrome. Work in molecular genetics has identified specific genes associated with LQTS.[4]

CLINICAL FEATURES

The congenital LQTS is characterized by recurrent syncope, QT-interval prolongation, and T- and U-wave abnormalities on the surface ECG (Fig. 18–2). There may be a positive family history of QT-interval prolongation, cardiac arrest, seizures, or sudden death. Children are frequently asymptomatic, but may present with a history of seizures, syncope, or cardiac arrest. Because of the marked variability in the clinical presentation, an accurate diagnosis may be overlooked, and syncope may be incorrectly attributed to a primary seizure disorder or a benign neurocardiogenic event.

The age at presentation varies and may range from *in utero* to adulthood. In the international collaborative study of the Pediatric Electrophysiology Society,[5] the average age at presentation was 6.8 ± 5.6 years (SD). The study defined QT prolongation as a corrected QT interval (QTc), using Bazett's formula, in excess of 440 milliseconds. The QTc at presentation was less than 440 milliseconds in 6% and more than 600 milliseconds in 13% of children with LQTS in this study. Five percent of children presented with atrioventricular (AV) block, 90% of whom had functional second-degree (2:1) AV block. The initial 12-lead ECG showed ventricular arrhythmias in 16% of patients, consisting of uniform ventricular premature contractions (4%), multiform ventricular premature contractions (5%), monomorphic ventricular tachycardia (1%), and torsades de pointes (6%). Congenital deafness was present in 4.5% of patients.

DIAGNOSIS

Criteria for Diagnosis

Patients with LQTS may not demonstrate classic changes on 12-lead ECG. As such, Schwartz in 1985 proposed major and minor criteria to aid in the diagnosis (Table 18–1).[6] Two major or one major and two minor criteria were necessary for diagnosis. As a greater understanding of the syndrome developed and experience in management progressed, a revised set of criteria was proposed

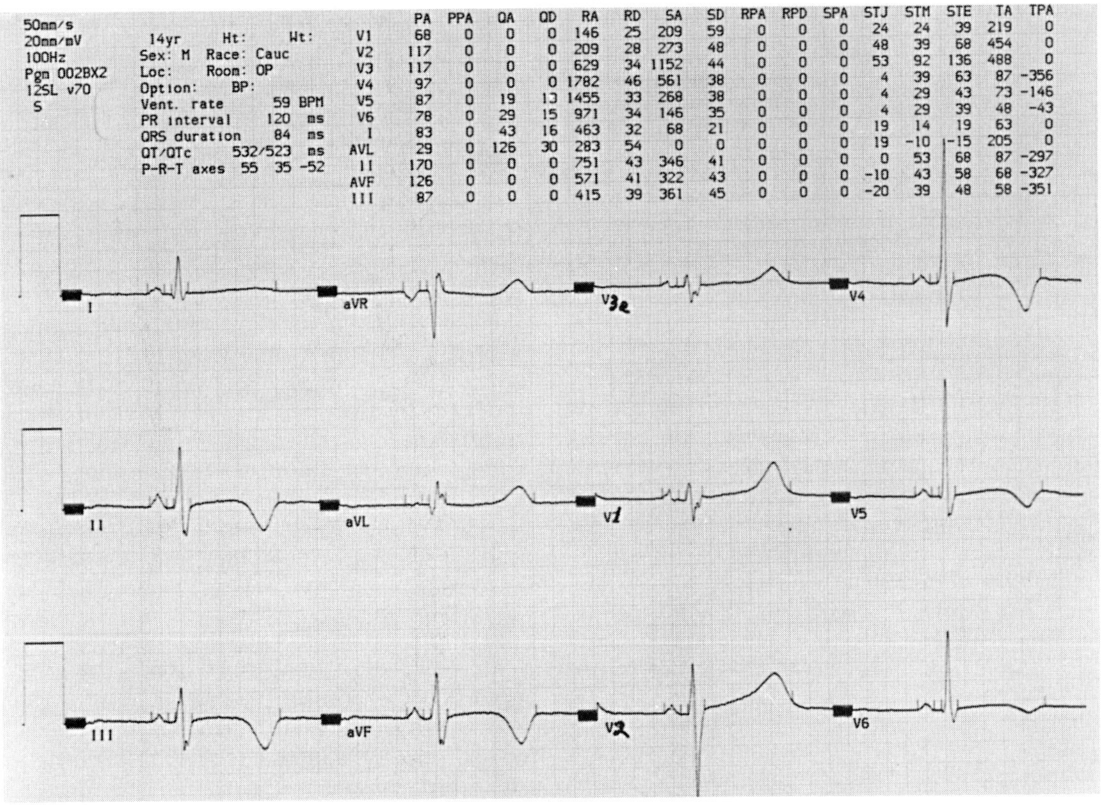

FIGURE 18–1. Prolonged QT interval documented by a digitally enhanced electrocardiogram. The digital program denotes the measurement points used to calculate the intervals printed on the report. In addition, the T-wave morphology is abnormal and the long ST segment is followed by a T wave that is long in duration.

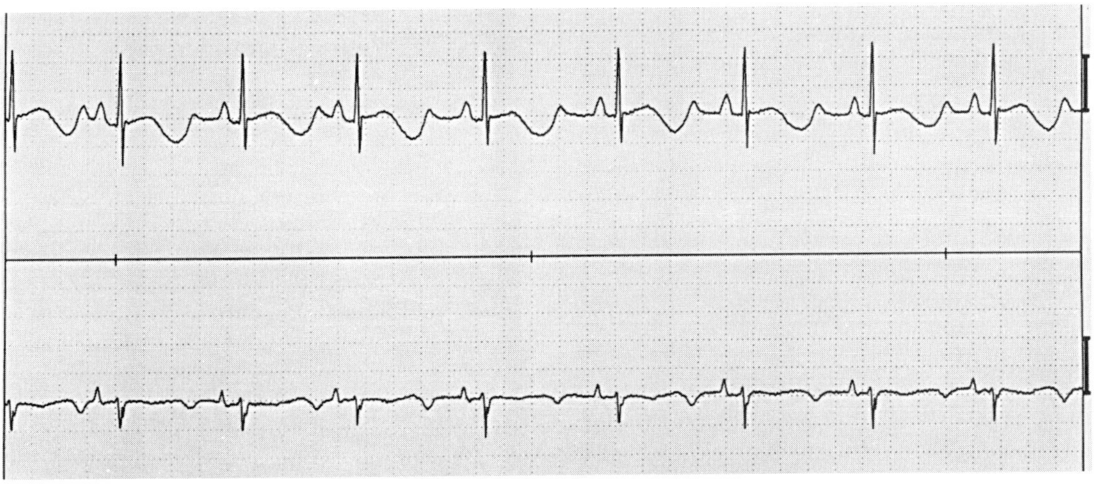

FIGURE 18–2. Twenty-four-hour ambulatory monitor recording from a patient with long QT syndrome and multifaceted T waves with a short ST segment.

Table 18–1. 1985 LQTS Diagnostic Criteria*

MAJOR	MINOR
Prolonged QT interval (Qtc > 440 ms)	Congenital deafness
	Episodes of T-wave alternans
Stress-induced syncope	Low heart rate (in children)
Family members with LQTS	Abnormal ventricular repolarization

*The diagnosis of LQTS is made in the presence of either two major criteria or one major and two minor criteria.

LQTS, long QT syndrome.

From Schwartz PJ: Idiopathic long QT syndrome: Progress and questions. Am Heart J 2:399–411, 1985.

in 1992 (Table 18–2).[7] The new system assigns points to diagnostic criteria based on clinical significance. The patient score may range from a minimum value of 0 to a maximum value of 9 points. The point scores have been arbitrarily divided into three categories with respect to probability of disease: category 1 = 1 point, low probability of LQTS; category 2 = 2 or 3 points, intermediate probability of LQTS; and category 3 ≥ 4 points, high probability of LQTS (Fig. 18–3).

Table 18–2. 1993 LQTS Diagnostic Criteria*

VARIABLE	POINTS†
ECG Findings	
QTc‡	
≥ 480 $ms^{1/2}$	3
460–470 $ms^{1/2}$	2
450 $ms^{1/2}$ (in males)	1
Torsades de pointes§	2
T-wave alternans	1
Notched T wave in three leads	1
Low heart rate for age‖	0.5
Clinical History	
Syncope§	
With stress	2
Without stress	1
Congenital deafness	0.5
Family History¶	
Family members with definite LQTS#	1
Unexplained sudden cardiac death < age 30 among immediate family members	0.5

*In the absence of medications or disorders known to affect these electrocardiographic features.

†Scoring: ≤1 point, low probability of LQTS: 2–3 points, intermediate probability of LQTS; ≥4 points, high probability of LQTS.

‡QTc calculated using Bazett's formula, where $QTc = QT/\sqrt{RR}$.

§Mutually exclusive.

‖Resting heart rate below the second percentile for age.

¶The same family member cannot be counted in A and B.

#Definite LQTS is defined by an LQTS score ≥4.

LQTS, long QT syndrome; ECG, electrocardiography; QTc, corrected QT.

From Schwartz PJ: Idiopathic long QT syndrome: Progress and questions. Am Heart J 2:399–411, 1985.

Diagnostic Tests

In patients with borderline QT prolongation, additional studies may help to confirm the diagnosis. Twenty-four-hour ambulatory monitoring may identify asymptomatic nonsustained ventricular tachyarrhythmias, transient profound sinus bradycardia, or episodes of T-wave alternans. The 24-hour ambulatory monitor may be helpful in documenting extreme QT-interval prolongation, such as that seen during marked bradycardia, which may not otherwise be documented. Additionally, the presence of ventricular arrhythmias may also be documented (Fig. 18–4). Exercise stress testing may also be helpful in evaluating the patient with borderline QT-interval prolongation. Failure of the absolute QT interval to shorten and exercise-related prolongation of the QTc are subtle indicators of LQTS. Isoproterenol or epinephrine infusions mimic the effects of endogenous catecholamines and may also be used in screening for latent QT prolongation and arrhythmic risk (Fig. 18–5).

MOLECULAR GENETICS

The primary abnormality in LQTS is a defect in cardiac ion channel structure and function.[8] Three of the genes responsible for these defects have been identified and isolated to chromosomes 11 (LQT1), 7 (LQT2), and 3 (LQT3). A fourth locus has been mapped to chromosome 4 (LQT4); however, the specific gene involved has not been identified. Additional families have been excluded from linkage at any of the identified sites, suggesting that at least one and possibly several additional LQTS loci exist.

Chromosome 11–Related LQTS (LQT1)

Despite the early identification of LQT1 via linkage studies, the specific gene locus was first identified only in 1997.[9] The gene, KvLQT1, encodes a protein that, when coexpressed with minK, produces an ion current with characteristics of IKs, the slowly activating component of the delayed rectifier.[8] The reduction in IKs seen in LQT1 may explain the prolonged T-wave duration observed in these patients. All parameters of QT duration (Qt_{onset}, QT_{peak}, and QTc) are markedly prolonged in this group. LQT1 appears to be the most prevalent subgroup; however, nearly all families genotyped demonstrate a unique mutation of the KvLQT1 gene.[10, 11] Mutations in the gene encoding minK, although not

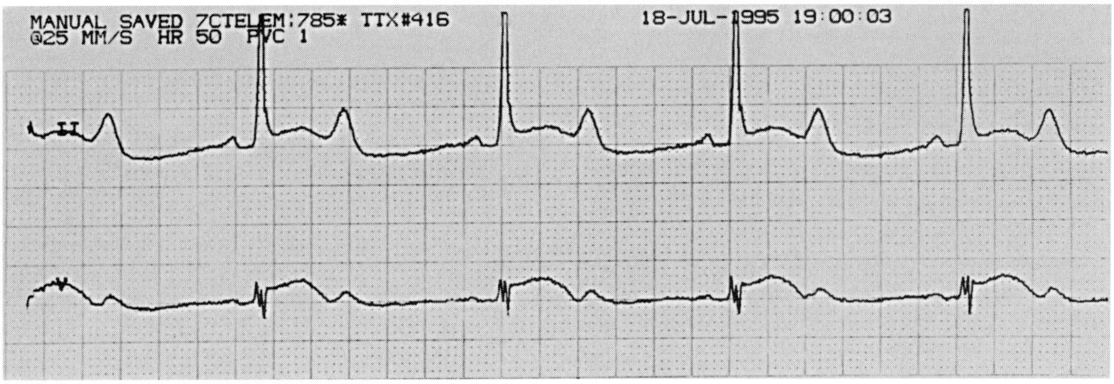

FIGURE 18–3. Telemetry monitor electrocardiographic recording from a patient with newly diagnosed QT syndrome; ventricular fibrillation was the presenting symptom. In lead II, the distal component of the TU segment is larger than the proximal.

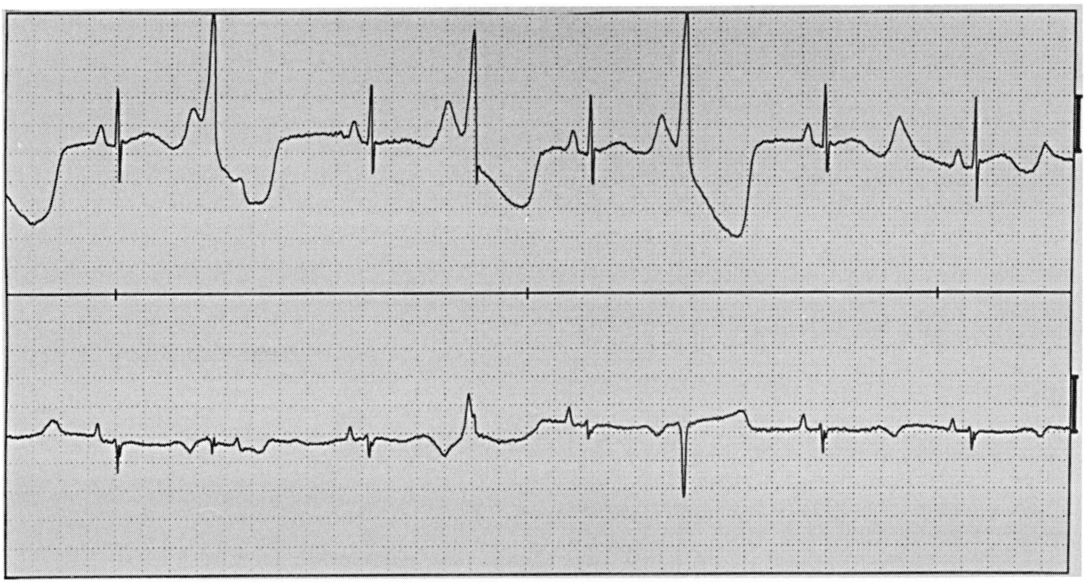

FIGURE 18–4. Telemetry monitor electrocardiographic recording from the patient in Figure 18–3 at a different time of day. Note that the second portion of the T wave has increased in amplitude and multiform premature ventricular contractions originate from the downward deflection of the T wave.

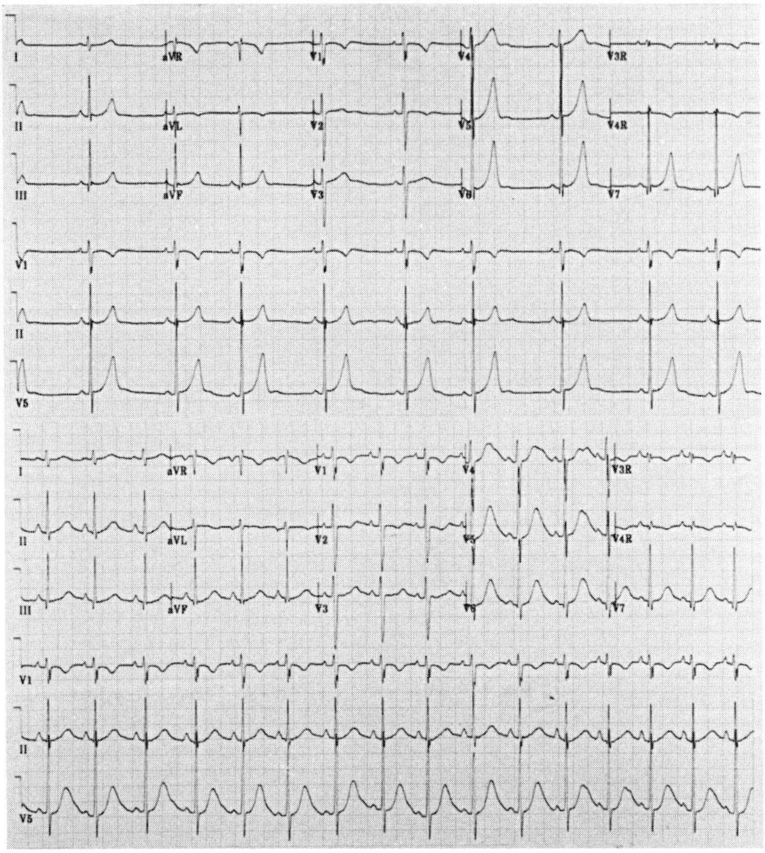

FIGURE 18–5. Enhancement of the QT interval with adrenaline infusion. The top six recordings of electrocardiographic complexes were taken with the patient at rest; the bottom recordings exhibit sinus tachycardia with prolongation of the corrected QT interval.

yet identified, could result in the altered IKs currently seen in LQT1. Thus, it is possible that the gene encoding minK may represent an additional locus for the LQT1 phenotype.[9]

Chromosome 7–Related LQTS (LQT2)

The gene identified in LQT2 is HERG, which encodes a potassium channel responsible for the rapidly activating delayed rectifier current IK.[12] Of the 14 LQT2 families identified, all display a unique mutation.[13–17] Priori et al reported two unrelated families with a distinct mutation at the same site (AA428), raising this as a possible critical locus for LQT2.[16]

The decrease in IKr current seen with the HERG mutation may account for the diffusely low-amplitude, broad T-wave characteristic of this defect (Fig. 18–6). To mimic the HERG mutation, Priori et al exposed guinea pig myocytes to the IKr blocker dofetilide.[18] The model showed no response to the sodium channel blocker mexiletine and demonstrated prolongation of the action potential duration with isoproterenol and rapid pacing. This suggested that patients with LQT2 lack the ability to adapt action potential duration to heart rate; therefore, they may demonstrate significant clinical benefit from antiadrenergic therapy. Compton et al showed that increasing extracellular potassium concentration results in a shortening of the resting QTc interval and a reduction in QTc dispersion.[19] This led to the hypothesis that LQT2 patients may demonstrate antiarrhythmic benefit from therapy aimed at increasing extracellular potassium concentration such as oral potassium supplementation and the potassium-sparing drug spironolactone.

Chromosome 3–Related LQTS (LQT3)

Wang et al demonstrated that a mutation of the cardiac sodium channel gene SCN5A results in an altered cardiac sodium current and is responsible for chromosome 3–related LQTS (LQT3).[20–22] Three mutations have been identified: a nine–base pairs deletion (ΔKPO, believed to be the most severe variant) and two point mutations (R1644H and N1325S).[9] The sodium channel encoded fails to inactivate normally,

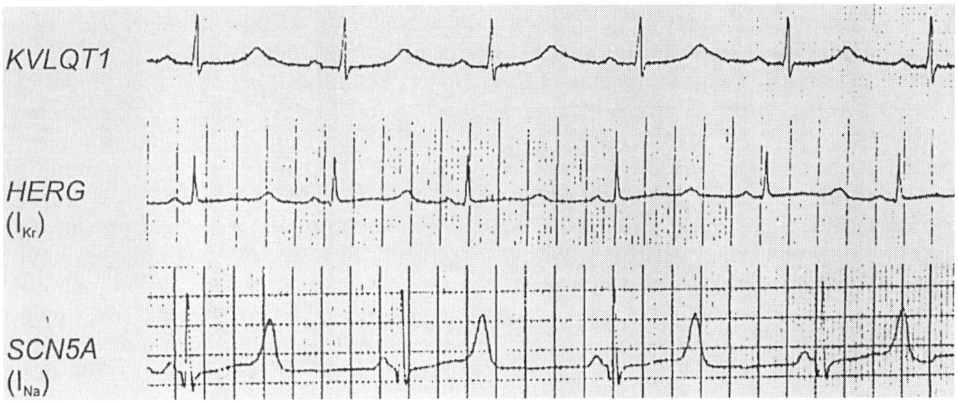

FIGURE 18–6. Lead II rhythm strip showing the distinctive T-wave patterns reported in the three types of long QT syndrome. (From Rhoden DM, Lazarra R, Rosen M, et al: Multiple mechanisms in the long-QT syndrome: Current knowledge, gaps, and future directions. Circulation 94:1996–2012, 1996. Used with permission.)

leading to intermittent reopenings throughout the action potential. The resultant sodium current prolongs the action potential duration and myocardial repolarization. This likely explains the prolonged and prominent late component of the T wave seen on the surface ECG in LQT3 patients (see Fig. 18–6).[23] The T wave is characterized by a late peaking, prominent terminal portion, displaying higher amplitudes than those seen with other subtypes of the disease.

Priori et al exposed guinea pig myocytes to the sea anemone toxin anthopleurin to mimic the SCN5A defect seen in LQT3 patients.[18] In contrast to the LQT2, the LQT3 model demonstrated a marked shortening of action potential duration on exposure to mexiletine. The same response was observed with isoproterenol and rapid pacing; thus, it was theorized that patients with LQT3 would exhibit shortened QT-interval duration as well as ventricular refractoriness in response to mexiletine and, possibly, less susceptibility to the arrhythmogenic effects of increased heart rate and endogenous catecholamine surges. Priori et al tested this hypothesis on a group of LQTS patients and confirmed that, unlike LQT1 and LQT2 patients, LQT3 patients shorten their QT interval in response to mexiletine and increased heart rate.[18] This raised the hypothesis that LQT3 patients may benefit from sodium channel blockade and bradycardia pacing and may actually be at increased risk for ventricular tachyarrhythmias at slower heart rates.

Jervell and Lange-Nielsen Syndrome

Neyroud[24] and Splawski[25] and their colleagues independently reported the findings of genetic analyses performed in two kindreds in which the proband had the Jervell and Lange-Nielsen syndrome form of the disease. Analyses revealed that asymptomatic family members were normal or had one mutant allele for KvLQT1, whereas both probands were homozygous for the gene. This suggested that parents of patients with the Jervell and Lange-Nielsen syndrome are obligate heterozygotes for KvLQT1. Congenital deafness, which is observed only in the homozygous state, is inherited as an autosomal recessive trait. Defects in the potassium channel IKs demonstrate an autosomal dominant pattern; however, the reduction of IKs may be more profound in the homozygous state, explaining the marked QTc prolongation observed in the Jervell and Lange-Nielsen syndrome variant. On the basis of this information, all family members of patients with the Jervell and Lange-Nielsen syndrome require extensive clinical and genetic screening because of the increased risk of an asymptomatic carrier.

Application of Molecular Genetics to LQTS

In an attempt to define prognosis, Priori et al reviewed the clinical history of all genotyped families in the LQTS registry.[9] The analysis revealed that LQT1 represents the highest number of gene carriers to experience symptoms, and LQT2 represents the highest number of patients experiencing syncopal events. With the analysis of larger sample sizes, it may be possible to delineate relatively benign LQTS genotypes from those carrying a more malignant prognosis.

Moss identified distinct genotypic variation in the T-wave morphology of LQTS patients.[23] The QT parameters (Qt_{onset}, QT_{peak}, and QTc) were most prolonged in the SCN5A mutation, T-wave amplitude was lowest in the HERG mutation, and T-wave duration was longest in the KvLQT1 mutation (see Fig. 18–6). These findings demonstrate a direct correlation between genotype and clinical manifestations of the disease, suggesting the potential for a genotype-directed approach to diagnosis and therapy. At present, the advantage of a molecular diagnosis lies in the ability to define the presence or absence of the mutation in asymptomatic family members and to provide genetic counseling.

ARRHYTHMIA MECHANISMS

Ion channels are formed by proteins within the myocardial cell membrane that control the entry and egress of specific ions. The gene mutations identified in LQTS involve the cardiac sodium current and the delayed rectifier current. These mutations prolong action potential duration by increasing net inward current (Na^+) or by decreasing outward (repolarizing) current (IKr and IKs). This prolongation of action potential duration generates deformities in the early (plateau) and late (phase 3) repolarization phases of the action potential, known as early afterdepolarizations (EADs). The mechanism by which EADs support the generation of torsades de pointes is not fully understood; however, several hypotheses have been proposed.

It has been demonstrated that pacing the heart rapidly from multiple sites reproduces the time-dependent shift in QRS axis observed in torsades de pointes. EAD-related, triggered activity arising from multiple foci at different rates could thus explain the mechanism supporting torsades de pointes. A second possibility is that torsades de pointes results from re-entrant excitation. Unidirectional block supporting re-entry may occur in the midmyocardium (M cell layer). The re-entrant pathway would vary as location of the functional zone of block varied, explaining the observed shift in QRS axis. Finally, torsades de pointes may occur as a result of the generation of EADs in the Purkinje cell layer, with conduction to the myocardium demonstrating beat-to-beat variability.

MANAGEMENT

Indications for Therapy

The estimated mortality of untreated symptomatic LQTS exceeds 20% in the year after presentation and approaches 50% within 10 years.[7] With effective therapy, this risk can be reduced to approximately 3 to 4% within 5 years,[8] emphasizing the importance of appropriate therapy. As a result of the findings of the International Study of the Pediatric Electrophysiology Society, in which the presenting symptom in 9% of children with LQTS was cardiac arrest, it is recommended that children with LQTS begin beta-blockade therapy independent of symptoms.[5] Because of the association of life-threatening ventricular arrhythmias during excessive catecholamine states, such as physical or emotional stress, children with LQTS are also restricted from competitive athletic endeavors.[26]

Specific Treatment

The modalities for therapy of LQTS include (1) beta-adrenergic blocking agents, (2) bradycardia pacing, (3) mexiletine, (4) left cervicothoracic sympathetic ganglionectomy, (5) pacemaker-cardioverter-defibrillator therapy, and (6) genotype-guided therapy. The goal of therapy is to prevent life-threatening ventricular arrhythmias and to reduce the risk of sudden cardiac death.

Beta-Adrenergic Blocking Agents

Beta-adrenergic blocking agents constitute the first line of therapy for patients with LQTS. It is likely that adrenergic blockade provides primary benefit in mutations involving the delayed rectifier current (LQT1 and LQT2). The benefit of beta-adrenergic blocking agents in sodium channel defects (LQT3) is less clear; however, currently, they remain first-line therapy for all LQTS patients except those with asthma. As clinical and molecular investigative work into the antiarrhythmic benefit of genotype-guided medical therapy advances, these recommendations may change.

Priori et al reviewed the significance of QT dispersion in patients responding to beta blockade and those requiring more aggressive therapy.[26] The authors found that QT dispersion was higher in nonresponders than in responders to beta blockade. A cutoff value of 100 milliseconds for QT_{max}–QT_{min} had an 80% sensitivity and an 82% specificity in discriminating between responders and nonresponders.[26] Although the use of cardioselective beta-adrenergic blockade has been advocated by some, Trippel and Gillette suggested that these agents may not provide adequate myocardial protection in LQTS patients.[27] The two most commonly used nonselective agents are propranolol (2–4 mg/kg/day) and nadolol (0.5–1.0 mg/kg/day). Adequate beta blockade is best assessed by exercise stress test, aiming for a reduction in the peak exercise heart rate by approximately 30% from the baseline study. It is important to adjust the medication dosage for growth during childhood while also periodically reassessing the effectiveness of therapy by clinical history, 24-hour ambulatory monitor, and exercise stress testing.

Bradycardia Pacing

Combination therapy with beta-blocking agents and bradycardia pacing has proven to be of benefit in patients who remain symptomatic on beta-blockade therapy alone.[6] A subgroup of LQTS patients, particularly those with sodium channel defects (LQT3), manifest slow sinus rates at baseline, which may be exacerbated with beta blockers.[8] If therapy leads to profound bradycardia or excessive sinus pauses, concomitant bradycardia pacing eliminates the pause-dependent triggers to life-threatening ventricular arrhythmias.

Moss et al demonstrated no difference in palliative benefit between dual- and single-chamber (either atrial or ventricular) pacing in high-risk patients.[28] Given the potential for delayed repolarization resulting in functional second-degree (2:1) AV block, dual-chamber pacing is recommended. Rate-adaptive pacing will provide palliative benefit of chronotropic incompetence, which may be exacerbated with beta blockade.

Left Cervicothoracic Sympathetic Ganglionectomy

The adrenergic dependence of arrhythmias led to the initial hypothesis that the primary abnormality in LQTS was an imbalance in cardiac sympathetic innervation.[29] A predominance of left stellate ganglion input was thought to occur as a result of decreased right stellate ganglion activity. On the basis of this theory, Moss and McDonald, in 1970, proposed left cervicothoracic sympathetic ganglionectomy as an antiarrhythmic measure.[30] The effectiveness of sympathetic ganglionectomy remains controversial. Although specific centers have reported high success rates,[31, 32] these results have not been universally reproducible. The optimal technique for the procedure involves removal of the lower half of the left stellate ganglion and the second and third thoracic ganglia.[33] It is generally reserved for individuals in whom aggressive therapy with beta blockade and pacing has failed and should be performed at an experienced center.

Implantable Cardioverter-Defibrillator Therapy

Advances in technology have led to progressive decreases in device weight and dimensions, making implantable cardioverter-defibrillators (ICDs) with both single- and dual-chamber bradycardia pacing capabilities a more practical therapeutic option for high-risk pediatric patients. In patients who remain symptomatic with beta blockade alone, the ICD is often an appropriate subsequent therapy, particularly in survivors of sudden death. Garson et al postulated a potential role for ICD therapy in children with extremely long QTc duration (QTc in excess of 550–600 milliseconds), because the risk of sudden death did not correlate with symptoms in this group of patients.[5]

Groh et al reviewed the outcome of 26 patients treated with ICDs for congenital LQTS.[34] Age at implant ranged from 2 to 64 years (mean, 29 years ± 17 years SD) with weights from 9 to 86 kg (mean, 57 kg ± 17 kg SD). Implant indications included aborted sudden cardiac death, syncope, and symptomatic episodes of torsades de pointes. Complications associated with device placement included infection (2 patients) and the need for epicardial patch revision in a 2-year-old child. Multiple discharges, which were determined to be appropriate, occurred in 2 patients. These episodes responded to increased beta blockade and dual-chamber pacing, respectively.

ICDs can potentially reduce the incidence of sudden death in high-risk pediatric populations. Use of devices that provide bradycardia pacing can eliminate bradycardia or pause-dependent triggers that lead to ventricular arrhythmias. Beta blockade or mexiletine therapy should be continued in patients after ICD placement to treat the underlying arrhythmogenic substrate, possibly reducing the frequency of delivered therapy. During childhood, this carries particular significance, given the deleterious effects that repetitive discharges may have on psychologic development.

Genotype-Directed Therapy

As clinical and molecular research progresses, the antiarrhythmic benefit of specific therapy directed by genotype may become common practice in the therapy of LQTS. Further prospective studies delineating the clear antiarrhythmic benefit of mexiletine in patients with SCN5A defects and the use of agents to maintain serum potassium levels in patients with defects in the delayed rectifier will be necessary before such interventions become common practice. However, it is clear that a more complete understanding of the clinical manifestations of the genetic subtypes of LQTS will impact dramatically on the diagnosis and management of the disease in the near future.

WOLFF-PARKINSON-WHITE SYNDROME

WPW syndrome refers to the condition of anomalous antegrade AV conduction mediated by an accessory conduction pathway. Speculation of anomalous muscle bands spanning the AV groove and supporting paroxysmal tachycardia were first alluded to by Kent in 1893.[35] In 1930, Wolff, Parkinson, and White described a clinical syndrome consisting of short PR interval, abnormal QRS morphology, and paroxysmal tachycardia (Fig. 18–7).[36] Subsequently, Holzmann and Scherf proposed that the QRS abnormality resulted from a bypass of AV nodal conduction in ventricular activation.[37] Since these early reports, our understanding of WPW syndrome has progressed tremendously. Most recently, the advent of radiofrequency catheter ablation has provided even further insight into the anatomic and physiologic substrates supporting the syndrome.

PREVALENCE

The prevalence of WPW syndrome in the pediatric population has been estimated at 0.15 to 0.3% (1.5–3 per 1000),[38, 39] with an incidence of approximately 3.96 per 100,000 persons per year for all age groups.[40] In children with structural cardiac disease, the prevalence has been estimated at 0.5%,[41] likely reflecting the increased association of WPW with specific congenital cardiac defects. The most notable of these defects is Ebstein's anomaly of the tricuspid valve, with an estimated prevalence of 5 to 20%.[42–44] There is also an increased association of WPW with L transposition of the great arteries, hypertrophic cardiomyopathy, and cardiac tumors, especially rhabdomyomas.[45] The male–female ratio in children with WPW syndrome is approximately 57 to 65%.[38]

DEVELOPMENTAL ASPECTS

During embryogenesis, the myocardium of the atrium and ventricle are contiguous. As the fetal heart progresses in development, the myocardium between the primitive atrium and ventricle involutes and the anulus fibrosus forms. Defects in the continuity of the anulus fibrosus allow bandlike bridges of muscle to persist between

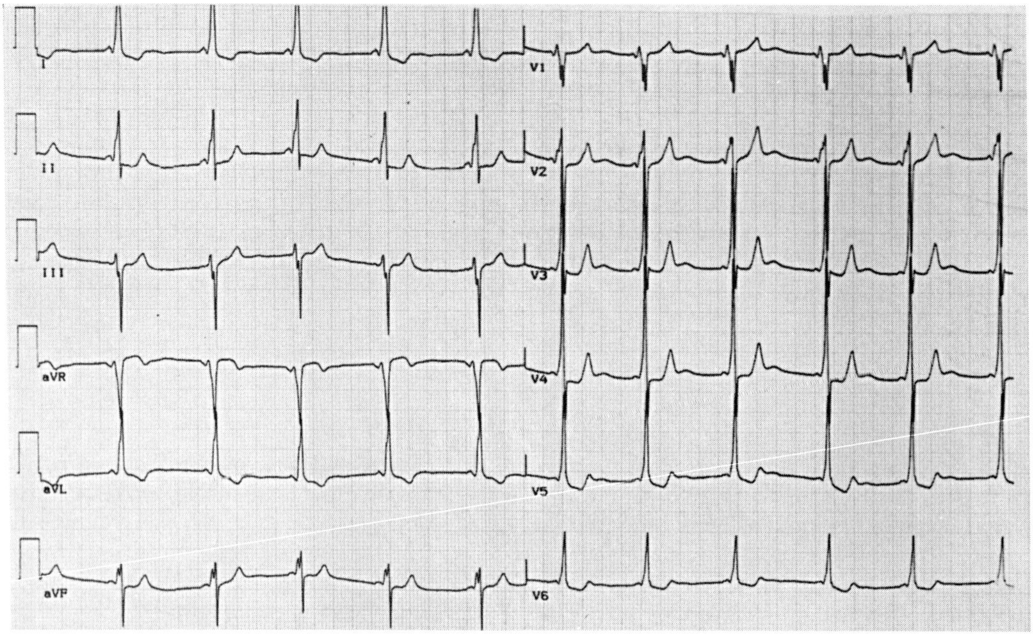

FIGURE 18–7. Wolff-Parkinson-White syndrome demonstrated by 12-lead electrocardiogram. The short PR interval and wide QRS are most obvious in leads I and II and the left precordial leads.

the atrium and ventricle. These bands are precursors to accessory pathways.[46] This accounts for the increased association of accessory pathways in structural defects involving the AV ring, such as Ebstein's anomaly and L transposition of the great arteries. A proportion of these bandlike fibers have no functional significance or resolve within the first months of life, explaining the observation by Deal and colleagues that up to 40% of manifest accessory pathways may resolve within the first year of life.[47]

ECG FINDINGS

In WPW syndrome, AV conduction occurs over both the AV node and accessory pathway, and the degree of pre-excitation manifested on the surface ECG reflects the relative contribution of each pathway to ventricular activation. Factors that influence this balance include pathway location and the conduction velocity and refractory periods of the atria, AV node, and accessory pathway, thus resulting in ECG variation from marked to subtle pre-excitation. It is not uncommon during childhood when AV nodal conduction is very rapid to have only a very subtle pattern of pre-excitation by surface ECG, especially in cases of left free wall accessory pathways, in which atrial conduction time to the accessory pathway may be much greater than that through the AV node. As such, left-sided accessory pathways in children may only manifest very subtle evidence of pre-excitation by ECG. Perry and colleagues showed that the surface ECG in such patients demonstrates the lack of a Q wave in the left precordial leads, a PR interval less than 100 milliseconds, and left axis deviation for age.[48]

Although WPW syndrome refers to accessory pathways that conduct in both the antegrade and retrograde direction, it is important to understand that accessory pathways may also conduct in a retrograde-only fashion supporting orthodromic tachycardia. These pathways are concealed pathways or unidirectional retrograde accessory pathways.

ARRHYTHMIAS

WPW syndrome has the potential for a wide range of varied arrhythmias, including ventricular fibrillation. The most commonly observed arrhythmia in the pediatric population is AV reciprocating tachycardia supported by a macro–reentrant circuit consisting of the atria, AV node, His-Purkinje system, ventricle, and the accessory pathway. In the more common form, the impulse traverses antegrade over the AV node and retrograde from ventricle to atrium across the accessory pathway. This is referred to as orthodromic tachycardia (*ortho*, meaning with; *dromis*, meaning node). In the less common, or antidromic (*ante*, meaning against; *dromis*, meaning node) form, the impulse travels antegrade over an accessory pathway and retrograde across the AV node or across a second accessory pathway. As such, orthodromic tachycardia inscribes a narrow complex QRS morphology, whereas antidromic tachycardia inscribes a wide complex (pre-excited) QRS morphology.

In up to 15% of pediatric patients with antidromic tachycardia, there is a second accessory pathway supporting ventriculoatrial conduction.[49] Pre-excited tachycardia occurs when the accessory pathway conducts in an antegrade-only fashion, such as in the case of Mahaim fibers. This may be a result of antidromic AV re-entry tachycardia or bystander pre-excitation with the tachycardia supported by re-entry or automaticity using an alternate substrate for tachycardia, such as AV node re-entry, primary atrial tachycardia, or atrial flutter.

Atrial flutter and fibrillation occur at a threefold increased incidence in patients with WPW syndrome compared with the general population.[50] These arrhythmias commonly develop as a result of degeneration of AV reciprocating tachycardia (AVRT) rather than as a primary event. The relative refractoriness and conduction velocities of the AV node and accessory pathway determine whether the resultant ventricular response is pre-excited, narrow complex, or fused in morphology. The ventricular refractory period and concealed penetration into the AV node and accessory pathway will also affect the degree of ventricular pre-excitation. The pathognomonic ECG during atrial fibrillation with WPW syndrome will demonstrate an irregularly irregular rhythm with varying degrees of fusion in antegrade AV node and accessory pathway conduction. It is of paramount importance to identify this rhythm readily, given the associated risk for degeneration to ventricular fibrillation. The incidence of sudden cardiac death in WPW syndrome during childhood has been estimated to be as high as 0.5%.[40]

MANAGEMENT

Various factors determine the need for therapy and the specific therapy indicated in children with WPW syndrome. These include presence of symptoms, severity of symptoms, age, and presence of underlying structural cardiac disease.

The approach to management of the asymptomatic child is confounded by the fact that sudden death may be the first clinical manifestation of the syndrome in a cohort of patients. In a multicenter study of children with WPW syndrome, 48% of patients who experienced sudden cardiac death had no prior documentation of an arrhythmia.[51] As such, our approach is to educate the patient and family in the signs and symptoms of supraventricular tachycardia (SVT), vagal maneuvers used to interrupt tachycardia, and medications and foods that might precipitate tachycardia episodes. An electrophysiology study is recommended to stratify risk in asymptomatic patients usually by the teenage years, and is required for clearance in all individuals who wish to participate in competitive athletic endeavors. This is supported by the findings of Bromberg et al in that the only truly sensitive predictor of sudden death in children with WPW is a shortest pre-excited RR interval during atrial fibrillation–flutter of less than 220 milliseconds.[52] At the time of the electrophysiology study, balanced by the location of the pathway and the relative risk demonstrated by the pathway conduction and refractoriness, radiofrequency catheter ablation of the pathway may be undertaken during this same procedure.

In patients with documented AV reciprocating tachycardia, first-line therapy is generally with a beta-adrenergic blocking agent. In children weighing less than 10 kg, propranolol is used at an initial dose of 2 to 4 mg/kg/day on a dosing schedule of four times per day. In children weighing more than 10 kg, a long-acting agent such as atenolol, on a once per day dosing schedule, is used. Both agents may be suspended in various diluents for younger children while still maintaining extended bioavailability. Digoxin is contraindicated in patients with WPW syndrome given the associated risk of an accelerated pre-excited ventricular response to atrial fibrillation and sudden death.[53]

In children younger than approximately 3 years in whom therapy with beta-adrenergic blocking agents fails, the next agent that is generally instituted is amiodarone. Some studies support using this class III agent as a first-line drug in infants with SVT.[54] In infants who have had fetal tachycardia, especially in association with nonimmune hydrops, it has become our practice to institute amiodarone as first-line therapy. These patients tend to have frequent episodes of AVRT in the first few months of life likely resulting from a component of systolic or diastolic dysfunction, which eventually resolves. As such, we have seen fewer breakthrough episodes of tachycardia in these patients as opposed to patients receiving beta-adrenergic blocking agents. Because amiodarone does have many noncardiac adverse effects, especially involving thyroid and liver function, blood work must be evaluated at frequent intervals to avoid unwanted sequelae. Some of these very young patients are refractory to any combination of antiarrhythmic drug therapy. Although drug therapy is the treatment method of choice in this age group, radiofrequency catheter ablation can be performed safely and successfully in select patients.[55, 56]

In children with structural cardiac disease and impending cardiac surgery, the practice of performing a complete electrophysiology study with the plan for radiofrequency catheter ablation of the accessory pathway before surgery has been adopted. As outlined by Van Hare,[57] the patient may experience episodes of SVT in the postoperative period, especially as a result of the administration of necessary inotropic agents. In addition, these episodes may be poorly tolerated as a result of altered hemodynamics in the immediate postoperative period. If catheter-guided attempts at ablation are unsuccessful, surgical interruption of the accessory pathway at the time of structural repair is highly recommended.

Although many children with WPW syndrome or LQTS are diagnosed and treated, a small percentage initially present with sudden cardiac death. A simple ECG may have prevented some of these deaths. In the case of the normal or borderline prolonged QT interval, a careful history, including a family history, may be the clinician's most useful tool. The advancements made in the diagnosis and treatment of children with either of these ECG abnormalities has been phenomenal over the past decade, and the future will most likely result in many more major developments.

REFERENCES

1. Jervell A, Lange-Nielsen F: Congenital deaf mutism, functional heart diseases, with prolongation of the QT interval and sudden death. Am Heart J 54:59–68, 1957.
2. Romano C, Gemme G, Pongiglione R: Artmie cardiache rare dell'eta pediatrica. Clin Pediatr 45:658–683, 1963.
3. Ward OC: New familial cardiac syndrome in children. J Irish Med Assoc 54:103–106, 1964.
4. Schott JJ, Charpentier F, Peltier S, et al: Mapping of a gene for long QT syndrome to chromosome 4q25–27. Am J Hum Genet 57:1114–1122, 1995.
5. Garson A Jr, Dick M, Fournier A, et al: The long QT

syndrome in children: An international study of 287 patients. Circulation 87:1866–1872, 1993.
6. Schwartz PJ: Idiopathic long QT syndrome: Progress and questions. Am Heart J 2:399–411, 1985.
7. Schwartz PJ, Moss A, Vincent GM, et al: Diagnostic criteria for the long QT syndrome: An update. Circulation 88:782–784, 1993.
8. Roden DM, Lazzara R, Rosen M, et al: Multiple mechanisms in the long-QT syndrome: Current knowledge, gaps, and future directions. Circulation 94:1996–2012, 1996.
9. Priori S, Napolitano C, Paganini V, et al: Molecular biology of the long QT syndrome: Impact on management. Pacing Clin Electrophysiol 20:2052–2057, 1997.
10. Towbin JA, Li H, Taggart RT, et al: Evidence of genetic heterogeneity in Romano-Ward long QT syndrome. Analysis of 23 families. Circulation 90:2635–2644, 1994.
11. Benhorin J, Kalman YM, Medina A, et al: Evidence of genetic heterogeneity in the long QT syndrome. Science 260:1960–1962, 1993.
12. Sanguinetti MC, Jiang C, Curran ME, et al: A mechanistic link between an inherited and an acquired cardiac arrhythmia: HERG encodes the IKr potassium channel. Cell 81:1–20, 1995.
13. Curran ME, Splawski I, Timothy KW, et al: A molecular basis for cardiac arrhythmia: HERG mutations cause long QT syndrome. Cell 80:795–803, 1995.
14. Schultze-Bhar E, Haverkamp W, Weibusch H, et al: Frequency and phenotype of HERG mutations in congenital long QT syndrome (LQTS). Circulation 94:719, 1996 (abstract).
15. Benson DW, MacRae CA, Vesley MR, et al: Missense mutation in the pore region of HERG causes familial long QT syndrome. Circulation 93:1791–1795, 1996.
16. Priori SG, Napolitano C: Impact of molecular biology on diagnosis and management of arrhythmogenic disorders. Revista Portuguesa de Cardiologia 17:323–327, 1998.
17. Sanguanetti MC, Curran ME, Spector PS, et al: Spectrum of HERG K^+- channel dysfunction in an inherited cardiac arrhythmia. Proc Nat Acad Sci 93:2208–2212, 1996.
18. Priori SG, Napolitano C, CantNu F, et al: Differential response to Na^+ channel blockade, β-adrenergic stimulation, and rapid pacing in a cellular model mimicking the SCN5A and HERG defects present in the long QT syndrome: Experimental basis for gene specific therapy. Circ Res 78:1009–1015, 1996.
19. Compton SJ, Lux RL, Ramsey MR, et al: Genetically defined therapy of inherited long QT syndrome: Correction of abnormal repolarization by potassium. Circulation 94:1018–1022, 1996.
20. Wang Q, Shen J, Splawski I, et al: SCN5A mutations associated with an inherited cardiac arrhythmia, long QT syndrome. Cell 80:805–811, 1995.
21. Wang Q, Shen J, Li Z, et al: Cardiac sodium channel mutations in patients with long QT syndrome. An inherited cardiac arrhythmia. Hum Mol Genet 4:1607, 1995.
22. Wang Q, Zhizhung L, Jiaxiang S, et al: Genomic organization of the human SCN5A gene encoding the cardiac sodium channel. Genomics 34:9–16, 1996.
23. Moss AJ: Clinical management of patients with the long QT syndrome: Drugs, devices, and gene-specific therapy. Pacing Clin Electrophysiol 20:2058–2060, 1997.
24. Neyroud N, Tesson F, Denjoy I, et al: A novel mutation in the potassium channel gene KVLQT1 causes the Jervell and Lange-Neilsen cardioauditory syndrome. Nat Genet 15:186–189, 1997.
25. Splawski I, Timothy K, Vincent GM, et al: Molecular basis of the long QT syndrome associated with deafness. N Engl J Med 336: 1562–1567, 1997.
26. Priori SG, Napolitano C, Diehl L, et al: Dispersion of the QT interval: A marker of therapeutic efficacy in the idiopathic long QT syndrome. Circulation 89:1681–1689, 1994.
27. Trippel DL, Gillette PC: Atenolol in children with ventricular arrhythmias. Am Heart J 119:1312–1316, 1990.
28. Moss AJ, Liu JE, Gottlieb S: Efficacy of permanent pacing in the management of high-risk patients with long QT syndrome. Circulation 84:1524–1529, 1991.
29. Swartz PJ, Locati E: The idiopathic long QT syndrome: Pathogenetic mechanisms and therapy. Eur Heart J 6:103–110, 1985.
30. Moss AJ, McDonald J: Unilateral cervicothoracic sympathetic ganglionectomy for the treatment of long QT interval syndrome. N Engl J Med 285:903, 1970.
31. Schwartz PJ, Locati EH, Moss AJ: Left cardiac sympathetic denervation in the therapy of congenital long QT syndrome. J Am Coll Cardiol 10:600, 1987.
32. Schwartz PJ, Locati E, Moss AJ, et al: Left cardiac sympathetic denervation in the therapy of the congenital long QT syndrome: A worldwide report. Circulation 84:503–511, 1991.
33. Ouriel K, Moss AJ: Long QT syndrome: An indication for cervicothoracic sympathectomy. Cardiac Surg 3:475–478, 1995.
34. Groh WJ, Silka M, Oliver RP, et al: Use of implantable cardioverter-defibrillators in the congenital long QT syndrome. Am J Cardiol 87:703–706, 1996.
35. Kent AFS: Researches on the structure and function of the mammalian heart. J Physiol 14:233–246, 1893.
36. Wolff L, Parkinson J, White P, et al: Bundle branch block with short P-R interval in healthy young people prone to paroxysmal tachycardia. Am Heart J 5:685–704, 1930.
37. Holzman M, Scherf D: Ueber Elektrokardiogramme mit Verkurzter Vorhof-Kammer-Distanz und positiven P-Zacken. Z Klin Med 121:404–422, 1932.
38. Gillette PC, Blair HL, Crawford FA: Preexcitation syndromes. In Gillette PC, Garson A, Jr (eds): Pediatric Arrhythmias: Electrophysiology and Pacing. Philadelphia: WB Saunders, 1990, pp 363.
39. Sorbo MD, Buja GF, Miorelli M, et al: The prevalence of the Wolff-Parkinson-White syndrome in a population of 116,542 young males. Giornale Ital Cardiol 25:681–687, 1995.
40. Munger TM, Packer DL, Hammill SC, et al: A population study of the natural history of Wolff-Parkinson-White syndrome in Olmstead County, Minnesota, 1953–1989. Circulation 87:866–873, 1993.
41. Porter CJ, Holmes DR: Preexcitation syndromes associated with congenital heart disease. In Benditt DG, Benson DW Jr (eds): Cardiac Preexcitation Syndromes. Boston, Martinus Nijhoff, 1986, pp 289–302.
42. Watson H: Natural history of Ebstein's anomaly of the tricuspid valve in childhood and adolescence: An international cooperative study of 505 cases. Br Heart J 36:417–427, 1974.
43. Giuliani ER, Fuster V, Brandenburg RO: Special review: Ebstein's anomaly: The clinical features and natural history of Ebstein's anomaly of the tricuspid valve. Mayo Clinic Proc 54:163–173, 1979.
44. Smith WM, Gallagher JJ, Kerr CR, et al: The electrophysiologic basis and management of symptomatic and recurrent tachycardia in patients with Ebstein's anomaly of the tricuspid valve. Am J Cardiol 49: 1223–1234, 1982.
45. Van Hare GF, Phoon CK, Munkenbeck F, et al: Electrophysiology study and radiofrequency ablation in patients with intracardiac tumors and accessory pathways: Is the tumor the pathway? J Cardiovasc Electrophysiol 7:1204–1210, 1996.

46. Lindsay BD, Crossen KJ, Cain ME: Concordance of distinguishing electrocardiographic features during sinus rhythm with the location of accessory pathways in Wolff-Parkinson-White syndrome. Am J Cardiol 59:1093–102, 1987.
47. Deal BJ, Keane JF, Gillette PC, et al: Wolff-Parkinson-White syndrome and supraventricular tachycardia during infancy: Management and follow-up. J Am Coll Cardiol 5:130–135, 1985.
48. Perry JC, Giuffre RM, Garson A Jr: Clues to the electrocardiographic diagnosis of subtle Wolff-Parkinson-White syndrome in children. J Pediatr 117:871–875, 1990.
49. Gillette PC, Garson A Jr, Cooley DA, et al: Prolonged and decremental antegrade conduction properties in right anterior accessory connections: Wide QRS antidromic tachycardia of left bundle branch block pattern without Wolff-Parkinson-White configuration in sinus rhythm. Am Heart J 103:66–74, 1982.
50. Morady F: The spectrum of tachyarrhythmias in preexcitation syndromes. In Benditt DG, Benson DW Jr (eds): Cardiac Preexcitation Syndromes. Boston, Martinus Nijhoff, 1986, pp 119–139.
51. Deal BJ, Dick M, Beerman L, et al: Cardiac arrest in young patients with Wolff-Parkinson-White syndrome. Pacing Clin Electrophysiol 18:815, 1995 (abstract).
52. Bromberg BI, Lindsay BD, Cain ME, et al: Impact of clinical history and electrophysiologic characterization of accessory pathways on management strategies to reduce sudden death among children with Wolff-Parkinson-White syndrome. J Am Coll Cardiol 27:690–695, 1996.
53. Byrum CJ, Wahl RA, Behrendt DM, et al: Ventricular fibrillation associated with use of digitalis in a newborn infant with Wolff-Parkinson-White syndrome. J Pediatr 101:400–403, 1982.
54. Villain E, Bonnet D, Iserin L, et al: Prophylaxis of supraventricular tachycardia in the first year of life: Digoxin or amiodarone? In Proceedings of the Second World Congress of Pediatric Cardiology and Cardiac Surgery, Armonk NY, Futura Publishing Co., Inc., 1997, p 24 (abstract).
55. Case CL, Gillette PC, Oslizlok PC, et al: Radiofrequency catheter ablation of incessant, medically resistant supraventricular tachycardia in infants and small children. J Am Coll Cardiol 20:1405, 1992.
56. Erickson CC, Walsh EP, Triedman JK, et al: Efficacy and safety of radiofrequency ablation in infants and young children $<$ 18 months of age. Am J Cardiol 74:944–947, 1994.
57. Van Hare G: Radiofrequency ablation of accessory pathways associated with congenital heart disease. Pacing Clin Electrophysiol 20:2077–2081, 1997.

CHAPTER 19

CHRONIC POSTOPERATIVE ARRHYTHMIAS

Seshadri Balaji, John Deanfield, Arthur Garson, Jr., and Paul C. Gillette

Late arrhythmia is an important cause of morbidity and mortality in patients who have undergone surgery for congenital heart diseases. Sudden death in these patients is thought to be secondary to arrhythmia in most cases. Late arrhythmia is, therefore, a major diagnostic and therapeutic challenge. This challenge is further compounded by the frequent presence of compromised hemodynamic function.

PATHOPHYSIOLOGY

The three major substrates for development of arrhythmias—scarring, hypertrophy, and dilatation—are all present to some degree in patients with postsurgical congenital heart disease. The more complex the initial defect, the more difficult the repair, the more extensive are the scars of surgery, and the more likely it is that, despite good surgery, residual hemodynamic problems are left behind. Also notable is that arrhythmias, when they do develop, are less well tolerated by those with residual hemodynamic problems. Furthermore, frequent arrhythmias can lead to worsening of myocardial function, as can most drugs used to treat such arrhythmias. Therefore, it is paramount that arrhythmias be viewed with an understanding of the hemodynamic problems of the patient. This is vital in terms of management, because management of the arrhythmia without giving thought to the hemodynamic problems usually is unsuccessful.

Although these concepts apply mainly to tachyarrhythmias, late development of bradyarrhythmia is also possible. Gradual deterioration of the sinoatrial node, the atrioventricular (AV) node, or the bundle of His as well as prolongation of conduction defects resulting from scarring, hypertrophy, or dilatation can lead to bradycardia requiring therapy.

BRADYARRHYTHMIAS

The two major bradyarrhythmias are sinus node dysfunction and complete AV block.

Sinus node dysfunction may be produced by operations in the atrium, such as repair of atrial septal defect,[1] Mustard or Senning operation for transposition of the great arteries,[2] and the Fontan operation.[3] In some cases, such as atrial septal defects, the sinus node injury may be due to the cannulation site for cardiopulmonary bypass and can be avoided by changing this to selective cannulation of the superior vena cava.[4] In other conditions, such as post-Mustard and post-Senning operations, the problem is not so easily resolved.[5]

In the study by Deanfield et al,[6] only 56% of Senning patients and 66% of Mustard patients were in stable sinus rhythm on Holter electrocardiogram (ECG) 7 years after surgery. In the study by Vetter et al,[7] only 14% had normal sinus node function at 6 years when examined by electrophysiologic (EP) study.

The incidence of sinus node dysfunction is just as apparent in patients after the Fontan procedure[3, 8] and also after its recent modification, the total cavopulmonary connection.[9] In these patients, the issue is further complicated by the presence of only one functioning ventricle, which makes the patient more susceptible to the hemodynamic compromise produced by chronotropic incompetence.

Late development of AV block is possible after operations around the AV node and bundle of His, such as repair of AV septal defect, closure of ventricular septal defect, and AV valve replacement. Patients usually present with tiredness, syncope, or presyncope on developing significant bradycardia. However, most are detected by routine checkups on the ECG or by ambulatory Holter monitoring.

Pacemaker insertion is indicated in all symptomatic (syncope, presyncope, exercise intolerance) patients and all those with severe bradycardia (< 60/m in children ≤ 2 years; < 50/m between 2 and 10 years; < 40/m > 10 years). Patients needing antiarrhythmic therapy other than digoxin for tachyarrhythmias should also be considered potential candidates for pacemaker implantation because the drugs used might depress sinus or AV node conduction. A dual-chamber pacemaker is indicated in all but those patients who have isolated sinoatrial node disease, who should be suitable for an atrial pacemaker.

ATRIAL TACHYARRHYTHMIAS

Atrial tachyarrhythmias are predominantly seen after complex atrial surgery, such as the Mustard/Senning operation or the Fontan procedure. The most common arrhythmia is atrial flutter. However, ectopic atrial tachycardia and atrial fibrillation can also occur.

Mustard/Senning Patients

Atrial flutter is the most common tachyarrhythmia after Mustard and Senning operations for transposition (Fig. 19–1). The incidence varies from 5 to 25% and increases with duration of follow-up. The occurrence of atrial flutter is related to sinus node damage and to the extensive atrial suture lines. Factors related to atrial flutter are loss of sinus rhythm, ventricular dysfunction, and venous pathway obstruction.[10] In the study by Gewillig et al,[10] there was a 20% (50 of 249 patients) incidence of late death; of these, 37 patients died suddenly (74%). Although not directly proven, these late deaths could have been due to atrial flutter because sudden death is a known complication of atrial flutter, particularly if an effective drug regimen is not found.[11]

Bink-Boelkens et al[12] studied 36 asymptomatic children 7 years after Mustard operation. Of these, only 3 had normal hemodynamic and EP studies. In the rest, the main electrical problems noted were abnormal sinus node and atrial muscle function; the AV node was nearly always normal. Vetter et al[7] reported similar findings. Half of their patients had inducible atrial flutter, and half of this subgroup went on to experience clinical episodes of flutter.

Fontan Patients

The risk of atrial flutter and of hemodynamic compromise and death as a result of atrial flutter seems greater in Fontan patients.[3, 8, 13–17] In Porter and Garson's[13] study, patients who had a supraventricular tachycardia before discharge from hospital after their Fontan operation had a 66% chance of experiencing a similar arrhythmia within 5 years. These increased risks are probably due not only to the extensive suture lines but also to the inevitable volume and pressure stresses experienced by the right atrium after this procedure. Because the loss of pulsatile flow seems to be unimportant to maintain pulmonary flow, and

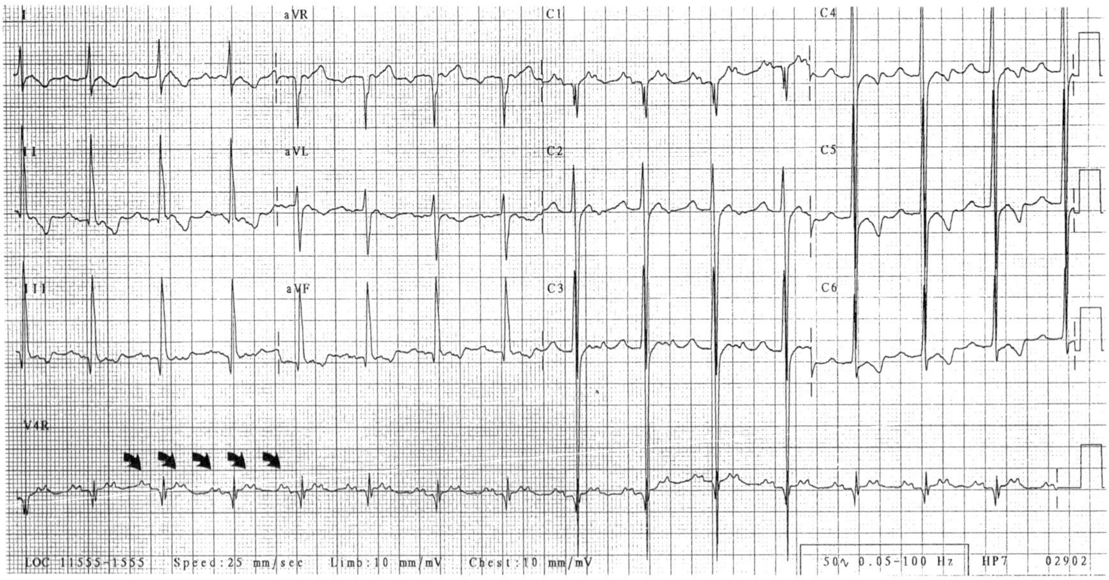

FIGURE 19–1. Atrial flutter with 2:1 block in a post-Fontan patient. The ventricular rate is about 88/min and the atrial rate twice that. Flutter waves *(arrows)* are best seen in the rhythm strip (at bottom).

tachyarrhythmias (and loss of sinus rhythm) predominantly depress cardiac output by the loss of left atrial augmentation of ventricular filling, de Leval et al[18] proposed the total cavopulmonary connection. Early results showed that, although the incidence of atrial flutter was similar in the two groups at follow-up, the total cavopulmonary group seemed better able to tolerate the arrhythmia.[15] Other groups[17] reported a lower incidence of atrial flutter after the total cavopulmonary connection. The incidence of late atrial flutter is related to the history of early (< 30 days postoperative) arrhythmias,[17] more complex anatomic subtype relative to tricuspid atresia, pulmonary artery pressure greater than 20 mm Hg,[3] and increased size of the right atrium.[3]

Other Patient Groups

Atrial flutter may develop late after many other operations, such as repair or replacement of an AV valve (particularly if residual valve stenosis or incompetence is present), repair of atrial and AV septal defects, Blalock-Hanlon septectomy, and repair of anomalous pulmonary venous drainage. Atrial flutter may also complicate operations that mainly involve ventricular surgery, such as tetralogy of Fallot (TOF) repair.[19] As a rule, most of those patients have a poor hemodynamic result with residual shunts, AV valve regurgitation, and ventricular dysfunction.

Evaluation of the Patient With Atrial Flutter

Because atrial flutter may be a feature of an underlying hemodynamic problem, all patients need a careful hemodynamic assessment. This may include a physical examination, chest radiographs, and echocardiogram. If the echocardiogram does not provide satisfactory information (as is often the case in patients after multiple surgeries), further assessment with magnetic resonance imaging or cardiac catheterization is indicated. From the arrhythmia point of view, other important questions to be addressed are as follows: Are there clinically unrecognized periods of arrhythmia, as shown by Holter monitor? Can the arrhythmia be precipitated by exercise, such as stress testing?

The cardiac catheterization may be combined with an EP study. The EP study will look specifically at sinus node, atrial muscle, and AV node function. It may also be used to test the prospective usefulness of an antitachycardia pacemaker (i.e., is the flutter reproducibly and reliably overdrive pace terminated?). If AV node function is suboptimal, the patient may need a ventricular pacemaker, particularly if strong antiarrhythmic drug therapy is being contemplated.

Another useful add-on to this evaluation may be an attempt at radiofrequency catheter ablation of atrial flutter. Although results are modest, this therapy is fast becoming an important addition to the options available to the cardiologist.[20]

Management of Atrial Flutter

The acute management consists of either direct current cardioversion or overdrive pacing (either transvenous or transesophageal). The first-line drug therapy for long-term prophylaxis is digoxin, but it may only provide ventricular rate control. A class Ic drug (flecainide or propafenone) or class III drug (amiodarone or sotalol) may be added to digoxin. Combination therapy using a class I and a class III agent may occasionally be necessary. Care must be taken to provide adequate ventricular rate protection using a pacemaker when powerful antiarrhythmics are used that may depress the AV node. The process of repeated admissions to hospital for cardioversion is not considered an adequate option.

Nonpharmacologic therapy has a major role in the management of atrial flutter. Overdrive pacing, using an antitachycardia pacemaker, can help reduce hospital and emergency room visits and is an important therapeutic advance in these patients.[21] Radiofrequency ablation of atrial flutter is fast gaining popularity.[20] Although currently long-term results are modest, the hope of permanent relief makes it an extremely attractive option. Concomitant pursuit of hemodynamic improvement by drug therapy (e.g., angiotensin-converting enzyme inhibition), interventional catheterization (e.g., dilating baffle obstructions; closing baffle leaks), or surgery, or a combination, may make flutter less likely and better tolerated.

All of these measures tend to be less effective in the control of atrial flutter in Fontan patients compared with Mustard or Senning patients. Last, we have had to resort to surgical excision of the right atrial wall (right atriectomy) in three patients after Fontan operation. Two of them went on to have a good result with resolution of atrial flutter, and one died postoperatively.[22] In two additional patients, modification of a classic Fontan procedure into total cavopulmonary connection (the lateral tunnel approach) did not prevent further flutter (BA Bubolz, PC Gillette, personal communication, 1995). Thus, once the atrial tissue is severely abnormal, it probably remains arrhythmogenic.

Ectopic Atrial Tachycardia

Ectopic pacemakers can develop within the atria long after surgery. The diagnosis is based on the presence of a tachycardia that is often incessant with abnormal P-wave morphology. If untreated, the incessant tachycardia leads to ventricular dilatation and failure. Drug therapy is usually with class Ic or class III drugs and is often ineffective. Catheter ablation is the best approach but can be technically difficult, depending on the anatomy of the patient.[23]

VENTRICULAR ARRHYTHMIAS

Ventricular tachycardia (VT) may be incapacitating and can lead to death (Fig. 19–2). Most cases of sudden death in postoperative patients are thought to be due to VT. Whether ventricular fibrillation (not preceded by tachycardia) can be the terminal event is unclear. This section focuses on TOF because it is the best studied lesion. However, the same general concepts can probably be extended to other lesions.

Sudden death can occur in up to 6% of patients late after TOF repair.[24, 25] Current evidence favors VT as a precursor of sudden death. Hence, prevention or treatment of VT is probably the best way to prevent sudden death. There is no accepted means of predicting patients at risk of VT and sudden death.

Initially, it was believed that ventricular ectopics in the setting of residual right ventricular outflow obstruction were the precipitating event in sudden death.[25] The emphasis has gradually shifted, and the current view favors volume overload secondary to long-standing pulmonary incompetence and consequent right ventricular enlargement as the most important factor in causing sudden death. The role of ventricular ectopics is unclear. Although conventionally complex or frequent ectopy on Holter monitor was thought to be an adverse predictor, this view has lately been challenged.[26]

Even TOF patients who have not undergone repair have ambient ectopy. Some have postulated that the right ventricular pressure overload and myocardial hypoxemia resulting from cyanosis may be arrhythmogenic. There is some evidence that earlier surgery may prevent this natural course of events.[27] Walsh et al,[28] in their report on a series of primary TOF repair at infancy, found a low incidence of arrhythmia, admittedly at relatively short follow-up.

Other factors that may play a role are residual hemodynamic problems, such as a residual ventricular septal defect, longer follow-up, and transventricular (as opposed to transatrial) repair.[29] Thus, surgical advances over the last few decades probably imply a lower incidence of sudden death for patients operated on in that time period.

There has been interest in three other meth-

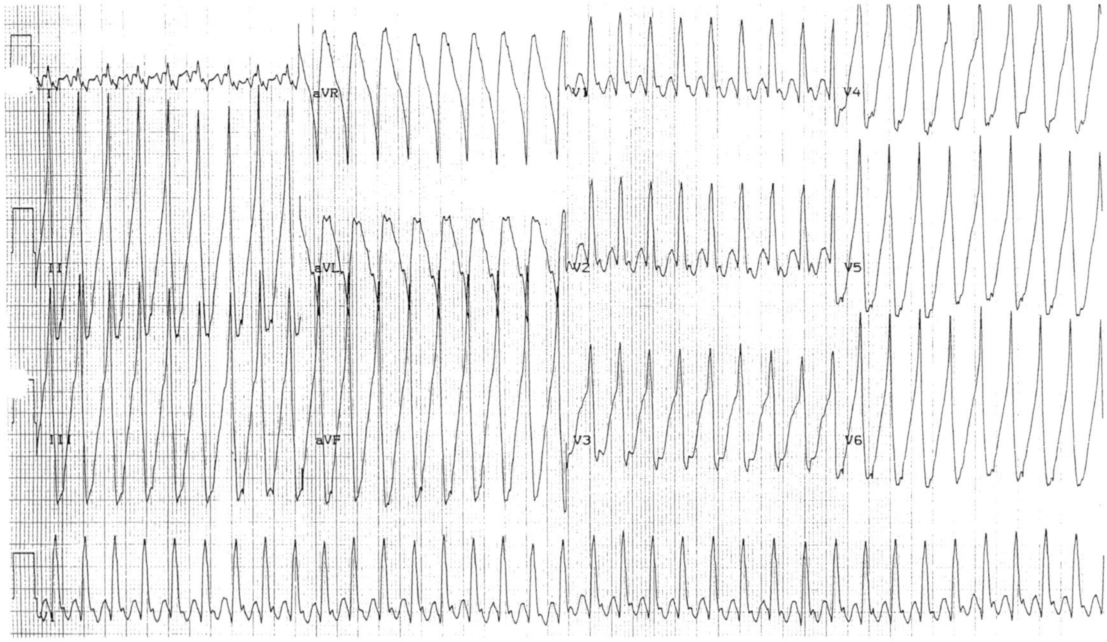

FIGURE 19–2. Ventricular tachycardia in a postoperative tetralogy of Fallot patient.

ods of noninvasively predicting the risk of sudden death: (1) the signal-averaged ECG, (2) QRS duration, and (3) QT dispersion.

The signal-averaged (or high-resolution) ECG finding of positive late potentials may imply an area of slow conduction within the heart and, thus, a risk of intraventricular re-entrant rhythms (i.e., VT). Although this is theoretically true, its practical use is not established and its role in risk stratification unclear.[30, 31]

QRS duration was shown to be related to right ventricular size, with good prediction of adverse events in patients with a QRS duration of greater than or equal to 180 ms (i.e., extremely prolonged).[32] There is also much interest in QT dispersion (defined as the difference between the maximum and the minimum QT interval between the various leads of a standard ECG). Some found it to predict ventricular arrhythmia independently,[33, 34] whereas others found that it adds to the sensitivity and specificity of risk stratification when used in combination with QRS duration criteria.[35]

The role of EP studies in risk stratification is unclear. EP study can reproduce clinical VT[36] and help identify a successful drug treatment regimen.[37] Whether it can prospectively identify a patient who may be a candidate for sudden death is contentious. We studied an unselected cohort (N = 135) of patients after TOF repair. All patients with clinically documented VT (N = 4) and half of those with symptoms (11/22) had induced sustained VT using an aggressive stimulation protocol. This protocol had been validated in 17 patients with structurally normal hearts undergoing EP study after previous successful ablation of accessory pathways or dual AV nodal pathways responsible for supraventricular tachycardia. None of those control patients had induced sustained VT (MC Sokoloski, PC Gillette, personal communication, 1996). In contrast to symptomatic post-TOF patients, only 11 of 113 (10%) asymptomatic patients had induced sustained VT. Thus, currently, the EP study identifies a subset of asymptomatic patients thought to be at risk. Whether this is a high false-positive rate is unknown because none of our patients has died suddenly. When a positive EP study was related to noninvasive tests (QRS duration, QT dispersion, and RV dimension), these simpler tests were highly specific but not sensitive in identifying a positive EP study. It is possible that a combined approach using noninvasive tests as a guide to recommending EP study will prove successful in risk stratification.

We believe that finding induced sustained monomorphic VT on EP study identifies the presence of a potential re-entrant circuit. However, whether this circuit will ever become clinically active will depend on modulating factors (e.g., right ventricular dilatation, electrolyte imbalance) and triggering factors (such as frequent ectopy). We currently treat all patients with induced sustained monomorphic VT with phenytoin. Phenytoin was chosen because it is good at suppressing ectopy,[38] has a low proarrhythmia rate,[38] and has shown direct promise in preventing sudden death in one study.[39]

The relevance of induced polymorphic VT is unclear. Although most regard it as an unwanted by-product of an aggressive EP study,[40] it must be noted that the dilated ventricle is at greater risk of polymorphic VT[41] and that mechanical stretch can be arrhythmogenic to cardiomyocytes.[42] One can easily speculate that, in patients with highly dilated ventricles, polymorphic VT or acute ventricular fibrillation is the cause of death. However, no proof exists for this hypothesis.

Evaluation

Again, as for atrial flutter, a thorough hemodynamic evaluation is recommended for all symptomatic patients and those with VT (sustained or not) on Holter monitor. For asymptomatic patients, periodic outpatient review with ECG, chest radiographs, and echocardiograms should suffice.

It is our view that all symptomatic patients need EP studies. We have not found hemodynamic catheterization to be of benefit because most residual problems are already known from the echocardiogram.

Management

The management of patients with clinical VT or documented near-miss sudden death is relatively straightforward. Drug therapy (usually class III or Ib and rarely Ic because of proarrhythmic potential), catheter or surgical ablation (the former with doubtful long-term results), and use of automatic implantable cardioverter-defibrillators are the choices to be made. In patients with documented near-miss cardiac death, drug therapy alone is unlikely to succeed unless a drug can be identified by repeated EP testing.

The prophylactic management of patients thought to be at risk of sudden death is fraught with controversy. Attention to improving the hemodynamic state is paramount. Once this is done to the best possible state, drug therapy may be considered. Class Ib drugs (phenytoin) are probably the best choice. There is some evidence that they may help decrease the risk of sudden death.[39] More important, the risk of proarrhythmia is low. The next alternative is beta blockers. Unless clinical or EP evidence of sustained VT is present, the use of class Ic or III drugs cannot be justified. The implantation of antitachycardia pacing defibrillators offers the surest form of protection and makes drug therapy safer.

The best hope for patients with TOF lies in the fact that better surgery, younger age of surgery, and better myocardial preservation at surgery may all decrease the risk of ventricular arrhythmia and sudden cardiac death in the long term.[28, 43]

Other congenital heart defect patients with a significant risk of sudden cardiac death are those with double-outlet right ventricle,[44] those undergoing Rastelli-type operations, and aortic or mitral valve replacement. All patients need careful follow-up and vigilance regarding arrhythmias. Also of note is the risk of sudden cardiac death and ventricular fibrillation in patients with Mustard/Senning operations for transposition of the great arteries. Here, too, the risk may be secondary to stretching of the right ventricle, just as in post-TOF patients.[45]

In summary, the current state of knowledge regarding ventricular arrhythmia and sudden cardiac death after repair of congenital heart disease leaves much to be desired. Prophylactic management to prevent sudden death is controversial until a test that specifically identifies the population at risk is found. Further studies in the coming years will, we hope, address this important issue in this difficult group of patients.

REFERENCES

1. Bink-Boelkens MTE, Velvis H, Homan van der Heide JJ, et al: Dysrhythmias after atrial surgery in children. Am Heart J 106:125–130, 1983.
2. El-Said GM, Gillette PC, Mullins CE, et al: Significance of pacemaker recovery time after the Mustard operation for transposition of the great arteries. Am J Cardiol 38:448–451, 1976.
3. Gewillig M, Wyse RK, de Leval MR, Deanfield JE: Early and late arrhythmias after the Fontan operation: Predisposing factors and clinical consequences. Br Heart J 67:72–79, 1992.
4. Bink-Boelkens MTE, Meuzelaar KJ, Eygelaar A: Arrhythmias after repair of secundum atrial septal defect: The influence of surgical modification. Am Heart J 115:629–633, 1988.
5. Duster MC, Bink-Boelkens MTE, Wampler D, et al: Long-term follow-up of dysrhythmias following the Mustard procedure. Am Heart J 109:1323–1326, 1985.
6. Deanfield J, Camm J, Macartney F, et al: Arrhythmia and late mortality after Mustard and Senning operation for transposition of the great arteries: An eight-year prospective study. J Thorac Cardiovasc Surg 96:569–576, 1988.
7. Vetter VL, Tanner CS, Horowitz LN: Electrophysiologic consequences of the Mustard repair of d-transposition of the great arteries. J Am Coll Cardiol 10:1265–1273, 1987.
8. Kürer CC, Tanner CS, Norwood WI, Vetter VL: Perioperative arrhythmias after Fontan repair. Circulation 82:IV190–IV194, 1990.
9. Kavey RW, Gaum WE, Byrum CJ, et al: Loss of sinus rhythm after total cavopulmonary connection. Circulation 92:II304–II308, 1995.
10. Gewillig M, Cullen S, Mertens B, et al: Risk factors for arrhythmia and death after Mustard operation for simple transposition of the great arteries. Circulation 84:III187–III192, 1991.
11. Garson A Jr, Bink-Boelkens MTE, Hesslein PS, et al: Atrial flutter in the young: A collaborative study of 380 cases. J Am Coll Cardiol 6:871–878, 1985.
12. Bink-Boelkens MTE, Bergstra A, Cromme-Dijkhuis AH, et al: The asymptomatic child a long time after the Mustard operation for transposition of the great arteries. Ann Thorac Surg 47:45–50, 1989.
13. Porter CJ, Garson A Jr: Incidence and management of dysrhythmias after Fontan procedure. Herz 18:318–327, 1993.
14. Weber HW, Hellenbrand WE, Kleinman CS, et al: Predictors of rhythm disturbances and subsequent morbidity after the Fontan operation. Am J Cardiol 64:762–767, 1989.
15. Balaji S, Gewillig M, Bull C, et al: Arrhythmias after the Fontan procedure: Comparison of total cavopulmonary connection and atriopulmonary connection. Circulation 84:III162–III167, 1991.
16. Peters NS, Somerville J: Arrhythmias after the Fontan procedure. Br Heart J 68:199–204, 1992.
17. Cecchin F, Johnsrude CL, Perry JC, Friedman RA: Effect of age and surgical technique on symptomatic arrhythmias after the Fontan procedure. Am J Cardiol 76:386–391, 1995.
18. de Leval MR, Kilner P, Gewillig M, Bull C: Total cavopulmonary connection: A logical alternative to atriopulmonary connection for complex Fontan operations. J Thorac Cardiovasc Surg 96:682–695, 1988.
19. Roos-Hesselink J, Perlroth MG, McGhie J, Spitaels S: Atrial arrhythmias in adults after repair of tetralogy of Fallot: Correlations with clinical, exercise, and echocardiographic findings. Circulation 91:2214–2219, 1995.
20. Lesh MD, Van Hare GF, Epstein LM, et al: Radiofrequency catheter ablation of atrial arrhythmias: Results and mechanisms. Circulation 89:1074–1089, 1994.
21. Rhodes LA, Walsh EP, Gamble WJ, et al: Benefits and potential risks of atrial antitachycardia pacing after repair of congenital heart disease. Pacing Clin Electrophysiol 18:1005–1016, 1995.
22. Balaji S, Johnson TB, Sade RM, et al: Management of atrial flutter after the Fontan procedure. J Am Coll Cardiol 23:1209–1215, 1994.
23. Walsh EP, Saul JP, Hulse JE, et al: Transcatheter ablation of ectopic atrial tachycardia in young patients using radiofrequency current [see comments]. Circulation 86:1138–1146, 1992.
24. Murphy JG, Gersh BJ, Mair DD, et al: Long-term outcome in patients undergoing surgical repair of tetralogy of Fallot. N Engl J Med 329:593–599, 1993.
25. Garson A Jr, Nihill MR, McNamara DG, Cooley DA: Status of the adult and adolescent after repair of tetralogy of Fallot. Circulation 59:1232–1240, 1979.
26. Cullen S, Celermajer DS, Franklin RCG, et al: Prognostic significance of ventricular arrhythmia after repair of

tetralogy of Fallot: A 12-year prospective study. J Am Coll Cardiol 23:1151–1155, 1994.
27. Deanfield JE, McKenna WJ, Presbitero P, et al: Ventricular arrhythmia in unrepaired and repaired tetralogy of Fallot: Relation to age, timing of repair, and haemodynamic status. Br Heart J 52:77–81, 1984.
28. Walsh EP, Rockenmacher S, Keane JF, et al: Late results in patients with tetralogy of Fallot repaired during infancy. Circulation 77:1062–1067, 1988.
29. Dietl CA, Cazzaniga ME, Dubner SJ, et al: Life-threatening arrhythmias and RV dysfunction after surgical repair of tetralogy of Fallot: Comparison between transventricular and transatrial approaches. Circulation 90:II7–II12, 1994.
30. Janousek J, Paul T, Bartáková H: Role of late potentials in identifying patients at risk for ventricular tachycardia after surgical correction of congenital heart disease. Am J Cardiol 75:146–150, 1995.
31. Stelling JA, Danford DA, Kugler JD, et al: Late potentials and inducible ventricular tachycardia in surgically repaired congenital heart disease. Circulation 82:1690–1696, 1990.
32. Gatzoulis MA, Till JA, Somerville J, Redington AN. Mechanoelectrical interaction in tetralogy of Fallot: QRS prolongation relates to right ventricular size and predicts malignant ventricular arrhythmias and sudden death. Circulation 92:231–237, 1995.
33. Daliento L, Caneve F, Turrini P, et al: Clinical significance of high-frequency, low-amplitude electrocardiographic signals and QT dispersion in patients operated on for tetralogy of Fallot. Am J Cardiol 76:408–411, 1995.
34. Shah MJ, Sweeten TL, Rhodes LA, Vetter VL: JTc and QTc dispersion in patients following surgical repair of tetralogy of Fallot. J Am Coll Cardiol 27:297A, 1996 (abstract).
35. Gatzoulis MA, Till JA, Redington AN: QT dispersion refines risk prediction for sustained ventricular tachycardia after repair of tetralogy of Fallot. J Am Coll Cardiol 27:296A, 1996 (abstract).
36. Horowitz LN, Vetter VL, Harken AH, Josephson ME: Electrophysiologic characteristics of sustained ventricular tachycardia occurring after repair of tetralogy of Fallot. Am J Cardiol 46:446–452, 1980.
37. Deal BJ, Scagliotti D, Miller SM, et al: Electrophysiologic drug testing in symptomatic ventricular arrhythmias after repair of tetralogy of Fallot. Am J Cardiol 59:1380–1385, 1987.
38. Moak JP: Pharmacology and electrophysiology of antiarrhythmic drugs. In Gillette PC, Garson A Jr (eds): Pediatric Arrhythmias: Electrophysiology and Pacing. Philadelphia, WB Saunders, 1990, pp 37–115.
39. Garson A Jr, Randall DC, Gillette PC, et al: Prevention of sudden death after repair of tetralogy of Fallot: Treatment of ventricular arrhythmias. J Am Coll Cardiol 6:221–227, 1985.
40. Wellens HJJ, Brugada P, Stevenson WG: Programmed electrical stimulation of the heart in patients with life-threatening ventricular arrhythmias: What is the significance of induced arrhythmias and what is the correct stimulation protocol? Circulation 72:1–7, 1985.
41. Meinertz T, Treese N, Kasper W, et al: Determinants of prognosis in idiopathic dilated cardiomyopathy as determined by programmed electrical stimulation. Am J Cardiol 56:337–341, 1985.
42. Dean JW, Lab MJ: Arrhythmia in heart failure: Role of mechanically induced changes in electrophysiology. Lancet 1:1309–1312, 1989.
43. Joffe H, Georgakopoulos D, Celermajer DS, et al: Late ventricular arrhythmia is rare after early repair of tetralogy of Fallot. J Am Coll Cardiol 23:1146–1150, 1994.
44. Judson JP, Danielson GK, Puga FJ, et al: Double-outlet right ventricle: Surgical results, 1970–1980. J Thorac Cardiovasc Surg 85:32–40, 1983.
45. Scagliotti D, Strasberg B, Duffy CE, et al: Inducible polymorphous ventricular tachycardia following Mustard operation for transposition of the great arteries. Pediatr Cardiol 5:39–44, 1984.

INDEX

Note: Page numbers in *italics* refer to illustrations; page numbers followed by t refer to tables.

ISBN-0-7216-6629-9

90038

9 780721 666297